THE COMPLETE HOME VETERINARY GUIDE

Chris C. Pinney, DVM

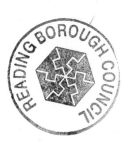

Third Edition

McGraw-Hill

New York ·Chicago San Francisco Lisbon London Madrid
Mexico City Milan New Delhi San Juan Seoul
Singapore Sydney Toronto

The McGraw-Hill Companies

Library of Congress Cataloging-in-Publication Data

Pinney, Chris C.
    The complete home veterinary guide / Chris C. Pinney.
        p.   cm.
        ISBN 0-07-141272-7
        1. Pets—Diseases. 2. Pets—Health.   3. Veterinary medicine.   I. Title.
    SF981.P558   2004
    636.089—dc21   2003052668

1 2 3 4 5 6 7 8 9 0   DOC/DOC   0 9 8 7 6 5 4 3

ISBN 0-07-141272-7

The sponsoring editor for this book was Scott Grillo, the editing supervisor was Caroline Levine, and the production supervisor was Pamela Pelton. It was set in Melior per the Mod. CMS design by Kim Sheran of McGraw-Hill Professional's composition unit, Hightstown, N.J.

Printed and bound by RR Donnelley.

This book is printed on recycled, acid-free paper containing a minimum of 50% recycled, de-inked fiber.

McGraw-Hill books are available at special quantity discounts to use as premiums and sales promotions, or for use in corporate training programs. For more information, please write to the Director of Special Sales, McGraw-Hill Professional, Two Penn Plaza, New York, NY 10121-2298. Or contact your local bookstore.

The Complete
Home Veterinary
Guide

CONTENTS

INTRODUCTION

Welcome to the Third Edition of *The Complete Home Veterinary Guide*, your one-stop resource for information on companion animal husbandry and health care. This Third Edition has been completely updated and contains many new and exciting features, including a newly formatted and expanded section on pet first aid, a glossary of veterinary terms, a listing of the most common drugs and medications prescribed for pets, a section on injured or orphaned wildlife, and much, much more!

It's no secret that pets are an integral part of our society today, as evidenced by the billions of dollars spent each year on food, supplies, housing, and pet care services. And of the over 60 million households that contain companion animals in this country alone, many are home to more than one pet, and oftentimes these pets are of differing species. Because of this, a resource was needed that contained information on a variety of companion animal species, all condensed into one easy-to-read volume. Hence, *The Complete Home Veterinary Guide*, a comprehensive, up-to-date guide to caring for companion house pets, was created.

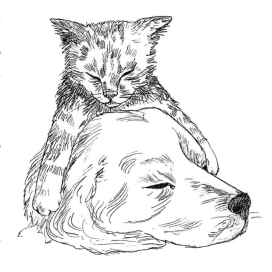

The Complete Home Veterinary Guide is loaded with illustrations and covers important topics concerning husbandry and health care for all popular species of pets. Written from a veterinary perspective, this book provides an objective "nuts-and-bolts" look at pet care. It doesn't matter if you own one pet or multiple species of pets, *The Complete Home Veterinary Guide* covers them all.

Here are just a few of the subjects presented and questions answered in this expanded Third Edition:

- Simple steps that you can take to improve your pet's mental health and well-being

- Matching clinical signs and complaints to disease conditions in dogs and cats

- Ten strategies for reducing pet care costs that you can implement today

- How to treat annoying behavioral problems in dogs and cats

- Complementary medicine and holistic approaches to pet care

- What to do if you find an injured or orphaned bird or wild animal

- The vaccination controversy: What is a pet owner to do?

- How to treat skin challenges without steroids

- The universal warning signs of illness in pet birds

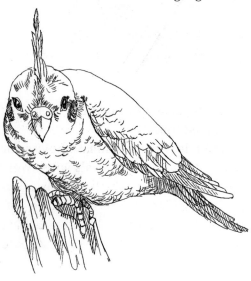

- Vital first-aid procedures, all of which could save your pet's life someday

- Seven ways to help our pets live longer and healthier lives

- Protecting your family and yourself from zoonotic (petborne) diseases

- The care and husbandry of exotic pets, from sugar gliders to tarantulas

■ How to maintain high water quality in aquariums

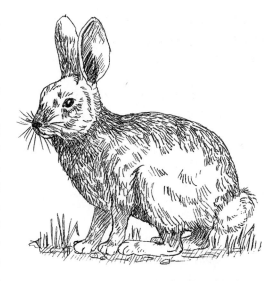

Part I of this book deals with dogs and cats. Information ranging from selecting a pet to preventing disease is covered in this section. Fighting fleas, managing allergies, and coping with various medical conditions such as arthritis and diabetes are just a few of the topics that will prove valuable to everone who owns one or more of these tried and true companions.

The popularity of pet birds is quickly closing the gap on that of dogs and cats. Part II covers important information regarding the selection, housing, feeding, and preventive health care of pet birds, as well as select diseases and disorders.

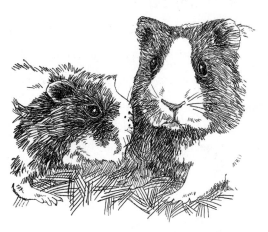

There are even sections on hand raising baby birds and on emergency and first aid procedures for our feathered friends.

For those pet fanciers who prefer less conventional choices for companionship, Part III is where it's at! This section deals with exotic or alternative pets, including rabbits, guinea pigs, small rodents, chinchillas, prairie dogs, hedgehogs, sugar gliders, ferrets, miniature pot-bellied pigs, reptiles, amphibians, and invertebrates. For tropical fish lovers, there's also a chapter on aquarium maintenance and disease prevention in fish.

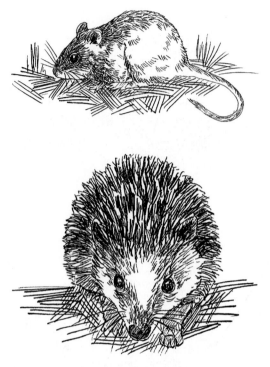

Part IV presents a variety of topics of interest to pet owners. You may have wondered how to administer cardiopulmonary resuscitation to a dog or cat, or what to do if your pet swallows a poison. Chapter 38 covers those and other important topics regarding emergencies and first aid procedures for dogs and cats. In fact, this could very well be the most important section of the book, since, in emergency situations, timing is of the essence. As a result, foreknowledge of the material presented in this chapter could very well save your pet's life one day.

Other interesting and useful information presented in this section includes caring for orphaned or injured wildlife, caring for the older pet,

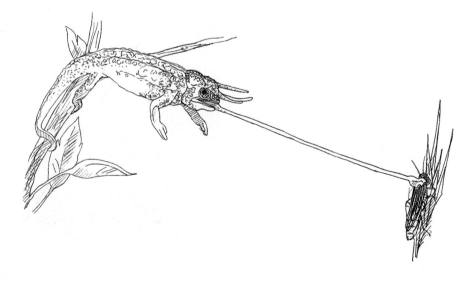

increasing your pet's longevity, reducing stress and promoting mental wellness in pets, and understanding cancer in dogs and cats. The chapter covering zoonotic diseases, or diseases that can be transmitted from pets to people, is sure to open some eyes! Although the chances of transmission can be minimized through good preventive health care, many pet owners fail to realize the importance of such care. As a result, they can inadvertently place their health and, indeed, that of their families, in jeopardy.

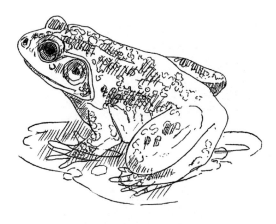

With the growth in popularity of holistic approaches to health care among people, it is no wonder that many satisfied followers are seeking such approaches for their pets. As a result, therapies such as acupuncture, herbal medicine, homeopathy, chiropractic, and nutritional medicine, as they relate to the health and well-being of our pets, are presented in Chapter 45. What you read may surprise you!

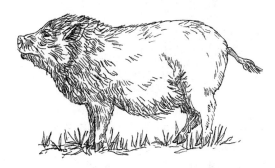

Saving money seems to be first and foremost on

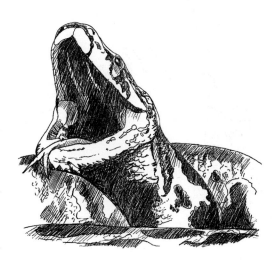

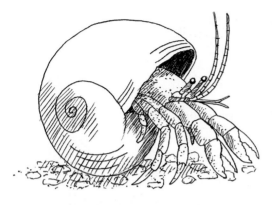

everyone's mind these days. And by following the 10 superstrategies suggested in Chapter 46 for reducing the cost of pet ownership, you'll quickly realize that this book is one of the best investments you'll ever make!

Of course, despite all the information mentioned above, this book is not designed to replace quality veterinary care for pets, but rather to supplement it. If your pet is exhibiting signs of injury or illness, always consult your veterinarian. Remember: The sooner a correct diagnosis can be made by a qualified veterinarian, the greater the chances are for a successful treatment.

Now get set for an informative voyage into the world of pets with *The Complete Home Veterinary Guide* as your tour leader. Regardless of your pet fancy, this book is sure to increase your "pet savvy" as well as enrich the relationship you have with your loving companion(s)!

DOGS AND CATS

According to a recent (as of 2003) study conducted by the American Veterinary Medical Association, there are over 110 million cats and dogs living in the United States alone. Pet owners spend billions of dollars each on veterinary medical services and supplies for their four-legged companions. And this figure does not even include the food they feed them! There is no doubt that, in American society at least, dogs and cats are here to stay.

History of the Dog

For over 10,000 years, the dog has been an integral player in man's social and cultural development. It's blood and toil have helped humans discover new lands and build civilizations, and its use in war has helped topple the same. It has hunted alongside humans for centuries and has been hunted by man for food. As eyes for the blind and ears for the deaf, the dog has become an indispensable member of our modern society. But what really sets the dog apart from all the rest? Millions of dog lovers will agree that it's the special loyalty and devotion the dog exhibits toward members of our own species—a characteristic that has justly earned it the proper title of "[hu]man's best friend."

The modern-day dog (*Canis familiaris*) descended from the wolf, with four distinct groups recognized. The first group, the *dingo group*, is descended from the wolves of Asia. Its members were dispersed throughout the Asian, African, and Australian continents. Modern-day descendants of this group include Rhodesian ridgebacks, basenjis, and the dingoes of Australia. One distinguishing characteristic of this group is that they don't like to bark too much.

A second group of dogs, the *greyhound group*, is believed to have evolved from wolves inhabiting the open plains of central Asia, Africa, and the Middle East. The oldest member of this group, the *saluki,* is thought to have originated prior to 1400 B.C.! Distinguishing features of the greyhound group include keen eyesight and incredible speed, two characteristics that the Egyptians found especially useful for hunting purposes. Besides the saluki, other modern representatives include the Afghan hound, the borzoi, and, of course, the greyhound.

The *Northern dog group* is believed to have evolved from the large gray wolf of northern Europe. Generally regarded as one-master dogs, descendants of this group have been used for a variety of functions, including pulling sleds (Alaskan malamutes, Siberian huskies), hunting game (Norwegian elk hound), and guarding flocks (collies).

A final group, the *mastiff group,* arose from wolves occupying the mountainous regions of Eurasia. Gifted with a keen sense of smell, members of this group were commonly used as war dogs and as hunting dogs. We still utilize the hunting skills of retrievers, setters, and pointers today. The mastiff, the St. Bernard, and the Great Pyrenees are a few of the more sizable members of this group.

History of the Cat

Like the dog, the cat is thought to also have wolflike ancestors. The modern cat, *Felis catus,* is a direct descendent of *Felis libyca,* the African wildcat, and *Felis sylvestris,* a European wildcat with a tabby-like appearance.

Interestingly, over the years, the domestic cat has undergone only limited selective breeding. As a result, it has the closest ties to its "wild" ancestors when compared to other domesticated animals. Evidence of this phenomenon can be seen in the similar size and anatomic features of all cats. Except for variations in characteristics such as muzzle and coat length and color, different breeds of cats generally look alike. Compare this, if you will, to the dog, which comes in a multitude of sizes, shapes, and varieties, all brought on by selective breeding.

Cats first associated with humans back in the Stone Age, where they probably hung around camp for food scraps and leftovers. It was not until ancient Egyptian times that humans and felines became true companions. Cats were used to hunt birds and catch fish for the Egyptians, and to rid their granaries of rats and mice. So revered did the cat become in early Egyptian society that goddesses were fashioned after its image, and separate burial grounds were set aside for the mummified remains of those felines that departed from this world.

As the world trade routes opened up and the high seas became an important means of interaction between countries and peoples, the cat spread throughout the civilized world. Longhaired varieties soon developed, and became highly favored in the European community until the Dark Ages, when superstition began to run rampant and cats became symbols of evil and witchcraft. They quickly lost their preferred status, and the European cat population fell into decline. Unfortunately, when the Crusaders returned from the Holy Land carrying plague-laden brown rats with them on their ships, there were few cats around to meet this threat. As the bubonic plague devastated Europe, the importance of the predatory nature of the cat increased, and numbers were soon back on the rise. As they regained their status in society, cats found their way back into the farmers' granaries and into the courts of royalty. To this day, in the eyes of millions of cat fanciers, they still command a royal status in our society!

DID YOU KNOW?

The first evidence of feline domestication dates back over 9000 years!

Choosing the Right Pet for You

Because dogs and cats come in all types of shapes, sizes, colors, coat lengths, and personalities, how do you know which one is going to be just right for you and for your particular situation? Here are several questions you should be asking yourself before you take the plunge:

Why do I want a pet and what type do I want?

Is it going to be an indoor pet or an outdoor pet?

How will this pet interact with my children or other pets in the household?

Am I willing to devote the time and money needed to raise this pet?

If you are simply looking for companionship, then you need only to choose a furry individual

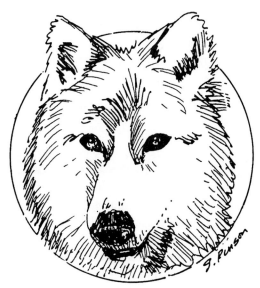

FIGURE 1.1 Dogs are believed to be descended from wolves.

that strikes your fancy. Both purebreds and those of "questionable ancestry" can make great pets, and the decision concerning genetic purity is entirely up to you (Figs. 1.1 and 1.2). If you choose to go the purebred route, expect to pay more up front for your purchase. In addition, you run greater risk of facing genetic disorders inherent to that particular breed. Being very cautious and prudent in your selection process can minimize this risk.

If you are like many pet lovers, you might be less finicky about a lengthy pedigree and instead prefer a pet with a more mysterious gene pool. In fact, there are several advantages to owning mixed-breed dog and cats (also known as *domestic shorthairs, domestic mediumhairs,* and *domestic longhairs*). First, because of their diluted,

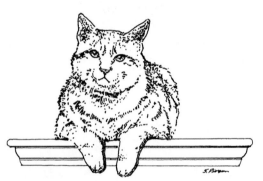

FIGURE 1.2 Cats can be just as social and loving as dogs.

colorful ancestries, they exhibit a unique genetic phenomenon known as *hybrid vigor.* Because of hybrid vigor, genetically blended pets, as a group, tend to be healthier and live longer than their purebred cousins.

Another obvious advantage of choosing a hybrid is that they cost less to purchase than do their papered peers. Ask yourself, "What type of purebred breed(s) do I like best?" Then start looking in newspapers, pet stores, and pounds and other animal shelters for crosses that contain the genes of your favored breed. In many instances, the genetic makeup of the parents is not known, yet you can usually guess the genetic background of the candidate by its anatomic features or by its behavior.

For instance, let's say you notice that a dog's ears stand erect, yet are folded halfway. There is a good chance that this mystery breed is part terrier. Does the dog enjoy lounging around in its water dish? It could contain some retriever blood. Does the cat appear to be slightly cross-eyed? No doubt it is part Siamese. Odds are that the individual you encounter will be a cross between one or more of this country's top 10 most popular dog or cat breeds.

Of course, space limitations will play an important role in the type of dog or cat you'll ultimately choose. For example, apartment dwellers will usually want to limit themselves to a cat or small dog, whereas those with larger living spaces will have more options. However, there are exceptions to every rule!

Are you looking for an exercise companion (Fig. 1.3)? If so, you will want to choose a dog breed with a stride length and aerobic capacity that won't slow you down. On the other hand, you might want a cute lap warmer just to keep you

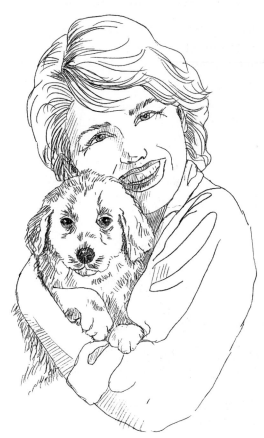

FIGURE 1.3 Companionship is the number one reason for dog ownership.

DID YOU KNOW?

The excellent tracking skills of hunting dogs arise in part from their ability to detect distinct volatile fatty acids located on the surface of game or left over on the ground, brush, and/or trees.

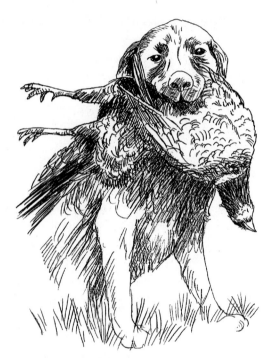

FIGURE 1.4 As hunting partners, dogs have no equals!

company. If so, a cat or toy poodle will fulfill that need quite nicely.

If you are in the market for a hunting dog, there are many from which to choose (Fig. 1.4). Setters, pointers, retrievers, hounds, and spaniels come in a wide variety of types, shapes, sizes, and abilities. For upland game hunting, setters, pointers, and spaniels fit the bill. For waterfowl, retrievers won't hesitate to plunge into the water to retrieve a fallen bird. For tracking larger game, one of the keen-scented hound breeds might be what you require. Some hunting dogs will do it all! Keeping your particular needs in mind, research your options thoroughly, and talk with local gun club, hunting club, and/or breed club members to assist you in the decision-making process.

Perhaps you want a dog for protection purposes. If you envision your new acquisition roaming your backyard, lunging and snarling at anyone or anything that approaches your gate, then forget it. Obtaining a dog under such pretenses is only asking for trouble (and a lawsuit), and is heartily discouraged. If, on the other hand, you plan to treat your dog as a true companion and household member, as well as protector, then your qualifications for ownership are acceptable.

It stands to reason that an 85-pound rottweiler with glistening white teeth would certainly be more imposing to an intruder than would an 11-pound Lhasa apso (not that the latter wouldn't tear into the former—Lhasa apsos were originally bred for this purpose)! However, it is instinctive that all dogs, regardless of breed or size, will actively defend pack members (and, like it or not, you are a pack member) or territory if threatened. If you want your dog to protect you, it is important that it recognize what does and does not constitute a threat. And this is where professional protection training will come in handy.

FACT OR *FICTION*

Cats are loners by nature. *FICTION.* Research has shown that feral cats, especially females, will actually exhibit pack behavior similar to dogs, grooming and taking care of one another! Only about 15 percent of cats will refuse to socialize at all with humans.

All dogs to be used for protection purposes must be properly socialized with people. Military and police dogs are perfect examples. These dogs are trained to attack on command only. Off duty, most are gentle as lambs. This is how your dog should be. This will not only ensure your safety and that of your family and friends but also might prevent a lawsuit! Remember: A socialized dog can be a great protector; an unsocialized dog is downright dangerous!

Unless you are planning to become (or are already) a professional breeder, don't purchase a dog or cat with visions of large profits from the sale of future litters. Most novices find out quickly that breeding operations, if done correctly and humanely (as they should always be), represent a considerable investment in time and money. Be sure to find out what these investments are prior to plunging into the pet breeding business.

If you are a novice, confine your efforts to one of the more popular breeds rather than to some exotic, delicate breed. As a rule, you'll be rewarded with larger litters and fewer problems with *dystocia* (difficult or complicated birthing). In addition, the more popular the breed, the greater the demand will be for the offspring, resulting in greater financial rewards.

But breeder beware: When selecting your initial breeding stock, closely scrutinize the pedigree of the dog or cat in question. All that it takes is one genetic defect to appear in one or more of the offspring, and your reputation as a breeder could be shattered!

For many, the pleasure of dog or cat ownership is compounded by the thrill of competition in the field or show ring (Fig. 1.5). Thousands of events are sanctioned each year by national, state, and local clubs

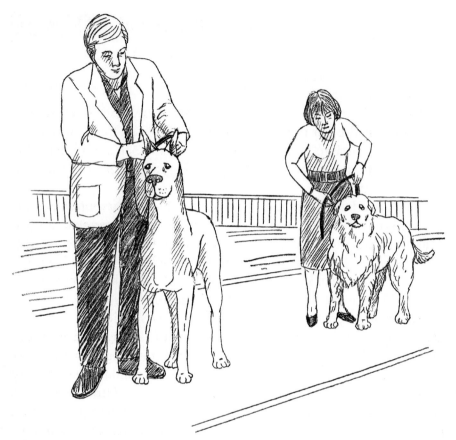

FIGURE 1.5 The thrill of competition.

that bring owners and their performers in from all over the country. Breeders are motivated by these events as well, for earning a reputation for producing show champions is rewarding not only to the ego but also to the pocketbook.

Housing Considerations

Where are you planning to house your new pet? Hopefully, your answer is "indoors." For some reason, many cat owners are under the false impression that a cat cannot be happy unless it is roaming free outdoors. Although this might have been the standard of thinking years back, it is time that cat owners change their attitudes toward this subject. Aside from the obvious health hazards to outdoor cats, such as car

DID YOU KNOW❓

The average cat will sleep well over half its life away.

fenders and fan belts, hostile dogs, hostile humans, and infectious diseases, there is another important reason: an increased threat of zoonotic disease transmission. As a result, although it is fine to allow your cat to spend some time outside, it should spend the majority of the day (and all of the night) inside.

Dogs raised as housepets will respond more favorably to training and generally have less behavioral problems than those that are perpetually banished to the backyard from day 1. This is because dogs crave the attention and company of people, and, in most instances, a backyard existence does not fulfill this need. Problem behaviors and disobedience frequently result from such discontent.

In decisions regarding the housing of dogs, excitability, size, and coat length are certainly three important considerations (Fig. 1.6). As a rule, the more excitable the dog, the more attention that dog will crave. Isolate an excitable dog in a backyard away from human contact, and you are just begging for behavioral problems. At the same time, selecting a large dog for a housepet and failing to housetrain or command-train it properly could lead to some very disturbing and destructive confrontations. If you are not willing to devote the time to properly train an indoor dog, you should stick to one of the smaller breeds in order to limit the damage that is bound to befall your carpet and furniture!

Depending on the type of climate in which you live, haircoat length becomes an important factor to consider when deciding on indoors versus outdoor housing. In colder climates, dogs with long coats and dense undercoats can withstand the outdoor chill much better than can their shorthaired counterparts. Conversely, dogs such as the Siberian husky and the chow chow may have a difficult time coping with southern heat without the benefits of air conditioning.

Outdoor dogs with long haircoats will also require more grooming time and effort to keep their coats healthy than if they were housed indoors. Are you willing to devote this time each day? If not, either select a dog with a shorter coat, or plan on housing your dog indoors.

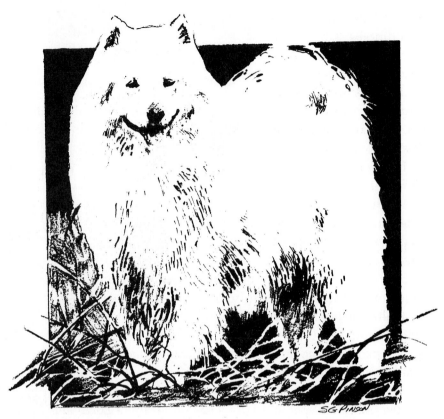

FIGURE 1.6 Dogs with long coats and/or thick undercoats should not be housed outdoors in hot climates.

If you plan on housing a dog outside when it becomes an adult, be sure that it is housetrained as a puppy. That way, if the need ever arises to bring the dog indoors, it will be easier (and certainly more sanitary) to accomplish such a conversion.

Pets and Children

Dogs and cats can serve as great teachers to educate children about responsibility and unconditional love! However, wait until your children are at least 5 years old before acquiring a new pet. Younger children, some of who might just be starting to crawl or walk, stand a greater chance of being accidentally hurt or scratched by a housepet than do older children. On the contrary, older children are better equipped to learn about and/or undertake responsibilities associated with pet ownership, and can become active participants in the care of the new family member.

When selecting a pet for a child, choose one with an outgoing personality, one that can stand up to the rigors of ownership by a child (Fig. 1.7). Shy, introverted puppies and kittens rarely satisfy the energy requirements of children. Such pets might be difficult to socialize and could turn aggressive if mentally traumatized by an overzealous child.

With dogs, medium to medium-large breeds are preferred for children. Small dogs and toy breeds,

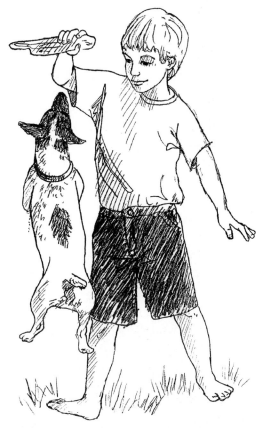

FIGURE 1.7 Dog ownership is an excellent way to teach children about responsibility and unconditional love!

because of their small stature, are more susceptible to accidental injury at the hands and feet of young ones. They are also more likely to become aggressive if mishandled. On the other hand, while one of the giant breeds can be gentle as a lamb, such a pet could still pose a significant health threat to your child because of its sheer mass.

Personality features to look for in dogs include low aggressiveness, high tolerance, and low excitability. Golden retrievers are a favorite among parents, owing to their reputation for gentleness with children. Basset hounds, Labrador retrievers, and collies are also popular picks for children. Finally, when purchasing a puppy or kitten, limit your selection to one that is between 8 and 12 weeks old. Because socialization naturally occurs during this time, a greater bond will form between it and your child.

New Pets and Other Pets

Before bringing home a new dog or cat, consider your other pets that are already in your household. Jealousies or incompatibilities (e.g., cats and birds) could arise that need to be anticipated ahead of time. Be sure the new addition has been properly socialized to other pets, and vice versa! For example, if your existing dog is the type that attacks anything that barks or moves on four legs, it might do the same to your new arrival. Unsocialized dogs and cats (and even some that are properly socialized) might refuse to accept another of their kind into their territory without a fight.

All newcomers should be gradually introduced to existing pets one day at a time. Keep your new pet in a separate room or enclosure, allowing initial interactions to take place only under your direct supervision. These gradual encounters should eventually help break the ice between the two and help establish a social pecking order within your furry family.

The Responsible Pet Owner

Pet ownership comes with major responsibilities in terms of both time and money. For instance, dogs are pack animals and crave attention from their human pack members (Fig. 1.8). Certainly one of the easiest ways to upset a dog is to habitually ignore it. In fact, this lack of owner attention underlies many of the problem behaviors seen in dogs. Regardless of whether you keep your dog indoors or outdoors, consider how much quality time you will be able to spend with it each day. If your projections are low because of your job or other commitments, two dogs are often better than one. The company that one provides the other while you are away can be an effective substitute for your affections.

Another factor to consider with a dog is how much time you will have to devote to training. It cannot be stressed enough how important this is to your future relationship with your dog. One major cause of

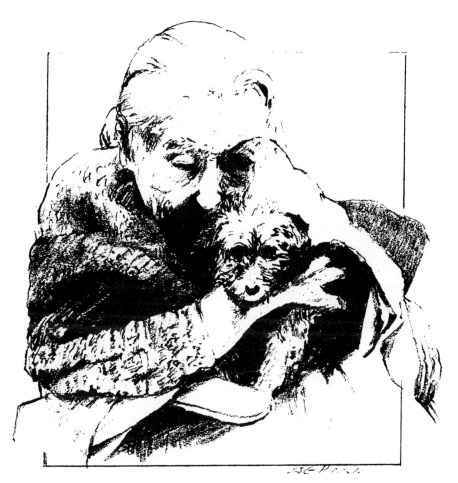

FIGURE 1.8 Dogs are pack animals, and they crave attention.

owner dissatisfaction is an unruly pet. As a result, training is definitely one aspect of pet ownership that should never be neglected.

Reduced time requirement is a major reason for the increasing preference for cats over dogs as pets. Cats are indeed fairly self-sufficient, seemingly needing only food, water, a clean litterbox, and very little training. While this is true in many instances, you are still not off the hook! All cats still need a daily dose of attention and grooming.

The financial aspects owning a dog or cat, including food, supplies, training, and veterinary care, can cost hundreds of dollars each year, and that's assuming that it stays healthy (see Chap. 46). Are you willing

DID YOU KNOW?

A dog and cat that are correctly socialized to one another can become best of buddies, whereas the same two animals, if socialization does not occur, often become bitter enemies!

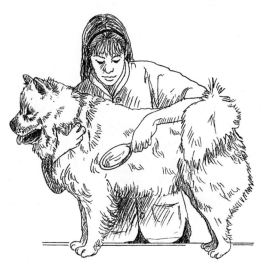

FIGURE 1.9 Plan on brushing your dog every day!

to accept financial responsibility for your pet's preventive health care or for treatment in an event of an injury or illness? If not, you are not ready for pet ownership.

On a final note, although your intentions might be pure, never surprise someone with a new dog or cat unless you are positively, absolutely sure that they want one in the first place. Think about it: Your gift to them includes not only that furry bundle of energy but also a hearty commitment to training, time, and money (Fig. 1.9). Unfortunately, too many people do fail to think about it that way, and as a result, our nation's pounds and shelters are overflowing with unwanted pets turned in by disgruntled or disinterested gift recipients. As a result, it is always best to allow other people to come to a decision about pet ownership by themselves, and not to force it on them by your good intentions. Believe me, everyone will be happier in the long run!

Finding the Right Dog or Cat for You

Once you have decided on a particular type of dog or cat, now is the time to start your search. Newspapers, pet stores, veterinary hospitals, the Internet, and word of mouth are all fruitful avenues for information. If you're not interested in a registered pet, check with the local humane society or animal shelter in your area. These are excellent places to start and are often jam-packed with canines and felines of all types, all eager to be adopted into happy homes. Usually, one can be yours to love for only a nominal adoption fee. As an added benefit, you will feel good knowing that you've saved an unwanted pet from an uncertain future.

> **DR. P'S VET TIP**
>
> To determine the age of a young kitten, use a scale. Kittens under 6 months of age will usually gain about a pound per month of life. For instance, a 3-month-old kitten usually weighs around 3 pounds, and a 4-month-old kitten will generally weigh in at about 4 pounds.

If a purebred fits your fancy, check pet stores or contact breeders, preferably within your area. Local veterinarians and groomers can often provide specific recommendations. Magazines catering to dog and cat owners can also be excellent reference sources for professional breeders. Finally, shows and other competitive events provide a means of giving you a firsthand glimpse of the cream of the crop and can give you the opportunity to meet prominent breeders in person.

Before you go shopping, do your homework. Find out what the going rate is for the particular breed you want. Beware of the small-time operator who advertises or offers you a great deal on a "registered" pup. These so-called great deals can end up costing you more in the long run in medical bills and emotional drain. Where quality counts, stick with reputable breeders who can provide you with the complete pedigrees of both parents and references of satisfied clients. This rule holds true for pet store purchases as well. Before buying from a pet store, ask where the puppy or kitten came from and who the breeder was. Ask to see the pedigrees of both parents. Reputable pet stores will have all this information readily available for your inspection. And don't hesitate to ask for references from satisfied customers. If the store is unwilling or unable to divulge such information, look elsewhere.

Whatever you do, don't rush your decision. Remember that you are making a long-term commitment. Take your time, and pick out that special individual just right for you!

The Prepurchase Exam

Once you think you've finally found the perfect companion, now what? For starters, you want to be sure you are getting a healthy specimen. Be sure to inquire as to vaccination and deworming history. You might be told that all of the "shots" and dewormings have been given. This might be true, but don't hesitate to ask for, in writing, dates and names of products used. Your veterinarian can then review this list for completeness during the professional prepurchase exam.

Even before your veterinarian gets involved, you should perform your own prepurchase exam on the prospect. It is easy to do on site and will help illuminate many problems that might otherwise elude the untrained eye.

1. *Environment.* For starters, take note of the surrounding environment in which the puppy or kitten is being kept. Does it look and smell clean, or is it filthy, with uncleaned litterboxes or urine and feces lying all around? If the latter is true, you should question the integrity of the seller. Observe all the individuals in the litter or group. Do any appear sickly, depressed, or otherwise unhealthy? An infectious disease can run rampant through such a congregation of young dogs and cats, and it could be just beginning to rear its ugly head within the group.

2. *Attitude.* Now focus your attention on the actual candidate. Start with overall attitude. Does it appear active and healthy, or is it lethargic and depressed? Are breathing problems evident? Does it seem friendly and outgoing to people and to the other animals in the group, or does it seem shy and introverted? Dogs and cats destined to be good pets should take an instant fancy to people, and should outwardly display this affection. At the same time, avoid those individuals with overbearing and domineering personalities. Observe how your favorite treats other members of its group. Domineering personalities are usually quite evident. As a general rule, choose one that is "middle of the road"—not too domineering yet not too shy.

3. *Skin and coat.* Once attitude and personality have been evaluated, check out the skin and coat. Any fleas or ticks present? How about any hair loss, scabs, or signs of infection? These could be indicators of diseases such as mange or ringworm, both of which can be zoonotic. Cats especially are meticulous self-groomers. As a result, an unkempt hair-coat could signify parasitism or some other underlying health disorder.

4. *Lumps, bumps, or swellings.* Run your hands over the umbilical area and, on both sides, over the points where the inner thighs connect with the abdominal wall. Do you notice any soft, fluctuant masses? These could be herniations. Run you hands over the entire body surface, feeling for other types of lumps and bumps. Note the location of any you find. Does the belly seem distended (swollen)? If so, it could be full of food, or it could be full of worms. Check beneath the tail, looking for tapeworm segments and for evidence of diarrhea. Soiling on and around the hair in this area should tip you off to a potential intestinal disorder.

5. *Other anatomical considerations.* Observe leg conformation and the way the puppy or kitten walks and runs. Any obvious deformity and/or lameness should be noted. In male dogs, check for descent of the testicles. Both testicles should be present at birth. If they aren't, be prepared to neuter at a later date, not only for health reasons but also to prevent the passage of this inheritable trait to future generations. Fortunately, cryptorchidism is rare in cats.

6. *Head region.* Now focus in on the head region. Using your eyes and your nose, check the ears for discharges or strong odors (usually a sign of infection). Both eyes should be free of matter, with no cloudiness or redness. Compare both eyes, making sure that they are of the same size, and that the pupils are of the same diameter. Glance at the nose, noting any discharges or crusts. Finally, look into the mouth. The gums should be pink. If they are white, the dog or cat could be anemic. Look for any severe underbites or overbites, or any missing teeth. Also glance at the roof of the mouth. Cleft palate is a serious birth defect (see Table 1.1), and unless it is surgically corrected, it will lead to secondary aspiration pneumonia and ultimately death.

Consulting a Veterinarian

Let's say you've completed the exam described above and have found some potential problem areas. What do you do next? First, don't get discouraged. Many of these conditions have quick, inexpensive solutions. This is where a veterinarian comes in handy.

Table 1.1 Congenital or Inherited Disorders in Dogs*

Eyes	Microphthalmia (small eyes)
	Juvenile cataracts
	Entropion/ectropion
	Glaucoma
	Prolapsed third eyelid
	Tear duct deformity
Ears	Congenital deafness
Nervous system	Epilepsy
	Brain underdevelopment
	Hydrocephalus
	Invertebral disk disease
Integument	Umbilical hernia
	Inguinal hernia
	Demodectic mange
Digestive system	Cleft palate
	Abnormal dentition
	Overbite or underbite
Musculoskeletal system	Dwarfism
	Joint dislocations
	Patellar luxation
Cardiovascular system	Blood-clotting disorders
	Heart murmurs
	Anemia
Respiratory system	Collapsed trachea
Reproductive system	Retained testicles (cryptorchidism)

*For ethical purposes, all pets with congenital or inherited disorders should be neutered.

Don't feel awkward about asking the seller to pick up the tab (pay) for a professional prepurchase exam [and for cats, feline leukemia virus (FeLV) and feline immunodeficiency virus (FIV) testing] by a veterinarian of your choice. Sellers who are confident in the quality of their pets should have no qualms about this. If they balk, a warning light should flash in your head. And don't get suckered into a "money-back" or "lifetime" guarantee on a pet as an alternative to a professional prepurchase screen. Such a guarantee doesn't protect you against the emotional distress caused by having to return a pet to which you've already grown attached.

Follow your veterinarian's recommendations as to the purchase quality of the dog or cat in question. If the one you have your heart set on does have medical problems that can be easily corrected, ask the seller to deduct these costs from the purchase price. They aren't obligated but by character to do so; as a result, you must decide on your next move if they refuse or fail to compromise. The extra expense (including cost of supplies and required documents in addition to initial purchase price of the pet; see Tables 1.2 and 1.3) out of your own pocketbook might be worth it if you think you have truly found the pet of your dreams! You be the judge.

Table 1.2 Supply Checklist for Your New Cat

Food and water bowl	Brush
Cat (kitten) food	Comb
Collar or harness	Bed or cathouse
Leash	Travel kennel
Claw trimmers	Flea control products
Identification tag	Scratching post
City license (if required)	Toothbrush/paste
Proof of rabies vaccination	Toys
Litterbox	Heartworm preventive agent
Litter	

Table 1.3 Supply Checklist for Your New Dog

Food and water bowls	Brush
Dog (puppy) food	Comb
Collar	Bed or doghouse
Leash	Travel kennel
Training lead and rope	Nail trimmers
Identification tag	Ear cleanser
City license (if required)	Toothbrush/paste
Proof of rabies vaccination	Toys
Heartworm preventative	Flea control products

Petproofing Your Home

If you choose to allow your new pet to have the run of the house, be sure to take proper steps to petproof your home. For instance, keep all electrical cords well out of reach. This might mean banishing your playful pet from certain areas of the house, but it is a minor inconvenience compared to a potentially fatal accident. Puppies especially love to chew, and electrical cords can be mighty appetizing.

Puppies explore with their mouths, and will pick up anything. Keep everything that's not a toy out of reach, including spare change. Also, be careful when putting out cockroach or rat poisons, as these can attract curious mouths.

You will probably want to confine unsupervised puppies to non-carpeted floors until proper housetraining has been accomplished. Even so-called stain-resistant carpets can buckle under the strain of repeated bombardments.

Keep all plants out of reach. Many dogs and cats love to chew on foliage, and if they decide to nibble on a harmful ornamented variety of plant, they could poison themselves. Cats will also enjoy using potting soil as litter, and cat urine has the unique ability to quickly dispatch even the heartiest of house plants!

F ACT *OR* *FICTION*

Cats love to play with strings and ribbons. **F** ACT. Unfortunately, string foreign body intestinal obstructions are relatively common feline medical emergencies seen by veterinarians. As a result, keep these items well out of reach of your cat!

Cats love to jump onto ledges, windowsills, and furniture. As a result, be sure all opened windows are screened, and that all lamps, pictures, and collectibles are secured. Open washers/dryers, drawers, high ledges or balconies, hot irons on ironing boards, and stovetop burners left on can all be insidious dangers to your cat's health.

Pins, needles, rubber bands, yarn, string, ribbons, aluminum foil, cellophane, and holiday tinsel are just a few items that could cause serious health problems if eaten by dogs or cats. Inquisitive cats have been known to get their heads lodged within open cans and jars, and because cats possess a strange attraction to bags of all types, plastic bags can become death traps if entered.

Your Dog's Outdoor Home

No doubt there will undoubtedly be special situations which prohibit the indoor dwelling of a grown dog. In these instances, outdoor accommodations provided for your pet must take into account its comfort and well-being. Remember that dogs get hot and cold just as we do, and when housed outdoors, need to be provided a means of protection against extremes in the weather. Your friend is entitled to a sturdy, well-insulated shelter. The doghouse should be positioned in a relatively shady area of the yard, and should also be elevated a few inches off of the ground using bricks or wood to prevent flooding in the event of a rainstorm. Ideally, the shelter should have a short, enclosed porch which leads into the main house. This will help keep wind drafts from penetrating into the main living area. The main living quarters should be large enough to allow your dog to turn around comfortably within, yet confined enough to provide it a sense of security and to concentrate heat during cold winter days. Finally, a ramp should be included to allow your dog easy access into its elevated home.

If you build the doghouse yourself, select sturdy building materials, remembering that they must be able to withstand constant punishment from teeth and claws. If fiberglass insulation is to be used, make certain that it remains well contained and sealed within the walls and roof, since such material can cause severe gastrointestinal upset if swallowed.

If you plan on further confining your dog to a pen or run, use a smooth concrete or quarry tile as flooring on which to place the doghouse. Although such surfaces may not be the most comfortable for your pet, they are the most sanitary and easy to clean. Floors consisting of grass, sand, pebbles, and/or just plain dirt only serve to trap and accumulate filth and disease, and should be avoided.

The fence surrounding the enclosure should be made of wire chain link and be tall enough to prevent escape. Exposed metal points from the chain links at the top of the fencing material should not extend above the metal support bar in order to prevent injuries if your dog does try to jump. The same rule applies for the bottom perimeter of the fence as well, just in case your dog tries to squeeze its way out.

Naming Your Pet

Naming your new pet should be fun and involve the entire family. You can even find entire books dedicated to choosing the right name for your dog or cat at your favorite bookstore. When deciding on a name, stick to one that has two syllables. This is especially important for dogs, enabling them to tell the difference between their name and those one-syllable commands they must learn. You can further set its name apart from potential commands or reprimands by adding a vowel sound to the end of it. Just be creative!

Introducing Your Pet to Its New Home

You will want to do everything in your power to make your new pet feel comfortable and secure in its new home. Establish an area in the house that your pet can call its own, and completely petproof it. When you first get your pet home, introduce it to its special room immediately. Allow it some time to scope out the new surroundings, including the sleeping accommodations you have provided. This should include a cushioned bed, basket, or travel kennel. For kittens, cardboard or plastic boxes work just fine, assuming that easy access into these enclosures is provided. Be sure that your pet's sleeping area is in a part of the house far from noise and other disturbances.

Special Considerations for Cats

Your cat's litterbox should also be placed in an area in the house where interruptions are not likely to occur. For very small kittens, an aluminum pan or shallow tray may be used; for larger kittens and adult cats, your standard plastic varieties available from a pet shop work just fine.

Avoid using boxes or other cardboard devices for a litterbox. Not only do they have a tendency to leak, but their porous nature is most unsanitary to your cat. Covered litterboxes have the advantage of keeping the litter from being strewn across the floor—assuming, of course, that your cat feels comfortable enough to enter such an enclosure!

Try to match the type of litter used in your cat's previous home, but be sure that it is dust-free. Also, avoid products containing chlorophyll to mask odors, as this substance can irritate your cat's nose and prevent it from using the box. Fill the box with about $1^{1}/_{2}$ inches of litter. For sanitation purposes as well as aesthetics within the house, make a habit of scooping out solids from your cat's litterbox on a daily basis. (*Note:* Pregnant women should pass this duty on to someone else, in order to reduce their risk of exposure to toxoplasmosis.) Both coarse-grained and fine-grained ("clumping") litters can be spot-cleaned daily without having to dump out the entire box. However, regardless of litter type used, litterboxes should be emptied completely and cleaned with soap and water at least once a week to maintain sanitary conditions and to control odor.

Unless you plan to have your cat declawed at a young age, you will also need to invest in a good scratching post to spare your furniture and fixtures from the ravages of your cat's claws. Clawing comes naturally to cats, which use such behavior to keep their nails in top condition and to mark their territory. The scratching post should be made of sturdy material and be heavy enough or braced so that it doesn't fall over when the cat attempts to scratch. A sturdy piece of soft wood is ideal for this purpose. Other commercial varieties can be obtained from a local pet store. Avoid those posts lined with thick, compliant carpet, as this might not satisfy your cat's needs, causing it to look elsewhere for a surface that will.

First Encounters

Your new pet's first encounters with the rest of your family are important. Be sure that initial introductions, be they with children or other adults in the family, turn out to be positive ones. Carefully supervise child-pet interactions, and stress to your children the importance of gentle play and handling. Instruct your children and other adults on the proper way to pick up and hold a new puppy or kitten. Pets should not be picked up solely by the front legs or by the neck. Instead, the entire body should be picked up as one unit, with the hind end supported, not left dangling in midair. Picking a cat up by grasping the skin over the back of the neck is acceptable as long as the hind end is supported as well.

If they had it their way, most children, and some adults, for that matter, would choose to play with a new puppy or kitten 24 hours a day. However, you need to stress the importance of a rest time after periods of play, and lay down strict ground rules against disturbing the pet during this downtime (Fig. 1.10).

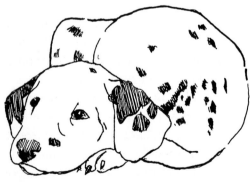

FIGURE 1.10 Puppies need their rest, too.

Rules of Play

Puppies and kittens love to play. In fact, it's part of their normal behavioral development. However, realize that there is a right way and a wrong way to go about it. Follow these "rules of play" to be sure that your approach is the correct one.

For dogs, toys should be made of nylon, rawhide, or hard rubber. Of the three materials, hard nylon or compressed rawhide is most desirable because it is most easily digested if swallowed. Regular rawhides, pig ears, and similar substances are fine if the dog takes its time and chews slowly. For those dogs that don't take the time to chew, avoid giving these items altogether because they can cause serious stomach upset and even intestinal blockage if swallowed whole. Also, some dogs have difficulty differentiating rawhide from refined leather, which could put your new pair of shoes in serious jeopardy! Rubber chew toys should be solid and sturdy so that they cannot be easily ripped apart by sharp puppy teeth. Avoid chew toys with plastic "squeaks" in them. Most dogs can extract these mechanisms too easily, only to swallow them or aspirate them into their airways Regardless of the type of chew toy you pick, choose it as you would a child's toy. If its design is such that it could cause suffocation or serious problems if swallowed, put it back and choose a safer one.

Avoid using old socks, shoes, or sweatshirts as substitute toys for your dog because it won't be able to tell the difference between old and new. Allow a puppy to chew on an old shoe or sweatshirt while still an adolescent, and you might find it fancying your expensive leather shoes or tennis warmups when it grows up.

When selecting toys for your new kitten or cat, be sure that they cannot be torn apart easily and that they do not contain small parts that could be swallowed. Wrinkled paper and shoeboxes are intriguing to most cats. Rubber balls or mice too large to swallow, as well as catnip toys (again, constructed for safety), are also considered safe toys. If a string is attached to a toy in order to entice a cat to play, always remove it after the play session is over. Along the same lines, never use ribbon or laces as play items. If a cat swallows such items, they could damage their intestines and have to be removed surgically.

It is fine to play intensely with a puppy or kitten, but overt roughhousing should be avoided. If a play session progresses from a friendly romp to an all-out frontal assault, end it immediately. Your pet needs to learn how to keep its activity level to a socially acceptable intensity. Also, be sure that the youngster gets plenty of time to rest after an especially active play period.

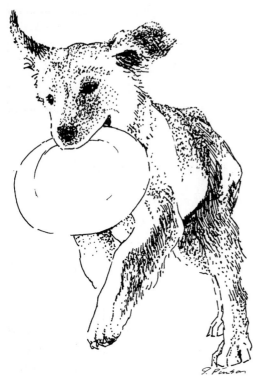

The same rules of moderation apply to chewing. It is perfectly natural for a puppy to want to explore its environment with its mouth. During play, there will be times when the pup will bite and nip too much or too hard. When this occurs, shout "No," pull your arm or leg away, and provide a chew toy as a substitute. In essence, what you want to tell your pup is that it is fine to use its mouth to explore, just as long as it knows its limits (Fig. 1.11). You'll be surprised how quickly they learn!

FIGURE 1.11 Make sure that your puppy learns the rules of play early!

Training Essentials

Proper training is definitely the key to a happy owner-pet relationship. It establishes your dominance in the relationship between you and your pet right from the start, and it can help prevent many behavioral challenges from rearing their ugly heads later on. Solid training can also keep your pet out of troublesome situations that could threaten both its health and yours (Fig. 2.1)!

There is one characteristic exhibited by every good trainer: patience. Without this virtue, you're going to have a tough time teaching your pet anything. You need to set aside time each day for training and resolve to stick to it. Keep in mind that it will only be a temporary dip into your time budget. After all, the more time you devote from the start, the quicker and more satisfying the results will be.

What about training school? Is it worth the time and the money? The answer is "Yes" if it will motivate you to devote the time for the task at hand. You still have to be physically present during the training (you can't have someone else train your dog, and then expect your star pupil to respond likewise to your commands). If you choose this route, enroll in an active-participation class in which an instructor directs you and your dog through the training session. However, keep in mind that such a class doesn't relieve you of your homework duties. You still need to practice with your pooch daily on your home turf.

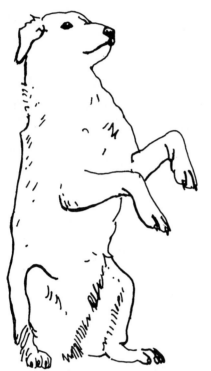

FIGURE 2.1 Proper training will enhance your relationship with your dog.

Main Principles of Training

For any training method to be effective, it must follow some basic principles to ensure its success. Some of these principles are described in the following paragraphs.

Consistency and Repetition

The magic success formula for all training endeavors is derived from two key concepts: consistency and repetition. Consistency provides the building blocks; repetition is the mortar that holds the program together. Without the two, you might as well try to teach a rock how to fetch. The results will be the same!

Consistency means more than just using the same commands over and over again. It also means using the same praises and corrections each time and keeping your voice tones consistently unique for each. Even your body language and postures used during training should remain uniform between sessions. As trivial as it might seem, pets pick up on stuff like that. Dogs and cats also like routine, so stick to it. Train at the same hour each day and for the same length of time for each daily session.

Just as important as consistency to a dog or cat's learning process is *repetition*. Repeating an action or training drill over and over will help reinforce the positive response you are looking for. Furthermore, the more

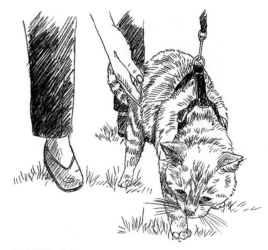

FIGURE 2.2 All cats should be trained to a harness and leash.

repetition you implement into training, the leaner and more refined your pet's learned skills become (Fig. 2.2).

Verbal Praise

Use verbal praise instead of physical pain in your training sessions. Food treats are fine as a reward supplement, but they should never replace verbal compliments. Punishment might be warranted if your pet purposely disobeys a command or commits an undesirable act, but this should never take the form of physical punishment. There are alternative means, each of which is at least just as effective as physical violence.

Punishment

Dogs and cats can be reprimanded effectively with a sharp verbal "No." Water sprayers, air horns, a can full of coins, handheld vacuums, and so on can all be used to gain your pet's attention quickly without inflicting any pain.

If you decide to use punishment, be sure to institute it quickly, preferably within 5 seconds of the act. If you

DR. P's VET TIP

When training, always end your session on a positive note. This will greatly accelerate your results.

> ### 🔍 **F**ACT *or* *FICTION*
>
> Sticking a dog's nose in its stool or urine is an effective form of punishment. **FICTION.** C'mon, who thought of this one! For some reason, this type of punishment is still quite popular among pet owners, even though it serves no useful purpose. Dogs are attracted to the smell of this stuff, anyway!

don't apply it before this time expires, any punishment thereafter might satisfy your anger, but it will serve no useful training purpose. Don't extend your punishment past a few seconds. Prolonged exhortations will only confuse your pet (and might cause you to lose your voice).

Never use your pet's name during the negative reinforcement. If you do, your pet might start to associate its name with the bad act and eventually become a basket case whenever the name is called. Reserve this name calling for positive, happy experiences only.

If you do punish, always follow it up shortly thereafter with a command or drill that will lead to a praise situation. Remember that the most effective training programs rely on praise more than on punishment. For some dogs, simply withholding praise from them is punishment enough to modify their behavior! By rewarding your pet for doing good rather than punishing it for doing bad, you'll get the positive results you are looking for much faster.

Other Suggestions

1. *Get the whole family involved.* In any training situation, always try to involve all members of the family. An all-too-common scenario is one in which a pet virtually ignores the commands of anyone but the one person who trained it. To avoid this, get the whole family involved. Just be sure to remain consistent within the family with regard to the training methods and commands used.

2. *Use short commands.* All verbal commands you employ need to be kept short and sweet. Using slightly different voice tones for each command will help prevent confusion. If verbal punishment is to be used, make certain that it is totally different in tone and in presentation than the other commands.

3. *Start young.* Always start your pet's training at an early age. While it is true that certain advanced training techniques can be best taught at around 6 months of age, basic training, including housetraining for dogs, should be started as early as 8 weeks of age. If basic command training is not taught this early in life, bad habits arise later on, some of which can put a damper on future training efforts.

4. *Keep training sessions short.*   Try to keep the training sessions short and to the point. For puppies and kittens 8 to 12 weeks of age, devoting 10 minutes two to three times daily will yield excellent results. As your pet matures, the length of each of these sessions can increase. Let your pet's attitude be your judge. If it seems bored or indifferent, or has become totally unruly, you have probably exceeded its attention span.

5. *End on a good note.*   Always end your training session on a good note. Doing so is very constructive in terms of your pet's mental development, and effectively sets the tone for the next session.

Socializing and Desensitizing Your Pet

There is no doubt that the most important time in a new puppy or kitten's life is between the ages of 3 and 12 weeks. During this short timespan, the adolescent will learn who it is, who you are, and who and what all of those other living, moving beings surrounding it are as well. This stage of life in which such vital learning takes place is called the socialization period (Fig. 2.3).

If for some reason a puppy or kitten fails to be properly introduced to members of its own species or to other species (including children) during this time, then there is a good chance that it will not recognize

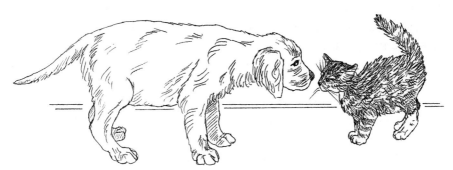

FIGURE 2.3   Dogs and cats can become best of friends if socialized at an early age.

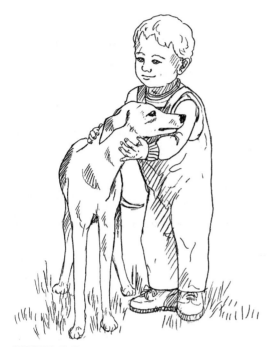

FIGURE 2.4 All dogs must be properly socialized to children.

these individuals for what or who they are, and it might even show aggressiveness toward them. For example, dogs intended for breeding purposes must be properly socialized to members of their own species if they are to be expected to breed with one of these members. Also, prime examples of dogs not properly socialized include those that show extreme aggressiveness to men only, or those aggressive to children. Dogs in particular see people as two species: big people and little people. As a result, while a dog might recognize an adult person as the one who feeds and commands it, it might not recognize a small toddler as one who commands the same respect if the pet is never properly socialized to small children (Fig. 2.4). Some dogs aren't fit for any type of human interaction at all. These have absolutely no socialization whatsoever and could pose a threat to humans.

Improper or negative socialization is even worse than no socialization at all. Any traumatic experience or physical punishment that occurs before 12 weeks of age could permanently scar a pet's personality to a specific group or species for life. For instance, dogs or cats that exhibit a fear of men were most likely abused by a member of this sex during the socialization period. This is one reason why all physical punishment should be avoided during this time in your pet's life. Such activity could damage its relationship with the person doing the punishing for life!

The existence of this socialization period is one reason why you should select puppies and kittens less than 12 weeks of age when choosing a new companion. If you don't, you have no way of knowing whether proper socialization has taken place, and you might be faced with behavioral problems in the future. Socializing a pet is not difficult if you remember to keep all interactions positive and to guard against any physically and emotionally traumatic situations (Fig. 2.5).

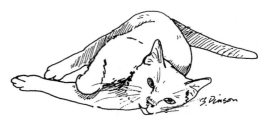

FIGURE 2.5 Socialization is just as important for cats as it is for dogs.

Before introducing a new puppy or kitten to other animals, be sure that it and the other animals are current on

DID YOU KNOW?

Cats may socialize to one breed of dog but not to another!

vaccinations and dewormings. In addition, always be sure that the animals you are planning to introduce it to are socialized themselves, or else you could have a battle on your hands.

Weekend excursions to a park and/or neighborhood strolls are some of the more opportune ways of introducing your new pet to other animals and to other adults and children. Allow children to freely interact with your puppy or kitten, but again, be sure that none gets too rough. For best results, you should repeat such encounters throughout its socialization period. And by all means praise your pet for good behavior during these interactions. It will leave a lasting impression on its personality (Fig. 2.6)!

One word of caution: Socialization, like any personality skill, can eventually be lost if it is not reinforced periodically. As a result, even as your dog or cat matures, don't just discard those trips to the park or strolls through the neighborhood. Remember: You have to use it or lose it!

Desensitization training is often overlooked by most new pet owners, yet it can be one of the most valuable tools for preventing stress

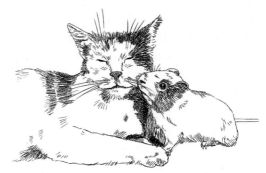

FIGURE 2.6 The power of socialization!

and behavioral problems as their dog or cat matures. There are three types of desensitization that need to be accomplished: (1) contact desensitization, (2) separation desensitization, and (3) noise desensitization. The first two types should be instituted at 8 weeks of age, and the third should commence at 16 weeks of age.

The first type, contact desensitization training, will condition your pet to allow its haircoat, feet, ears, and mouth region to be handled. This is vitally important for your pet's preventive health care program, for it will allow you to brush hair, trim nails, brush teeth, and clean ears without a fight! When interacting with your puppy or kitten, make a special effort to gently touch these regions with your fingers several times a day. Don't attempt to perform any of the grooming procedures mentioned above with the actual utensils; instead, simply go through the motions with your hands and fingers. Soon, your puppy or kitten won't think twice when you reach out and grasp a paw or an earflap. Once it has been desensitized to your touch, then you graduate up to actual grooming utensils. Just remember to temporarily discontinue your efforts if a struggle ensues. Any negative or painful experience involving these regions during your initial training efforts can produce the exact opposite effect and create an individual that will struggle vehemently when attempts are made to perform these simple procedures.

The goal of separation desensitization training is to desensitize a pet to being left alone by itself. This is especially important in dogs because of their "pack" mentality; however, it can apply to cats as well. As far as dogs are concerned, separation desensitization training will help prevent one of the most common behavioral disorders seen in the species: separation anxiety. You can start by placing your puppy in its travel kennel and leaving the house for a predetermined period of time (a few minutes at a time for the first day, then gradually working up over several weeks to 20 to 30 minutes departures each day), being careful not to make a fuss over your puppy or respond to its protests before you leave. In addition, when you reenter the house, wait several minutes before you let your pet out of its kennel, doing your best to ignore its pleas. When you do finally let it out, take it immediately outside to use the bathroom. Act as though your arrivals and departures are "nothing special," and your puppy will soon acquiesce to being left alone (see discussion of behavioral disorders).

Desensitization to strange or loud noises should also be performed when a puppy or kitten is still young. The easiest method for accomplishing this training is to regularly expose your young pet to recordings of various sounds, such as thunder, lightning, and fireworks. Compact disks containing these sounds and others are available at most book and record stores, or can be tracked down over the Internet. Playing these recordings while in the presence of your pet for 15 minutes daily, adjusting the volume up over a 3- to 6-week period, will usually achieve the desired desensitization

Basic Training for Dogs

Some tools of the trade you'll want to acquire to assist you in your canine training efforts include a leash, a 20- to 25-foot rope with an end clasp attached, and a sturdy collar or harness. If you decide to use a slip or choke chain collar, read the package directions and make certain that you know how to use it properly; otherwise, serious damage to your pet's neck and trachea could result. Because this device can be easily misused, many veterinarians recommend not using them unless you are a seasoned trainer. A better alternative is to use a head collar (i.e., a Gentle Leader®). This device applies pressure to the back of the neck and to the muzzle (without inflicting pain or pressure on the trachea), allowing you to effectively control your dog's head during training.

If your new puppy or dog is not used to wearing a collar (halter), harness, or leash, you must get it accustomed to them prior to any training efforts. Start by placing a collar, halter, or harness on your dog and allowing it to wear it around the house for several days. Once you think your dog feels fairly comfortable with it on, attach a leash to the clasp and allow your dog to walk around with the leash dragging behind. To protect your dog from snagging furniture or other objects with the leash and hurting itself, you should supervise these sessions. After about six to eight sessions over the course of 2 days, your dog should feel more comfortable with its leash being attached to its collar, halter, or harness, and should be ready for further instruction (Fig. 2.7a).

Heel

The first command you will teach your four-legged student is to heel, or walk at your side (Fig. 2.7b). To begin, position yourself on your

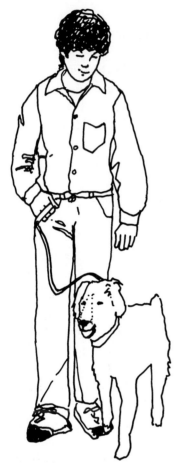

FIGURE 2.7a All dogs should be taught to walk on a leash.

dog's right side facing forward, with its shoulders even with your left knee. Take up the slack on the leash to prevent your dog from becoming entangled in the excess. Now, in simultaneous fashion, give a quick forward tug on the lead, say "heel," and start forward with your left foot leading. As your dog follows, keep its head level and in control using the leash. Start out by going 5 yards at a time, then stopping to praise for a job well done.

If your dog refuses to move on your initial command, go back to the starting line and set up again. This time, if needed, follow the quick tug with an encouraging pull on the lead to initiate movement. Start and stop frequently, praising as you go. As your dog starts to catch on, increase the distance you go each time. The ultimate goal is to have your dog walk briskly by your side until a command is given to do otherwise.

If your dog gets too far out in front of you, a quick, backward tug on the lead should be used to correct the discrepancy. For those trainees more interested in playing rather than learning, stop the training session temporarily until your dog settles down. Don't scold or show any other acknowledgment of its antics. It will soon learn that you mean business!

Once your dog has become comfortable walking in straight lines by your side, take it through some turns both to the right and to the left. During the turns, your dog's shoulder should remain aligned with your knee.

Stop

Once your dog responds favorably to the heel command, it is time to teach it the command "stop." With your dog heeling at your side, give a sharp backward tug on the leash as you say "stop," and halt your forward motion. (The verbal exclamation differentiates this from the backward tug used to slow an overenergized heeler.) Hold the stop for 3 seconds, then praise heavily for compliance. Afterward, have your dog heel again, and repeat the process over and over again, gradually increasing the amount of time you require your pet to remain still.

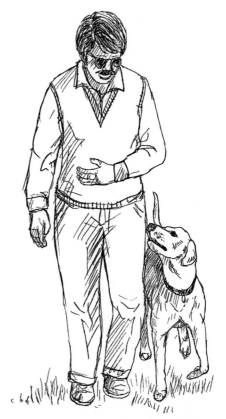

FIGURE 2.7b Teaching your dog to "heel."

Sit and Stay

From the "stop" position, pull upward on your dog's lead while at the same time saying "sit," and pushing down on its rear end to achieve the sitting position (Fig. 2.8). Have your dog maintain this posture for a good 5 seconds, then break into a heel. Gradually increase the sitting interval as your training progresses.

When your dog has learned what "sit" and "stop" mean, it's time to teach the "stay" command (Fig. 2.9). This is where your 20-foot rope lead comes in handy. Attach this to the collar and walk your dog again through the heel-stop-sit routine. Once your dog is in the sitting position, place your left hand in front of its face and say "stay." Now slowly walk about 3 yards away, keeping your back to your dog. If it breaks its "stay" when you move, reel your dog in with the lead, and make it immediately return to the sitting position. Then try again.

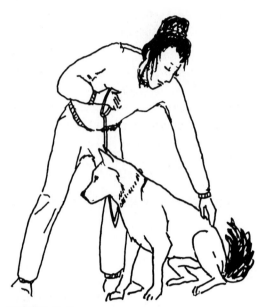

FIGURE 2.8 The "sit" command.

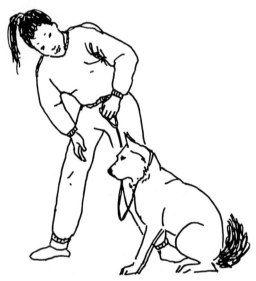

FIGURE 2.9 The "stay" command.

If the student stays in place even for 3 seconds after you walk away, heap on bundles of praise. If your dog still disobeys, walk it through your heel-stop-sit routine a few more times before returning to the "stay" command. As your pet starts to catch on, you can begin increasing the distances you go and time intervals for it to stay put.

Other Commands

"Heel," "stop," "sit," and "stay" are the basic obedience commands that you should start teaching your dog as early as 8 weeks of age. Two other commands that are optional, yet could come in handy in certain instances, are "down" and "come."

"Down" should be included as an adjunct to the "sit" command. After your dog is in the sitting position, utter the command while applying downward pressure with your free hand to its shoulder region. Note the difference from the "sit" command, in which downward pressure is applied to the hind end. Now, from this down position, you can proceed into the "stay" drill.

"Come" can be taught as a continuation of the "stay" command. With your dog sitting or lying at rope's length, give a quick forward tug while saying the command "come." Again, use the lead to reel it in if it decides to wander off track. Praise your dog only if it comes directly to you from its original starting position.

When, and only when, your dog has mastered these commands and responds to them consistently can you discard the leash or lead. For off-leash training, repeat each command sequence as before. Don't hesitate to put the lead back on if your dog fails to cooperate. At first, it is especially important to hold all off-leash training sessions in fenced-in yards or other enclosed areas to prevent you star pupil from dashing off into the sunset!

Housebreaking Your Puppy

Puppies should be housebroken at an early age, preferably as close to 8 weeks old as possible (Fig. 2.10) because this is when the period of stable learning begins in adolescent dogs. Their minds are wide open to suggestions, and they learn quite quickly at this early stage of life.

If you expect to yield successful results, you must be willing to devote some quality time to the task. Recognize that puppies have four fairly predictable elimination times:

1. After waking

2. After eating

3. After exercising

4. Just before retiring for the night

Make a concerted effort to take your puppy outside at these times, and every 3 to 4 hours in between. When you suspect that it has to go, take your pup outside and set it down in the grass.

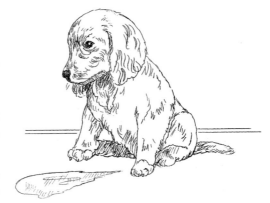

FIGURE 2.10 When housebreaking a puppy, use lots of praise and avoid punishment.

If elimination takes place, praise your puppy, and then take it immediately back inside the house. By doing so, you will help it associate the act with the location.

If a minute passes and your puppy hasn't gone, take it back inside. Don't leave it outside to play or roam. Puppies trained in this manner soon realize that their primary business for being outside is to eliminate, not to play. What happens if you catch your puppy in midact? If this is the case, go ahead and rush it outside. The puppy might finish what it started before you make it out the door, but don't get upset. Again, praise it immensely for going outside, and then bring it immediately back inside.

If you happen to miss an accident altogether, don't fret. If you saw it happen, a verbal punishment is warranted. On the other hand, if you didn't see it happen, do nothing. Simply try to be more attentive next time.

Other housetraining tips to remember are

1. Be sure that your puppy is current on its vaccines (since it will be going outside) and is free of intestinal parasites. The latter is very important because the presence of worms in the intestinal tract will cause unpredictable urges to eliminate.

2. Always use lots of praise; never physically punish. Again, remember that puppies crave praise, and if they don't get it, they feel punished. Give plenty of praise when they deserve it; hold it back when they don't.

3. When verbal punishment is indicated, avoid associating your puppy's name with the reprimand. For instance, simply say "bad," instead of "bad dog, Sugar." By leaving names out of it, the puppy won't associate its name with the bad behavior.

4. Establish a regular feeding schedule for your new puppy. Feed no more than twice daily, and take your puppy outside after it finishes each meal. It is preferable to feed the evening portion before 6:00 P.M. in order to help reduce the number of overnight accidents that can occur otherwise.

5. To help prevent accidents, keep your puppy in a confined area at night. It should be puppyproofed and have a floor that won't

be damaged if a slipup occurs. Utility rooms and half-bathrooms work well for this purpose, as do kitchens if they can be cornered off. If accidents occurs during the night or while you are away, don't get upset. As your training sessions progress, you'll find that this will become less and less of a problem. A natural instinct of any canine is to keep its "den" clean. These inherent instincts, combined with correct housetraining efforts on your part, will help fuel the success of your training efforts.

6. When cleaning up an accident, always use an odor neutralizer rather than a deodorizer on the area in question. These are available at most pet stores, and will usually eliminate any lingering scents that can lure your pet back to the same spot. Avoid using ammonia-based cleaners, since ammonia is a normal component of canine urine. Such cleaners might serve to attract, rather than to repel, repeat offenders.

Basic Training for Cats

Contrary to popular belief, some cats can be just as trainable as dogs. Keep in mind, though, that the independent nature of cats can make certain training procedures a bit tricky, but if you maintain an understanding attitude toward your task, your frustrations will be minimal and your rewards plentiful.

As with dogs, all cats should be trained to walk on a leash at an early age. Why? By teaching your cat to accept a leash and harness, you will be able to institute a daily exercise program for it, keeping it fit and healthy. In addition, since allowing a cat to roam freely outdoors these days is becoming more dangerous, a leash-trained cat can enjoy the same benefits of the great outdoors, yet without the risks. Finally, many travelers find that leash training comes in quite handy at rest stops during lengthy trips.

Before you attach a leash to your kitten or cat, it must become accustomed to a halter. Because halters provide more control and security than do collars, the latter should not be used to walk a cat on a leash. Place the new halter on your cat and allow it to wear it around the house for 10 to 15 minutes at a time. Then take it off, and repeat the process at 3-hour intervals throughout the day. Eventually lengthen the time you leave the halter on until your cat will wear it all day without a fuss.

At this point, attach a leash to the halter and allow your cat to drag the leash around for 10 to 15 minutes at a time before removing it. Repeat this procedure throughout the day for a week or so. Do not allow your cat to walk around unsupervised with the leash dangling free. If the leash becomes snagged, your cat could seriously injure itself.

Once you feel that your cat has become accustomed to the leash, practice walking with it indoors using the lead for a week or two. Only after your cat gives you total compliance should you attempt the same maneuver outdoors. If everything goes as planned, be sure to reward your cat for a job well done. A scratch behind the ears or under the chin, or a favorite food treat, does wonders to help solidify and promote such desired behavior.

If you so desire, teach your cat commands as you would a dog. Remember: Because of the very nature of the feline, you can't always expect 100 percent compliance; simply take all successes and run with them! One helpful tip is to hold your training sessions when your cat is hungry. If you do so, food rewards become powerful motivators for good behavior.

Litter Training Your Kitten

Kittens will be instinctively drawn to litter or dirt in which to eliminate as early as 4 to 6 weeks of age. As a result, housebreaking a kitten usually involves minimal effort on an owner's part (Fig. 2.11). Allowing access of your new kitten to its litterbox after eating, playing, waking up, or just before bedtime will help encourage repeat use. If your cat doesn't seem to catch on, there might be some reason for its reluctance to use the litterbox. If so, it is your job to find out why.

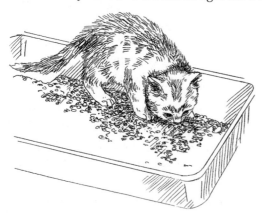

FIGURE 2.11 Most kittens will learn to use a litterbox without your help.

Solving Challenging Behaviors

When searching for the leading cause of dissatisfaction among pet owners, problem behaviors top the list. Each year, a multitude of dogs and cats are abandoned, evicted from their homes, or even put to sleep because of annoying behavioral activity. However, by understanding and employing special training techniques and/or therapy to correct such vices, and by allowing veterinarians to play active roles in the treatment process, pet owners can often avoid such drastic actions.

Canine Behavioral Disorders

The most common behavioral disorders you may encounter with your dog include separation anxiety, nuisance barking, inappropriate elimination, digging, destructive chewing, jumping, fear of loud noises, and aggressiveness.

Separation Anxiety

It has happened to many of us: We leave the house, sometimes for only a few minutes, and our "best friend" proceeds to chew up the furniture, bark or howl, and/or eliminate in the house. If your dog behaves this way when you leave your home, it is probably suffering from the behavioral problem known as *separation anxiety*. (*Note:* Medical problems can be the cause of such aberrant behavior; these must be ruled out before you can safely assume that you are dealing with a case of separation anxiety.) Before you can successfully treat a problem like separation anxiety, it is helpful to know what causes it.

Dogs are considered pack animals; that is, they prefer to associate in groups rather than act as loners. Because you are its owner, a dog will consider you part of its "pack" and will constantly want to associate with you. When you leave, you separate the dog from its pack, and this creates separation anxiety (Fig. 2.12). This behavior will be magnified if you tend to make a big fuss over the dog when leaving or returning

> ## Dr. P's Vet Tip
> For cases of separation anxiety that are refractory to conventional management, veterinarians can prescribe specific antianxiety medications to help effect a cure.

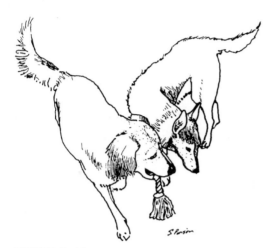

FIGURE 2.12 Dogs enjoy spending time with other members of their "pack."

to the house. Furthermore, certain other behavioral patterns on your part, such as rattling the car keys or turning off the television, can be associated to your departure by the dog.

When treating separation anxiety, you must remember that it is an instinctive behavior; it is not due to disobedience and/or lack of training. As a result, overt punishment for the act tends to be unrewarding. In fact, most of these dogs would rather be punished than left alone! The key to treating this problem lies in planning short-term departures, then gradually lengthening them until your dog gets used to your absence.

Begin by stepping out of the house for 10 seconds at a time for the first few days or so. Hopefully this will allow your dog to get used to you leaving the house, since it will learn that you will return soon. Vary your training session times throughout the day. The idea is to gradually lengthen your absences (30 seconds at first, then 1 minute, then 2 minutes, etc.) so that your departures soon become second nature to the dog.

Points to keep in mind when attempting to break your dog of this annoying behavior are as follows:

1. Don't make a fuss over your dog within 5 to 10 minutes of your arrival to or departure from home. This will help keep the excitement and anxiety levels in your dog to a minimum. During your training sessions, try not to reenter the house while the dog is performing the undesirable act. Doing so will only serve to encourage the dog to repeat the act.

2. Eliminate any behavior that might key the dog off to your departure, such as rattling your car keys or saying "goodbye" to your dog.

3. For the dog that likes to chew a lot, provide plenty of nylon chew bones to occupy its time.

4. Leaving the television or radio on while you're gone seems to help in some cases.

For severe cases of separation anxiety that fail to respond to desensitization training, an antianxiety medication, prescribed by a veterinarian, may be necessary.

Excessive (Nuisance) Barking

Let's face it: Some dogs just love to hear their own voices! Unfortunately, most owners and their neighbors hardly share the same adoration. There is no doubt that dogs that bark excessively are a nuisance and can cause many a sleepless night. For this reason, correction of the problem is essential to your sanity, and that of those who live around you.

A dog might bark excessively for a number of reasons. The first is boredom. Dogs that have nothing else to do might simply "sing" to themselves to whittle time away.

Another potential cause is territoriality. Outsiders, whether human or animal, will almost always elicit a bark out of a dog if threatening to encroach on its territory. Dogs can also use the bark indiscriminately as a communiqué to other outsiders to stay away. In such instances, the far-off bay of a neighborhood dog or the slamming of a car door down the street can trigger a barking episode.

Separation anxiety is another common source of nuisance barking. Some dogs have it so bad that they bark continuously when their owner leaves them, even for a short period of time. Often, owners return home to find their dogs hoarse from so much barking.

When attempting to break your dog of this annoying habit, always remember this one principle: If you respond to your dog's barking fit by yelling at it or physically punishing it, you will make the problem worse. Dogs that are isolated from their owners for most of the day don't care about what kind of attention they receive (positive or negative), as long as they get some. Dogs that are barking because of boredom or separation anxiety will soon learn that their actions will eventually get them attention, and they'll keep doing it. Even dogs that are barking for other reasons can catch on quickly that such vocalization will bring them a bonus of attention from their beloved owners. As a result, no matter how mad you get, or how sleepy you are, avoid the urge to punish your dog for its barking.

The first thing you need to determine is whether separation anxiety has anything to do with the problem. If you think it does, treat it as you would any other case of separation anxiety. In many cases, dogs that bark for this reason alone can be cured of their habit.

Keep in mind, though, that the source of the barking might involve a combination of the factors, not just one. Dogs that bark for reasons other than separation anxiety need to be given more attention throughout the day. A dog that tends to bark through the night should be given plenty of exercise in the evening to encourage a good night's sleep. A nylon or rawhide chew bone can be helpful at diverting its attention. Feeding the dog its daily ration later in the evening can also promote contentment for the night.

For those times of the day or night when the barking seems the worst, consider bringing the dog inside the house or the garage. This, of course, will not be possible if you failed to instruct your dog as to the ways of household living when it was a puppy. Nevertheless, removing your dog from its primary territory and/or increasing the amount of contact with members of its pack can help curb the urge to bark. Also, if possible, encourage your neighbors to keep their pets indoors at night, since nighttime roaming of neighborhood dogs and cats is a major cause of nuisance barking.

Inappropriate Elimination

It has happened to all of us: the early morning encounter in the family room or the unexpected (or sometimes expected) surprise awaiting our arrival home from work—house soiling. It is a dirty habit, yet one that millions of pet owners have to put up with each day. In many of these cases, the problem has an origin traceable to puppyhood; for others, it results from developmental behavioral and/or health problems. Regardless of the cause, pet owners can take an active role in most cases to minimize or stop completely this annoying habit.

Don't think that you will break your dog of this nasty habit by sticking its face and nose in the excrement after the fact. Not only is this action illogical and inappropriate for the particular situation; some dogs might even enjoy it! Instead, pet owners need to take a more rational approach to identifying the cause and solving the problem. To do that, you must first determine what is causing it.

LACK OF OR INADEQUATE HOUSETRAINING

The most common cause of house soiling is undoubtedly the failure of an owner to housetrain the dog prop-

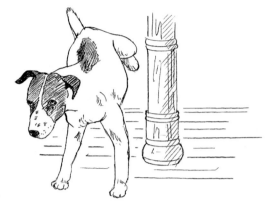

FIGURE 2.13 The cause of house soiling must be determined before effective treatment can be instituted.

erly during its puppyhood (Fig. 2.13). Many pet owners can't understand why their puppy has no problems going on newspaper, but just can't get the knack of going outside. They seem to forget that, to a puppy, newspaper and grass are two different surfaces with different smells. To paper-train a puppy and then expect it to switch easily to another type of surface is asking a lot, and this often presents a confusing dilemma to the poor creature.

Puppies need to be taught right from the start to go outside to use the bathroom instead of encouraging them to go within the confines of the home. At the same time, dogs that will be spending a great deal of time outside need to be housetrained as puppies, in case the need arises later in life to bring them indoors for whatever reason. If you miss this chance when it is a puppy, you could be in for trouble later on.

Contrary to popular opinion, you can teach an old dog new tricks; it just takes longer! With older canines that weren't properly potty-trained, proceed with training or retraining as you would with a puppy. Along with lots of praise, a favorite treat or snack can also be used to reinforce desired behavior. For those times you can't be at home to monitor indoor activity, confine your dog to a travel kennel or small bathroom, since dogs are less likely to have premeditated accidents in such confined spaces. Just be reasonable as to the amount of time you make it wait between eliminations.

SEPARATION ANXIETY

Inappropriate elimination activity can, as do many other behavioral problems, result from separation anxiety. Dogs left alone may become frustrated and soil one or more parts of the house. Some dogs can even become downright spiteful, targeting favorite furniture, bedding, and, if kept in the garage, even the roofs of automobiles. If your dog is truly suffering from separation anxiety, most of its adverse behavior will occur within 15 to 20 minutes of your departure. This predictability can assist in efforts to correct the problem. Treat this as you would any other case of separation anxiety.

DESIRE TO DELINEATE TERRITORY

The desire to delineate territory is another reason why a dog may choose to urinate (or sometimes defecate) indiscriminately. Certainly, intact (nonneutered) male dogs are more prone to this instinctive activity. Dogs have such a keen sense of smell that the mere presence of a canine trespasser around the perimeter of the home can set off a urine-marking binge. Owners who move into preowned homes often find out the hard way that the previous owners had a poorly trained or highly territorial pet housed within.

Neutering your pet may or may not help solve this problem, depending on its age. In many older males, house soiling has become more habitual than hormonal, and neutering does little to prevent it.

Use of a pet odor neutralizer on the carpet and baseboards is warranted if you suspect that a previous occupant is to blame. Use of fencing or dog repellent (not poison!) around the perimeter of the house may also help keep persistent urine-markers away from your house.

EXTREMELY SUBMISSIVE BEHAVIOR

Extremely submissive behavior often results in a cowering dog that urinates whenever anyone approaches. This type of adverse elimination is common in dogs that have been abused as puppies or have spent most of their growing years in a kennel or pound facility.

Management of such behavior depends on your actions and body language when approaching or greeting such a dog. Try to avoid direct eye contact and sudden physical contact with such dogs, for by doing so, you can send them into immediate submissiveness. If you've been gone from the house for a while, avoid sudden and exuberant greetings when you get home. By ignoring your dog initially, you'll lower its excitement level, reduce the immediate threat, and give it no reason to urinate.

One trick you can try is to immediately and casually walk over to your dog's food bowl and place some food or treats in it. The idea is to distract your dog's attention away from the excitement of your arrival and create a more comfortable, pleasing situation for it. Once you've been home a while, then you can (and should) offer more of your attention.

ILLNESS OR DISEASE

Finally, don't forget that some diseases or illnesses can cause a pet to urinate or defecate indiscriminately. For instance, dogs that tend to defecate inside the house should be checked for internal parasites. Diets with increased fiber content can also increase the number of trips your pet will need to take outdoors.

Certainly if the stools are semiformed or seem to differ from normal appearance or consistency, an underlying medical reason should be suspected. In addition, some of the conditions that can increase the frequency and/or urge to urinate include urinary tract infections, kidney disease, and diabetes mellitus. Urinary incontinence, characterized by the inability of the bladder to retain urine because of poor sphincter function, is common in older dogs. For these reasons, don't just assume that your dog's soiling problem is purely mental. Have the potential medical causes ruled out first; then you can concentrate on behavioral modification.

Just a word about cleaning up an accident in the house. When using cleaners to tackle the initial mess, be sure that they don't contain ammonia. Dog urine contains a form of ammonia, and such products might actually attract your dog back to the same spot later on. Along this same line, after the initial manual cleaning, your next job is to ensure that residual smell doesn't attract your pet back to the same spot. To accomplish this, you need to employ a product containing odor neutralizers specifically targeted for dogs. These products are available at grocery stores or pet shops. Deodorizers should not be used, for it is virtually impossible to completely mask or hide a scent from the keen canine nose.

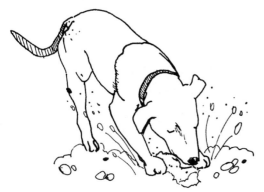

Digging

Although separation anxiety can cause digging episodes, its influence on this behavior is much less than with other problem behaviors. Instead, sheer boredom and/ or instinctive behavior are the two common states of mind that compel a dog to dig (Fig. 2.14).

FIGURE 2.14 Digging behavior is often caused by instinct or by sheer boredom.

Dogs with nothing else to do might opt for yard excavation just to help pass the time or to use up extra energy. The urge to break out of confinement and roam the neighborhood can also compel a dog to start digging. Finally, as you might have already experienced, many dogs like to bury personal items such as bones or toys for exhumation at a later date. Such instinctive behavior, although aggravating, can hardly be considered abnormal, and is difficult to totally eliminate.

Increasing your dog's daily dose of exercise could be just what the doctor ordered to help resolve its boredom and release any pent-up energy. Diverting the attention of a chronic digger is another plausible treatment approach. For instance, some troublesome cases have responded very well to the addition of another canine playmate. Rawhide bones and other chewing devices can also be used as attention-grabbers, but only if they don't end up underground themselves. If most of the digging occurs at night, overnight confinement to the garage might be the answer to spare your yard from the ravages of claws. Finally, if you haven't already done it, neutering can sometimes help snuff out the strong urge to dig in those dogs wanting to escape the yard and roam the neighborhood.

Destructive Chewing

Many canines are literally "in the doghouse" with their owners because of their destructive chewing. No one wants a pet that seeks and destroys any inanimate object into which it can sink its teeth. However, the urgency for dealing with such behavior is not governed merely by personal property damage. Many of these chewers also end up in veterinary hospitals suffering from gastroenteritis or intestinal obstructions. Hence, such adverse activity can cost more than just replacement value of furniture or fixtures. It can even sometimes cost the life of a pet!

In puppies, destructive chewing can easily arise from lack of training and from inappropriate selection of toys (Fig. 2.15). Although puppies are naturally going to explore their environment with their mouths, they need to learn at an early age what is and isn't acceptable to chew on. Solid command training is a must in these little guys.

Avoid providing normal household items such as old

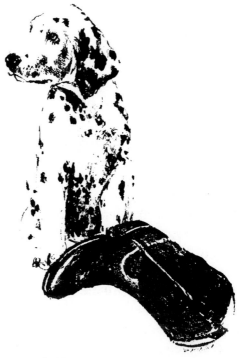

FIGURE 2.15 Destructive chewing is an annoying behavior that can lead to serious health challenges.

shoes, T-shirts, or sweatshirts as toys to play with. Puppies can't tell the difference between old and new shoes, and they might decide to try out your new pair for a snack one afternoon!

Objects that repeatedly bear the brunt of your dog's teeth should be placed as far out of reach as possible. For furniture or immovable objects, special pet repellents should be sprayed around their perimeters to make a mischievous puppy think twice before sinking its teeth into the item.

In young to middle-aged adults, separation anxiety is probably the number one cause of destructive chewing. As with all cases of separation anxiety and the behavior it provokes, correction of the problem should focus on correction of the anxiety attack. Finally, as with problem barking, boredom plays a leading role in destructive chewing in some adult dogs. If you think this might be the case, increase your dog's daily activity, and provide it with plenty of alternative targets, such as rawhides or nylon bones, on which to chew. Divert its attention, and most likely it will divert its chewing.

Other Causes and Forms of Aberrant Behavior

JUMPING

Talk about annoying behavior! Jumping is right up there with house soiling and incessant barking. Jumpers are usually right there at the door when visitors call and have this innate tendency to spoil a perfectly cordial greeting. After all, nobody wants a dog with dirty paws to jump on their nice, clean clothes, especially if the dog weighs 50 pounds or more (Fig. 2.16)!

This is one challenging behavior that should never be allowed to gain a firm root in a puppy. Probably the best way to assure this is through strict command training, starting at an early age. Until it learns its commands, be sure to discourage your dog from jumping on you or family members when the occasion arises. When it does jump at or on you, quickly push it off with your hands and shout "No!" Or, as an alternative, flex your knee and make sudden contact with its chest, making it fall backwards. Just don't overdo it and hurt your pet!

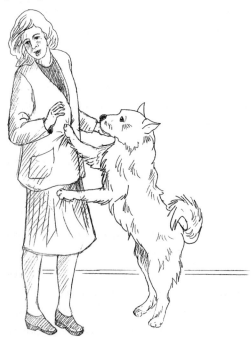

FIGURE 2.16 Proper obedience training is the key to curing the "jumper."

For adult dogs that never learned their manners, a refresher course in command training is the most effective method of curing the chronic jumper. Sometimes dogs that jump are simply trying to tell their owners that they want more attention. In such cases, a few more moments of your time devoted to your furry friend each day is an important adjunct to therapy.

FEAR OF LOUD NOISES

Fear induced by loud noises such as thunder or gunshots can be a common cause of aberrant behavior in canines.

Many people argue that because of the ultrasensitive hearing of dogs, pain induced by the noise or a pressure change might play a bigger role than fear itself. Regardless of the reason, when confronted with the disturbing sound, these dogs often become hysterical and quite destructive in their attempts to escape. Many might even injure themselves or their owners in the process.

In the case of the hunting dog that shies away when a gun is fired, training sessions involving repeated, gradual increases in exposure to the sound of gunfire are an effective method of ridding the dog of its fear. For dogs that fear the sound of thunder, fireworks, and other loud noises, owners must avoid direct attempts at comforting the pet, since doing so would be indirectly rewarding the undesirable behavior. If your dog is the type that comes unglued in these situations, consider letting it "ride out the storm" in a travel kennel. In addition, playing a radio or television loudly in the room where your pet is present might help muffle some of the fearful sounds, as well as make your dog feel more at ease.

Your veterinarian can prescribe antianxiety medications for your dog if it has an exceptional fear of loud noises. In any event, these should be used sparingly and only as needed. The best treatment is prevention through the use of proper desensitization training.

AGGRESSIVENESS

Of all the undesirable behaviors a dog can exhibit, this one is certainly the most disturbing and the most unacceptable. Aggressiveness can be directed toward other dogs or toward other species, including humans. Certainly dogs harboring an uncontrollable inherent aggressiveness toward the latter pose special problems to their owners in terms of liability as well.

DOMINANCE

This certainly plays an important role in canine aggressiveness. Some dogs refuse to submit to authority and will lash out at anyone or anything that attempts to exert such. In many instances, these dogs were not properly socialized and/or trained when they were young. In others, sex hormones—namely, testosterone—can exert a strong influence as well.

Treatment for such aggressiveness consists of a return to basic command and obedience training. In addition, exercises designed to reestablish dominance should be performed as well. If the aggression is directed toward a particular person, that person should be included in these exercises. Remember: Extreme caution and a good, strong muzzle are both advised before any attempts at such dominance assertion are made! For domineering male dogs, neutering is recommended prior to any attempts at retraining.

FEAR AND PAIN

These are the two other common causes of aggressive showings in canines. If a dog feels threatened or overwhelmingly fearful, it naturally experiences a "fight or flight" syndrome, and might choose the former option over the latter, depending on how it perceives its situation. In addition, dogs have been known to naturally lash out in fear at humans or other animals on being startled, or more frequently, when they are experiencing pain. For this reason, sudden aggressive changes in personality with or without other signs of illness warrant a complete checkup by a veterinarian.

Treating fear-induced aggression is aimed at reducing the threat you or others pose to your pet. If fear aggression is induced by some outside stimulus, such as thunder, then proper restraint and isolation are recommended while the stimulus lasts. If a dog suffers from a vision or hearing deficit, attempts should be made to capture the dog's attention prior to approach. Also, remember that physical punishment not only is a useless tool for training but it also, by itself, can lead to natural, aggressive backlashes due to pain (and fear). This is just one more reason why such punishment should be avoided. Finally, for those dogs suffering from injuries or illnesses, owners should remember to always approach and handle them with caution, for although they might not mean to, they could exhibit aggressive tendencies due to the pain associated with the disease.

TERRITORIAL DEFENSE

Dogs, male or female, will certainly defend that property they deem theirs, and they might not hesitate to fight for it. Territorial aggressiveness toward unwelcome animals or people is not uncommon, as any utility-meter reader would attest to! Such aggressive behavior can be just as easily sparked by a perceived encroachment while the dog is eating, or while it is playing with its favorite toy. Many bite wounds to humans have been inflicted because of such actions.

Again, a return to the basics of command training should help curb some of the territorial aggressiveness that might be exhibited by some canines. Certainly, showing some respect for a dog's "private property" (toys, bowls, etc.) and its eating privacy is a commonsense way to avoid this type of aggressive behavior. It is important to impress this concept on children, too, because they are often the most frequent violators of this rule. If a dog seems particularly possessive over toys, bones, and other objects, then the number of these objects should be reduced to only one or two items. Also, consider feeding the dog in an isolated area of the home, free from interruptions.

"MEAN STREAKS"

Finally, certain breeds and canine family lines can have inherent "mean streaks" in them. For instance, chow chows are notorious among veterinary circles for their aggressiveness toward strangers. In addition, pit bull terriers, because of selective breeding, pose a real threat to any other dog that might cross their paths.

In many instances, this inherent aggressiveness can be harnessed by way of proper socialization and by strict command training. Neutering can be of assistance as well in select instances.

TREATMENT

The best treatment for most types of aggression is prevention. By adhering to the principles of proper socialization and by proper command training, most behavioral problems related to aggressiveness can be controlled or avoided altogether.

However, for any dog exhibiting aggressiveness, a thorough physical examination and consultation with a veterinarian is warranted. Ruling out underlying medical causes is certainly one reason for this; the other is that your veterinarian might choose to prescribe medications to assist in retraining efforts or as a direct attempt to curb the psychological aspects of your dog's aggressiveness. Antianxiety medications and behavior modification drugs are now commonly used in veterinary medicine to help assist in the correction of many behavioral problems, including aggressiveness. Don't hesitate to ask your veterinarian for more details.

Feline Behavioral Disorders

Among cats, the three most common behavioral disorders seen include inappropriate eliminations, destructive scratching, and aggressiveness.

Inappropriate Elimination

Cats exhibit two types of normal elimination behavior. The first involves urine spraying to delineate territories (the typical feline territory encompasses over one-tenth of a square mile) and to attract members of the opposite sex (see Fig. 2.17). The second type is called covering behavior, in which a cat digs a hole in the soil (or litter), eliminates in it, and then covers it to mask the scent. Most inappropriate house soiling that occurs with cats involves indulgences or deviations in one or the other.

The most frequent cause of house soiling deals with the first type, territoriality and sexual behavior. Both male and female cats, neutered or not, can spray urine. A new cat in the neighborhood or a female in heat can quickly set off instinctive behavior in a male cat kept indoors and lead to inappropriate markings. Even moving into a new house or apartment in which a cat previously lived might entice your cat to go around the dwelling and mark those areas in which a scent from the previous inhabitant is picked up.

Neutering might help control urine spraying in the repeat offender, yet, as mentioned before, it is not necessarily a cure-all. If there is a particular area in the house that your cat fancies the most for its spraying activities, do your best

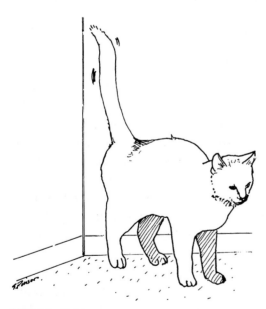

FIGURE 2.17 Cats will often spray urine to mark their territories.

to prevent its access to that part of the house. Or if you can, catch your cat in the act and punish it using a squirt from a water sprayer or a blast of air from a compressed air canister. Then leave the sprayer or canister sitting beside the soiled object or in the room for a few days. Chances are that your cat will get the drift and will abandon its tendencies to repeat the action. [*Note:* If plain water from your spray bottle seems to have little impact with your cat, adding a small amount of vinegar or lemon juice (2 tablespoons per cup of water) to it will impart to it an odor that is offensive to most cats.]

Feline odor neutralizers can be used on carpets and furniture to help eliminate those lingering odors that might be causing the problem behavior. They should also be used anytime an elimination accident occurs outside the litterbox. These odor neutralizers are available from a veterinary clinic or a pet supply store. Household cleaners designed to simply mask odors or those containing ammonia are of no use; in fact, the latter might actually attract your cat back to the same spot.

For those tough cases of urine spraying in which nothing seems to work, special drug therapy prescribed by a veterinarian might provide a satisfactory solution to the problem. However, such agents should be used only after other training methods have failed.

REFUSAL TO USE THE LITTERBOX

What about the cat that has stopped using the litterbox? There could be a number of reasons for this behavior. Some cats may not like the type or brand of litter that was put in the box. Have you changed brands lately? If so, switch back to the brand you were using before the house soiling started. Remember that the texture and scent of a litter are two factors that can influence your cat's reaction to it.

Some cats become upset if too much litter is placed in the box. Cats should be able to reach the bottom of the pan when digging. If you have one of these fickle cats, restocking the box with just a 1-inch layer of litter might do the trick.

Still other cats will refuse to use a litterbox that, in their minds, is dirty. Check your frequency of litter changes. If the litter is not being replaced every day, this could be the problem. If so, step up the frequency. Also, do not use strong cleansers when doing your weekly litterbox cleaning, as the residual scents from these might be just enough to send your cat off searching for another place to do its business.

Refusal to use a litterbox may also be linked to some traumatic incident, emotionally or physically, that occurred while your cat was using the box on a previous occasion. Because of this, it now associates the box or its location with the unpleasant incident. Obviously, the best way to find out if this is indeed the cause is to move the litterbox to a different location, one that is quiet and away from disturbances. For those cats that are especially emotional, buying new litterboxes might be required.

Not all causes of house soiling are psychological in nature. For instance, the presence of feline lower urinary tract disease can be the underlying cause of abnormal elimination behavior in felines. Since some of the diseases causing abnormal elimination can be life-threatening, always let a veterinarian rule out any medical causes before concentrating on behavioral causes.

Destructive Scratching

Scratching comes naturally to cats, which use this behavior to keep their retractable claws manicured and to mark their territories. As a result, scratching, though it might become destructive and annoying, should be viewed as a perfectly natural behavior.

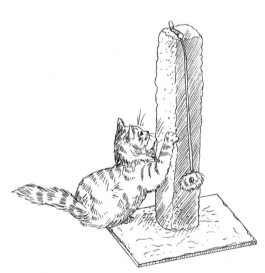

If your cat is engaged in destructive scratching, you haven't satisfied a basic need. A scratching post is a required tool for anyone who owns a cat (Fig. 2.18). In fact, it is preferable to train a cat on a scratching post right from the start instead of bringing one in to offset problem scratching activity. If your cat seems to

FIGURE 2.18 A scratching post can be used to spare you furniture from the ravages of your cat's claws!

fancy one or more particular pieces of furniture in your home, see if you can catch it in the act. If you do, use a blast of water or compressed air from a sprayer or canister to reprimand it, then leave the sprayer or canister sitting beside or on top of the piece of furniture for several days. Most cats will avoid that piece of furniture like the plague from that point on. Some persons recommend commercial cat repellents or vinegar be used on furniture to discourage scratching, but these can be messy and could stain your furniture.

For that feline that seems refractory to punishment, try placing the scratching post near its favorite piece of furniture and allow it to make a choice. Make the scratching post as plush and tempting as possible. Catnip attached to the post can help lure a reluctant cat to its new scratching post. Be sure to reward your cat for making the switch.

Special nail covers are available through veterinarians and pet stores and can be applied to the nails of your cat to prevent scratching. Surgical removal of its front claws can also be considered to spare your house from total destruction.

Aggressiveness

Because of the inherent nature of the cat, a display of aggression toward another member of its own species, especially if a territory has been violated, is somewhat common. Aggressiveness toward humans, on the other hand, can be influenced by a number of factors, including personality defects, fear, play activity, and medical disorders. Cats that have not been properly socialized to people can be expected to show some degree of aggressiveness when feeling threatened. It is also a well-known fact that even some socialized cats just want to be left alone at times and may become aggressive if disturbed.

PERSONALITY DEFECTS

Personality defects can lead to true aggressive tendencies in cats. These are cats that have been poorly socialized to humans, or have experienced negative socialization. Nervous or hyperexcitable cats or those with extremely domineering personalities can also show aggressiveness at times as well. An agitated or angry cat will flag its tail and flatten its ears against its head when approached or touched. A low-pitched growl or hiss is usually heard as well.

All aggressive cats, especially males, should be neutered or spayed. If neutering doesn't eliminate the problem, then antianxiety medications can be used to help "take the edge off" the pugnacious feline.

FEAR-INDUCED AGGRESSION

Fear-induced aggression rarely responds to training or reprimand. In fact, if such actions are attempted while the cat is in such a state, serious injury to an owner could result! The self-defense posture caused by fear-induced aggressive behavior is characterized by piloerection (hair standing on end), arched back, flattened ears, and hissing or spitting. Cats that feel threatened will lash out with their claws, and make short, sharp lunges at their adversaries. If they really sense danger, they often roll over on their backs, and assume a defense posture that will allow them to utilize the claws on all four feet.

Obviously, eliminating the source of fear is the first step in managing such aggression. Afterwards, give your cat plenty of time alone to calm down and relax. A special food treat can be offered as well to help take its mind off the incident.

PLAYFUL AGGRESSION

Playful aggression must be differentiated from the two previous types of aggression, since it is by far the easiest to address. This type of aggression is seen primarily in younger cats filled with youthful energy and curiosity. These cats may stalk house guests or ambush unexpecting owners when they arrive home. This behavior provides them a way to release excess energy and to practice their instinctive hunting skills. Most bites inflicted during this type of play are not meant to break the skin; however, this can certainly be a function of the game's intensity. One physical characteristic of a mischievous cat or kitten is that they often carry their tail arched up over their back or in an inverted "U" position during these play episodes.

Playful aggression can be managed by allowing your cat greater access to toys such as paper bags, ping pong balls, or windup, moving figures. If you play action games with your cat using strings attached to toys, be sure to remove these strings following a play session. Finally, taking your cat out for more walks during the day can help expend some of its pent-up energy.

Negative reinforcement utilizing water sprayers or compressed-air canisters can also be used to break overzealous cats of their bad habits. As a last resort, simply isolating your rambunctious feline in another room while you have guests over will ensure that they are not met with any unexpected surprises!

MEDICAL CAUSES

Let us not forget about medical causes for aggressiveness in cats. Cats that don't feel good often just want to be left alone, and if they are disturbed, they may show aggressiveness. Diseases that affect the nervous system (including rabies), metabolic disorders, and pain can all have a negative effect on a cat's personality. If your cat has experienced a gradual or sudden change in personality, have it examined by a veterinarian in order to rule out possible medical causes for the change.

Traveling with Your Dog or Cat

As a rule, most pets are good travel companions. Rarely do they become hysterical or sick to their stomachs when placed inside a moving object! However, whenever you plan on traveling with your dog or cat, be it on an extended vacation or a short trip to the local grocery store, there are some guidelines that you should follow to ensure a safe, pleasant experience.

Traveling by Car

When traveling with your pet by automobile, always keep the safety and comfort of both driver and passenger in mind. As a result, always use a travel carrier when transporting your four-legged friend by car (Fig. 3.1). Not only will your pet feel more secure in a carrier, helping to reduce stress associated with the ride, but it will help minimize jostling and jolting movements that could injure your pet. If you have a dog that is too large to fit comfortably into one of these carriers, or if the carrier is too big for your car, then the backseat is the place to be, not the frontseat! An excited or stressed-out, unrestrained pet in the passenger seat of an automobile creates a very dangerous driving condition. In addition, dogs and cats allowed to ride in frontseats can suffer serious or even lethal injuries should airbags deploy in an accident.

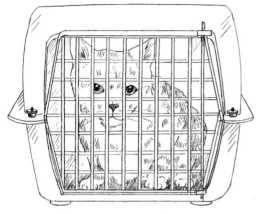

FIGURE 3.1 Cats should always be transported in sturdy carriers.

Special restraint harnesses or seatbelts are available commercially and should be used to secure your pet to its assigned seat.

Even though most dogs love to stick their heads out of car windows while cars are in motion (it reminds them of the wind in their face while they are chasing prey), don't let yours do it. Dogs with long, floppy ears can suffer trauma to their earflaps. Also, both ear and eye injuries from insects and flying road debris can easily occur in dogs allowed such freedoms.

For truck owners, never allow any dog to ride in the bed of a pickup truck unless it is confined to a carrier. Many of the dogs you see lying dead along the highway met their fate as a result of owners failing to heed such commonsense advice!

Keep the interior of your car cool and well ventilated. Dogs and cats that are excited and forced to travel in hot stuffy cars or those filled with cigarette smoke can hyperventilate and overheat. Cigarette smoke in itself can be quite irritating to the eyes, nose, and mucous membranes of your pet, and has even been linked to cancer in cats! Also, car exhaust fumes can quickly overcome a pet left inside an idling car. If you become stuck in traffic, be sure to crack the windows and keep the air circulating within the car. And never leave a dog or cat unattended in a parked car if outside temperatures exceed 72 degrees Fahrenheit or drop below 55 degrees Fahrenheit (Fig. 3.2). If you do, your pet could succumb to heat stroke or hypothermia, respectively.

DID YOU KNOW?

Second-hand cigarette smoke, either inhaled or licked from the fur, has been linked to cancer in cats!

For trips over 2 hours, be sure to take plenty of breaks to give your pet water and to relieve itself (for felines, keep a clean absorbent towel lining the floor of the carrier,

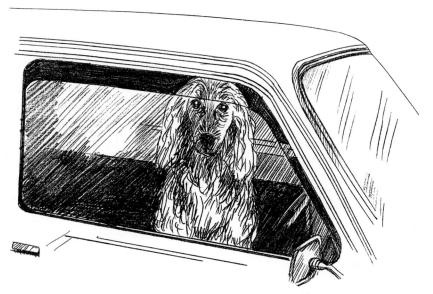

FIGURE 3.2   Leaving your dog in a parked car even with the windows cracked can be hazardous to its health.

since many cats on long trips will refuse to use a litterbox if offered one). Crushed ice is a neat and spillproof way to quench a thirsty traveler's thirst.

If your pet gets car sick, try feeding a small amount of food about 30 minutes prior to your trip. Often, an empty stomach coupled with stress can predispose a pet to motion sickness. If this fails to work, an antihistamine may be administered prior to travel. Contact your veterinarian concerning the various over-the-counter medications you can use and their dosages.

For those pets absolutely terrified of the car, a stronger tranquilizer prescribed by a veterinarian may be needed. Although this should be used only as a last resort, it can be an effective tool for taking the edge off your phobic friend and thereby making the ride much less stressful for everyone concerned.

Traveling by Air

If you are planning to transport your pet by plane, consult a veterinarian before your trip to determine whether your pet has any medical conditions that may prohibit such travel. For example, should significant temperature and/or pressure fluctuations occur during flight, they could be harmful to a pet suffering from an underlying heart condition.

Since different companies may have different policies, check ahead of time with the airline concerning its travel rules and requirements for pets. Many airlines will allow you to take a cat or small dog into the cabin with you; however, realize that for the comfort of you and fellow passengers, it must be well behaved and silent during the trip. If you fear that these two criteria will not be met, your pet should travel cargo.

If your dog or cat is to travel cargo, book either an early evening or early morning flight during the summer months and midday flights during winter months to protect it from exposure to temperature extremes. Also, book direct flights only so that there's no chance of "lost baggage." If possible, plan on arriving early enough at the gate so that you can observe your pet being loaded onto the plane.

If you own a pet carrier that is not fit for air travel, most airlines have carriers for rent; however, be sure that the carrier selected for your pet is the proper size for its safety during the flight. Call ahead of time to confirm carrier availability.

You will want to pad the inside of the carrier liberally with large blankets and/or towels. And don't forget to throw in one of your dog or cat's favorite toys! A "live animal" sticker, as well as your name, address, and phone number, should be attached conspicuously to the outside of the carrier.

Avoid feeding your pet solid food within 6 hours of the plane trip. Provide a constant source of water during the flight by freezing water in a water bowl the night prior to your trip and placing this in your pet's carrier prior to the flight.

Dr. P's Vet Tip

When transporting your pet by air, book nonstop flights to reduce the chances of your pet becoming lost luggage. In addition, during the summer, book flights early in the mornings or late in the evenings to avoid exposing your pet to midday heat.

Vacation Planning

Prior to leaving on a vacation, there are certain items that need to be taken care of first. To begin, be sure you are aware of all the requirements necessary for taking your dog or cat to its intended destination, including required health certificates, quarantines, and customs. When traveling domestically and interstate with your pet, two items you should always have with you are your pet's vaccination record and a current health certificate. A licensed veterinarian must issue this health certificate within 10 days of your trip. If traveling overseas, the embassy of the country of destination can inform you of all the necessary requirements for the safe and legal transport of your pet.

Be sure that the carrier you have for your dog or cat is sturdy and in good condition. Also, make sure that your pet's collar has identification tags, including a phone number, if possible, of where you'll be staying just in case your pet gets lost. Of course, you'll want to take a leash along for daily exercise, as well as your pet's brush and/or comb for daily grooming. Finally, plan on taking plenty of your pet's food along with you, just in case the brand you normally feed your pet is not available at your destination.

Consult travel guides or travel agents to find listing of those motels, hotels, and campgrounds that accept pets, and plan your overnight stops around these locations. Finally, when you arrive at your destination, look in the local phone directory for the name and number of a local veterinarian in the area, in case of emergency.

Try not to leave your pet unattended in your motel or hotel room. If you do, be sure to place the "Do not disturb" sign on the front door so that your pet doesn't accidentally escape if housekeeping comes to clean your room while you are away.

When camping with your pet, don't allow it to roam or to interact with wild animals. Cats especially, being the natural-bred hunters that they are, could get themselves in trouble real quick! It's also a great idea to have your pet checked out by a veterinarian following these camping trips to be sure that it didn't pick up any unwanted parasites from the local fauna.

Finally, there will be times when your dog or cat will be better off staying at home rather than traveling with you. In these instances, choose a kennel facility for your dog or cat as you would a hotel for yourself, making sure that it is clean, well ventilated, and staffed by a caring group of people. Many newer facilities are equipped with interactive cameras attached to each run or pen that can be accessed over the Internet, allowing you to check in on your pet even if you happen to be on the other side of the world! Although it costs more to board a pet at such a facility, many owners feel it is well worth the price.

Another great alternative is to let your dog or cat stay home and hire a pet sitter to check in on it throughout the day. If you can't find a neighbor or friend to oblige, check your phone book for a reliable professional pet sitter near you, or ask someone at a local veterinary clinic to recommend one to you.

Preventive Health Care

When it comes to health, pets are just like people. Some will go through their entire lives without any health problems along the way; others just seem to be prone to every illness that comes along. A number of factors play a role in the susceptibility of dogs and cats to illness, including genetics, environment, nutrition, immune system competence, and, very importantly, the extent of preventive health care provided to them by their owners. In fact, for a pet that is genetically prone to illness, this latter factor can do wonders to help counteract some of these inherent effects. Unfortunately, many pet owners fail to realize the importance of preventive health care; as a result, their pet can ultimately pay the price later in life.

At-Home Physical Exam

Do you worry about your pet's health even when it appears healthy? Your veterinarian can ensure that your dog or cat is thriving by performing a thorough checkup, but what can you do between visits? Pets cannot verbalize their discomforts, and people often worry that they'll miss the early signs of illness. If you learn to examine your pet at home, you can have that all-important peace of mind between visits to the vet (Fig. 4.1).

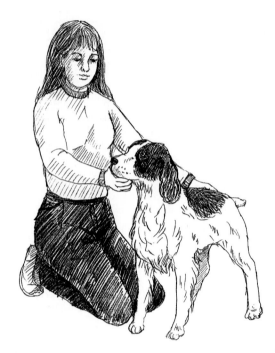

FIGURE 4.1 Periodic physical exams performed at home are a vital part of your pet's preventive health care program.

During your next visit to pet clinic, the veterinarian will probably begin with an examination of your pet. Watch how your veterinarian performs the exam and ask to participate in the process. Discuss your desire to supplement the vet's exams with at-home checks that you will make. The veterinarian should be pleased with your desire to provide such attention to your pet's health and should be happy to help develop your skills (Fig. 4.2). Your teamwork will provide the consistent attention to details that could prevent a tragedy.

At-home examinations are no substitute for a veterinary checkup, but doing them might one day give you a jump on treating a minor or serious condition. For convenience, these exams can be combined with regular grooming sessions. Use the physical exam checklist in Table 4.1 as your guide. Also, see Fig. 4.3 for instructions on how to take your pet's temperature (see also Table 4.2), pulse, and respiratory readings. Finally, get into the habit of weighing your pet every 3 months and recording your readings. Unexplained weight loss or weight gain or a pattern of continual loss or gain should prompt you to contact your veterinarian. Also check for other signs of illness, such as a visible "third eyelid" in cats (Fig. 4.4).

Vaccinations and the ABCs of Immunity

The theory behind vaccinating any pet is to provide artificial exposure to certain disease-causing organisms, thereby priming the body's immune system before actual exposure occurs (Fig. 4.5). Doing so will

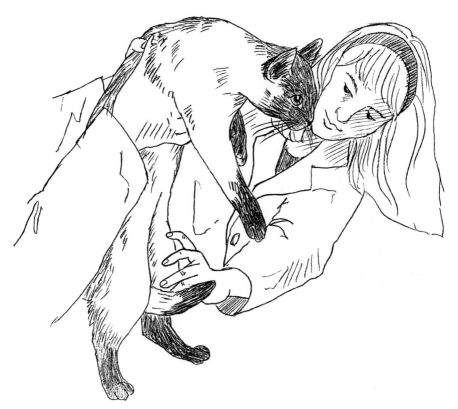

FIGURE 4.2 Preventive health care can help your cat live a happy and healthy life.

allow for a rapid, effective immune response if this exposure does happen, without the lag time associated with a first exposure.

If the mother has been properly vaccinated prior to pregnancy, most puppies and kittens receive protective antibodies from their mother through nursing, primarily during the first 24 hours of life. These "passive" antibodies are important, since the immune system of a neonate less than 6 weeks of age is incapable of mounting an effective response to any antigen (foreign organism or substance). Around 8 weeks of age, levels of these antibodies begin to taper off, leaving the pet to fend for itself.

If a puppy or kitten that still has adequate levels of passive antibodies present in its system is immunized, the vaccination will be rendered ineffective. For this reason, initial vaccinations are usually given around

Table 4.1 Physical Exam Checklist for Dogs and Cats

Date _____ Temperature _____ Weight _____

General evaluation

—Alert	—Disinterested
—Active	—Lethargic
—Healthy appetite	—Poor appetite
—Playful	—Weight loss/gain
—Lameness	—Abnormal posture
—Abnormal aggressiveness	

Skin and haircoat

—Appear normal	—Shedding
—Hair loss	—Mats
—Dull; unkempt	—Tumors or warts
—Scaly	—Parasites
—Dry	—Abnormal lumps under the skin
—Oily	—Crusts on neck and head
—Itching	

Eyes

—Appear normal	—Haziness/cloudiness
—Clear discharge	—Unequal pupil size
—Mucus discharge	—Discoloration
—Redness	—Squinting
—Eyelid abnormalities	—Protruding third eyelids

Ears

—Appear normal	—Hair loss on pinnae
—Red; swollen	—Bad odor

Table 4.1 Physical Exam Checklist for Dogs and Cats (*Continued*)

—Itchy	—Masses
—Creamy, yellow discharge	—Tender
—Brown to black discharge	—Head tilt
—Head shaking	
Nose and throat	
—Appear normal	—Ulceration on nose
—Nasal discharge	—Crusty nose
—Enlarged lymph nodes (feel on either side of the neck just under the jaw)	
Mouth, teeth, and gums	
—Appear normal	—Tooth loss
—Broken, discolored, or loose teeth	—Inflamed gums
—Foul odor	—Excess salivation
—Tartar accumulation	—Pale gums
—Growths or masses	—Ulcers
—Base of tongue inflamed	—Foreign body noted
Miscellaneous	
—Abdominal tenderness	—Increased water consumption
—Coughing	—Decreased water consumption
—Breathing difficulties	—Genital discharge
—Abnormal stools	—Mammary lumps
—Straining to urinate	—Swollen limb

8 weeks of age, when levels of passive antibodies begin to decrease. Vaccination as early as 6 weeks of age may be indicated in those instances where the mother has not been vaccinated, or if lack of passive antibody absorption is a possibility (i.e., inadequate nursing during the first hours of life).

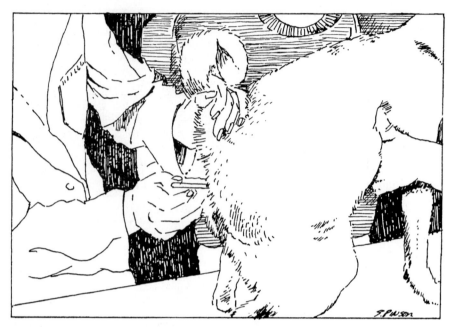

FIGURE 4.3   Use a digital thermometer to obtain your pet's temperature.

Table 4.2 Potential Causes of Elevated Body Temperature in Dogs and Cats

Fear or excitement

High environmental temperature

Exercise

Infection

Tissue inflammation or trauma

Autoimmune disease

Cancer

Drug reactions

Endocrine disorders (e.g., hyperthyroidism)

Vaccinating Your Dog

Four core vaccines should be administered to all dogs. These include those protecting against distemper, parvovirus, adenovirus (infectious canine hepatitis), and rabies. Other vaccines, including those against parainfluenza, canine contagious respiratory disease (kennel cough; *Bordetella*), leptospirosis, coronavirus, lyme disease, and *Giardia* are optional, and should be administered only upon the recommendation of your veterinarian. See Table 4.3 for current recommendations.

Vaccinating Your Cat

Five core vaccines should be administered to all cats. These include vaccines against panleukopenia (parvovirus), herpesvirus (viral rhinotracheitis), calicivirus, feline leukemia (FeLV), and rabies. Other vaccines, including those for the feline immunodeficiency virus (feline AIDS), feline infectious peritonitis (FIP), ringworm, *Chlamydophila,* and *Bordetella* are optional, and should be administered only on veterinary recommendation. Table 4.4 lists current vaccination recommendations for cats.

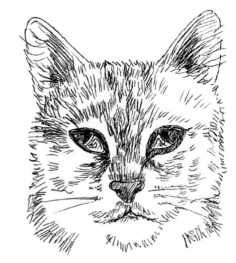

FIGURE 4.4 Protrusion of the third eyelids is a sign of illness in cats.

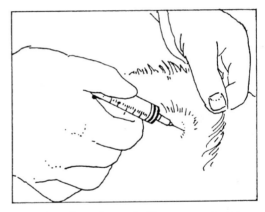

FIGURE 4.5 Immunizations are an important line of defense against disease.

As you can see from Tables 4.3 and 4.4, the school of thought regarding canine and feline immunizations has changed. Many veterinary practitioners and veterinary schools are using extended vaccination schedules in lieu of the traditional "yearly booster" approach. These changes in traditional protocol are based on research findings indicating that

■ Certain vaccines may provide extended immunity and, in some cases, lifelong immunity after an initial series of immunizations.

FACT OR FICTION

Vaccines given to puppies 8 weeks of age or younger are generally ineffective. **FACT.** Vaccines administered before a puppy is 8 weeks old are rendered useless by antibodies that the puppy received from its mother while nursing. In addition, even if the puppy did not receive such antibodies, its immune system is often too immature at 6 weeks of age to respond effectively to antigenic stimulations.

- Vaccines administered after this immunity has been established may be neutralized and rendered ineffective by the pet's immune system.

- Repeated immunization using certain vaccine agents, especially those that contain adjuvants (chemical compounds designed to increase the effectiveness of the vaccine), has been linked to allergic reactions, autoimmune disease, and feline sarcoma, a deadly form of cancer in cats.

Discussion

Research also suggests that individual vaccines that provide protection against a single type of disease ("univalent" vaccines) should be administered in lieu of those containing multiple agents that stimulate immunity against more than one type of disease ("multivalent" vaccines). The traditional "5-way" and "7-way" vaccines used in pets for years are examples of multivalent vaccines. Even though it may mean more needles for your pet, the protection conferred by univalent vaccines is deemed superior to that of the multivalent varieties.

Regardless of types of vaccines used and frequency of immunizations, such a protocol must be one that provides maximum protection with minimum risk to the pet. One option that many veterinarians are now offering prior to vaccinating a pet is antibody titer testing. With such testing, levels of antibodies to the various disease agents are measured in a blood sample. If a specific antibody titer (the level of antibodies in the blood) is deemed protective, no vaccination is necessary. However, if this level is too low, then a vaccine can be given to stimulate the body to produce a protective level once again. Be sure to ask your veterinarian about titer testing and about the latest research findings regarding canine and feline immunology. Your pet's health depends on it!

Table 4.3 Canine Vaccine Schedule

Vaccine	Initial series	Booster interval
Core group		
Rabies	16 weeks	Every 1–3 years, depending on the state in which you live
	1 year + 4 months	
Distemper	8 weeks	Every 3–7 years or as recommended by veterinarian
	12 weeks	
	16 weeks	
	1 year + 4 months	
Parvovirus	8 weeks	Every 3–7 years or as recommended by veterinarian
	12 weeks	
	16 weeks	
	1 year + 4 months	
Adenovirus	8 weeks	Every 3–7 years or as recommended by veterinarian
Noncore group		
Bordetella (intranasal)	10 days prior to boarding, grooming, and dog shows	Every 6 months as needed
Parainfluenza	As recommended by veterinarian	
Leptospirosis	As recommended by veterinarian	
Lyme disease	As recommended by veterinarian	
Giardia	As recommended by veterinarian	
Coronavirus	As recommended by veterinarian	

Table 4.4 Feline Vaccine Schedule

Vaccine	Initial series	Interval for boosters
Core group		
Rabies	16 weeks	Every 1–3 years, depending on state
	1 year + 4 months	
Herpes/calicivirus	8 weeks	Intranasal vaccine an nually or as recommended by veterinarian
	12 weeks	
	16 weeks	
	1 year + 4 months	
Panleukopenia	8 weeks	As recommended by veterinarian
	12 weeks	
	16 weeks	
	1 year + 4 months	
Feline leukemia	9–12 weeks	As recommended by veterinarian
	12–16 weeks	
Noncore group		
Chlamydophila	As recommended by veterinarian	
Bordetella	As recommended by veterinarian	
Feline infectious peritonitis (FIP)	As recommended by veterinarian	
Feline immuodeficiency virus	As recommended by veterinarian	

Controlling Internal Parasites

Left undetected and untreated, intestinal parasites can rob your dog or cat of much-needed nutrients, can cause severe gastrointestinal upset, and can predispose it to secondary disease. Internal parasites are widespread throughout the pet population. To make matters worse, many internal parasites of dogs and cats are also classified as *zoonotic diseases*; that is, they can be directly communicable to humans, especially children. As a result, controlling intestinal parasites is a vital part of any preventive health care program.

Management of intestinal worms should begin when a puppy or kitten is as young as 3 weeks of age. At this age, these infants can harbor immature hookworms and roundworms without any evidence of eggs shed in the stool. Puppies and kittens should receive medications for these parasites at 3, 6, and 9 weeks of age, regardless of whether eggs are detected in their stool.

Stool Examinations

More treatments might be necessary for those puppies or kittens found to be actually harboring worms. Stool examinations on such a pet should be performed by a veterinarian at 6, 9, and 12 weeks of age to ensure that it is indeed free of these parasites and is not shedding eggs into the environment.

Frequent stool checks such as these will also assist in the detection of two other common intestinal parasites: tapeworms and coccidia. The latter parasite can especially cause severe gastroenteritis and sometimes even neurological problems in puppies and kittens if left undetected and untreated.

Most heartworm preventives available for dogs also contain medication to protect against common canine intestinal parasites. As a result, if your pet is taking such medication (and it should be!), it does not need to be routinely dewormed. However, your pet's stools should still be examined for parasite eggs at least once a year, just to be safe. Stool exams should also be conducted on any ill animal, regardless of clinical signs. Even when the worms do not directly cause the illness, their mere presence and effect on the host's immune system can exacerbate any disease, regardless of cause.

Environmental Sanitation

Aside from routine stool checks, good environmental sanitation is another way to lessen the impact of intestinal parasites. Many parasite eggs that are shed into the environment via feces take days of sitting in the sunlight or in other favorable environmental conditions before becoming infective to other pets. As a result, keeping all fecal matter (either your pet's or that of an unwelcome visitor) cleaned up out of your pet's environment (or litterbox) on a daily basis is a very effective way of protecting your pet (and yourself) from these worms.

Controlling Fleas and Ticks

Much confusion exists about the proper approaches to external parasite control and prevention in pets. Many different products are now available for external parasite control. The key to successful control is to choose and properly use the products that provide the best possible results for the specific external parasite and environment involved.

Flea Control

Fleas are by far the most common external parasites with which your dog or cat will have to contend. Effective flea control entails not only treatment for fleas on the pet but environmental control as well (Fig. 4.6). Consult with your veterinarian concerning the best approach to take to relieve your pet of these pesky parasites.

INSECTICIDE SPRAYS, POWDERS, COLLARS, AND DIPS

Once serving as the vanguard in the war against fleas and ticks, these products are being replaced by newer, more effective agents. However, some can still be helpful in certain situations, and warrant mention here.

Flea and tick sprays, available in both liquid and aerosol forms, are useful for spot treatments. Sprays containing natural chemicals

DID YOU KNOW?

Not only can their annoying bites produce extreme discomfort and even allergic reactions, fleas are also the source of the most common tapeworm that affect cats, *Dipylidium caninum*.

called *pyrethrins,* derived from chrysanthemums, are the preferred products over others for flea control because of their safety and efficacy if used properly. The major advantage of natural pyrethrins is that they are relatively safe for use on pets of all ages. The disadvantage is that they have poor residual flea-fighting activity, lasting only a day or so. Newer, synthetic pyrethrin products available on the market today have improved this residual activity while still maintaining a good safety mar-

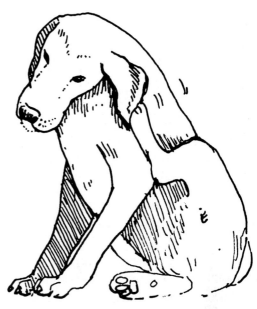

FIGURE 4.6 With the advent of sophisticated methods and products, flea control has never been easier!

gin. If pyrethrin products are used, frequent spray application, both on the pet and in its environment (bedding, carpeting, etc.), is imperative for effective flea control. In some instances, this means on a daily basis. Just be sure before doing so to check the label on the particular product you are using to confirm the safety of this practice. If you are in doubt, always follow label directions!

As with the sprays, pyrethrin-containing powders are preferred over others because of their low toxicity potentials. Powders do not evaporate like liquid products; therefore, under dry conditions, powders stay active on the hair and skin somewhat longer than do sprays. Again, frequent application is required for best results. Exposure to water inactivates most insecticide powders.

> ## Dr. P's Vet Tip
>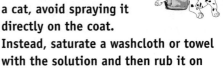
> When applying any type of spray to the haircoat of a cat, avoid spraying it directly on the coat.
> Instead, saturate a washcloth or towel with the solution and then rub it on the haircoat. Your cat is much less likely to object to treatment that way.

Insecticide shampoos and collars are common items in both retail stores and in most veterinary clinics. However, since frequent shampooing can lead to excessively dry skin, and collars are of little use to begin with, these products are not recommended for flea control. Dips, which are simply highly concentrated preparations of insecticides, are also no longer recommended for flea and tick control, because of their highly toxic nature and the advent of newer, safer products.

SECOND-GENERATION (ONCE-A-MONTH) PRODUCTS

When treating for parasites on your dog or cat, a number of products designed to be administered only once per month are now available. For instance, fipronil (Frontline®) kills adult fleas on pets and helps to break the flea life cycle by killing immature fleas before they can lay eggs. This product is also effective against ticks that your pet may encounter in the woods or field. Applied as a spray or topical drops, fipronil collects within the hair follicles and sebaceous glands of the skin, providing good residual action after initial application. Imidacloprid (Advantage®) is yet another addition to the flea-control arsenal that can be incorporated into a comprehensive flea-control program. Imidacloprid works by killing adult fleas on contact, before they can lay eggs. Applied as topical drops on the back, according to the manufacturer, this product retains its effectiveness even after shampooing or repeated swimming. Lufenuron (Program®, Sentinel®) is a product designed to be taken internally by your dog. Available in tablet form, lufenuron exerts its flea control action by sterilizing the fleas that bite the dog. Since they cannot reproduce, fleas are eventually eliminated (in a contained environment) via attrition. It is important to remember that lufenuron does not actually kill fleas. As a result, products that kill adult fleas must be used in conjunction with this treatment in order to achieve effective flea control. As one might expect, many veterinarians recommend this product only for those dogs kept in an indoor (contained) environment.

DID YOU KNOW?

Since the advent of newer, safer flea-control products, the incidence of insecticide-related poisoning in cats has decreased dramatically!

NATURAL REMEDIES

Throughout the years, countless natural remedies

for parasite control have been touted as effective alternatives to insecticides. Some of these substances or devices are worn or applied externally; some are designed to be taken internally.

Products such as brewer's yeast, garlic, and B vitamins have all been implicated at one time or another as flea-control remedies. Unfortunately, controlled scientific studies indicate little to no benefit in flea control with these products. In addition, some natural substances can be highly toxic to cats. Check with a veterinarian before giving any natural remedy to your cat.

Certain products containing abrasive-type ingredients (e.g., silica gel and diatomaceous earth) are available for external flea control. These noninsecticidal products act by damaging the chitin exoskeleton of the flea, leading to desiccation (drying up) and death of the flea.

Moderate success has been reported with these abrasive-type products. Drying and/or mild irritation of the pet's skin may occur with these products. Frequent application (four to seven times weekly) is required if these are to be used.

Electronic flea collars have limited popularity, as well as limited benefits. Although manufacturers may stand by their efficacy, scientific studies have shown that their worth in controlling external parasites is minimal. The idea behind them is that the device emits a high-pitched sound that can't be heard by humans or pets, yet it drives fleas away. Unfortunately, aside from their relative ineffectiveness, some models might indeed deliver an audible pitch that can be heard by—and might be quite discomforting to—the dog or cat wearing the collar.

ENVIRONMENTAL CONTROL

Environmental control of fleas begins in the home (Fig. 4.7). You can use insecticidal foggers to get the job done, or you can employ a professional exterminator. For excellent results, you can also use polymerized borate compounds, available under various brand names from a veterinary clinic or pet supply store. Sprinkled on the carpets, baseboards, and/or furniture, these compounds will kill all fleas that come in contact with them. Noticeable results are usually obtained within a week after application. Best of all, these powders are odorless, easy to use, and safe for pets and children. Under normal conditions, application of this product must be performed every 6 to 12 months. Carpets must remain dry for continued efficacy; if the carpet becomes damp or is shampooed, reapplication will be necessary.

Your yard should be treated with insecticidal granules every 6 to 8 weeks during the warm months of the year. Alternating the types of insecticidal granules used with each treatment (several different types are available commercially) can improve effectiveness of your overall control program.

Tick Control

Besides fleas, the next most prevalent external parasite that your dog or cat will likely encounter is the tick. Dogs are more likely than cats to be parasitized by ticks, since cats, because of their meticulous grooming habits, rarely afford a tick the time it needs to attach itself. Regardless, controlling ticks on your pet and in your environment is important not only for your pet's health but for yours as well. These unsightly parasites, which attach themselves to their host via sucking mouthparts, can transmit serious diseases such as Rocky Mountain Spotted Fever and Lyme disease to pets and to people. As far as their four-legged hosts are concerned, untreated infestations can also lead to skin irritation and in severe cases, blood-loss anemia.

Female ticks lay their eggs in and under sheltered areas in the environment, such as wood stumps, rocks, and wall crevices. Once hatched, the larvae, called "seed ticks," will crawl up onto grass stems or bushes and attach themselves to a host that may happen to pass by. Depending on their life cycle, immature ticks may seek out one to three different host animals to complete the maturation process into an adult.

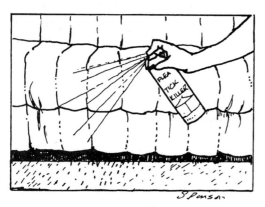

FIGURE 4.7 Environmental treatment is required for effective flea control.

Since ticks are sensitive to the same type of chemicals as are fleas, treatment and control are basically the same. Certain topical once-a-month treatments for fleas in dogs and cats can be effective in controlling ticks as well. Ask a veterinarian for details. Flea and tick collars can be effective at keeping ticks out of the ears. Just be sure that if you plan to use one on your cat, it is of the "breakaway" variety that is designed to snap apart in case it gets snagged on a fence or tree branch. A pyrethrin spray or powder can also be applied to your pet's haircoat prior to a trip outdoors to discourage ticks from attaching.

Certainly a thorough and consistent treatment of the yard (and sometimes the house) with an approved insecticide is the cornerstone of an effective control program. Since ticks can live for months in their surrounding habitat without a blood meal, treatment should be performed every 2 to 4 weeks during the peak tick seasons in your area.

If a tick happens to attach itself to your pet, use a pyrethrin spray to kill it. Never attempt to remove ticks from your dog or cat by applying manual pressure alone, or by applying a hot match or needle to the tick's body. Most ticks first killed by the application of a pyrethrin spray will fall off with time once they die. In some cases, you may need to manually remove the dead tick after spraying. When picking them off your pet, never use your bare hands, in order to prevent accidental exposure to disease. Instead, use a pair of gloves and tweezers to grasp the dead tick as close to its attachment site as possible, then pull straight up using constant tension. Once the tick is freed, wash the bite wound with soap and water and then apply a first aid cream or ointment to prevent infection. Again, be sure that the tick is completely dead before removal; this will ensure that the tick's mouthparts come out attached to the rest of the body. If left behind, the mouthparts can cause an irritating localized skin reaction.

Preventing Heartworm Disease

Heartworm disease is a devastating illness of dogs, responsible for tens of thousands of deaths each year. Most of these occur due to the destruction that these worms do to not just the heart, but the lungs, liver, and kidneys as well. In some cases, the worm burden within the heart and blood vessels can become so great that circulation of blood is actually compro-

Dr. P's Vet Tip

Even if the heartworm preventive medication is not required year-round in your area, you should still give it to your pet all throughout the year. The reason: Most preventives sold on the market today also prevent infestations with intestinal parasites (some of which can be zoonotic, including roundworms), providing an important source of continual protection not only for your dog but for you and your family as well.

mised, resulting in sudden death. Other infected dogs can go years without showing any signs of heartworm disease, seemingly forming a symbiotic relationship with the parasites. Regardless of its presentation, the presence of heartworm disease puts a tremendous burden on the body's organs and immune system (Fig. 4.8). (For more information regarding canine heartworm disease, see Chapter 7.)

The good news is that this destructive disease is completely and easily preventable! The most popular heartworm preventive medications come in tablet form or as topical "spot-ons" and are designed to be given just once a month. If your dog is not currently on a heartworm prevention program, call right now and schedule an appointment with your veterinarian to start one (Fig. 4.9). As a responsible pet owner, you owe it to your companion! In warmer clients where mosquitoes are present nearly year-round, the heartworm preventive must be given 12 months out of the year. In contrast, in those regions that experience seasonal changes and lower temperatures, the preventive need not be given for the entire year but only during the warmer mosquito season. Be sure to consult your veterinarian as to the proper preventive schedule to follow in your particular area.

Before starting a dog on heartworm preventive medication, a simple blood test needs to be performed to determine if exposure to heartworms has already

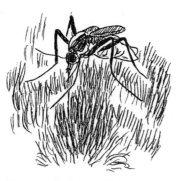

FIGURE 4.8   The mosquito is the vector for both feline and canine heartworm disease.

occurred (Fig. 4.10). If the test results are negative, then your dog may be started on a preventive. However, if the test returns positive for heartworms, then treatment options must be discussed. Furthermore, if you are currently giving your pet preventive medication and you miss a scheduled administration, consult a veterinarian before resuming the treatments. Depending on how late you are on the treatment, retesting may be recommended. For those dogs

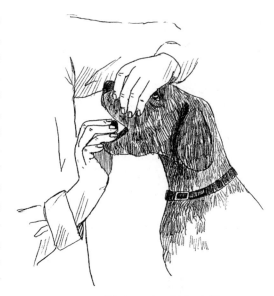

FIGURE 4.9 All dogs should be taking heartworm preventive medicine.

on a seasonal prevention program, blood retesting should be performed before the first preventive medication of the season is given.

Although cats are not the natural host of heartworms, they can infest the heart and vessels of this species as well, with serious consequences. Even though the number of worms typically found in an infected feline's heart is usually small, these worms still take up a lot of space and interfere with proper heart function. The challenge is that cats afflicted with this parasitism are difficult to treat, because killing the adult worms in the relatively small heart and lungs of cats (when compared to dogs) can cause life-threatening blockages to proper blood circulation. As a result, preventing this disease from the start is the key. And the good news is that, as in dogs, it is easy to do so. Feline heartworm preventive medication comes in tablet form, and is designed to be given just once a month as well. Ask a veterinarian for details.

Dental Care

Periodontal disease, or tooth-and-gum disease, is one of the most common diseases affecting pets today. In fact, most dogs and cats show

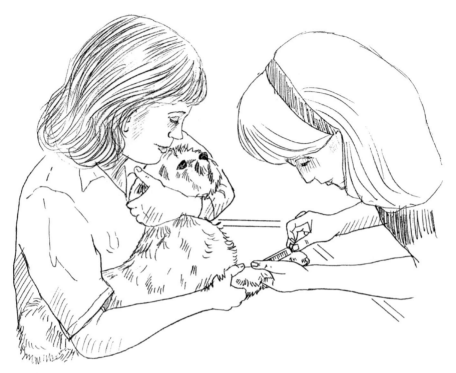

FIGURE 4.10   Drawing blood for a heartworm test.

some signs of this disease by 3 years of age. Signs can include tender, swollen gums, excessive drooling, loss of appetite, and bad breath.

A complete dental exam should be performed on all pets at least once a year. For smaller breeds more prone to periodontal disease, these exams should be done every 6 months. If dental calculus is present at the gumline, the veterinarian should professionally clean the teeth (Fig. 4.11). Because this cleaning can be a painful procedure, especially if periodontal disease already exists, a short-acting sedative or anesthetic is essential for your pet's comfort and safety. An ultrasonic dental scaler, combined with manual scaling instruments, is used to break apart and remove the hard calculus and deposits from the tooth surfaces. Afterward, the teeth are polished with a special paste to restore their natural smooth surfaces.

Your pet's dental care doesn't stop there, though! At-home aftercare is a vital part of your pet's dental health. Toothpaste, gels, and rinses formulated for use in pets are readily available from pet stores or from veterinary offices. Choose one that contains chlorhexidine, as this antibacterial compound can remain effective for up to 12 hours after application. Human toothpaste should not be used, as it can cause stomach upset if swallowed by your pet. Also, the much-advocated home formula mixing baking soda and

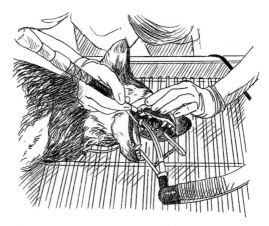

FIGURE 4.11 Professional cleaning will be needed to effectively remove dental calculus from your pet's teeth.

salt in water can be effective as a toothpaste alternative, yet, because of the high sodium content of this mixture, it should not be used in older pets or in those pets suffering from heart ailments. A regular, soft-bristled, human toothbrush can be used to apply the dental product. For cats and smaller dogs, a child's toothbrush can be substituted. However, for best result, purchase a special "finger" brush that fits on the end of your finger (Fig. 4.12). These can be purchased at any pet supply store. Apply the paste, gel, or solution to the brush, and proceed to brush as you would your own teeth, concentrating on the gumline as well as the outsides of the large premolars and canine teeth. No rinsing is necessary.

What about flossing? Yes, you can floss your dog's teeth, but not in the conventional way. Flossing devices in the form of chew toys have been developed to assist in dental hygiene (Fig. 4.13). Don't laugh; such devices can have a significant impact on dental health, assuming, of course, that your pet will play with them.

Rawhides, nylon chew bones, and urethane chewing devices can also prove helpful in mechanically removing plaque from canine dental surfaces. Contrary to popular belief, feeding hard chew biscuits does little by itself to prevent periodontal disease; in fact, the starchy nature of such food items can promote plaque formation. The same holds true for most hard dry foods, although most contain substantially less

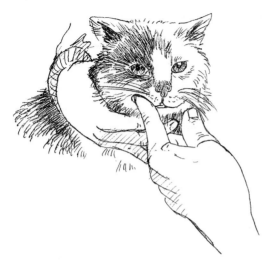

FIGURE 4.12 You can use your finger to apply dental paste along the gumline to help prevent periodontal disease.

plaque-promoting sugar than do their moist counterparts. Special diets do exist that contain ingredients to help control tartar buildup in dogs and cats. Ask a veterinarian if such a diet would be right for your pet.

Remember: Good dental hygiene is important to the health of your pet. In fact, it can help it live a longer, happier life. If you have any questions concerning your pet's dental health, don't hesitate to confer with a veterinarian.

Feeding Your Pet

There can be little doubt that proper nutrition is the cornerstone of a long, healthy life for all pets. As our understanding of the link between diet and health increases each day, so does the quality of foods that are available to feed your pet. Not long ago, the diet of most dogs and cats consisted primarily of table scraps, supplemented by whatever other

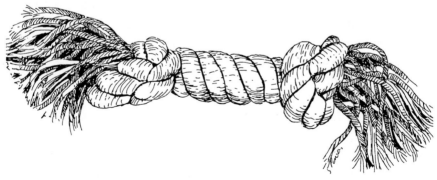

FIGURE 4.13 Dental floss for dogs.

foods they could find while roaming freely. Today, our pets more often than not live indoors with us, and it is much more practical to feed them commercially prepared food that is complete and balanced for the particular stage of life of each pet.

While the quality of nutrition for dogs and cats has improved considerably with the increasing use of prepared pet foods, there remains a great deal you should know about choosing the proper diet for your pet from among the many thousands of brands available in this country alone. Because dogs and cats move through several "life stages" as they age, it is easiest to discuss the nutritional needs of these different life stages separately and in the order in which the pet experiences them.

Nutrition for Puppies and Kittens

For most dogs and cats, childhood lasts for about 1 year, although very large breed dogs (Great Danes, Newfoundlands, St. Bernards, etc.) may continue to grow rapidly until they are 18 to 24 months of age. During this time, puppies and kittens requires higher levels of minerals such as calcium and phosphorus, protein, vitamins, and energy (calories) than they will as an adult. Therefore, foods fed to young, growing pets should contain these higher levels in balance with each other and with all other dietary nutrients. Such a pet food will carry a designation such as "canine growth," or "kitten food," to distinguish it from diets that contain levels of nutrients that are right for other stages of life.

Please note that the commonly held belief that if "a little is good, more must be better" is not true when it comes to feeding pets. Diets that contain very high levels of minerals, protein, and some vitamins are not superior to those that contain only the amounts required for growth. Excesses can actually be harmful to the growing pups and kittens, as can the practice of supplementing a good growth diet with various human foods or vitamin/mineral preparations.

> ## Dr. P's Vet Tip
>
> Be careful not to overfeed growing puppies, especially fast-growing large breeds. To do so could lead to arthritis later in life. As far as how much to feed, follow the manufacturer's recommendation for the particular food you are using.

For instance, scientific studies have shown that high calcium and phosphorus intake by young dogs can lead to a variety of bone problems, especially in large, rapidly growing dogs. In addition, research has also shown that allowing your puppy to overeat even a high-quality, well-balanced growth diet can lead to some of these same problems because the pup grows too rapidly as a result of the increased food intake.

To be sure that your puppy or kitten gets all the good nutrition it needs for good growth and development, but never too much, follow these simple guidelines:

1. Feed a high-quality, balanced commercial puppy food for puppies or kitten food for kittens. A veterinarian can recommend an appropriate brand. Remember that your pet's nutrition will influence its lifelong health and happiness. It is very important that you invest in good nutrition at this crucial life stage.

2. If you own a large breed puppy that will have an adult weight exceeding 55 pounds, consider feeding it a diet specially designed for its growth needs. These diets contain controlled levels of fat, calories, and minerals when compared to conventional puppy foods in order to promote a proper growth rate, thereby guarding against bone and skeletal disorders that can be caused by extrafast growth in large breed puppies. Ask a veterinarian to recommend such a diet for your dog.

3. Do not supplement a quality, balanced food; you will almost certainly create an imbalance in your pet's diet if you do. Avoid giving table food, table scraps, or treats and snacks to your puppy or kitten for the same reason (Fig. 4.14).

4. Kittens can be fed free-choice; however, follow the daily recommendations given on the food bag or can and don't offer more than these amounts. Do not feed puppies free-choice. Most pups are very eager eaters and will tend to eat too much of a high-quality, highly palatable (good-tasting) diet. It is much better to put down one-half of the recommended daily ration amount (as stated on the bag or can) for a limited time period, say, 30 minutes. Allow your pup to eat all that it wishes to eat in that time, and then pick up any uneaten food and save it until the next feeding. Later on in the day, feed the second half of the daily ration, along with the food not eaten at the first sitting.

5. Keep fresh, clean water (preferably filtered) available at all times (Fig. 4.15).

Nutrition for Adults

At about 12 months of age, switch your pet to a maintenance diet for adults. Once your puppy or kitten is grown, its nutritional needs are reduced considerably from those during the rapid development of that first year. Continuing to feed your adult pet high levels of minerals (particularly calcium and phosphorus), protein, and energy (calories) could lead to problems later in life. Just as we are finding that excess intake of certain dietary nutrients (like phosphorus, sodium, and fat) are harmful for humans over long periods, certain excesses might also contribute to diseases such as kidney failure, heart failure, obesity, and diabetes in adult and senior pets. Also, we know that reducing the level of key nutrients in the adult's diet to meet but not greatly exceed its needs is never harmful. Good quality, scientifically designed,

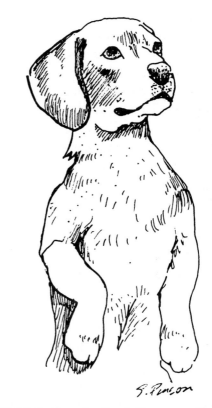

FIGURE 4.14 Feeding table scraps will promote an annoying begging habit.

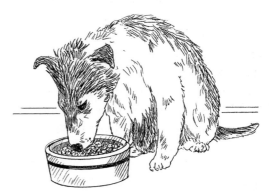

FIGURE 4.15 For better health, consider offering your dog filtered water instead of plain tap water.

adult-maintenance diets always contain these reduced and balanced nutrient levels.

Guidelines for feeding adult dogs and cats include

1. Feed a high-quality, complete, and balanced diet specifically designed for adults. Be aware that foods that say they are "complete and balanced for all life stages" are actually designed for puppies and kittens, since they have been formulated to meet the needs of the most demanding life stage, namely, growth. They contain excesses of most nutrients for adults and seniors.

2. It is best not to give supplements or treats to your adult dog or cat. If you must give an occasional food snack, use either a small amount of the regular food, or fresh, unsalted vegetables cut up in bite-size pieces.

3. Most dogs can receive their allotted daily ration at one sitting. Adult cats can be fed free-choice. Use the manufacturer's recommended feeding amounts as a starting point only. If your pet gains weight, reduce the portion offered. If your pet starts to lose weight, increase the amount you feed. A veterinarian can help you decide what your pet's optimum weight should be. Once you know this, weigh your pet periodically to prevent weight loss or gain from becoming a problem.

4. Some pets show a pronounced tendency to gain weight as they grow older, despite eating only moderate amounts of an adult maintenance diet. For these, follow the instructions for overweight pets in this chapter.

DID YOU KNOW?

Cats can starve themselves to death. Whereas otherwise healthy dogs will eventually give in to hunger pressures, cats can be more stubborn. If they go without food long enough, they can develop life-threatening malnutrition and hepatic lipidosis!

5. Dogs that are very active, work regularly, have nervous dispositions, or are simply not eager eaters should be fed a ration that contains extra calories. In

addition, pregnant dogs and cats will need extra nutrition during the last few weeks of pregnancy and throughout lactation (Fig. 4.16). Growth diets fulfill this role well. Feed such a food starting in the last trimester of pregnancy and continue it until all puppies or kittens are weaned. Also, feed her free-choice, and do not add vitamin/mineral supplements unless your veterinarian recommends it.

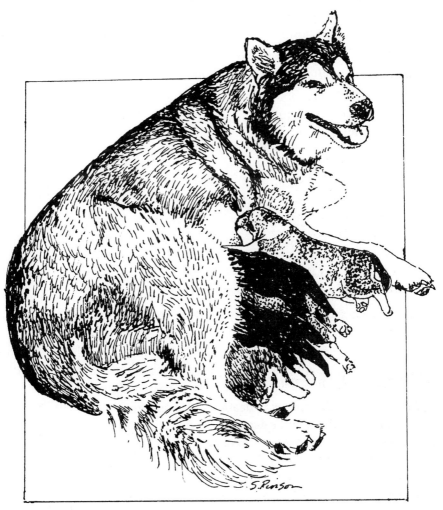

FIGURE 4.16   Pregnant and lactating females should be fed a "growth" formula to provide added nutritional support.

6. Keep fresh, clean water (preferably filtered) available at all times.

A word about bones: To get to the point, natural bones should not be fed to dogs. Now some might scoff at this, saying that dogs have been surviving on bones for centuries. While this is true, we still don't know how many of those dogs succumbed to impactions and to intestinal perforations. Why take a chance?

Bones, regardless of type, can splinter, causing penetrating wounds within the gastrointestinal tract. They can also add unwanted amounts of minerals to the diet. Nylon and/or compressed rawhide substitutes more than adequately satisfy that bone-chewing urge and are much safer (Fig. 4.17).

Nutrition for the Older Pet

Once your pet is 7 years old (5 years old for large breed dogs), another dietary change becomes necessary. As people and animals age, many organ systems begin to show the effects of wear and tear. The kidneys especially begin to lose the ability to handle waste materials that must be removed from the bloodstream and excreted in the urine. Even older dogs and cats that appear to be in perfect health could have kidneys that function much less effectively than they used to.

Guidelines for feeding the older pets include

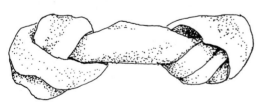

Dr. P's Vet Tip

Feeding your cat a high-quality, highly digestible diet will cut down on litterbox odor as well as litterbox mess.

FIGURE 4.17   Rawhide bones are relatively safe alternatives to real bones.

1. Feed a high-quality pet food specifically designed for the senior pet. A veterinarian can advise you of any special health problems that your pet already has and any other dietary changes that might be necessary. In many cases of "old age" diseases, special foods can be prescribed along with medication to help manage these conditions. For instance, studies have shown that feeding a diet rich in antioxidants can help lessen age-related senility.

DR. P's VET TIP

Food palatability can be enhanced by increasing a food's odor or changing its texture. Odor can be enhanced by warming the food or by adding bouillon or gravy to it. The texture of a ration can be changed by blending it or cooking it further.

2. If you notice your older pet gaining or losing weight, consult with a veterinarian about any changes in diet that can correct the problem. At the same time, the vet will check for any medical problem that might be contributing to the change in weight.

3. Do not supplement your older pet's diet with anything unless a veterinarian specifically recommends it. Senior digestive systems are even more sensitive than younger ones to the unbalancing effects of frequent snacks, treats, and table food added to the diet.

4. Take your "senior" for regular (at least once a year) medical checkups to catch problems early or prevent them altogether. The right diet throughout life is an important part of a sound preventive medicine program to safeguard the health and long life of your treasured pet.

5. Keep fresh, clean, filtered water available at all times.

Dietary Management of Disease

For years, medical research has been telling us about the benefits of eating a well-balanced diet for good health. In addition, we also know that special modification of the dietary intake in the presence of a disease state can be helpful in the treatment and/or long-term management of the condition. This same nutritional health concept can be applied to dogs and cats as well.

Many disease conditions in dogs and cats, such as obesity (yes, obesity is a disease!), heart disease, kidney disease, and gastrointestinal disease, can be effectively controlled, and sometimes even cured, through diet modification alone.

For example, obesity, constipation, certain types of colitis, and diabetes mellitus all warrant an increase in the amount of fiber present in the ration. Dogs suffering from diarrhea, excessive gas production, and/or pancreatic problems can benefit from diets that are more easily digestible than standard maintenance rations. Cats suffering from certain types of feline lower urinary tract disease benefit from diets that acidify the urine and contain low levels of magnesium and other trace minerals. Finally, recommended management of dogs and cats suffering from kidney disease includes diets low in phosphorus and containing only the highest quality proteins.

These special diets or rations aimed at fighting or counteracting diseases can be purchased through a veterinarian, or can be prepared at home via veterinary-supplied recipes. In general, the commercially prepared products are preferred over the homemade rations. The cost of these diets is negligible when compared to continuing veterinary bills and the poor quality of life that would result by not feeding them. Just remember to follow the veterinarian's directions closely as to amounts and frequency of feeding of these diets if they are indeed used.

Battling Obesity in Dogs and Cats

Obesity is certainly one of the most prevalent diseases affecting the pet population today. For years, the frequency of this health disorder was skyrocketing at an alarming pace, owing primarily to improper feeding practices and inadequate time spent exercising due to owners' perceived lack of time (Fig. 4.18). Sounds a lot like the cause of most obesity in humans, doesn't it? In fact, dogs and cats are not much different from us in this respect. The problem, however, is that most overweight pets were made that way not by themselves, but by their owners! Unfortunately, few owners realize that by encouraging their pet to get fat, they are at the same time endangering its health and unfairly reducing its quality of life.

The health-related ramifications in dogs and cats are the same as in people. Although pets don't suffer from atherosclerosis and "heart attacks" as we do, obesity does place a great strain on their cardiovascular systems. Other internal organs suffer the consequences as well. For instance, obesity promotes pancreatitis in dogs and liver disease in cats. Obese canines seem to suffer from more skin ailments and coat disorders than do their slim and trim counterparts. Musculoskeletal disorders, including intervertebral disk disease, occur with greater frequency in dogs carrying around excessive weight. In summary, it is safe to say that the overall quality of and length of life for these pets is reduced, owing to these side effects of obesity.

Visually, dogs that are overweight will sport a waist that is barely discern-

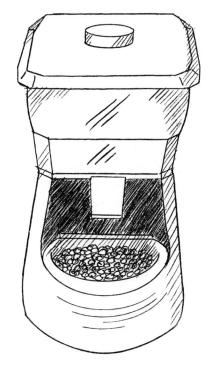

FIGURE 4.18 While automatic feeders may be convenient, they can predispose dogs to obesity.

able. In addition, their ribs can barely be felt when their chest is touched, and their abdomens may be noticeably distended. Finally, fat dogs will carry prominent fat deposits along the hips and at the base of their tails.

The average adult cat weighs anywhere from 8 to 15 pounds. Not only will fat cats tip the scale to the heavy side, but they will usually appear round and their bellies may sag under the weight of their excess adipose tissue.

Causes of Obesity

The causes of obesity in dogs and cats are numerous, but the first and foremost of them is plain, old dietary indiscretion [aka (also known as) too many table scraps]! Realize that when you feed 10-pound Ginger that tiny piece of hot dog, that is equivalent to you eating two to three hot dogs! In other words, it won't take many of these tiny pieces to make Ginger fat. Feeding one innocent cheese curl to a dog or cat might be the same as eating half a bag ourselves, depending on the pet's size! Table scraps do nothing but promote obesity and create an annoying beggar out of your pet.

Feeding table scraps is no doubt the biggest culprit causing obesity in pets, but simply feeding the wrong type of food can do the same. Most pet food manufacturers produce products geared for different stages of a pet's life. For instance, on the market today you have growth formulas, high-protein rations, "light" formulas, adult-maintenance formulas, geriatric formulas, and so on. The choices are so numerous that pet owners often become confused as to which type their particular pet should be on, and this could lead to improper feeding practices and obesity.

The only pets that need to be on a growth formula of food are puppies and kittens under 1 year of age, pregnant and lactating pets, and, in certain instances, dogs and cats that are recovering from or fighting off illness. Because energy requirements drop considerably as a pet matures, feeding high-energy, high-calorie growth formulas to an otherwise healthy adult dog or cat can inadvertently cause obesity. The same holds true for geriatric pets over 8 years of age. These pets should be fed "less active" or senior-type diets containing higher fiber and fewer calories instead of the regular adult-maintenance rations.

Failure to adjust dietary requirements to specific individual needs is another predisposing cause of obesity. As far as how much you should be feeding your pet, the first place to start is to consult a breed book or a veterinarian and find out what the ideal weight should be for your pet. Then look at the recommendations printed on the label of the pet food you are using. Even these printed guidelines should be considered averages, since the needs of each individual will vary, depending on individual metabolic rates, exercise levels, and eating habits.

For adult and senior dogs, the best approach is to feed the recommended amount of food over a 3-week period, monitoring your dog's weight each week. If weight gain is noted, cut back on the rations fed. If the opposite is true, then increase the rations slightly.

For puppies and kittens, follow the manufacturer's recommendations as to how much to feed. When your pet is still an adolescent, instilling solid feeding habits is more important than worrying about how much to feed.

Weight Reduction

If your pet is overweight, simply cutting back on the amount you feed will not do the trick. In fact, doing so could conceivably lead to a mild state of malnutrition and cause your dog or cat to be constantly hungry (and begging!). Many dogs that are not receiving adequate nutrition will try to eat anything, which in itself can lead to a serious case of gastroenteritis. Cats that are malnourished can develop serious liver disease as a result.

Instead of cutting back on its ration, switch your pet's feed to one that is specially formulated for weight loss. Studies have shown that a high-protein, low-fat diet can promote weight loss while maintaining lean body mass. Such diets are readily available from a veterinary clinic. They might cost a bit more than what you are accustomed to paying for pet food, but the switch is only temporary and the benefits to your pet are immense. Also, most of these "diet" foods have a high fiber content, which allows for calorie reduction while still giving your pet that feeling of fullness after eating.

A veterinarian can assist you in determining how much and how often to feed your pet. For dogs, spreading out the total daily food amount over two to three feedings during the day might help satisfy your pet even more. Be patient with the results. You might not realize it, but even 1 pound of weight loss is significant for both a dog or a cat.

It is vital that during the weight reduction period that you remain consistent with the feedings and avoid giving any snacks (a few kibbles of the special diet now and then can make for an excellent snack substitute). For dogs, nylon or compressed rawhide bones are okay to give to chew on during this time, but keep in mind that hungry dogs may gulp down these items without properly chewing them, leaving them susceptible to gastritis and intestinal blockage.

Make sure that your pet gets enough exercise. As with people, lack of exercise does its part to promote obesity. House dogs kept indoors most of the time are the ones at greatest risk. Many are lucky if they just get acknowledged when their owner steps in the door from a hard day's work. When they do get to go outside, it is often just to go to the bathroom, then back inside.

Regardless of whether your dog is kept indoors or out, make it a habit to devote a specific amount of time each day to social activity and exercise with your dog. It is important not only for its peace of mind but also to keep its body fit and keep the fat away.

A brisk, 15-minute aerobic walk or jog twice a day is all that should be needed. When exercising your dog, just be sure not to overdo it. Stride for stride, most dogs need to work twice as hard to keep up with the pace you set. Avoid exercising during those times of the day when the heat and humidity are at their worst. And remember to keep plenty of water available for your dog. Drinking water prevents these dogs from becoming dehydrated, and provides a cooling mechanism for their body.

Cats kept indoors rarely get enough exercise, unless, of course, they are leash-trained and can be taken for daily walks. However, simply playing with your cat more when you get home from work can do its part to help burn those calories!

You should also rule out medical reasons for obesity. Finally, just to be fair, the pet owner can't be saddled with the blame for his or her pet's obesity in all cases. There can be medical reasons behind a pet's weight challenge. For instance, hypothyroidism is a common condition in dogs, and it can lead to weight gain and lethargy by lowering the body's metabolic rate. One unique finding in hypothyroid dogs is that these dogs will gain weight despite a poor appetite. The signs associated with this condition can be quite subtle and might lead you to believe that improper diet is the cause of your dog's weight problem. For this reason, thyroid function tests should be administered to all dogs that have a weight problem. Most veterinarians now offer a simple, inexpensive in-house thyroid screen that can detect problems if they exist. In these cases, supplementing thyroid hormone by mouth not only makes the pet feel better but also helps conquer the weight disorder.

In summary, follow these guidelines to protect your pet from the health risks caused by obesity:

1. Be strict when it comes to your pet's diet. Keep it regular and feed a formulation suited for your pet's stage of life and physical activity level. Avoid feeding table scraps! If your pet needs to lose weight, don't just cut back on its ration. Switching to a specially formulated high-fiber diet is a must. Slow, steady weight loss is the goal. Eliminate all treats and special snacks during the weight reduction period, and never feed free-choice.

2. If you haven't already done so, implement an exercise program for your dog or a regular playtime for your cat. Not only will you be helping control your pet's weight, you'll also be preventing potential behavioral problems. Don't overdo the exercise, and keep plenty of water available at all times.

3. Always have a medical checkup performed on your pet before embarking on any weight-loss program. A veterinarian can tell you if your pet is actually overweight and can give you specific guidelines for weight reduction in your pet if needed.

Caring for the Canine Ear

Because of the unique anatomy of the canine ear, routine preventive ear care, involving cleaning, drying, and, when applicable, plucking is recommended.

Cleaning

Many different types of ear cleansers and drying agents are available from pet stores, pet supply houses, and veterinary offices (Fig. 4.19). Liquid cleansers are preferred over powders; powders can become quickly saturated with moisture, trapping them within the ear canal. Most liquid ear cleansers contain wax solvents as well as built-in astringents (drying agents) that help promote a healthy environment within the ear.

Cotton balls, cotton tip applicators, and tissues are also helpful accessories to have available. These are used to clean around the outer portions of the ear canal and surrounding structures. In no instances should a cotton-tipped applicator be placed down into an ear canal; you'll only serve to pack wax and debris down deep next to the eardrum or actually rupture the eardrum itself.

Be sure to consult a veterinarian before putting any medications or solutions into your pet's ears. This is especially important if those ears are inflamed or infected, since many solutions designed for use in

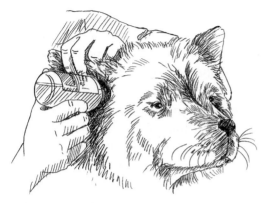

FIGURE 4.19 When cleaning your dog's ear, pull the pinna straight out (not up) to allow the medication to get down deep into the ear canal.

healthy ears can cause serious problems if used in ears with unhealthy or ruptured eardrums.

Restraint during Cleaning or Treatment

The most important part of any preventive or treatment program for the ears is proper restraint of the patient. This is essential for effective application of medications, as well for the safety of both owner and dog. If necessary, don't hesitate to use a muzzle. Unfortunately, many dogs object to having their ears medicated, especially if the ears are already sore from inflammation.

If at all possible, obtain assistance from a friend or family member for that extra set of hands. Smaller dogs can be placed atop tables or washing machines for a better working angle. This unfamiliar ground usually serves to pacify a fidgety protester.

Use good judgment: If it looks like all-out war is likely, abandon your efforts and seek the assistance of a veterinarian. Having to make repeated weekly trips back and forth from the veterinary office might be inconvenient, but try to keep the benefits afforded to your pooch's ears in mind. If your dog is suffering from an ear infection, consider leaving it at the hospital or clinic for a few days to make sure that those ears are treated properly.

Recommended Procedure

The procedure for cleaning and/or applying medication to the ears is easy. To begin, the pinna (earflap) should be pulled gently toward the handler in an outward, not upward, direction. By extending it in this fashion, the external ear canal will be straightened, allowing easy access of the cleanser to the deep portions of the canal. On the other hand, if the pinna is pulled upward, the ear canal will become flattened against the skull, rendering cleansing efforts ineffective.

Now carefully place the cleanser or medication into the external ear opening and squeeze a liberal amount of solution into the ear. The next step is to feel for the cartilage supporting the ear canal and, keeping the pinna extended outward, gently massage the ear canal for a good 15 to 20 seconds. Once this time is up, the dog should be allowed to shake its head before proceeding to the next ear.

After both ears have been treated, cotton balls, cotton applicators, or tissue can be used to wipe up excess cleanser, medication, or waxy debris stuck to the inside folds of the pinnae and the very outer portions of the ear canals. Again, never stick anything down into the ear canal itself. Serious injury could result! Most commercial ear cleaners contain or come with drying agents, which makes manual drying of the ear canals unnecessary.

HAIR IN THE EAR CANAL

In some breeds, hair can occlude the ear canal, predisposing to inflammation and infection. Poodles, terriers, and schnauzers are notorious for this. In cases where excessive hair is visualized in the ear canal, the veterinarian should perform an ear pluck (Fig. 4.20).

Why not do it yourself? Well, there are three good reasons not to. First, ear plucking is a painful procedure, especially if inflammation is already a factor. As such, it requires effective restraint. In some instances, sedation might even be required to do the job. Second, if done properly, an ear pluck should be focused not just on the hair visibly occluding the outside of the ear canal, but on the hair down deep within the canal as well. Special instruments are needed for this, the kind used by a veterinarian. Finally, if done improperly, ear plucking can lead to infection within an ear canal. Since the act of forcibly removing hairs from their follicles causes inflammation, the entire length of the plucked canal needs to be medicated afterward to reduce this inflammation and prevent a secondary infection from occurring.

> ### DR. P's VET TIP
> A 50:50 mixture of iso-propyl alcohol and white vinegar can be used as a routine ear cleanser for healthy ears or those with mild yeast infections. (*Caution:* Alcohol will sting an inflamed ear.)

The bottom line is this: Ear plucks done improperly and without proper medication afterward can actually do more harm than good!

Routine weekly application of an ear solution can help keep ear canals healthy. In addition, using a drying agent in the ears after a pet goes swimming or receives a bath is also a good idea. Daily or every-other-day (alternate-day) preventive treatment is not needed unless prescribed by a veterinarian; in fact, such frequent application could conceivably alter the normal flora and environment within the ear enough to allow disease-causing bacteria to proliferate.

Routine ear plucks should be performed on an as-needed basis. In most cases, this means every 4 to 6 weeks.

If the ears are being treated for an infection, follow the dosage and frequency guidelines prescribed by your veterinarian for the particular medications you are using. See Chapter 15 for more information regarding diseases and disorders that can affect the canine ear.

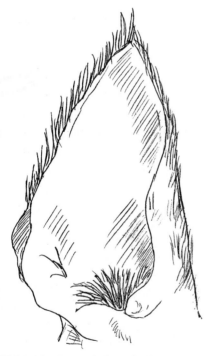

FIGURE 4.20 **Excess hair occluding the external ear canal should be plucked.**

Maintaining a Healthy Skin and Coat

Routine grooming is essential for maintaining healthy hair and skin in dogs and cats. Be sure to allot some time each day to this task (Fig. 4.21).

Brushing

Whether your dog or cat has short or long hair, brushing the coat thoroughly on a daily basis will aid in its appearance as well as promote healthy skin. It does this by

- Removing telogen (dead) hairs from the coat, making way for new ones to grow in.

- Preventing tangles and mats

- Stimulating sebaceous gland activity, which keeps the skin moisturized and the haircoat shiny. Brushing also helps to spread these oils across the entire skin and coat.

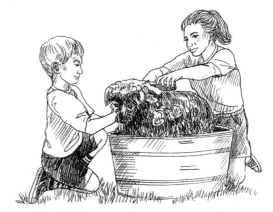

FIGURE 4.21 Contrary to popular belief, dogs do not need to be bathed on a regular basis.

- Removing scale (excess keratin), which could lead to itching.

- Increasing owner awareness of the presence of external parasites or other skin-related problems.

Long-haired and/or thick-coated breeds require more diligent brushing than do shorter-coated dogs. Minor shedding is normal year-round in all breeds. However, because the shedding cycle in dogs and cats is stimulated by changes in day length, most will occur during the spring and fall months, when the days become longer and shorter, respectively.

Be sure to choose the right type of brush for your pet. In general, the wider the bristles or pins are placed on the brush, the longer the coat it is designed to be used on. Brush medium- and long-haired dogs, as well as those breeds with thick coats, using a wire-pin brush. For dogs with short haircoats, brushing with a bristle-type brush will work best (Fig. 4.22). Long-coated cats should be brushed using a wire-pin brush or

DID YOU KNOW?

Dogs can't sweat like people do; thus they pant to dissipate heat via the mouth and tongue.

🔍 FACT OR FICTION

Dogs should be bathed at least once a week FICTION. Dogs with healthy skin and haircoats rarely require routine bathing. Daily brushing and application of a coat conditioner will accomplish the same results! In fact, indiscriminate bathing can dry out the skin and predispose an otherwise healthy skin to disease.

comb. For shorthaired cats, a bristle-type brush or rubber curry comb will do the trick.

In addition to the wire-pin brush, the slicker brush is another very popular type of device used on dogs. Most of these consist of a square head containing lots of tiny wire projections, and they can be used on almost any type of haircoat for removing shed hair and tangles.

Purchase of a comb is optional, unless you own a cat or one of the silky-fur breeds with a coat that might be too delicate for many standard brushes. Combs can also come in quite handy for removing tangles and mats when used in conjunction with scissors. Like brushes, the teeth of combs are set at different widths apart for different types of coats: widely spaced for thicker coats and closely spaced for longer, silkier hair. Just keep in mind that using the wrong type of brush or comb can be painful to your pet and actually damage the haircoat. For this reason, choose grooming tools with care.

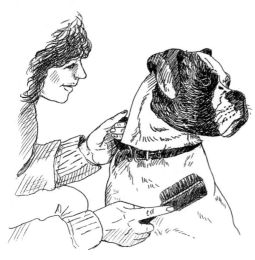

FIGURE 4.22   Be sure to use the right type of brush for your pet's particular haircoat.

Always use firm, short strokes when brushing, never forcing the brush through the coat. For dogs with short- to medium-length hair and all cats, brush with the grain of the hair. To help in the removal of shed hair, use towels or disposable gloves to buff the coat after brushing. For those canines with thick undercoats, the initial direction of brushing should be against the grain of the hair. Once the undercoat has been groomed, you can brush the outer coat with the grain.

If you encounter a mat, don't try to forcefully remove it with the brush. Instead, try to work it free with your fingers, using one hand to free the tangle and the other to stabilize the tuft of hair to keep it from pulling the skin. If the mat or tangle still can't be freed, insert a comb between the mat and the skin surface; then take a pair of blunt-nosed scissors and snip as much of the mat off as you can between the comb and the free end of the hair. Don't worry about cosmetic appearances. It will grow back! Mats that are left in place can promote infection involving the skin beneath. And always remember: If you brush your pet as often as you should, you won't have a problem with matting!

Bathing

Dogs and cats should be bathed when one or more of the following situations develop:

- Accumulation of excessive dirt, grease, or other foreign substances on the skin and coat
- Buildup of waxy sebum (seborrhea), which often leads to body odor
- Accumulation of skin scale (dandruff)
- Skin infections

Dogs and cats with normal, healthy skin and haircoats really do not require routine bathing. As far as cats are concerned, that's welcome news, since most cats abhor bathing!

If a bath is indicated for your dog or cat, a hypoallergenic shampoo is recommended. For medical conditions involving skin

Dr. P's Vet Tip

To remove skunk odor, mix one quart of 3% hydrogen peroxide with $1/4$ cup of baking soda and 1 teaspoon of mild liquid dish soap. Apply liberally to the coat, and then rinse thoroughly.

infections and seborrhea, use only those shampoos prescribed by a veterinarian. Using the wrong type of shampoo on such skin disorders will yield poor results and might even exacerbate them.

Before you put your pet into the tub, brush its coat out thoroughly and remove any mats and tangles. In addition, always apply some type of protection to both eyes to prevent accidental soap burns. Mineral oil has been used for this purpose; however, a sterile ophthalmic ointment is preferred. Such ointment is readily available from a veterinary clinic or pet store, and provides greater eye protection than does plain mineral oil.

After you've treated the eyes, stick some cotton balls into the outer portion of each ear canal to keep bath water out. If the nails need trimming or the anal sacs need emptying (dogs), do this before the bath as well. If you are bathing your cat, place a window screen or rubber mat in the tub to give your feline something to hold onto while getting scrubbed. Once these preparatory measures have been taken, you can proceed with the shampoo and rinse.

If you are using a medicated shampoo, allow it to remain in contact with the skin for a good 10 minutes prior to rinsing. After rinsing, a towel, chamois cloth, or brush and blow dryer (dogs only—on the low heat setting only) can be used for drying.

Nail Trimming

As part of a routine grooming program, you should perform a nail trim on your dog every 4 to 6 weeks and for cats, every 2 to 3 weeks (Fig. 4.23). The procedure itself is easy, assuming you have the right equipment and that your pet agrees to cooperate. If your pet refuses to hold still for its manicure, let a veterinary assistant perform the deed. It will be less stressful on both you and your pet.

There are many types and styles of nail trimmers on the market today. The preferred choice is the guillotine-type nail trimmers with replaceable blades. These are available at pet stores everywhere.

The procedure itself is simple on clear nails. Observe the nail to be clipped and identify the endpoint of the blood supply, or the quick. Then, staying just in front of the quick, snip off the end portion of the nail.

On dark nails that don't have readily identifiable quicks, start snipping back the end of the nail in small portions at a time. Stop when the nail is short enough as to not contact the ground when weight is placed on the paw (Fig. 4.24).

Invariably, the time might come when you accidentally "quick" your pet's nail, causing it to bleed. If this occurs, there is no cause for panic. Using a clean cloth or gauze pad, apply direct pressure to the bleeding nail for 5 minutes to stop the bleeding. Alternatively, you can apply clotting powder or clotting sticks, both of which can be purchased at pet stores, to the end of the affected nail to quickly stop the bleeding. If none of these are handy, ordinary flour can be used as an effective substitute.

Occasionally, a dog's nails might have grown so long that the quick has extended far down the nail, making it virtually impos-

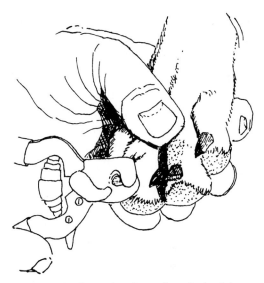

FIGURE 4.23 When trimming nails, trim back just far enough so that when your dog's paw is flat against a surface, the nails are just off the surface.

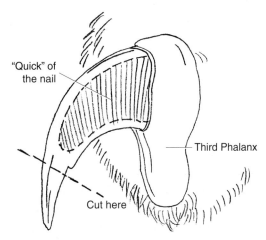

"Quick" of the nail

Third Phalanx

Cut here

FIGURE 4.24 Keeping a cat's nails trimmed short is one alternative to declawing.

sible to clip without making it bleed. In these instances, you might wish to employ the help of a veterinarian, who can sedate your pet and perform a short nail trim.

Expressing Anal Sacs

The anal sacs are structures located on either side of the anal opening in dogs and cats. Filled with a foul-smelling fluid that is used for intraspecies identification, these sacs normally empty with each bowel movement. Contrary to popular belief, these do not have to be manually emptied on a routine basis whenever a dog is bathed. In fact, by manually expressing healthy anal sacs, you could inadvertently cause inflammation and predispose to secondary impaction. Anal sacs require attention only if a dog is showing signs of impaction or anal sac irritation (Fig. 4.25). These signs usually appear in the form of scooting the rear end across the floor or excessive licking of that region. Fortunately, cats rarely have trouble with their anal sacs.

Mildly impacted anal sacs can be expressed by applying gentle, inward and upward pressure at the four o'clock and eight o'clock positions surrounding the anal opening, using your thumb and forefinger, respectively. If this fails to empty the sacs, or if the sacs are especially tender, stop what you are doing and call the veterinarian. In these instances the procedure is better performed at the vet's office.

🔍F ACT OR FICTION

A dog that scoots its rear end on the floor has worms **FICTION**. A dog that scoots its rear end on your floor has distended anal sacs and is trying to empty them on your floor or carpet!

(*Note:* If you happen to get anal sac secretion on your skin or clothes, you might lose your friends quickly unless you take appropriate action to neutralize the odor. Isopropyl alcohol can be used to get rid of the smell. Better yet, many commercial odor neutralizers that are available at your favorite pet stores can do the job even more effectively.)

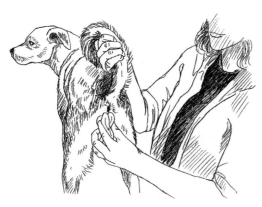

FIGURE 4.25   Anal sacs should be expressed only if they are impacted.

Elective Surgeries in Dogs and Cats

Some of the more common elective surgeries (surgeries not prompted by disease or illness) performed in dogs and cats include neutering (ovariohysterectomy, castration), ear crops (dogs), tail dock/dewclaw removal (dogs), and declawing (cats). While there is sound medical and sociological reasoning behind neutering dogs and cats, many other elective surgical procedures commonly requested by pet owners offer no benefits whatsoever. As a result, ear cropping, tail docking, and even feline declawing have come under increasing public scrutiny as to their necessity and humaneness.

Whether you decide to have an elective procedure performed on your pet is up to you (and current laws governing such practices), but before making a final decision, you are encouraged to communicate with your veterinarian, who will be able to answer your questions regarding benefits, risks, and controversy surrounding any particular elective surgery (Fig. 5.1).

The Facts Concerning Anesthesia

Anesthesia is a word that tends to inspire uneasiness and fear in many people. In actuality, though, anesthesia is an indispensable tool in veterinary medicine (and human medicine, as well!). It is required for

115

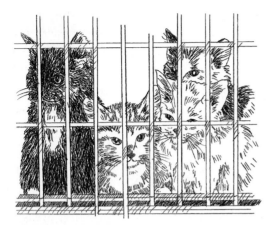

FIGURE 5.1 With animal shelters overflowing with so many unwanted pets, neutering your pet is highly recommended.

the painless performance of many important procedures, including surgery, dentistry, diagnostics, and restraint.

There are basically two types of anesthetics that are used alone or in combination in elective and non-elective surgeries. Injectable anesthetics are used quite often for procedures lasting for only a short period of time. For longer procedures, inhalation (gas) anesthesia is used for maintenance.

Newer, safer anesthetic agents are now available for use in pets. However, regardless of the type of anesthetic agent used, it is important to remember that none are totally risk-free. It is difficult to predict how each pet will react while under anesthesia, yet with strict monitoring and adherence to basic anesthetic principles, many problems can be avoided.

Ideally, animals should be as healthy as possible prior to undergoing anesthesia. For this reason, laboratory work is often required to confirm the health status of your pet. Of course, certain situations will require the use of anesthesia in sick animals. It is easy to see how the risks of anesthesia tend to be greater in these patients. Older animals also tend to be at greater risk. Yet, again, with the proper laboratory workup and a good physical exam performed by a veterinarian prior to anesthesia, as well as close monitoring during the procedure, the risks associated with the anesthesia can be greatly minimized.

Owners, too, have a responsibility to help ensure the safety of a pet undergoing anesthesia. Be sure to inform the veterinarian of all medications that your pet is currently taking, as well as any changes you have noted regarding your pet's behavior (more frequent urination, exercise intolerance, etc.). Don't hesitate to review your pet's past medical history with the veterinarian and to ask questions concerning the anesthesia to be used.

If the pet is to stay at home the night before the surgery, it is imperative that all food be taken away at least 12 to 18 hours prior to the scheduled procedure. Water, on the other hand, may usually be offered up to 4 hours before the scheduled anesthesia. Be sure to check with the veterinarian regarding this subject. If for some reason your pet does eat food or drink water when it's not supposed to, it is important that you relate this information to your veterinarian.

Neutering

Ovariohysterectomy (OHE) involves the surgical removal of the ovaries and uterus from an intact female dog or cat. The common term assigned to this procedure is "spaying." OHE is a preferred method of birth control in pets, since it is easy to do and ensures 100 percent sterility. Most veterinarians require a dog or cat to be at least 6 months of age before undergoing such an operation, although some will perform the procedure as early as 12 weeks of age.

> **DID YOU KNOW?**
>
> The feral cat population in the United States is estimated at over 50 million!

Aside from birth control, there are many other reasons for performing an OHE on your female dog or cat. For instance, it can be lifesaving as treatment for or prevention of pyometra (accumulation of pus within the uterus) as an animal matures. In addition, it has been used as a behavioral modification tool to calm excited or overly aggressive pets (Fig. 5.2). Finally, and very importantly, research has actually shown that in dogs, spaying at an early age can reduce the risks of that individual developing mammary cancer in the future.

> **FACT** OR *FICTION*
>
> Having a female dog spayed (OHE) when she is young will help prevent mammary cancer as she gets older. **FACT.** In fact, the most protection is afforded if the procedure is performed prior to a dog's first heat cycle. With each consecutive cycle a dog undergoes, this protective nature of an OHE declines until, by 2½ years of age, this potential benefit is lost altogether.

The entire surgery takes anywhere from 10 to 20 minutes, depending on the skill of the surgeon and certain patient factors. For instance,

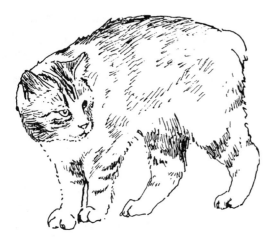

FIGURE 5.2 Castrating tomcats can sometimes help curb aggressive tendencies.

the procedure normally takes longer if the pet is in heat at the time of surgery, owing to an increased blood supply to the reproductive tract, requiring additional care and ligatures. The same holds true for pregnant pets. Dogs and cats that are excessively overweight are more difficult to spay because increased fatty tissue within the abdomen obstructs the surgeon's view. Finally, in the case of an OHE because of pyometra, the operation can take two to three times longer than it normally would, as the surgeon must use delicate care not to rupture the pus-filled uterus.

For whatever reasons, veterinarians often are asked if they could just remove the ovaries and leave the uterus intact (or vice versa). While the intentions of such a request may be good, it lacks medical reasoning. Pets whose ovaries are removed without the uterus are still at risk of developing pyometra in the future. Similarly, pets whose ovaries are left intact, but have had their uterus removed, can still develop a pyometra in the stump of the uterus left behind. In addition, such an operation does little to reduce the risk of mammary cancer in that particular individual.

The technical term for neutering a male canine is *castration,* which involves the surgical removal of the testicles. This procedure is commonly employed for birth control, and for reducing territoriality and aggressiveness in male dogs and cats. Castration is also employed in dogs as treatment for medical disorders that are directly influenced by testosterone, namely prostate disease, perineal hernias, and certain tumors. Retained testicles (testicles that have failed to descend into the scrotum) are also candidates for removal, since they have high incidence of becoming cancerous. In general, castrations can be safely performed on a dog or cat as early as 6 months of age.

Rather than having to have surgery performed at all, pets may soon be sterilized with a series of special injections. Chemicals that render the reproductive organs nonfunctional have been developed, and offer a safer, more affordable way to neuter a pet. Ask the veterinarian for details.

Common Concerns about Neutering

One common misconception about spaying a dog or cat is the belief that a female needs to go through at least one heat cycle or have at least one litter before the deed is performed. Many feel that this is necessary for the proper emotional development of their pet, but in fact, it isn't. On the contrary, spaying before the first heat cycle will have no adverse effect on a pet's's mental well-being, and, as mentioned earlier, can offer significant medical benefits, especially in dogs.

Another concern that many pet owners harbor is that neutering will cause their pets to gain weight. However, poor feeding practices, lack of exercise, or certain medical conditions (such as hypothyroidism) cause obesity, not the act of neutering. By addressing these issues, you can keep your neutered pet slim, trim, and healthy!

Tail Docking and Dewclaw Removal (Dogs)

Established conformational standards dictate that select breeds of dogs have artificially shortened tails and be free of dewclaws. Tail docking originated in centuries past as a way to prevent hunting and sporting dogs from traumatizing their tails while working in thick woods or underbrush (Fig. 5.3). Even as certain sporting dogs have evolved into lap dogs, tail docking still remains in vogue as a cosmetic standard for many of these breeds. Medical necessities might also warrant amputation of the tail. Trauma, infections, and tumors involving the tail may best be resolved by partial or complete amputation.

Dewclaws are actually functionless remnants of the first digit on each paw. Many puppies are born without any dewclaws at all; others are born with them on the front paws, but not the back, or vice versa. Conformational standards are not the only reason for removing these structures when a puppy is young. Dewclaws have a nasty habit of getting snagged and torn on carpet, furniture, and underbrush. Secondary

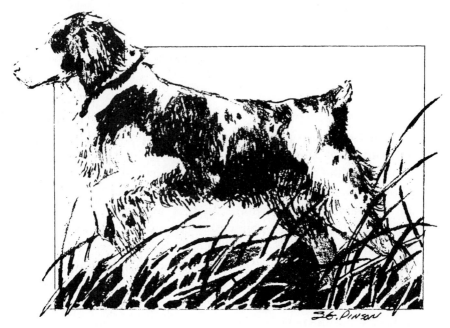

FIGURE 5.3   Tails are docked on many hunting breeds to prevent injury in the brush.

infections can develop if this trauma is repeated. For this reason, removal of dewclaws is a good idea if this is the case.

Tail docking and dewclaw removal are best performed within the first week of life (Fig. 5.4). The operations simply involve snipping off the dewclaws and the desired length of tail (per breed standards) with surgical scissors. One to two sutures are usually placed in the tail; the site of the dewclaw removal is often cauterized and left open.

If tail docking/dewclaw removal is not performed within 7 days after birth, anesthesia will be required for the surgery. As a result, the procedures must be postponed until the pet is 5 to 6 months of age.

Cosmetic Ear Trimming (Dogs)

Cosmetic ear trimming, or ear cropping, is the surgical alteration of the normal anatomy of the ear pinnae in dogs to conform to accepted breed standards. Many people feel that ear trimming puts a dog through needless pain and suffering. Veterinarians and veterinary organizations are even joining the bandwagon and are advising against cosmetic ear trims, since they serve no useful purpose. In certain countries, cropped ears are no longer considered an acceptable breed standard, and cosmetic ear trimming has been officially banned (Fig. 5.5).

The choice of whether to have it done or not is strictly up to you. If your pet's breed standard calls for it and you plan on competing on the show circuit, then you'll need to have your dog's ears cropped. In these cases, the surgery is best performed between 12 and 14 weeks of age. If, on the other hand, your dog is strictly for companionship, then such a procedure is not necessary.

Declawing (Cats)

The decision as to whether to have a cat declawed is certainly a controversial one, yet it is one that needs to be made based on individual circumstances. For indoor cats that refuse to stick to their scratching post, declawing is certainly a better

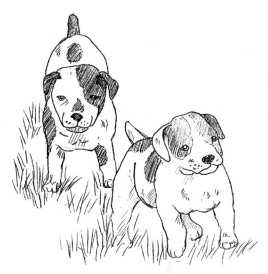

FIGURE 5.4 If desired, tails should be docked and dewclaws removed prior to 1 week of age.

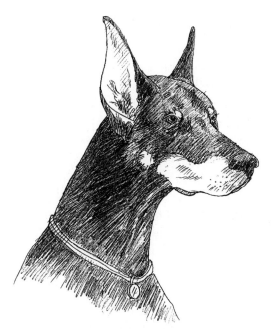

FIGURE 5.5 Cosmetic ear trimming has sparked much controversy among the dog-owning population.

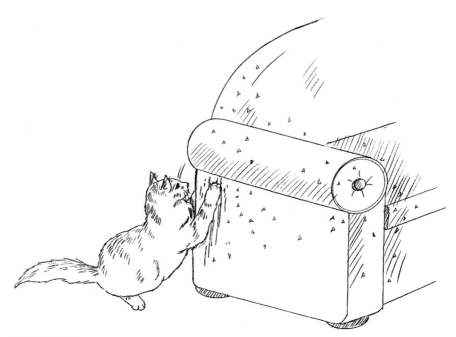

FIGURE 5.6 Declawing your cat may become necessary if it refuses to limit its scratching activities to its scratching post.

solution than drug therapy or worse yet, eviction from the home. Also, for predominately outdoor cats that spend their time indoors destroying the furniture with their claws, declawing might be the answer (Fig. 5.6). It is important to remember, however, that cats without their front claws cannot climb as well (although they can still climb!) as they could with them, and they might have trouble avoiding hostile dogs or fellow cats that they might encounter.

Declawing can be performed as early as 12 weeks of age. In fact, younger cats seem to recover much faster from the surgery than do older cats, primarily due to the immature development of the blood supply and other supporting structures to the nails at a younger age.

Before the decision is made to declaw your cat, try to train it to a scratching post first. If done correctly, you might find that it just may solve the problem. Also, consider keeping your cat's nails clipped short to minimize the damage caused by its scratching activity. Since the nails of cats are somewhat fragile, be sure that the nail clippers you use are sharp. Guillotine-type clippers available from pet stores work best.

When clipping the nail back, be sure to stop short of the pink "quick," which contains the blood supply to the nail. However, if an accident does happen, the bleeding can be controlled with direct pressure to the site through the use of clotting powder, again available at a local pet store.

> ## ⓕACT OR *FICTION*
>
> Cats that are declawed in front can't defend themselves. **FICTION.** A cat in true defense mode will utilize its back claws with utmost efficiency! What renders a feline truly defenseless is to remove these rear claws, which will also take away its ability to climb. As a result, remove only the front claws, never the back ones.

Finally, special nail covers are also available to minimize the damage associated with scratching activity. However, if none of the aforementioned options work, then removal of the front claws might be the only choice left to preserve that happy owner-pet relationship.

Postsurgical Care for Dogs and Cats

Following any type of surgery, you should receive specific instructions from your veterinarian as to the type of postsurgical care your pet requires. It is important to follow these instructions closely to ensure an uneventful recovery. Postsurgical instructions include

- Do not give your pet food or water for 30 minutes after arriving at home. To do so can cause nausea and vomiting.

- Restrict your pet's activity for 8 to 10 days or until the sutures are removed. Protect your pet from stress, such as extreme exertion, excitement, temperature fluctuations, and drafts. Traveling should be kept to a minimum.

- Check incision sites twice daily for any swelling and/or discharge. Keep them clean and dry at all times. Avoid bathing your pet until all sutures have been removed.

- Unless otherwise instructed, return to your veterinarian in 8 to 10 days for suture removal.

- If medications are dispensed, follow all label directions closely.

- Don't hesitate to call the veterinarian if any problems arise or if you have any questions regarding your pet's recovery.

Infectious Diseases

nfectious diseases are those diseases directly communicable between pets. They are certainly among the most common canine illnesses seen by veterinarians. Infectious organisms responsible for diseases in dogs and cats include a multitude of viruses, bacteria and bacterialike organisms, and fungi. Multiple organ systems (see Figs. 6.1 and 6.2) can be affected when an infectious disease is involved, resulting in a potpourri of clinical signs.

INFECTIOUS DISEASES IN DOGS

Viruses certainly account for the majority of infectious disease seen in dogs. Treatment for these agents is usually supportive in nature, owing to a lack of specific antiviral medications. Fortunately, most can be prevented through proper vaccination. As far as bacterial and fungal infections are concerned, most can be treated effectively with antibiotics and antifungal medications if recognized soon enough.

Canine Distemper

This infamous viral disease of dogs used to be one of the leading causes of death in unvaccinated puppies throughout the world.

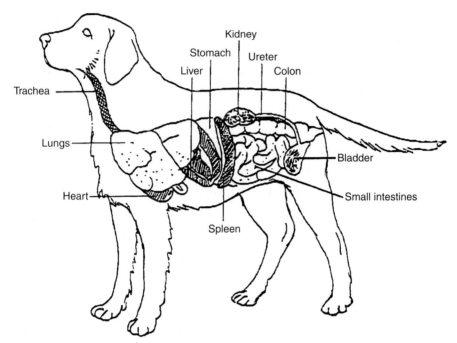

FIGURE 6.1 The internal organs of the dog.

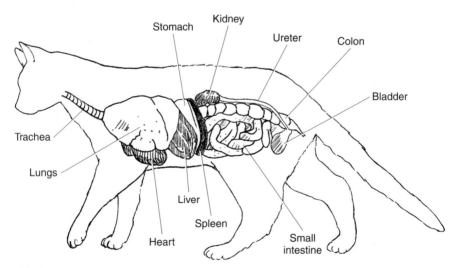

FIGURE 6.2 The internal cat.

Although the incidence of this disease has decreased dramatically over the years because of vaccination programs, the distemper virus is still out there and can strike without warning.

The virus itself is related to the human measles virus and can produce a number of different disease patterns in canines. Infected dogs shed the disease in all body excretions, and transmission usually occurs via airborne means. As a result, like canine cough, it is highly contagious and can travel some distance on an air current.

Distemper is considered a multifaceted disease; that is, it can affect a number of different body systems, including the respiratory, gastrointestinal, and nervous systems.

Early signs of the disease include fever, loss of appetite, and a mild conjunctivitis (eye inflammation). These signs can come and go, lasting only a few days. As a result, pet owners often miss or ignore this early phase of the disease.

As the disease progresses, signs become more serious and extensive. They can include coughing, breathing difficulties, eye and nose discharges, vomiting and diarrhea, blindness, paralysis, and seizures. The seizures associated with this disease often have their own unique presentation, called "chewing gum fits." As the name implies, pets stricken as such will look as if they are chewing gum during the attack. In fact, many owners, when they see this, immediately think of rabies.

The final outcome of an infection with the canine distemper depends on the extent of exposure, the strain of the virus involved, and the ability of the dog's immune system to mount a defense against the virus (with the help of supportive treatment). Depending on these factors, the outcome of such an infection can present itself in one of four ways:

1. Death

2. Recovery with no lasting side effects

3. Recovery, with non-life-threatening side effects

4. Recovery, with life-threatening sequelae

Outcomes 1 and 2 are fairly self-explanatory. Non-life-threatening side effects that can result from distemper can include such conditions as hard pad and enamel hypoplasia. The former is characterized by a prominent thickening and proliferation of the pads of the feet; hence the name. Enamel hypoplasia is a term used to describe the lack of normal enamel covering the tooth surfaces. This occurs in puppies stricken with distemper at an early age, before their permanent teeth have erupted. What happens is the virus attacks and kills off those cells responsible for manufacturing the tooth enamel; hence the new teeth grow in lacking this vital component. Needless to say, teeth lacking enamel are not very strong and tend to erode quickly, becoming brownish in color.

These innocuous side effects might be all that linger, or they might be coupled with more serious sequelae. One such side effect that could become life-threatening to some recovered cases is a degeneration of the nervous system, which can occur slowly or very rapidly. Dogs so affected sometimes show a progressive deterioration of both their motor skills and mental abilities. Rhythmic muscle twitching can become so bad that it totally disables the unfortunate pet. Seizures, paralysis, and incoordination can also become factors as progression proceeds.

A diagnosis of canine distemper is based on a history of exposure, the absence of proper vaccination, and classical clinical signs associated with the disease (eye and nasal discharges, chewing gum fits, enamel hypoplasia, hard pad, etc.). In addition, direct microscopic evidence of the virus within blood cells, or within scrapings of the conjunctiva of the eye or tonsils, can help the veterinarian in the diagnosis.

There is no specific treatment for the canine distemper virus; as a result, supportive care with antibiotics, fluids, and anticonvulsants is indicated. Unfortunately, the overall prognosis is poor, with over 50 percent of dogs that exhibit severe signs dying in spite of good supportive care. Of those dogs that do recover, about 50 percent of them can be expected to develop some form of nervous system complication down the line.

With recent advancements in veterinary dentistry, enamel restoration with artificial compounds has become available for those cases suffering from hypoplasia, and it is a viable way to prevent further tooth deterioration.

Immunization at an early age with a canine distemper vaccine is the cornerstone for preventing this disease. Any puppy or dog suspected of having the disease should be immediately isolated from its pack members. Disinfection of the contaminated premises with bleach (1 part bleach to 30 parts water) will also help reduce spread.

Parvovirus

First identified in 1977, this virus, which is related to the feline panleukopenia virus, usually strikes young, unvaccinated puppies under the age of 6 weeks, although all ages can be susceptible to infection. It is highly contagious, spreading from host to host via oral contamination with infected feces. Parvovirus affects the intestines, the immune system, and/or the heart of infected canines and can quickly be fatal if neglected.

The parvovirus is attracted to those areas of the body in which normal cells are actively dividing and multiplying. In dogs, the lining of the intestines, lymph nodes, and bone marrow are targeted areas. In addition, in puppies less than 6 weeks of age, the virus can infect heart cells, causing irreparable damage to this organ.

The intestinal form of the disease is by far the most common. Signs seen include loss of appetite, persistent vomiting, and profuse, odiferous diarrhea, often streaked with blood (Fig. 6.3). In severe cases, the actual lining of the intestines may be shed in the stool. As these signs develop, dehydration and secondary bacterial infection can rapidly occur, especially in the young pup. If not treated immediately, both conditions can lead to organ failure and death.

The cardiac, or heart, form of the disease is usually characterized by sudden death for no apparent reason, and often with no outward signs to indicate involvement of the virus. In a few

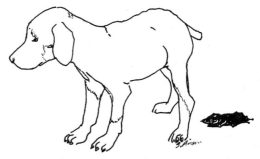

FIGURE 6.3 Bloody diarrhea accompanies acute parvovirus infections.

cases, severe breathing problems may arise as the heart is attacked, which may then be followed up by vomiting and diarrhea as the disease progresses into its intestinal stage.

Diagnosis of parvovirus infection is based on clinical signs, vaccination history, and laboratory tests. A declining white blood cell count, which reflects the virus's invasion into the bone marrow, is one of the most consistent signs seen with parvovirus. In fact, this parameter is used as a prognostic indicator by veterinary clinicians for determining the severity of a particular infection. In general, if this white cell count continues to fall even after 3 days from the onset of clinical signs, the prognosis for recovery is poor. On the other hand, if the count rebounds, and starts its way back up by day 3, recovery can usually be expected, provided, of course, supportive treatment is continued.

Because there are no specific antiviral agents available for this disease, treatment for parvovirus infection involves supportive care and the prevention of secondary complications. Success of treatment depends on many factors, including how quickly it is instituted after the onset of signs, how aggressively treatment is applied, and which strain of the virus is involved.

Intravenous fluids are a must in treating existing dehydration and preventing further dehydration from occurring. Supplementation with potassium, a substance vital to the normal motility of the intestinal tract, is also used to replace the amount that was lost from vomiting and diarrhea.

Since an infected puppy or dog cannot keep any food down, a dextrose or sugar supplement and vitamins may be given intravenously as well. Antibiotics and drugs designed to control vomiting are also part of the support plan. Good nursing care to maintain an adequate body temperature and reduce stress is also a must. Finally, injections with special preparations of antibodies (immunoglobulin injections) that actively fight the parvovirus are showing great promise in the active treatment of parvovirus infections. Whole-blood transfusions with blood from vaccinated dogs can help achieve a similar effect.

Starting immunizations at a young age is the most effective way to prevent serious complications associated with parvovirus exposure and infection. To help reduce the chances of puppies coming down with the heart form of this disease, bitches should be current on vaccinations prior to breeding in order to ensure that optimum amounts of protective maternal antibodies will be passed on to the offspring.

Minimizing exposure is also an important control measure for parvovirus. This virus survives relatively well in the environment outside its host, so its contagiousness can last for weeks. All puppies and dogs, even those vaccinated, should be kept well away from dogs infected with the virus. Owners should also realize that some of these infected dogs can even shed the virus in their stools for weeks after clinical recovery. Puppies should be restricted in their contact with other dogs and with stressful situations until their vaccination program is complete. Contaminated environments can be cleaned with a 1:30 dilution of bleach to help inactivate the virus.

Coronavirus

Coronavirus infection is a highly contagious disease of puppies that can cause minor gastrointestinal illness. The virus is transmitted via contact with shed fecal material containing the virus. This can present a problem when large groups of puppies are housed together, since viral shedding from one infected animal can continue for several weeks even after clinical signs have abated.

Coronavirus causes mild, self-limiting diarrhea and occasional vomiting in affected puppies. However, if a puppy contracts parvovirus, the resulting immune suppression can allow the coronavirus to replicate unchecked and exacerbate the clinical signs seen as a result of the parvovirus.

Diagnosis is afforded by a thorough history, clinical signs seen, and laboratory tests. There is no specific treatment for coronavirus itself. If coupled with parvovirus, treatment approaches will be the same as those for the latter disease.

The need for vaccination against coronavirus is questionable. As a rule, puppies that are properly vaccinated against parvovirus rarely suffer from coronavirus enteritis.

Infectious Canine Hepatitis (ICH)

This disease is caused by the canine adenovirus 1, an organism found worldwide and known for its stability outside its host environment (it can survive for up to 2 weeks!). The virus is shed in all body excretions, and can be found in the urine of a recovered dog for up to 6 months. Direct contact with such secretions by an unsuspecting dog, usually under 1 year of age and unvaccinated, is the method of disease transmission.

As the name implies, once the organism enters the body, it can set up a severe inflammation of the liver, or hepatitis. ICH does not, however, stop there. Other organ systems, including the eyes and kidneys, can be affected as well.

Loss of appetite, depression, and fever, sometimes reaching 106 degrees Fahrenheit, are initial symptoms seen. Enlargement of the tonsils and other lymph nodes occurs as the virus multiplies in these regions. As the liver is attacked, abdominal pain and jaundice become evident. In addition, inflammation of the blood vessels within the body can lead to clotting problems and internal bleeding.

One characteristic lesion of infectious canine hepatitis that can develop later as the disease progresses is called "blue eye." In this condition, one or both eyes can take on a blue appearance due to fluid buildup and inflammation within the eye(s).

Diagnosis of infectious canine hepatitis is based on the age of the animal involved, vaccination history, and laboratory data. Such data will reveal elevated liver enzyme levels, a lowered white blood cell count, and increased clotting time. Biopsy samples might reveal the actual presence of the virus within the tissue itself.

Treatment aims are preventing secondary complications, such as bacterial infections, and giving intravenous fluids to combat dehydration. In severe cases, blood transfusions could be required. Even when vigorous therapy is instituted, prognosis for recovery remains very guarded in the majority of cases.

Vaccination is the best way to prevent this disease.

Canine Contagious Respiratory Disease (CCRD)

CCRD (also known as "canine cough" and "kennel cough") is a highly contagious disease transmitted by air and wind currents contaminated with cough and sneeze droplets from infected canines. It occurs with high frequency in boarding kennels, dog shows, and other areas where dogs may be congregated. There is no one organism on which to solely place the blame for this disease. In fact, over six different causative agents have been isolated, including several types of adenoviruses and reoviruses, the canine herpes virus, the parainfluenza virus, and a bacterium called *Bordetella bronchiseptica*. All of these agents can cause disease by themselves or in combination with the others. The *Bordetella* organism is related to the bacterium that causes whooping cough in humans, and can cause permanent damage to the airways of affected dogs if not detected and treated soon enough.

The classic clinical sign associated with an uncomplicated case of CCRD includes a relentless dry, hacking cough, usually nonproductive (Fig. 6.4). Occasionally, a clear discharge from the nose might appear. Gagging or retching might be noted at the end of a coughing spell and is often mistaken for vomiting. Affected dogs rarely run a fever or seem to "feel bad," nor is it common for them to lose their appetite—that is, if the case doesn't become complicated with secondary infections.

Complicated cases of CCRD are characterized by a greenish eye and nasal discharge, and by obvious breathing difficulties as pneumonia rears its ugly head. In these instances, affected animals do run fevers, do lose their appetites, and do appear sick.

Diagnosis of CCRD is based on the presence of the classic clinical signs, plus a recent history of exposure to other dogs. Radiographs might be required to evaluate the extent of the lung and airway involvement in complicated cases. Bacterial cultures are also indicated in these latter instances.

Treatment of the disease consists of antibiotic therapy, and, in the case of non-productive coughs, cough suppressants. Owners need to realize that coughing can persist for up to 3 weeks, even after treatment.

If complications exist, more specific therapy will be

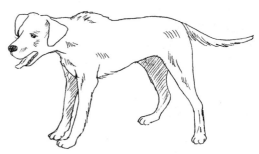

FIGURE 6.4 A dry, hacking cough is characteristic of "kennel cough."

needed to battle the pneumonia and fever and to prevent dehydration. Vaporizers are often used to liquefy secretions in the airway, allowing for greater ease of passage. A similar effect can be obtained by placing the affected pet in a steam-filled bathroom for 10 to 15 minutes. Just be sure that the temperature within the room doesn't get too hot; drinking water should be provided to the dog to help prevent overheating.

An intranasal vaccine can be administered to provide some protection against CCRD. If a dog has not been vaccinated within the past 6 months, it should be administered no later than 1 week prior to a scheduled boarding or event.

Herpes Virus

This virus poses no real threat to adult dogs. In fact, it is thought to be a natural inhabitant of the respiratory tract and sometimes the reproductive tracts of these adults. Its main importance rests in the disease it causes in puppies under 2 weeks of age.

As it turns out, this herpes virus does not multiply well in the higher body temperatures normally found in adult dogs. However, neonatal puppies, whose ability to maintain this body temperature is poor, are prime targets for the virus. They can become infected with it directly inside the mother's uterus, or they can become exposed after birth. Unfortunately, once clinical signs appear in these young puppies, there is not much that can be done to save them.

The time from exposure to the appearance of clinical signs is about 7 to 10 days. Afflicted puppies will cry constantly, become depressed, and stop nursing. Death usually occurs within 24 hours after the signs begin.

Because of its age specificity, herpes virus infection should be suspected anytime puppies under 2 weeks of age become ill and cry constantly. Further diagnostics performed on tissue samples after death can help confirm the diagnosis and shift focus on saving the remaining members of the litter.

As mentioned before, once signs appear in an individual, death is inevitable. However, there are steps owners can take to try and spare the other puppies in the litter from the same fate. Be sure to provide a source of heat (*remember—never* allow a heating pad to come in direct contact with the body surface, and always keep heating pads on their low setting!) to the puppies to maintain their body temperatures above 100 degrees Fahrenheit. This will help slow the multiplication of the virus. If indicated, supportive fluids and forcefeeding can be helpful as well.

There is no vaccine available to help combat this disease.

Leptospirosis

Canine leptospirosis is a bacterial disease of dogs characterized by jaundice, vomiting, and kidney failure. At least four different groups of leptospirosis organisms, all belonging to the genus *Leptospira,* have been implicated in this disease in dogs. Remarkably, most infections are subclinical; that is, few show clinical signs of disease. When clinical signs do arise, however, the results can be serious, even life-threatening. Leptospirosis becomes more of a problem in kennels where animals are kept together under poor sanitary conditions. Animals become infected with the organisms through contact with infected urine.

Leptospirosis is found primarily in young animals between the ages of 1 and 4 years. In addition, males seem to be more commonly affected than females. Signs associated with the disease reflect the damage done by the organisms to the body's blood, liver, and kidneys. Fever, depression, vomiting, and diarrhea might be early signs that become noticeable. Anemia might set in as red blood cells are destroyed by the invading organisms, and distinct bruising on the skin surface becomes evident as the body's blood clotting mechanisms are impaired. In severe cases, liver failure and/or kidney failure appear, leading to rapid dehydration and to a urine with an orange-brown color, a feature characteristic of this disease. Left untreated, this disease will often result in death.

To diagnose this disease, veterinarians rely on a thorough history (including potential exposure to livestock), clinical signs, and special laboratory tests. The white blood cell count is usually elevated, in contrast to those seen with viral diseases. Blood and urine cultures might be used to confirm a diagnosis. Antibody levels measured at 2-week intervals have been used as well for this purpose.

Treatment of leptospirosis consists of high levels of specific antibiotics, combined with fluid therapy to combat dehydration and medications to stimulate kidney function. Unfortunately, unless treated early enough, the kidneys could suffer irreparable damage, leading to unavoidable failure.

Because of the serious nature of this disease, dog owners need to focus their attention on prevention. Since cross-protection against this disease is not afforded by most leptospirosis vaccines, prevention is aimed at limiting access to potentially infected livestock and the water sources they may frequent.

Rabies

If there was ever a disease to strike fear into the hearts and minds of pet owners everywhere, this is it! Rabies is a deadly viral disease that can infect any warm-blooded mammal, including domesticated animals such as dogs, cats, horses, and cattle. As a disease to be avoided, rabies is one of the earliest to ever be recorded, dating back to almost 2000 B.C. It is found worldwide, except in a few countries, such as Great Britain and Japan, which have strict laws designed to keep the countries rabies-free.

The incidence of rabies within the United States varies with each state, depending on the normal fauna found in that state and on existing vaccination laws. It is estimated that over 86 percent of all rabies cases occur in wildlife species of animals, with about 14 percent spilling over into the domestic pet and livestock population. It is certainly these latter groups that pose the greatest threat to public health. Species that are commonly culprits of spreading wildlife rabies include skunks, raccoons, coyotes, foxes, and bats. Opossums are noted for their resistance to this virus, and they rarely become infected. Rodents, such as rats and mice, are not significant carriers of the disease, either, since few survive encounters with rabid animals in the first place.

Skunk rabies is most prevalent in the midwestern and southwestern states and California; raccoon rabies, in the mid-Atlantic and southeastern United States; fox rabies, in the eastern

DID YOU KNOW?

Contrary to popular belief, a bite wound or direct contamination of an open wound isn't the only way a person can be exposed to the rabies virus. Aerosol transmission has been known to occur as well (e.g., breathing air in caves heavily populated by bats).

states; and bat rabies—well, it's found in all states. Most cases seem to occur during the spring and fall months of the year.

The rabies virus is usually transmitted via the infected saliva of affected animals through a bite wound or contamination therewith of an open wound or mucous membranes. The disease is uniformly fatal once contracted.

Dogs are a leading host for this killer, and serve as a major vector for transmission of the disease to humans. Studies have shown that rabies occurs in higher incidence in younger dogs; the median age is about 1 year. In addition, due to hormonally related roaming and territorial instincts, male dogs are at greater risk of exposure than are females.

Traditionally, when speaking of rabies, most people visualize a snarling, frothing dog snapping at anything in sight. While this is true in some instances, pet owners should understand that this represents only one of three stages that are part of the overall disease process. Depending on each individual case, viciousness might take on a prominent role, or might not occur at all. These three stages of rabies include the prodromal stage, the furious stage, and the dumb or paralytic stage.

The first stage, which might last for 1 to 3 days, is characterized by a change in the overall behavior of the animal. Normally friendly dogs might suddenly exhibit aggressive tendencies toward their owners or toward other pets in the household. Affected individuals might also hide a lot, preferring to be left alone, and becoming upset when disturbed. Loss of appetite might become apparent, and owners might notice an increased sexual arousal and/or frequency of urination.

Once the prodromal stage is complete, the victim then enters into the "furious" stage. This is the stage most persons equate with a traditional rabies presentation. Dogs in this stage often become quite restless, excitatory, and aggressive, losing fear of natural enemies. They might wander about aimlessly, snapping and biting at anything that moves. The character of the animal's vocalizations might noticeably change. In dogs especially, *pica,* or an abnormal desire to eat anything within reach (rocks, wire, dirt, feces, etc.), might become apparent. As the disease enters the third stage, the swallowing reflex becomes paralyzed, making it impossible to eat, drink, or swallow saliva. This is what accounts for the excessive drooling seen in rabid animals.

The furious stage might last for up to a week before progressing into stage 3, the paralytic or "dumb" stage. Pet owners should be aware of the fact that some animals, especially dogs, might skip the furious stage entirely, going directly from the prodromal stage into the paralytic stage. When this happens, the disease can be easily mistaken for other nervous system disorders if the diagnostician is not careful. Because this quick transition can occur, the risk of human exposure is greatly increased. The paralytic stage presents itself as a general loss of coordination and paralysis. A droopy lower jaw with the mouth just hanging open is often characteristic. A general paralysis and death usually overtakes the unfortunate animal in a matter of hours.

Rabies should be suspected anytime a dog exhibits behavioral changes with unexplained, abnormal nervous system signs. Unfortunately, the only way to definitively diagnose a case of rabies is to have a laboratory analysis performed on the animal's brain tissue, which means of course, euthanasia of the animal in question.

There is no known treatment for this fatal disease; as a result, stringent control and vaccination measures are a must. All puppies should receive a rabies immunization between 3 and 4 months of age. In most states, a licensed veterinarian must administer this vaccine. Depending on the vaccine used and on the state in which you live, a booster immunization is required every 1 to 3 years. Owing to the public health implications of this disease, dog owners who fail to keep their pets current on this immunization are putting their own health at risk!

Other preventive control measures that can be taken include discouraging night roaming and keeping all pets restrained on a leash when walking outside. Repairing or constructing fences and enclosures to help keep wild animals out of a pet's play area or living area will also help reduce chances of exposure.

If a stray or wild animal bites a dog, the wound needs to be seen immediately by a veterinarian, and, depending on when the last one was given, a booster rabies immunization should be administered. The animal should also be placed in quarantine for a minimum of 90 days, unless the particular animal that did the biting can be found and its rabies status confirmed as negative.

If the dog that was bitten by a known carrier of rabies has never been vaccinated before, immediate euthanasia is warranted. If an owner of such a pet refuses to do so, then, for safety reasons, the pet should be quarantined for at least 6 months before it is declared uninfected.

Laws in most states spell out regulations concerning vaccinations, bites involving humans, and the ownership of wildlife in order to curb the impact of this disease. Any vaccinated dog that bites a human being needs to be placed in quarantine for a minimum of 10 days to observe for signs of rabies. If suspicious signs appear, the animal is then euthanized, and samples are sent to the laboratory. If there is no history of the dog ever having a rabies vaccine in the past, or if a wild animal is involved, euthanasia and prompt laboratory examination of the brain tissue are warranted to expedite the diagnostic process.

Euthanasia should be carried out only by veterinarians or other public health and/or wildlife officials to ensure that the sample that reaches the lab has been properly handled and stored. Certainly any person bitten by an animal should contact a physician immediately. If the situation warrants it, prophylactic rabies treatment should commence on the bitten individual until the quarantine period is over or until the specific laboratory test results are in.

It is interesting to note that because the concentration of the rabies virus in the infected dog's saliva might be low or even absent in some cases, less than 50 percent of all bites from rabies-positive animals will result in the transmission of the disease. Yet because there is no way of knowing which fall into this category, prophylactic treatment is a must, just to be on the safe side!

Finally, ownership of wild animals, especially skunks (descented or not) and raccoons, should be avoided for a number of reasons. First, there are no licensed vaccines available for these wild animals. Second, because the incubation period of rabies can last for months, owners might be exposing themselves to rabies right from the start without knowing it. Finally, in many states, it is outright illegal to own such animals without a permit.

Parents should always discourage children from interacting with stray animals or wildlife. Their natural curiosity could lead to a serious bite wound and much anxiety, especially if the offender is not found.

Bacterial Disease

Dogs most often develop bacterial infections and abscesses secondary to traumatic wounds and dietary indiscretions. However, in most instances, bacterial infections occur secondarily to other disease conditions, such as periodontal disease, stress, viral infections, and parasites. As a result, whenever a bacterial disease rears its ugly head, all underlying problems that may exist must be identified and addressed at the same time.

Higher Bacterial Disease

A special group of bacteria, called "higher bacteria," which share characteristics of both standard bacteria and fungi, can cause significant disease in exposed dogs.

Two of the more prevalent organisms in this class are *Nocardia* and *Actinomyces.* These agents, found in soil, are transmitted primarily via traumatic wounds. Draining, painful skin lesions, and severe pneumonia are consequences of higher bacterial infections in dogs. Diagnosis and treatment for these diseases are similar to those for standard bacterial infections; however, surgical removal of infected tissue is often required to afford a complete cure.

Ringworm and Fungal Disease

Along with viruses and bacteria, fungal organisms can cause disease in dogs. Probably the most common one pet owners are familiar with and have heard about is dermatophytosis, or ringworm. In addition, yeast infections can be a common problem in the ears of dogs. These types of yeast and fungi that affect mainly the outer skin surfaces are termed *superficial mycoses.*

The most prevalent fungal disease that afflicts dogs is ringworm. Three different organisms—*Microsporum canis, Trichophyton mentagrophytes,* and *Microsporum gypseum*—can actually cause ringworm (Fig. 6.5). The first two are contracted from infected animals; the third, from contaminated soil. In dogs, ringworm causes patchy hair logs with or without an accompanying lesion on the skin beneath. Since humans can be susceptible to the same type of ringworm, reddened, circular lesions occurring on the owner as well might support a diagnosis. Diagnosis of ringworm is confirmed by a fungal culture. Treatment can consist of iodine or chlorhexidine shampoos and topical and/or oral antifungal medications.

In contrast to ringworm, fungal and yeast infections involving the deeper tissues of the body are termed *subcutaneous* or *deep mycoses,*

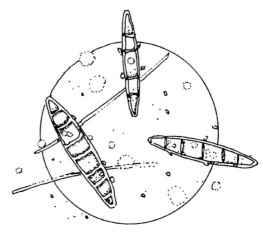

FIGURE 6.5 Microscopic appearance of ringworm spores.

depending on the depth of tissue involvement. These diseases, including sporotrichosis, aspergillosis, blastomycosis, histoplasmosis, coccidioidomycosis, and cryptococcosis, can be quite severe, and even life-threatening at times. Spores from these organisms are inhaled, are ingested, or penetrate the skin via wounds. Depending on the organism involved, clinical signs can include weight loss, coughing, breathing difficulties, draining skin lesions, tender skin masses, lameness, diarrhea, and nervous system impairment (i.e., blindness).

History, physical exam findings, and laboratory tests, including radiographic X rays, and biopsies of affected regions can lead the veterinary practitioner to a tentative diagnosis of a fungal infection within the body. Microscopic examination of body fluids or drainages for fungal spores or yeast can also be helpful. In most cases, a definitive diagnosis is made by testing a blood serum sample for antibodies against the fungal organisms in question, or, less commonly, by culturing for growth.

A number of antifungal medications are available and can be used to treat such infections in dogs. Depending on which agents are used (many are used in combination with one another), duration of treatment required is often 1 to 3 months to afford a complete cure.

Radiographs and special immunologic tests can be used to monitor the response to treatment. In many cases, surgical excision of those regions infected with the fungus can afford faster recovery. The prognosis for dogs is good when fungal infections are detected and treated in their early stages but guarded to poor if dissemination throughout the body has occurred.

INFECTIOUS DISEASES IN CATS

As with dogs, viruses cause the majority of infectious disease seen in cats. Again, treatment for these agents is usually supportive in nature, owing to a lack of specific antiviral medications. The best treatment is prevention using proper immunization procedures. With those infections caused by bacteria and fungi, most can be treated effectively with the early use of antibiotics and antifungal medications.

Parvovirus (Panleukopenia; Feline Distemper)

The feline parvovirus is found worldwide, affecting cats in much the same way as parvovirus affects their canine counterparts. The feline parvovirus causes severe gastroenteritis in affected cats, and can be fatal unless treated with haste. This highly contagious disease primarily affects unvaccinated cats less than a year old.

Spread by oral contact with infective feces, urine, or saliva, the feline parvovirus strikes the intestines with a fury, causing fever, depression, vomiting, diarrhea, abdominal pain, and dehydration. The disease can be complicated even further as bacteria within the gut proliferate as a result of the virus and release toxins into the bloodstream. The virus itself can even spread to the bone marrow and interfere with the body's ability to mount an effective immune response to the disease. If a queen becomes infected with the parvovirus while pregnant, abortions or weak kittens could result. In many instances, these newborn kittens suffer from underdeveloped brains, causing permanent incoordination.

Diagnosis of a parvovirus infection in cats is based on history, clinical signs, and a marked reduction in the circulating number of white blood cells (Fig. 6.6).

Treatment is supportive, involving antivomiting drugs and intravenous fluids to correct and prevent further dehydration, and antibiotics to keep the secondary bacterial infections at bay. Recovery will depend on how rapidly this supportive treatment is instituted.

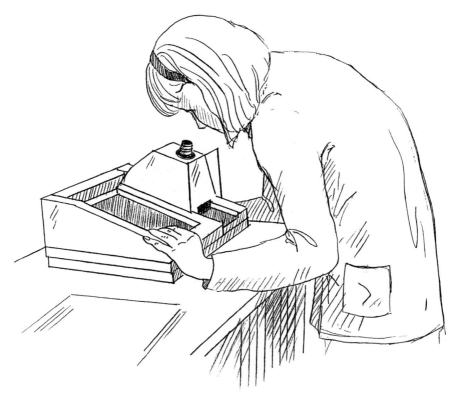

FIGURE 6.6 Laboratory analysis of a blood sample can help confirm a diagnosis of panleukopenia.

Feline parvovirus can be prevented through vaccination. Queens should be current on vaccinations prior to becoming pregnant to protect unborn offspring from the virus. Finally, this virus is relatively stable in the environment, so it is a good idea to wait 3 to 4 weeks before introducing any new kittens or cats into a house where the parvovirus has been.

Feline Infectious Peritonitis

Feline infectious peritonitis (FIP) is a unique viral disease of cats, unique in that the actual organ damage resulting from infection is not directly caused by the virus itself, but from the immune response to the invader.

The FIP organism is classified as a *coronavirus,* belonging to same group of viruses that cause gastrointestinal disease in dogs. Cats actually can be infected with two types of coronavirus: the feline enteric coronavirus and the feline infectious peritonitis coronavirus. Although the former can cause severe gastroenteritis in affected cats, most cases are subclinical; that is, there are no apparent clinical signs caused by the infection. The importance of these enteric coronaviruses is not only that their presence in a feline can interfere with some standard testing procedures designed to diagnose FIP but also that the FIP coronavirus may actually be a mutation of the enteric coronavirus. If this is true, then all cats could be at risk of this disease.

Cats less than 4 years and over 12 years of age seem to have a higher preponderance for this disease than do other age groups. Inhalation or ingestion of infective secretions and excretions is the primary way in which this highly contagious disease is spread from cat to cat. The virus can even be passed via the uterus from an infected queen to her kittens.

Interestingly, most cats that contract this potentially deadly viral disease rarely show signs of infection, and may actually eliminate the infection soon after exposure occurs. If they are to appear, clinical signs usually show up 2 to 3 weeks after exposure, although this can vary by months to years. Upper respiratory signs can appear for a few days, then subside without any further problems until other clinical signs appear years later.

Another interesting fact about cats infected with FIP is that many are also concurrently infected with the feline leukemia virus. Since the leukemia virus suppresses the immune system, this paves the way for clinical FIP if exposure occurs.

FIP infections are unique in that the actual virus itself does not cause specific damage to the body's organs or tissues. It is the cat's exaggerated immune response to the virus that damages the organs, tissues, and blood vessels within the body. Clinical signs that are seen depend on where this damage is done. Almost all affected cats run persistent, low-grade fevers. Insidious weight loss and appetite loss are common as well.

Clinical FIP presents itself in three forms:

1. Wet or effusive FIP

2. Dry or noneffusive FIP

3. A combination of forms 1 and 2

Wet FIP. When the immune system attacks the blood vessels in response to FIP, wet FIP results. Fluid that leaks out of the damaged vessels accumulates within the chest and/or abdomen, causing nonpainful abdominal distension and/or breathing difficulties.

Dry FIP. With dry FIP, many small nodules and regions of inflammation appear in various areas of the body, including the gastrointestinal tract, the lungs and heart, the brain and spinal cord, the kidneys, and/or the eyes. Obviously, with so many organ systems potentially affected, a wide variety of clinical signs, including coughing, vomiting, diarrhea, seizures, and blindness, can result.

In an effort to diagnose a suspected case of FIP, a veterinarian will rely initially on clinical signs seen, physical exam, blood samples, and perhaps microscopic examination of any abnormal fluids within the chest or abdomen. A persistent nonresponsive fever in a cat may point to FIP infection. As mentioned, diagnosis of the FIP coronavirus using certain tests designed to detect antibodies to FIP can be obscured by the presence or absence of the enteric coronavirus.

Unfortunately, there are no effective treatments that can eliminate the FIP virus from the feline body. Modulating the immune response with steroids and certain chemotherapy drugs can help provide temporary relief from clinical signs, but will do nothing to afford a cure. Survival time for cats exhibiting clinical signs can vary from days to weeks, depending on the degree of organ involvement.

Because of the lack of an effective treatment, prevention is the key with this disease. A vaccine is available for FIP. Also, owners should take alternative steps to protect their cats from the deleterious effects of this disease. Because FIP can gain a foothold in cats with unhealthy immune systems, it is important to keep the immune system in top-notch shape. This includes keeping cats on a good plane of nutrition and being sure that they are current on their feline leukemia vaccinations. Keeping cats indoors, restricting their interaction with stray felines, is another excellent way to limit potential exposure. Finally, all new cats brought into a household should test negative for the feline coronavirus.

Enteric Coronavirus (EC)

As a disease entity itself, EC can cause fever, vomiting, and diarrhea in kittens; however, if supportive care is provided, the gastrointestinal tract of these kittens usually recovers in a few days. Yet, the primary importance of this virus is not in the disease it causes, but in the confusion it often generates when trying to diagnose a case of feline infectious peritonitis.

Feline Upper Respiratory Disease (URD)

At least six infectious agents are responsible for upper respiratory disease in cats, including *Bordetella,* the same bacterium that causes kennel cough in dogs. The primary agents in the majority of cases include the feline herpes virus (rhinotracheitis) and the feline calicivirus. Vaccinations against these two organisms are routinely administered to cats at the time of their yearly checkup. In many parts of the country, veterinarians also routinely vaccinate for *Chlamydophila felis,* a bacterial agent that causes a condition known as *feline pneumonitis.* However, because many other less common organisms can cause feline respiratory problems, vaccination is not a guarantee against a cat coming down with respiratory disease.

Feline Rhinotracheitis

Feline rhinotracheitis is caused by a herpes virus that infects the nasal passages and upper airways of the affected individual. The virus itself is very contagious, with the incubation period (the period from exposure to the appearance of clinical signs) ranging from 2 to 20 days. Kittens are usually more severely affected by acute disease than are adults. The presence of the feline leukemia or AIDS (FIV) virus can also significantly increase the susceptibility to rhinotracheitis. Clinical signs associated with rhinotracheitis include sneezing, loss of appetite, conjunctivitis, oral ulcers, and nasal discharge (Fig. 6.7). The discharges might start out as clear, but turn thick and mucuslike as secondary bacterial infection sets in. Severe infections can result in corneal ulcers of the eye, and pregnant queens might even abort their fetuses. Rhinotracheitis in newborn kittens can be deadly, with infected kittens dying within hours to days after birth. This syndrome is better known as "fading kitten syndrome."

Many cats, especially those infected when young, will suffer continued recurrences of this disease as they mature if the virus decides to set up housekeeping within the bones of the nasal passages. Purebreds such as Siamese and Himalayans are especially predisposed to

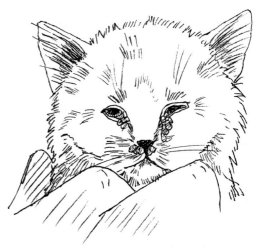

FIGURE 6.7 Conjunctivitis is often caused by upper respiratory viruses.

these chronic, recurring infections and become effective carriers of the virus. Recurring episodes are brought on by stress due to shipping or boarding, pregnancy, or other illnesses.

Feline Calicivirus

As with rhinotracheitis, the feline calicivirus is a very contagious organism that can create both acute upper respiratory disease and chronic carriers in all ages. The incubation period of the calicivirus is anywhere from 2 to 10 days. Sneezing, fever, nasal discharge, oral ulcers, and conjunctivitis are all characteristic signs of the acute disease. The chronic form of the disease can be responsible for recurring gingivitis and oral infections in infected individuals.

The feline calicivirus has also been implicated in the disease syndrome of kittens known as "limping kitten syndrome" (LKS). LKS is seen in kittens less than 14 weeks of age and appears as a generalized arthritis (hence the name), especially affecting the back legs. This presentation of the disease will usually run its course without causing any permanent joint damage.

Chlamydophila

Chlamydophila felis does not limit itself to the airways of cats; humans and birds are also susceptible to infection by this organism. Although this organism is not a virus, *Chlamydophila* behaves very similarly to the herpes virus and the calicivirus in causing disease and clinical signs. The incubation period for this organism is approximately the same as that for the calicivirus.

Chlamydophila felis is susceptible to antibiotic therapy and can be brought under control with rapid treatment. Unfortunately, as with the viruses, carrier states can occur, and recurrence of clinical signs might result secondary to stress.

Diagnosis and Treatment of Upper Respiratory Disease

Because viruses cannot be readily identified microscopically or cultured, diagnosis of URD in cats relies on history of occurrence and clinical signs seen. Laboratory findings from blood samples are usually nonspecific as well. If *Chlamydophila* is suspected, microscopic examination of some of the cells lining the conjunctiva and/or nasal passages might reveal characteristic inclusions created by this organism. Also, because of its effect on the immune system, all cats suffering from URD should be concurrently tested for feline leukemia and the feline immunodeficiency virus.

Any sign suggestive of upper respiratory disease in cats warrants prompt veterinary examination and treatment to prevent serious sequelae. In the case of rhinotracheitis and calicivirus, there are no specific drugs to combat these agents; however, with good supportive care, life-threatening situations can be avoided. Antibiotic therapy is usually implemented to prevent any secondary infections from setting up; antibiotics are also indicated for combatting *Chlamydophila* and *Bordetella* infections. If eye manifestations are present, antibiotic-containing eyedrops or ointment will help protect the eyes and speed healing.

In addition to oral and, if needed, ophthalmic antibiotics, it is vital that the nose and airways be cleared of discharge and fluid as soon as possible. Because a feline's appetite is dependent on its ability to smell its food, cats with URD will show a marked reduction in appetite, which could conceivably lead to secondary complications from malnutrition and dehydration.

Nasal discharges should be manually removed as often as possible. Human nasal decongestant sprays might be used to help break up any mucus buildup that might be present (contact a veterinarian as to types and dosages).

Humidifying the cat's room air using a vaporizer or by placing it in a misty bathroom where hot water has been running in the shower will also assist in the breakup of mucus within the airways. If dehydration is a factor, intravenous fluid replacement performed by a veterinarian might be necessary.

Finally, good nursing care can do wonders to assure a positive outcome. Keep the ill cat warm and dry and free from stress. If required, forcefeeding or tube feeding can help provide the nutrition necessary to boost the effectiveness of the cat's own immune system and shorten the convalescent period.

Prevention of URD

Owners can help prevent URD in their cats by making sure that they remain current on vaccinations. Both intranasal (Fig. 6.8) and injectable vaccines are available to combat respiratory viruses. In multicat

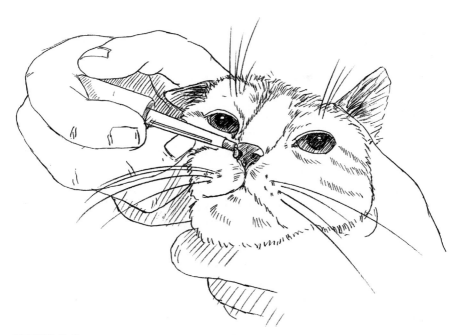

FIGURE 6.8 Administering an intranasal vaccine to a cat.

households, prompt isolation of sick and sneezing cats might help prevent its rapid spread to other cats in the household.

Feline Leukemia Virus (FeLV)

Certainly one of the most devastating diseases affecting cat populations around the world is feline leukemia. The feline leukemia virus belongs to a group of infectious agents known as *retroviruses,* and it shares some characteristics with the human AIDS virus. It can occur by itself, or in combination with the feline immunodeficiency virus (FIV), a deadly AIDS-like virus that in itself has been spreading at an alarming rate in cats in recent years.

DID YOU KNOW?

Susceptibility to feline leukemia decreases with age. Cats over 1 year of age appear to be resistant to the virus.

Like the human AIDS virus, both of these feline diseases wreak havoc on the cat's immune system, predisposing it to a wide variety of infectious diseases and to cancer.

The feline leukemia virus can be transmitted via all bodily excretions from an infected cat (Fig. 6.9). Infected queens can transmit the disease to their offspring through the placenta prior to birth or through the milk during lactation. As a result, even newborn kittens can test positive for this disease. For other cats, close contact is required for

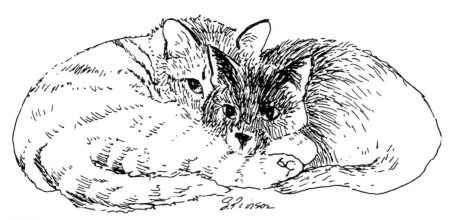

FIGURE 6.9 The feline leukemia virus is easily spread through close contact.

effective transmission. As a result, feline leukemia is most prevalent in multiple-cat households and catteries. Interestingly, cats over 1 year of age that have otherwise healthy immune systems seem to develop a natural resistance to the feline leukemia virus.

Because of the ability of the feline leukemia virus to suppress the cat's immune system, infected felines are prone to cancer (especially lymphosarcoma and leukemia), anemia, kidney disease, and a wide variety of secondary infections such as feline infectious peritonitis, hemobartonellosis, cryptococcosis, and upper respiratory viruses. Pregnant queens might abort their kittens, or give birth to weak, unthrifty offspring that die soon after birth.

Even cats suffering from seemingly innocent lesions on their skin and mucous membranes could actually be suffering from an underlying infection with feline leukemia. Finally, in some affected individuals, the only apparent signs might be lethargy, weight loss, and/or chronic gingivitis.

Diagnosis of feline leukemia is accomplished by a simple test that can be performed in a veterinarian's office. Tears and saliva can be used for initial screening purposes, but for definitive answers, a blood test should be performed.

Once bone marrow penetration has occurred, permanent infection is likely, and the majority of these cats will become active carriers and shedders of the disease. FeLV has the ability to incorporate itself into the genetic material within host cells and remain dormant (not causing disease) for long periods of time. As a result, an infected cat might not show any adverse signs for years. However, if the immune system becomes stressed in any way, the FeLV will become active, and clinical signs appear. In general, cats with permanent FeLV infections usually succumb to FeLV-related disease within 3 to 5 years after initial exposure.

Currently, there is no cure for the FeLV virus. Treatment is directed at relieving any clinical signs seen and eliminating secondary infections or managing cancerous conditions present. Unfortunately, however, recurrences of such diseases are common after treatment. Many experimental agents, such as interferon, antiviral drugs, and medications designed to modulate the immune system, have been employed in an attempt to eliminate the feline leukemia virus itself. Unfortunately, to date, these have met with limited results. Bone marrow transplant, although helpful in some experimental instances, is not as yet a proven or practical means of treatment. The bottom line: The best treatment for feline leukemia is prevention!

Vaccines that can help protect a pet against this deadly disease are available from veterinarians. Kittens in high-risk households can be vaccinated as early as 9 weeks of age. These kittens should receive two initial boosters 3 weeks apart.

Prior to receiving the vaccine, all kittens should be tested for the leukemia virus. While such testing is not mandatory before the vaccine is given, it is always a good idea to prevent a false sense of security in an owner's mind. Remember: Because they can be born with this disease, even kittens that have no other history of exposure should be tested.

There are other control measures that you can implement to protect cats from FeLV. Testing all new cats before introducing them into a household is one. In addition, when boarding a feline or taking one to cat shows, be certain that the facility or event requires that all cats be tested free of leukemia and vaccinated prior to admission. Finally, keeping a cat indoors at night and, if it is a male, having it neutered, will help reduce potential interactions with neighborhood carriers of the disease.

A question frequently asked concerning a cat that has tested positive for FeLV is "Is feline leukemia transmissible to humans?" To date, no antibodies to FeLV have ever been found in human individuals in high exposure–risk groups such as veterinarians, cat breeders, and laboratory handlers. In addition, the incidence of cancer in humans seems to show no correlation with exposure or nonexposure to FeLV-positive cats.

However, the ultimate decision governing whether a FeLV-positive cat is to be kept in a household rests on the cat owner. Many veterinarians and researchers do recommend segregating children, pregnant women, the elderly, and immunocompromised persons from cats that have FeLV, primarily because of the other zoonotic organisms that these immune-depressed cats may be harboring. Certainly other cats within the household, even if fully vaccinated, are at risk of contracting the disease from an infected cat. However, in those situations in which none of the above apply, the difficult decision on whether to keep a FeLV-positive feline is a personal one, and should be influenced by an owner's individual feelings on the matter and the cat's overall health status.

Feline Immunodeficiency Virus (FIV)

Until the late 1980s, the feline leukemia virus was the only agent linked to acquired immunodeficiency syndrome in cats—that is, it was until the feline immunodeficiency virus (FIV) (also known as "feline AIDS") was identified. This organism is unlike the feline leukemia virus in that it belongs to the same subfamily of retroviruses as the human AIDS virus (HIV). FIV is now known to be widespread among the cat population across the United States and around the world.

> ## DID YOU KNOW?
>
> It is believed that up to 15 percent of all sick cats presented to veterinarians are infected with the feline leukemia and/or feline AIDS virus.

FIV behaves the same way in cats as HIV does in humans; that is, it attacks the host's immune system and debilitates it, leaving the body wide open to secondary invaders and disease. The disease does not appear to be readily sexually transmitted in cats, and rarely is it passed on through casual contact with saliva, urine, or other body fluids, as the feline leukemia virus can be.

Instead, the main mode of transmission of FIV between cats is through penetrating bite wounds that introduce infected saliva deep into the tissues. This method of transmission is said to be analogous to the use of a dirty hypodermic needle in humans as a means of spreading HlV between people. Needless to say, nonneutered male cats between the ages of 3 and 10 years that are allowed to roam about the neighborhood and fight with other cats are at greatest risk of contracting this deadly disease (Fig. 6.10).

Clinical signs associated with FIV in cats can be quite variable because of the immunosuppressive nature of the disease. Some cats might be carriers of the disease, not showing any clinical signs of illness whatsoever. In others, the only subtle signs noticed might be recurring infections (abscesses and skin infections, respiratory infections, bladder infections, etc.), weight loss, or chronic gingivitis and bad breath. Chronic, unresponsive diarrhea is another sign commonly seen in cats harboring FIV. Lymph node enlargement, loss of appetite, cancerous growths, and/or bizarre behavioral changes might also be present in an active infection. Finally, FIV makes the affected cat more

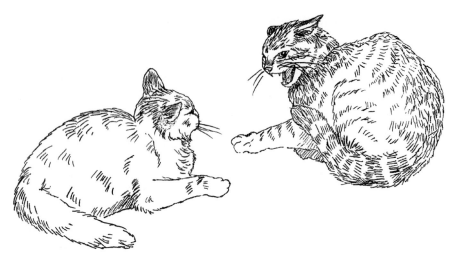

FIGURE 6.10 Cats that fight are at high risk of contracting the feline immunodeficiency virus.

susceptible to parasitic infections, such as toxoplasmosis, hemobartonellosis, and demodecosis, and their associated clinical syndromes.

Diagnosis of FIV can be made in a veterinarian's office using a quick, easy test similar to the one used to test for feline leukemia. In fact, it is common to test for both diseases at the same time, since they can occur concurrently.

All cats presented with acute illnesses or those with chronic, recurring disorders are prime candidates for testing. In addition, all new cats should be tested for both feline leukemia and FIV prior to their introduction into new households.

> ### *DID YOU KNOW❓*
>
> **Kittens under 6 months of age can test positive for FIV if they received antibodies to the virus from their mother's milk. However, this does not mean that they are necessarily infected with the virus. They should be retested at 6 months of age to ascertain their true status. The test will usually turn up negative.**

Kittens under 6 months of age can test positive for FIV if they received antibodies to the virus from their mother's milk. However, this does not mean that they are necessarily infected with the virus. As a result, they should be retested at 6 months of age to ascertain their true status.

As with feline leukemia, there is no known cure for FIV in cats. In the early stages of the disease, many infected individuals will respond well to treatments geared specifically toward any secondary problems of infections, yet as the disease progresses, even these treatments become less and less effective. Medications used to treat AIDs in humans have been used to treat FIV, yet such therapies are cost-prohibitive for most pet owners and have achieved limited success at prolonging life in these cats.

Felines exhibiting pronounced clinical signs are usually in the terminal stages of the illness, yet even then they might slowly deteriorate over months to years. Euthanasia should be a consideration in these instances.

A vaccine is now available for FIV. However, the most effective ways to protect a cat from the ravages of FIV are to have it neutered and to keep the cat indoors during the evening hours (the time when it is most likely to get into a fight with another cat). Cat owners should report all stray cats in the neighborhood to animal control because such animals are the most likely carriers. Finally, as mentioned above, have all new cats tested for the disease prior to their induction into a new household.

As with feline leukemia, the question arises, "Is FIV transmissible to humans?" The general consensus of veterinary and medical researchers is that it is not. Studies analyzing individuals at high risk of exposure to FIV (veterinarians, lab technicians, multiple-cat owners) have failed to show any link between FIV and human illness. Furthermore, viruses belonging to the same subfamily as HIV and FIV are quite species-specific, rarely crossing species lines.

The decision governing whether an FIV-positive cat is to be kept in a household rests on the cat owner. Many veterinarians and researchers agree that owners should consider segregating children, pregnant women, the elderly, and immunocompromised individuals from cats that are carriers of FIV, primarily because these immunosuppressed cats can be carriers of other zoonotic diseases that would not otherwise be found in a healthy cat.

Rabies

The incidence of rabies in cats has increased in recent years, actually surpassing that of dogs (Fig 6.11). Many attribute this to the nocturnal hunting

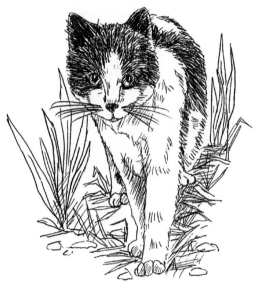

FIGURE 6.11 Because of their nocturnal and predatory behaviors, cats are at relatively high risk of exposure to the rabies virus.

DID YOU KNOW?

Not all pets stricken with rabies will exhibit aggressive behavior. In fact, some cats might skip the furious stage entirely, going directly from the pro-dromal stage into the paralytic stage. When this happens, the disease can be easily mistaken for other nervous system disorders, thereby increasing the risk of human exposure.

DID YOU KNOW?

Ringworm is not a "worm" at all, but a skin fungus.

behavior of this species; however, the tremendous increase in the number of homeless cats in recent years puts them at greater risk of exposure to this deadly disease. The disease in cats is the same as that in dogs.

Bacterial Disease

Cats develop bacterial infections and abscesses secondary to traumatic wounds (usually bite wounds from other cats) and by eating something they shouldn't be eating. However, in most instances, bacterial infections occur secondarily to other disease conditions, such as allergies, stress, viral infections, and parasites. As a result, as with dogs, all underlying problems must be identified and addressed before treatment can be administered effectively.

Higher Bacterial and Fungal Disease

Higher bacteria and fungi affect cats with clinical signs and disease similar to those found in dogs (see page 140). In cats, ringworm is certainly the most common fungal infection seen. Interestingly, many ringworm-infected cats display only subtle signs of infections, making them ideal transmitters of the disease to other pets in the household and to people! A vaccine does exist for ringworm, yet its efficacy is questionable. Consult a veterinarian for recommendations regarding this mode of prevention.

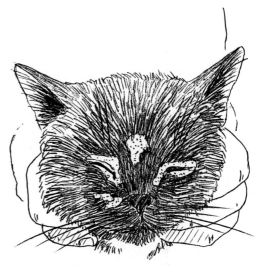

FIGURE 6.12 Ringworm often causes facial lesions in cats.

Parasitic Disease

long with infectious diseases, internal and external parasites are
responsible for the vast majority of illnesses and disorders seen in
dogs and cats. As a result, timely diagnosis and treatment for these
pests is vital to the health of the pet.

Fleas

Ctenocephalides canis (common dog flea) is by far the most common
external parasite seen on dogs and cats (Fig. 7.1). As most pet owners
will attest to, these pests are the number one health problem facing
these pets. However, aside from causing relentless chewing and
scratching, fleas are also disease carriers, and can threaten the pet
owner's health as well. For these reasons, the development of a good
control program to combat these irritating pests is a must.

It is important to understand that fleas spend the vast majority of
their time off of the pet, reproducing and maturing in the pet's environment. As a result, environmental control measures are essential for
successful flea control.

The flea life cycle includes four major stages: egg, larva, pupa,
and adult stages. Both the egg and pupa stages are very resistant to
insecticides, which can make complete flea control difficult. During

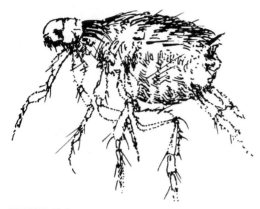

FIGURE 7.1 The flea is the most common parasite of dogs and cats.

DID YOU KNOW?

For every flea seen on your pet, there are nine more in your house or yard!

summer months, the entire flea cycle (egg to adult) might be completed in 16 to 21 days. Heat and humidity tend to shorten this cycle period. In addition, fleas are most prolific during hot humid weather.

A complete approach to flea control should always involve three steps:

1. Treating the home
2. Treating the yard
3. Treating the pet

Because fleas, on average, will only spend about 10 percent of their time on dogs and cats, treating the surrounding environment is probably more important than treating the actual pet. For more information regarding flea control, see Chapter 4.

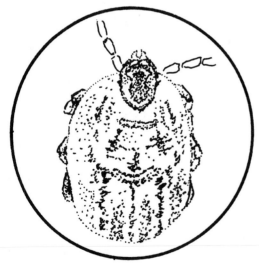

FIGURE 7.2 Female ticks engorged on blood can reach relatively enormous sizes!

Ticks

Ticks, unlike fleas, attach themselves to the pet's skin via their mouthparts. Ticks generally remain attached in one spot for long periods. The head, neck, and interdigital (between the toes) areas of the pet are the most common sites of severe infestation. Ticks produce local irritation and even anemia in heavy infestations (Fig. 7.2). Ticks might serve as intermediate hosts for disease-producing microorganisms and might transmit these "germs" (such as Lyme disease) to the infested pet. For more information on tick control, see Chapter 4.

Mites

Mite infestation, commonly known as *mange,* requires the diagnostic and treatment expertise of a veterinarian. The common mites infecting dogs and cats are microscopic, requiring skin scrapes and subsequent microscopic examination by the veterinarian for diagnosis. The most common forms of mange and pertinent facts concerning each are described below.

Sarcoptic Mange (Dogs)

Caused by the organism *Sarcoptes scabiei* var. *canis,* sarcoptic mange is characterized by a sudden onset of severe itching. Direct exposure to an infected animal is required for transmission (Fig. 7.3).

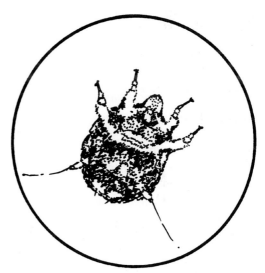

The mite burrows into the host's epidermis and tunnels. Severe itching results, particularly on the abdomen, chest, legs, and ears. Thickening and scaling of elbows, hocks, and eartips might be

FIGURE 7.3 The sarcoptic mange mite.

noted. Hair loss and skin irritation often result from the almost constant scratching and biting (Fig. 7.4).

Scabies is highly contagious to other dogs. In addition, it might temporarily produce chiggerlike bites and itching on exposed human family members.

Pet treatment consists of proper diagnosis, miticidal dipping, and/or systemic miticides. All dogs in the household should be treated because of the highly contagious nature of the scabies mite. If pet to human transmission occurs, contact your physician.

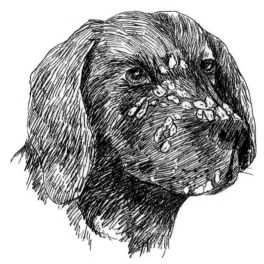

FIGURE 7.4 Facial crusting caused by sarcoptic mange.

FACT OR FICTION

Mange is always contagious from pet to pet. *FICTION.* Although many types of mange mites are indeed contagious, one of the most infamous, *Demodex,* is not. This type of mange causes problems only in pets with compromised immune systems.

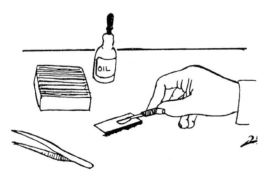

FIGURE 7.5 Skin scrapings can be used to detect mite infestations in pets.

Cheyletiella Mange

The mange mite *Cheyletiella* can cause skin scaling, intense itching, and hair loss in affected dogs and cats. The common name for this parasitism is "walking dandruff," since the flakes and scales produced by the disease, when observed closely, appear to be in motion. Like sarcoptic mange, this mite can temporarily infest people who become exposed. Diagnosis and treatment of *Cheyletiella* mange is the same as that for sarcoptic mange.

Notoedres Mange (Cats)

The most common mange mite infecting cats, *Notoedres cati,* is microscopic, and it requires special skin scrapes for its detection (Fig. 7.5). Direct exposure to an infected animal is required for its transmission.

The major symptom of *Notoedres* mange is a sudden onset of severe itching. As the mite burrows into the host's epidermis, itching, hair loss, and scaly skin result, initially on the face, neck, and ears, and then to other areas on the body. The haircoat on these cats often takes on a "mousy" odor as well.

Treatment for *Notoedres* mange consists of special miticidal dipping and/or systemic miticides. If dips are used, they should only be performed by a veterinarian, since toxicity can be a problem if they are not used correctly. All other cats in the household should also be treated due to the highly contagious nature of this mite.

Demodectic Mange

Demodectic mange is also called *follicular* or *red mange.* The demodectic mange mite, *Demodex canis,* might be found in the hair follicles of normal dogs in low numbers (Fig. 7.6). However, in cases where demodectic mange develops, normal immunity to the mite either fails to develop or is suppressed resulting in pathogenic proliferation of the mite within the hair follicles.

The majority of demodectic mange cases occur in dogs less than 2 years of age with immune systems that are immature or temporarily suppressed. The first symptom observable is usually small areas of hair loss. The lesions might occur anywhere on the body but often begin in the head area. Diagnosis requires a skin scraping and microscopic exam by a veterinarian.

The lesions (areas of hair loss) might be localized to one area or generalized over the body. Secondary bacterial hair follicle infections (folliculitis) are common sequelae to some localized and most generalized cases. The inflammatory skin reaction that ensues might result in the reddened skin referred to by the term *red mange.*

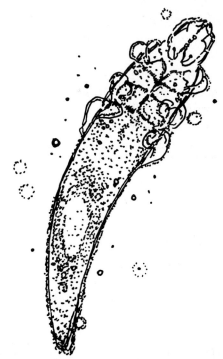

FIGURE 7.6 The demodectic mange mite.

With correct diagnosis and appropriate treatment, 80 to 90 percent of young dogs with demodicosis will recover. Maturation of the immune response plays a vital role in cases of complete recovery. Relapse might occur but is infrequent. However, unlike sarcoptic mange, demodicosis often requires long-term therapy

Demodectic mange in older dogs might reflect immunologic suppression elicited by an underlying disease. Liver disorders, viral infections, malnutrition, heat cycle changes, neoplasia, hypothyroidism, diabetes, and other problems might lead to impaired immune responses and demodicosis. A thorough physical examination is important in such cases. The success of the treatment is dependent on the cause of immunodeficiency.

Special insecticidal medications, both topical and systemic, are available for demodectic mange through a veterinarian.

Factors concerning a dog's immunologic ability to protect it from developing demodectic mange are considered hereditary. However, since most cases of demodicosis resolve when the dog matures, the significance of its inheritable nature is questionable.

The *Demodex* mange mite can also affect cats, yet its occurrence rate in felines is quite low. If present, it causes scaly, bald regions on the skin of the head, legs, and feet. As in dogs, this type of mange infestation is caused by a poorly functioning immune system. As a result, gaining a complete cure with treatment can be difficult.

Tapeworms

Tapeworms (Fig. 7.7) are considered segmented flatworms, belonging to a class of organisms called *Cestoda.* One important characteristic of this class is that all utilize intermediate hosts in their transmission cycle. Intermediate hosts can include rodents, fleas, and other insects, rabbits, sheep, swine, cattle, and in some instances, even humans!

Tapeworm segments containing eggs are shed in fecal material. When these eggs are accidentally or voluntarily consumed by an intermediate host, they hatch and the resulting larvae migrate into the body tissues and begin their development. Yet they won't reach their adult stage inside the tissues of this intermediate host. Instead, the life cycle is completed when this host or portions thereof are consumed by another, called the *definitive host.* Inside this new host environment, the larvae then proceed to develop into adult tapeworms, which attach to the intestinal wall, eat, and repeat the life cycle all over again.

The extent of disease caused by tapeworms depends on the type of worm involved, and if the affected individual is an intermediate or final host. As a rule, adult tapeworms living within the intestines of a definitive host are seldom life-threatening, causing varying degrees of gastroenteritis and malnutrition. Larval forms, on the other hand, tend to do more damage, simply because they migrate through the body tissues. Fur-

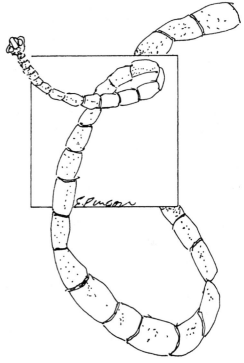

FIGURE 7.7 Tapeworms can grow to enormous lengths!

thermore, if these larvae gain entrance into the tissues of an animal (or human) that is not a normal intermediate host for that tapeworm, the results can sometimes be deadly.

By far the most prevalent species of tapeworm seen in dogs and cats is *Dipylidium caninum,* the double-pored tapeworm. It is so common because it uses the flea as an intermediate host (the dog louse can also be a carrier).

Segments from the tapeworm are passed in the feces or actually "crawl" out onto the haircoat of an infested animal. Once outside, the segments dry out and release egg baskets into the environment. Flea larvae looking for food then ingest these eggs, and a new tapeworm begins its development. If the flea happens to be ingested by a pet during chewing or self-grooming episodes, the tapeworm larvae will continue to develop into adult worms within the pet's small intestine.

Although less frequently, dogs and cats can become infected with other types of tapeworms besides *Dipylidium,* depending on potential exposure to intermediate hosts. For instance, dogs fed raw meat or garbage are at risk. *Echinococcus granulosus,* the tapeworm responsible for hydatid cyst disease, is often transmitted to dogs in this way. The hunting habits of outdoor domestic cats put them at high risk of exposure to this parasite as well.

Dogs and cats infested with adult tapeworms may or may not exhibit the typical signs associated with gastroenteritis, such as vomiting and diarrhea. Weight loss certainly can occur as the worms absorb nutrients from within the gut. Often, scooting and other signs related to anal sac discomfort might also tip off an owner as to the presence of these pesky parasites.

Diagnosis of a tapeworm infestation can be confirmed by actually seeing the white, moving, wormlike segments in fresh fecal material or on the haircoat around the hind region. Segments might also be seen on anal sac expression. If dried, the segments will take on a brownish, "ricelike" appearance.

Microscopic examination of the stool might be helpful as well; however, because the shedding of the segments is sporadic, a negative finding cannot totally rule out an infestation.

Tapeworms can be difficult pests to treat and totally eliminate. Praziquantel and epsiprantel are two effective medications used by veterinarians to eliminate tapeworms from the intestines. Other drugs are available as well. Repeating the treatment in 2 to 3 weeks helps ensure thorough elimination.

Flea control is the best way to prevent *Dipylidium caninum.* Other tapeworms, including *Echinococcus,* can be prevented by denying access to garbage and/or raw meat, and discouraging the hunting habits of felines.

Roundworms

Roundworms (Fig. 7.8), known as *ascarids* or "spool worms," are thick-bodied, whitish-to-cream-colored worms that can inhabit the small intestine of dogs and cats. This is one of the most common intestinal parasites affecting dogs and cats and young puppies and kittens. In fact, research has demonstrated that over 95 percent of all neonates are born with roundworms.

Adult worms exist unattached within the intestinal lumen and can grow up to 8 inches in length. If present in sufficient numbers, adult roundworms can cause prominent malnutrition and gastroenteritis. In some severe instances, rupture of an intestine jam-packed with roundworms has been known to happen. Immature roundworms can cause problems, too, since they might migrate throughout the lungs, liver, and other tissues of the body before settling down as adults within the intestines.

Unlike tapeworms, roundworms do not require an

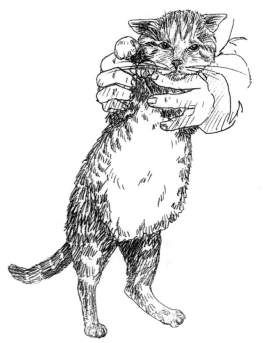

FIGURE 7.8 **A bloated abdomen in a kitten is caused by roundworms.**

intermediate host for their transmission. Each female worm sheds thousands of eggs into the environment by the way of feces. These eggs, which are covered by a thick shell, are very resistant and might remain viable in an environment for years prior to being consumed by an unsuspecting pet.

After consumption of a roundworm egg, it is possible for the hatched larvae to develop into adults without ever leaving the intestine. However, this is the exception rather than the rule. Usually the larvae penetrate the bowel wall and migrate to the liver and the lungs, maturing and growing along the way. Once inside the lungs, they can enter the airways, then be coughed up and swallowed again, allowing them to finish their development into adults within the intestines.

Alternatively, from the lungs, these larvae can enter the bloodstream and circulate throughout the body. In female dogs and cats, these larvae might settle down and become dormant within the mammary tissue until such time as lactation begins. In this way, newborns can ingest roundworm larvae through their mother's milk. But this isn't the only reason for the high incidence of roundworms in neonatal puppies and kittens. They can also be exposed to the circulating roundworm larvae via the umbilical cord while they are still in the womb, and actually be born with active infestations!

The clinical signs seen with a roundworm infestation depend on the age of the pet affected, the stage of maturity that the worms are in, and their location within the body. As a general rule, the younger the pet, the more severe the signs tend to be. In fact, some older dogs and cats can actually develop a resistance to these parasites. If adult worms are within the intestines, signs often include stomach pain with a prominent "bloated" appearance to the abdomen, vomiting, and diarrhea. In many instances, actual adult worms might be revealed within the vomitus or stool. Ruptured bowels and intestinal obstructions can result if not treated promptly.

Because of the migration through the lungs, coughing, breathing difficulties, and other signs of pneumonia might be present. In severe cases, seizures and other nervous system problems can occur.

Veterinarians can diagnose roundworms by using a microscope to look for eggs in a stool sample. Clinical signs and the pet's history are helpful in those cases where eggs might be absent from such a sample.

There are a wide variety of deworming drugs effective at removing roundworms from the intestines. You can buy relatively inexpensive dewormers at supermarkets and pet supply stores. Be sure, however, to consult a veterinarian before using one of these to be certain that it contains the correct ingredients for your pet's particular problem. Repeat deworming should be performed 3 weeks later to ensure that any migrating larvae that reached the intestines since the first deworming are killed.

Young puppies and kittens suffering from roundworm-induced pneumonia require intensive veterinary supportive care to prevent life-threatening complications from arising. Most will recover with such care.

All puppies and kittens should be dewormed for these parasites, even if parasite eggs are not seen on an initial stool exam. These dewormings should commence at 3 weeks of age, and should be repeated at 6 and 9 weeks of age. Periodic stool exams are warranted to confirm a puppy or kitten's negative status.

Good sanitation procedures will help prevent reinfections and spread to other dogs and cats. Realize, however, that once roundworms enter an environment, they are almost impossible to totally eliminate because of the hardy nature of the eggs. As a result, annual stool checks by a veterinarian are indicated to ensure that pets remain parasite-free.

Visceral larva migrans, a human disease syndrome caused by migrating roundworm larvae, does pose a serious public health threat. As a result, good personal hygiene after handling pets plus routine stool exams and treatments are a must to minimize the threat from this disease.

Most heartworm preventive medications on the market today also help prevent roundworm infestations if given on a regular basis. In those instances where environmental contamination is difficult to control, administering such a preventive year-round is one way to keep a pet free of these parasites.

Hookworms

The hookworm (*Ancylostoma, Uncinaria*) is another type of parasite that inhabits the small intestine of dogs and cats. Unlike the roundworm that floats unattached within the intestinal lumen, absorbing nutrients through its skin, the hookworm actually has teeth, which it uses to attach itself to the wall of the intestine. Once attached, it begins to suck blood from vessels within the wall. In fact, the infestation can become so severe that anemia and eventual death of the host animal could result if the hookworms are left unchecked.

Compared to roundworms, hookworms are fairly small and threadlike, measuring up to 1 inch in length. Their life cycle begins with adult worms within the gut laying eggs, which are then passed out in the stool. If environmental conditions are warm and humid enough, the eggs hatch and give rise to larvae, which then search for a host.

Once a host comes along, the larvae can gain entrance into the body in a number of ways. They can be picked up by way of the mouth, or they can actually penetrate the skin (usually the footpads) and migrate through tissue before reaching the small intestine. Like roundworms, some of these migrating larvae might decide to stop and settle for a while within the tissues, making it possible for offspring of such females to become infected while still in the womb, or through nursing infected milk. As a result, puppies and kittens can be born with these blood-sucking parasites.

The severity of clinical signs depends largely on the amount of worms present in the gut and the age of the pet infected. Generally speaking, the young suffer from more severe disease than do adults.

Lethargy, loss of appetite, and pale mucous membranes due to loss of blood are not uncommon in pets harboring a large worm burden. A dark, tarry diarrhea may be present. If skin penetration has taken place, the footpads or other areas might be reddened, bleeding, and/or infected because of the larvae. Intense itching can also be noted as a result of this penetration.

Diagnosis of a hookworm infestation is based on an examination of a stool sample for the presence of hookworm eggs.

There are a number of safe dewormers available from veterinarians that can help eliminate a hookworm infection. After the initial dose is given, a follow-up deworming should be administered 2 to 3 weeks later to kill any migrating larvae that have since reached the intestines.

In dogs and cats suffering from anemia, supportive veterinary care is needed. This might include blood transfusions if the loss of blood is severe enough. Intravenous fluids and antibiotics might also be used to combat dehydration and secondary infections. Vitamin and iron supplements, combined with a high-quality diet, are fed to provide building blocks within the body for new blood to be produced.

It is known that some dogs and cats can actually develop an immunity to hookworms after an initial infection has taken place. However, this does not preclude routine periodic stool checks by a veterinarian, since those individuals that actually develop immunity can be difficult to identify.

Hookworm eggs are not as hardy as their roundworm counterparts; hence, environmental control can be an effective way to prevent reinfection or spread to other dogs and cats. Since the eggs require optimum environmental conditions before hatching will occur, keeping fecal material picked up daily in and around the premises will reduce chances of exposure. Studies have also shown that outdoor dogs kept on concrete stand less chance of infection than do dogs housed in kennels with dirt or grassy floors. Again, this is assuming that daily removal of contaminated fecal material is performed.

Deworming female dogs and cats prior to pregnancy will help reduce the chances of puppies and kittens being born with hookworm infections. However, because deworming will not eliminate larvae within the mother's tissues and mammary glands, all neonates should be routinely dewormed for these parasites starting at 3 weeks of age.

Most heartworm preventive medications on the market today also help prevent hookworm infestations if given on a regular basis. In those instances where environmental contamination is difficult to control, administering such a preventive year-round is one way to keep a pet hookworm-free.

Some hookworm larvae have the ability to penetrate human skin, causing severe itching and dermatitis. This condition in humans is known as *cutaneous larva migrans,* or "creeping eruption." It is seen most often in tropical climates and in the southeastern portions of the United States. Since hookworm larvae thrive in warm sandy soils, this disease is one major reason why pets are denied access to most public beaches.

Whipworms (Dogs)

Trichuris vulpis, the dog whipworm, is a slender parasite that can reach 4 inches in length. Unlike tapeworms, hookworms, and round-worms, which inhabit the small intestine, whipworms colonize the large intestine, particularly the cecum (this structure corresponds to the human appendix).

The life cycle of this parasite is fairly simple. Eggs are passed in fresh feces into the environment. These eggs are then swallowed by an unsuspecting dog, and hatch within the dog's gut. From there, they set up housekeeping within the large intestine and grow to maturity, sometimes taking up to 3 months to do so. Adult females then produce more eggs, and the cycle is repeated. Note that unlike hookworms and roundworms, whipworms are not known to undergo tissue migration.

Light to moderate infections with whipworms might not give any outward hints of their presence. Sometimes dogs so affected might develop rough, unkempt haircoats and lose weight. Diarrhea might be a clinical sign. When it does occur, the stools are often blood-tinged.

Like other intestinal parasites, definitive diagnosis of a whipworm infestation is made by identifying whipworm eggs in stool under a microscope. Whipworms don't seem to be as prolific as other gut parasites; as a result, multiple samples might need to be examined before any eggs are seen.

Since whipworms are a common cause of chronic colitis in dogs, many practitioners opt to deworm for these parasites in such cases, even if eggs are not seen on a fecal exam. In those instances where whipworms are indeed to blame, the condition responds quite favorably to this empirical therapy.

Several different types of dewormers are effective at expelling whipworms. Some require only a single treatment; others need to be repeated months later.

As seen with hookworm infections, many heartworm preventive medications on the market today also help prevent whipworm infestations if given on a regular basis. In those instances where environmental contamination is difficult to control, administering such a preventive year-round might be useful.

Warbles (Cats)

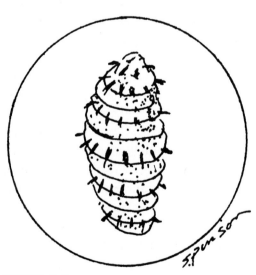

FIGURE 7.9 *Cuterebra* larva (warble).

Warbles (*Cuterebra* fly larva) are an unusual type of parasite that can be found on, or living within, the skin of cats (Fig. 7.9). They usually appear as nodules or lumps around the head or neck region. Often, these nodules are mistaken for plain abscesses, yet on close inspection inside, an actual fly larva, sometimes the size of a grape, will be visible living within a fibrous cavity.

In rare instances, depending on their location, these parasites can adversely affect the brain, leading to severe neurological signs.

Needless to say, such unwelcome guests need to be manually extracted by a veterinarian. In addition, the open cavity left over in the skin after extraction will usually require antibiotics in order for fast healing to take place.

Heartworms

Heartworms in Dogs

When we hear of parasites or worms, our natural inclination is to think of those that inhabit the gastrointestinal tract. However, there is one parasite that, instead of residing within the gut, prefers the heart. That parasite is *Dirofilaria immitis,* the canine heartworm.

Heartworm disease is a devastating disease of dogs, responsible for tens of thousands of deaths each year. Most of these deaths occur due to the destruction that these worms cause not only to the heart but the lungs, liver, and kidneys as well. In some cases, the worm burden within the heart and blood vessels might become so great that circulation of blood is actually compromised, resulting in sudden death. Other infected dogs might go years without showing any signs of heartworm disease, seemingly forming a symbiotic relationship with the parasites.

Regardless of its presentation, heartworm disease puts a tremendous burden on the body's organs and immune system. The good news is that this destructive disease is completely preventable!

Heartworm disease is transmitted through the use of a vector, the mosquito. When a mosquito feeds on a dog infected with heartworms, it picks up heartworm larvae (microfilariae) through its blood meal. Inside of the insect, the microfilariae begin to undergo primary development. Now when the mosquito gets hungry again, the larvae exit the feeding mouthpart of the mosquito and are deposited on the skin of the new host canine. From here, they gain access into the dog's tissue through the feeding port created by the mosquito, and begin a 100-day migration to the heart, growing and developing along the way.

Once they reach the heart, the worms set up housekeeping within the heart and blood vessels of the lungs and mature into sexually active adults within 2 to 3 months. Some of these can reach up to 14 inches in length! Once mature, they start reproducing and the new larvae produced are deposited into the bloodstream, just waiting to be picked up by a hungry mosquito.

Heartworm disease is found worldwide, anywhere mosquitoes are found. In North America, the southeastern and Gulf Coast regions of the United States have a greater prevalence of the disease than do other areas. However, infections have been documented as far north as Canada. The incidence of this disease seems to be higher in dogs between the ages of 4 and 7 years. Males are more likely to contract the disease than are females. Larger breeds that, as a general rule, spend more time outdoors are also more susceptible to heartworms. Of course, this does not mean that small, indoor lap dogs are safe from exposure, since they can't be totally shielded from the wayward mosquito that happens to find its way indoors. Interestingly, the length of a dog's haircoat does not figure in when determining a dog's risk of contracting heartworm disease.

Canines are the primary host of *Dirofilaria immitis*; however, other mammals can become infected, including cats and foxes. Humans have even been known to become accidental hosts for this parasite. In these instances, the larvae will migrate into the lungs, where they are sealed off by the body and subsequently cause no clinical problems. The lung lesions created, however, might be easily confused with tuberculosis or cancer, causing some consternation in physicians and in the patients so affected.

Clinical signs of heartworm disease can include exercise intolerance, coughing and breathing difficulties, or sudden death. The worms primarily reside in the right portion of the heart and in the lungs. Heartworms cause thickening of the lung's blood vessels, causing an increase in blood pressure and the workload on the heart (Fig. 7.10). Congestive heart failure is not an uncommon sequela in these individuals as the heart eventually becomes unable to compensate for such an increased workload. This in itself has a "snowball" effect, causing fluid buildup within the lungs and a disruption of blood circulation to the vital organs. Damage to the liver and kidneys is an ultimate consequence (Fig. 7.11).

Occasionally, the number of heartworms becomes so great that they can actually block the return flow of blood from other parts of the body to the heart. This condition and the resulting clinical signs are termed *caval syndrome.* Whereas the onset of clinical signs with a typical heartworm infection might be slow and gradual, the signs seen with caval syndrome occur abruptly and with fury. Dogs so affected might suddenly collapse, unable to breathe and in advanced organ failure. Actual surgical removal of the offending heartworms can be used to save the life of some of these dogs; in most, however, the disease is too far advanced to even attempt treatment.

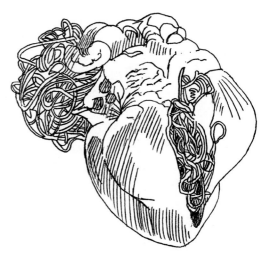

FIGURE 7.10 As one might imagine, heartworms can drastically reduce the heart's ability to pump blood effectively.

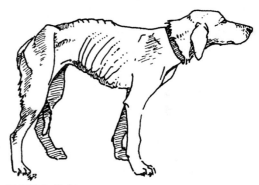

FIGURE 7.11 Dogs with advanced heartworm disease often appear emaciated.

Diagnosis of an active heartworm infestation can be made utilizing blood tests, radiographs, and/or ultrasound results. The blood tests are designed not only to detect microfilariae that may be in the blood but also to detect occult infections (infections characterized by the absence of circulating microfilariae, even though adults are present within the heart) (Fig. 7.12). These types of infections can occur in up to 50 percent of all heartworm-infected dogs. They can result from a number of factors, including the presence of immature adult worms in the heart that are not yet reproducing, infections involving worms of all the same

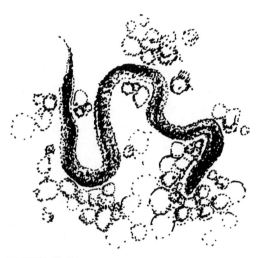

FIGURE 7.12 Larval forms of the heartworm, not adults, are found circulating in the bloodstream.

DID YOU KNOW?

Microfilariae can live for up to 2 years in a dog's bloodstream!

sex, the destruction of those microfilariae that are produced by the dog's immune system, and/or the elimination of larvae as a result of giving heartworm preventive medication to an infected dog.

Safe and successful treatment of a heartworm infection depends on prompt diagnosis in the early stages of the disease, before secondary organ damage has occurred. A special drug can be administered to a dog to kill the adult worms within the heart and lungs.

Prior to treating a dog for heartworms, a complete laboratory workup, including radiographic X rays and/or ultrasound, should be performed to determine the status of the internal organs, especially the heart, lungs, liver, and kidneys. If potential problems do exist, pretreatment with supportive medication might be needed to prepare the body for treatment. Then in a month or so, if all looks well, standard treatment is attempted.

FACT OR FICTION

Dogs kept indoors and dogs with long hair do not need to take heartworm preventive medication. **FICTION.** If you have ever been bitten by a mosquito in your house, then your pet is at risk! Also, research has yet to uncover a link between haircoat length and resistance to heartworm disease.

Because of the high potency of the drug used to treat heartworm disease, complications from the drug therapy can arise, prompting immediate cessation of the treatment series. These can include loss of appetite, vomiting, and/or the development of icterus, indicating liver inflammation. As the adult worms die, pieces of them might lodge within the blood vessels of the lungs, and if extensive, protracted coughing and lung hemorrhaging can result.

If all goes well with the treatment series, patients are usually discharged from the hospital 2 to 3 days after treatments are started to begin convalescence at home for the next 4 to 6 weeks. During this time, supportive treatments consisting of antibiotics, anti-inflammatories, and/or special diets might be prescribed.

It is of the utmost importance that a strict limitation of exercise and stress be employed during this convalescent period. In addition, preventive heartworm medication is not to be administered during this time.

Depression, loss of appetite, bleeding, and/or protracted coughing during this time should alert dog owners to potential posttreatment complications and warrant prompt veterinary attention.

Four to six weeks after treating the adult heartworms, special medication is administered to eliminate any circulating microfilariae that are present in nonoccult cases. Once this is performed, preventive medication can then be given on a routine basis. At 12 weeks posttreatment, another heartworm test should be done to be certain that the infection was

> ### Dr. P's Vet Tip
> Even if heartworm preventive medication is not required year-round in your area, you should still give it to your pet all throughout the year because most preventives sold on the market today also prevent infestations with intestinal parasites (some of which can be zoonotic, including roundworms), providing an important source of continual protection for not only your dog, but for you and your family as well.

completely eliminated by the treatment. If not, the treatment series might need to be repeated, generally 6 to 8 months after the first.

Heartworms in Cats

As frightening as it might seem, the incidence of this disease, once thought limited to canines, is on the rise in cats as well. *Dirofilaria immitis,* the same mosquitoborne organism that causes canine heartworm disease, also causes the feline disease. Most cats that become infested with heartworms develop less than 10 worms within the heart, yet even this low number can damage the heart and lead to lung and kidney disease as they do in the dog. The main reason for this is that cats produce a more potent immune response to the parasites than do dogs, which can result in greater damage to the tissues involved.

Male cats allowed to roam outdoors are at greatest risk of contracting this disease. Many cats infested with heartworms will show no clinical signs whatsoever, and the disease will be identified incidentally when these cats are brought to the veterinarian for other reasons. In more advanced cases, lethargy, breathing difficulties, coughing, vomiting, and sometimes even blindness can occur.

Special blood tests can be used to help detect heartworm disease in cats. However, because the worm burden in some cats is so low, some infections may be missed by these tests. As a result, many veterinarians base their diagnosis on chest radiographs (X rays) and ultrasound findings, which usually reveal changes in the heart and lungs characteristic of heartworm disease.

Treatment, if performed, is similar to that used for dogs. However, because of the comparatively small size of the feline heart and lungs and the intense feline immune response to these parasites, killing the adult worms contained within the heart can actually do more harm than good. As a result, cats diagnosed with this disease, yet not showing any clinical signs, are often not treated but placed on heartworm preventive instead to prevent additional infestation. Unfortunately, those cases exhibiting clinical signs of heartworm disease carry with them a poor to grave prognosis for recovery.

Because of the difficulty in safely treating heartworms in cats if they come down with the disease, cat owners should consider giving their pets preventive heartworm medication on a monthly basis. Such medication is available through veterinarians.

For information on preventing feline heartworm disease, see Chapter 4.

Coccidia

Coccidia belong to a group of microscopic parasites called *protozoans.* These organisms primarily inhabit the small intestine of affected dogs and cats. The disease caused by coccidia (coccidiosis) is rarely severe, yet the resulting diarrhea it causes can rapidly dehydrate a young puppy or kitten. Overcrowding and poor sanitation greatly contribute to the spread of these organisms within a group. Eggs passed in fecal material can be directly ingested by another pet, leading to the development and maturation of the organisms within the gut of their new hosts.

If coccidia are ingested by animals other than their normal host (e.g., if the feline *Toxoplasma* coccidia is ingested by a dog), tissue migration might occur, similar to that seen with roundworms. In most cases, this migration causes no problems, and the infection is quickly eliminated by the animal's immune system. However, if a neonate is involved, or an animal with a compromised immune system, severe disease might result.

In younger pets, diarrhea, abdominal pain, and weight loss are the most consistent clinical signs seen in an overwhelming case of coccidiosis. Older pets might not show any signs at all. If tissue migration has occurred (toxoplasmosis), other signs might be seen, including fever, muscle soreness, and convulsions.

A microscopic examination of a stool specimen will detect coccidia eggs if present. Treatment consists of administering an anticoccidia drug in proper dosages. If dehydration is present, intravenous fluids are indicated to correct the disorder.

Good sanitation practices are the best ways to prevent exposure to coccidiosis. Routine stool checks performed by a veterinarian should also be utilized to ensure that dogs and cats remain parasite-free. As a zoonotic disease, toxoplasmosis is of significance, especially in pregnant women. For more information, see Chapter 44.

Ehrlichiosis

Ehrlichiosis, also known as *canine typhus,* is caused by the bacterial organism *Ehrlichia canis.* One of many tickborne diseases, ehrlichiosis is primarily a disease of dogs, although cats can be affected in rare instances. The disease is spread from dog to dog by the bite of the brown dog tick, *Rhipicephalus sanguineus.* First reported in the United States in 1963, this disease is most prevalent in the midwestern and southern states. Left undetected, ehrlichiosis can be quite devastating and ultimately fatal to its host.

Once they gain entrance into the body, these parasitic bacteria set up housekeeping in various organ systems throughout the body within a week or two. As a result, clinical signs can be quite variable once they start to appear.

Acute signs of infection include general depression, weakness, fever, weight loss, eye and nose discharges, and swollen lymph nodes. As the disease progresses over time and the organisms colonize the bone marrow, dogs will often become anemic and immunosuppressed. As a result, secondary pneumonia is a frequent finding in infected canines. Nosebleeds and bruising of the skin might also become apparent as the body's blood clotting mechanisms are interfered with. Finally, in severe instances, the kidneys and brain might become affected, leading to kidney failure and nervous system disorders.

Noticeable drops in the total number of white blood cells, red blood cells, and platelets (structures that play a vital role in the body's blood clotting mechanism) within an obtained blood sample are usually the first parameters that tip veterinarians off to a possible infection with *Ehrlichia*. In fact, in many cases, the *Ehrlichia* organisms can be seen microscopically within the actual white blood cells themselves. Clinical signs related to a bleeding disorder or involving a high fever also provide clues leading to such a diagnosis. Specific *Ehrlichia* antibody detection tests are also available through veterinarians, and can help confirm what is already suspected.

Current treatment of ehrlichiosis in dogs employs high doses of special antibiotics until clinical signs go into remission. Owing to the organism's ability to hide within blood cells and bone marrow, ehrlichiosis is difficult to treat. The sooner treatment is instituted after the appearance of clinical signs, the better the chances are for a complete recovery.

Chronic long-term infections, however, might never clear up totally with antibiotic therapy. Drugs such as doxycycline and imidocarb dipropionate have shown some promise in many of these cases. Continuous low-dose administration of antibiotics, combined with supportive therapy, including occasional blood transfusions, might be needed to keep these long-term infections controlled.

To date, there is no vaccine available to protect against ehrlichiosis. As a result, a good tick-control program is still the best way to prevent this disease.

Lyme Disease

Lyme disease has come to the forefront in public awareness because of its ability to cause human illness. The disease, caused by the bacteria *Borrelia burgdorferi,* is spread to dogs and to humans primarily through the bite of an infected tick. The disease is fairly rare in cats. Many different species of ticks can be involved, including the deer tick, the black-legged tick, and the western black-legged tick.

Ticks, however, are not the only vehicles for spreading the disease; fleas and other biting insects are capable of spreading it as well. In addition, there have even been incidents in which Lyme disease has been transmitted via direct contact with infected body fluids. Because of this ease of transmission, Lyme disease is one of the most commonly reported tickborne diseases, and it has been diagnosed in many states across the country.

Clinical signs of Lyme disease in dogs include loss of appetite, lethargy, high fever, swollen lymph nodes and joints, and/or a sudden onset of lameness. This lameness often resolves on its own accord, only to recur weeks to months later. In untreated dogs, kidney disease and heart disease can be unfortunate sequelae.

Diagnosis of Lyme disease is based on a history of exposure to ticks and of recurring lameness. Veterinarians now have the ability to test for this disease in house.

Rapid treatment of a diagnosed case of Lyme disease is essential to prevent permanent damage to the joints or internal organs. Many different types of antibiotics can be used to treat this disease, and acute signs will usually disappear within 36 hours of instituting such therapy. Longstanding infections might not respond as well and require a more vigorous treatment approach.

A vaccine against Lyme disease is available for use in dogs living in endemic areas. Tick control is another important control measure to prevent Lyme disease. Since a tick must feed for about 24 hours before spread of the disease will take place, prompt removal of ticks will help break the transmission cycle.

The signs of this disease in humans are similar to those found in dogs. Vaccination of the family dog should help prevent it from becoming a source of human infection. In addition, prompt removal of ticks from the skin will help afford the same protection in people as in dogs.

Cytauxzoonosis (Cats)

Cytauxzoonosis is found mainly across the southeastern portion of the United States in cats allowed to roam in heavily wooded areas. Ticks are thought to transmit this protozoal organism, which attacks the host's red blood cells and causes anemia. As a result, clinical signs associated with cytauxzoonosis include those related to anemia, such as loss of appetite, lethargy, breathing difficulties, and pale mucous membranes.

Veterinarians can diagnose this disorder by observing specially stained blood smears under the microscope. Unfortunately, once a diagnosis is made, there is no known effective treatment and infected cats invariably die from the disease. Good tick control and limiting access to high-risk environmental areas are the two best ways to protect a cat from this fatal disease.

Hemobartonellosis

Hemobartonellosis is a disease seen primarily in cats, although dogs that have been splenectomized or suffer from immunosuppression can be at risk as well. This disease, which causes a profound anemia, occurs most often in young, male cats around 4 to 6 years old. Insects are thought to be the mode of transmission between these organisms and cats.

Clinical signs of hemobartonellosis include a sudden onset of depression, loss of appetite, and fever. Because of the anemia the disease causes, the gums and mucous membranes of these cats are often quite pale. The skin and whites of the eyes may appear jaundiced as well.

Diagnosis of this disease in cats can be made in a veterinary setting from the microscopic examination of fresh blood from suspected cats. Many felines suffering from hemobartonellosis also concurrently have feline leukemia. As a result, a feline leukemia test should be preformed on all cats with hemobartonellosis. Hemobartonellosis is treated with blood transfusions if the anemia caused by it is severe, and with special antibiotics and medications.

The prognosis for recovery from the anemia and associated symptoms is good if treatment is instituted quickly. Unfortunately, a total cure is rarely possible with this disease, and owners should be on the lookout for stress-induced relapses, and seek prompt treatment for their felines if they should occur.

The Immune System

Without a functioning immune system, our pets would easily fall prey to every hostile organism that came around. Immunity is designed to protect against such infectious invaders and eliminate any foreign matter or cells that somehow gain entrance into the body. Preventing the growth of cancer cells and tumors is also in its job description.

Although the immune system serves a rough and rugged function, a delicate balance does exist as far as its activity is concerned. Stress, poor nutrition, and hormone fluctuations are only some of the many factors which can deleteriously alter this activity, leading to a weakened defense system. As if this weren't enough, certain viruses, such as the canine parvovirus and the feline leukemia virus, have the ability to suppress the immune system. Such an overwhelming upset of the body's natural defense mechanisms can only lead to one outcome, and it isn't good.

This balance can be thrown the other way as well. There are certain disease conditions that can be caused by an overactive, overworking immune system. Allergies are a good example of this. Allergic reactions can even turn deadly if the response is exaggerated enough.

At other times the immune system, in carrying out its duties, will destroy or damage normal healthy tissue in the process. These autoimmune diseases usually result from the body's inability to turn off the immune response, with disastrous consequences.

Anatomy and Physiology

The immune system itself is a complex network of cells, organs, and special chemicals. No one division overshadows another; each team member relies on the others for support. In this way, they all work in unison toward a common goal.

Cells of the Immune System

Special cells, called *stem cells,* located within the bone marrow give rise to all the cells of the immune system. The cells that are produced by these stem cells are referred to as *white blood cells.* This general category comprises numerous types, each serving distinct functions.

The *neutrophil* functions to gobble up bacteria that gain entrance into the body. Also assisting in this function are white blood cells called *macrophages.* These cells usually come after the neutrophils are already engaged. In addition to bacteria, macrophages also have the capability to eat viruses, fungal organisms, and foreign matter.

When a dog or cat is vaccinated, special immune cells called *lymphocytes* are stimulated. B lymphocytes are responsible for producing actual antibodies in response to the vaccine or foreign organism; T lymphocytes don't produce antibodies per se, yet they assist the B lymphocytes in doing so, and help modulate the immune response. They also have the ability to attack and kill cells within the body that are cancerous or infected with viruses.

Both B and T lymphocytes are said to possess "memory"—that is, they remember the various organisms and invaders that they're fighting against. That way, if they show up again at a later date, they will be attacked without hesitation. Yet even with memory, this response can become slower and weaker over time if the immune system remains idle. This is why certain vaccination boosters are needed periodically.

Another important lymphocyte of the immune system is called the *natural-killer cell,* which searches for and destroys tumor cells and cells infected with viruses. Unlike their T-cell counterparts, natural-killer cells do not possess memory, yet at the same time, few of them require a previous exposure to a foreign agent to respond effectively.

Organs of the Immune System

The organs of the immune system include the bone marrow, the thymus, the spleen, and the various lymph nodes and aggregates of lymph tissue spread throughout the body.

BONE MARROW

As mentioned before, all cells of the immune system originate within the bone marrow. Many stay put and undergo maturity right where they are; other cells are shuttled off to the thymus.

THYMUS

The thymus is an organ located in the neck region of young animals. As that individual ages and the immune system undergoes a mature development, the thymus gland gradually disappears. It is in this organ that most of the T cells undergo their maturation.

LYMPH NODES AND TISSUE

From the thymus and the bone marrow, the cells of the immune system are then shipped to the front-line defenses, including the lymph nodes, tonsils, and other lymph tissue lining the gastrointestinal and respiratory tracts. This latter tissue, owing to its strategic location, provides a first line of defense against organisms that try to gain entrance into the body. B lymphocytes in this tissue produce special antibodies that coat the surface of the tract, and block such access.

Lymph nodes and tissue are responsible for filtering the body's blood and lymph for foreign agents and cells. *Lymph* is a special type of fluid that circulates throughout the body within its own separate channels or vessels, called *lymphatic vessels.* Fats that are absorbed via the intestinal tract enter into this lymphatic system, as do lymphocytes on their way to and from the front-line defenses.

THE SPLEEN

The spleen is an organ most have heard about; its various functions include filtering blood and providing a storehouse for blood cells.

Chemicals of the Immune System

Special chemicals produced by the cells of the immune system serve to assist them in their protective function. Among those chemicals generated are interferon, interleukins, and complement.

Interferon is a protein that is produced and released by cells that have been invaded by or come in contact with a virus. Released within 2 hours after the cell is invaded, it acts as a messenger to surrounding healthy cells and stimulates the immune system to respond. It even has antitumor effects, preventing tumor cell replication in some instances.

Interleukins are chemicals produced by macrophages that help control and modulate the activity of the T cells during an immune response. Interference with the release of interleukins, which can occur with many viral diseases, can lead to immunosuppression.

Complement is a special protein produced by the body that attaches itself to the surface of antibodies. When these antibodies bind to a bacterium or infected cell, the complement serves to "burn" a hole in the cell membrane, leading to the cell's destruction. In some instances, complement doesn't need the help of antibodies to fulfill this function.

Antigens

An *antigen* is defined as any substance capable of eliciting an immune response. Infectious organisms—such as bacteria, foreign matter, and even tumor cells—have antigens within their makeup and lining their outer surfaces. Since the body does not recognize such an antigen as one of its own, it mounts an immune response against it to try to eliminate it.

On initial exposure to an antigen, B lymphocytes start to divide and differentiate into their antibody-producing form. It might take up to 7 days before antibody production can be achieved. Even then, production is only moderate, and adequate levels generally last only about 3 weeks. In the meantime, however, other immune components, such as neutrophils, macrophages, and killer cells, are called in to fight off the invader.

If the invader is a tumor cell, foreign body, or an organism that lives and multiplies within body cells (such as viruses do), then the T lymphocytes start to multiply and prepare themselves for battle as well. As with the B lymphocytes, they are specific for each antigen; that is, a lymphocyte that responds to one type of antigen will not respond to any others. As a result, each different antigen that enters the body will stimulate its own group of antagonistic B and T lymphocytes.

Following this initial exposure, the lymphocytes that have been primed to the antigen retain "memory" of the experience. Sent to the front-line defenses, they simply wait for the antigen to show up again. If it ever does, the lymphocytes are ready for it, without the 7-day lag time. Antibodies are produced in high levels almost immediately, and the T cells are primed and sent into action with minimal delay.

Immunosuppression

As pointed out previously, the immune system is a complicated and delicately balanced system that performs a vital function within the body. If this balance is disrupted, serious trouble can develop.

A suppressed immune system leaves the body wide open to invasion by foreign organisms and cancer cells. This immunosuppression can occur secondarily to viral infections (such as parvovirus or distemper virus in dogs, and the feline leukemia and feline AIDs viruses in cats), drug therapy (including steroid treatments), severe stress, and disorders of the bone marrow. In addition, pets can actually inherit poorly functioning immune systems. For instance, the incidence of an underactive immune system seems to be higher in Doberman pinschers and rottweilers than in other breeds.

Allergies and Autoimmune Disease

Both allergies and autoimmune diseases are characterized by an overactive immune system that can irritate or damage its host's own tissues in response to an antigen invasion within the body. For example, atopic (allergic) dermatitis in dogs and cats results from an overactive immune response to inhaled pollens. Lupus erythematosus and pemphigus are two autoimmune disorders that, aside from causing significant skin lesions, can damage other organs of the body as well. With autoimmune hemolytic anemia, the immune system actually destroys the body's own red blood cells, leading to anemia. Myasthenia gravis, a disease characterized by profound muscle weakness after only minimal exertion, is also classified as an autoimmune disease. Immunity-mediated kidney disease and arthritis can also afflict pets stricken with a genetic predisposition for these disorders. Many cases of hypothyroidism in dogs are caused by an overactive immune system attacking and inactivating the thyroid hormone produced within the body. Finally, in cats, the classic example of an immune system gone awry is feline infectious peritonitis. In this disease, it is not the virus itself but rather the exaggerated immune response to it that actually proves fatal to the cat.

Allergies and most autoimmune reactions can be controlled with corticosteroid medication, which, at high enough dosages, has a suppressive effect on the immune system. However, because these steroids can have significant side effects, such treatments should only be performed under the close, continual supervision of a veterinarian.

The Cardiovascular and Hemolymphatic Systems

The systems responsible for the effective transmission of oxygen and/or nutrition to all organs and tissues of the body are the cardio-vascular and hemolymphatic systems. These systems are composed of the heart (Fig. 9.1) and blood vessels, located within the chest or thoracic cavity, and the vessels that carry blood and lymph throughout the body.

Anatomy and Physiology

The *heart* is a hollow organ that serves as a double pump and is located approximately in the center of the thoracic cavity. Its walls consist of muscular tissue called *myocardium.* The pumping action of the heart causes blood to flow through the circulatory system, supply-ing oxygen and nutrients to the body tissue. Inside the heart a wall of tissue separates the heart into two sections of pumps: the "right heart" and the "left heart."

Each side of the heart is made up of two hollow chambers: the upper chamber is the *atrium,* which receives blood; the lower chamber is the *ventricle,* which pumps blood from the heart. The cavities of the atrium and ventricle on each side of the heart communicate with each other, but the right chambers do not communicate directly with those

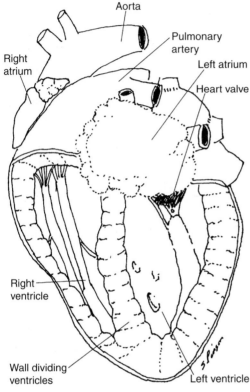

Aorta

Pulmonary artery

Right atrium

Left atrium

Heart valve

Right ventricle

Wall dividing ventricles

Left ventricle

FIGURE 9.1 **The heart.**

on the left. Thus, right and left atria and right and left ventricles are distinct.

Blood flow is directed by a series of valves that have nothing to do with the initiation of flow. The driving force for blood comes from the active contraction of cardiac muscles. The valves only prevent the blood from flowing in the opposite direction. Heart murmurs are caused by the backflow of blood through defective or diseased heart valves.

A drop of blood that is in the right atrium is first pumped through a valve into the right ventricle. The ventricle then pumps the droplet to the pulmonary arteries and lungs. In the lungs, the blood takes on oxygen and releases the waste product carbon dioxide. The oxygen-rich droplet is now ready to nourish cells of the body, but first it must return to the heart. This time the droplet enters the pulmonary veins and goes into the left atrium. The atrium pumps it through a valve into the left ventricle. The left ventricle then pumps it out to the cells, tissues, and organs of the body.

Arteries are blood vessels that carry oxygen-rich blood from the heart to the tissues. As these vessels approach their targets, they progressively branch out, creating smaller arterioles. Actual exchange of oxygen, nutrients, and waste products between the blood and the tissues occurs through microscopic, thin-walled vessels that originate from the arterioles called *capillaries*. Once this exchange has taken place, the capillary beds coalesce to form venules, which eventually empty into even larger veins. Blood is carried back to the heart via these veins.

The walls of arteries are much thicker and more elastic than those of veins primarily to compensate for the increased blood pressure within the arterial system caused by the pumping heart. Pets can suffer the same ill effects from high blood pressure as do humans. Although stress can cause the blood pressure to rise, some type of impedance to normal blood flow—such as heart failure, liver disease, and/or kidney disease—is the most common cause of its occurrence in animals.

Blood consists of a variety of cellular elements, including *erythrocytes* (red blood cells), which transport oxygen with the help of hemoglobin molecules contained within; *leukocytes* (white blood cells), which fight infections and foreign invaders; and tiny cell fragments called *platelets,* which initiate the blood clotting cascade.

Plasma is the noncellular portion of the blood. It consists of water, nutrients, waste products, and a wide variety of hormones, enzymes, and electrolytes. Plasma also contains three special plasma proteins: albumin, globulin, and fibrinogen.

Albumin is a transport protein that escorts large molecules, including some hormones, through the bloodstream. *Globulins* include antibodies formed by the immune system and certain proteins needed for normal blood clotting. *Fibrinogen* is a plasma protein also involved in the body's blood clotting scheme. *Serum* is plasma from which this clotting component has been removed.

The lymphatic system is an entirely different type of circulatory system found within the body. Lymphatic vessels that course throughout the body carry not blood, but a special substance called *lymph,* a plasmalike substance derived from fluid and protein that normally leaves the bloodstream at the capillary level to enter the tissues. Lymph components that are not used by the tissues enter the special lymphatic vessels, which carry them back into circulation. Lymph also contains fats absorbed from the small intestine.

Lymph nodes are special structures found all along the lymphatic chain that serve to filter bacteria and contaminates out of the lymph, while at the same time adding special immune cells called *lymphocytes* to the fluid for transport to the blood circulatory system. In dogs and cats, *edema,* or fluid retention within the tissues, can be caused by parasites or tumors obstructing normal lymph flow through the lymphatic vessels.

Heart Disease and Heart Failure

Heart disease, with subsequent heart failure, is one of the most frequent problems in small-animal medicine. Because the heart functions to supply oxygen and nutrients to the rest of the body via the blood, serious ramifications result if this function is interfered with by disease. In addition, the decreased movement of blood through the circulatory system caused by a faulty heart leads to high blood pressure, and fluid buildup within the abdomen and/or the lungs (congestive heart failure), depending on which side of the heart is involved. If the latter structures do become waterlogged, oxygen exchange is reduced even further.

Mitral Insufficiency and Other Valve-Related Disorders

Different diseases involving the heart valves or heart muscle can lead to heart failure. By far the most common type of heart disease seen in dogs, aside from that caused by heartworms, is *mitral insufficiency,* which involves the heart valve separating the left atrium from the left ventricle. If this valve becomes diseased and fails to close properly when it is supposed to, blood is allowed to flow back into the left atrium when the left ventricle contracts.

This has two effects: (1) The amount of blood pushed forward into circulation by each heart contraction is greatly reduced, which means that the heart (which, remember, is diseased) must work harder than it did when it was healthy to keep up with the body's demand for blood; and (2) the backup of blood that occurs as a result of the inefficient heart contraction leads to fluid buildup within the lungs, interfering with oxygen exchange between the blood and the lungs. As a result, a vicious cycle develops.

Mitral insufficiency can result from normal wear and tear associated with age, or—more importantly—it can appear secondary to other diseases, namely, periodontal disease. Bacteria from the diseased teeth and gums can enter the bloodstream and attach to the heart valve, setting up infection and inflammation. Over time, the heart valve becomes damaged and scarred, making it unable to function properly. The end result is often heart failure.

> **DID YOU KNOW?**
>
> Atherosclerosis, characterized by a buildup of fat, calcium, and cellular debris within the vessels, is not as significant a problem in pets as it is in people.

Although their frequency is much less, diseases involving the other valves in the heart can nevertheless occur. Disease of the tricuspid valve, which separates the right chambers of the heart, can occur secondary to age or infection and can interfere with the normal return of blood to the heart from the body. Defects in the pulmonic or aortic valves, which separate the ventricles from the pulmonary vessels and aorta, respectively, are usually congenital (present at birth) and might not be detectable when the dog is young. However, as the dog matures and the requirements placed on the heart increase, signs of heart disease or failure could become apparent.

Cardiomyopathy

Changes in the thickness and/or contractility of the muscles making up the heart are termed *cardiomyopathies.* The two main types of cardiomyopathies that dogs and cats can suffer from are hypertrophic cardiomyopathy and dilated cardiomyopathy.

In *hypertrophic* cardiomyopathy, the muscular heart walls become excessively thickened, shrinking the chambers of the heart and disrupting normal filling of the heart with blood. With *dilated* cardiomyopathy, the opposite occurs: The heart walls become thin and weak, making normal contractions difficult. Regardless of the type, a cardiomyopathy can lead to overt heart failure if progression occurs.

Cardiomyopathies are more prevalent in cats than they are in dogs. Middle-aged male cats seem to be affected the most. In addition, Siamese, Burmese, and Abyssinian cats appear to have a higher incidence of this disorder than do other breeds. The causes of hypertrophic cardiomyopathy in cats remain unknown; however,

> **DID YOU KNOW?**
>
> Over 75 percent of cats that develop heart disease are male!

researchers have found a link between dilated cardiomyopathy and dietary deficiencies in the amino acid taurine.

An increased lethargy and loss of appetite might be the initial signs seen in cats with cardiomyopathies. Other more advanced clinical signs can include coughing, difficulty in breathing, and overt collapse. Vomiting can also become a factor, especially if there is secondary kidney damage caused by poor blood circulation. In addition, hind-end weakness and muscular pain due to aortic thromboembolism can be seen in these cats.

These clinical signs can help lead a veterinarian to a diagnosis of cardiomyopathy in a cat. Using a stethoscope, the veterinarian can detect rapid heart rates, abnormal rhythms, and heart murmurs as well. Radiographic X rays and ultrasound show abnormal heart shapes, abnormal heart wall thickness, and, if heart failure is present, fluid buildup within the thorax in these cats.

Electrocardiograms are useful in determining the extent of any heart enlargement and to assess the electrical conduction occurring within the heart walls. If a taurine deficiency is suspected, measuring blood levels of this amino acid can prove or disprove such suspicions.

Treatment of cardiomyopathy consists of medications designed to reduce blood pressure and to increase the efficiency of heart contractions. Drugs designed to move fluids out of the lungs might also be prescribed. In cats with advanced heart failure, oxygen therapy might be necessary. Obviously, for those cats with taurine-deficiency cardiomyopathy, taurine supplementation should also be used to normalize cardiac function.

Unfortunately, little can be done to reverse the anatomic changes to the heart seen in most cardiomyopathies. With supportive treatment, however, the quality of life of affected felines can be maintained at a good level for months, even years.

Birth Defects

Birth defects involving the heart wall (septal defects), the heart valves (valvular stenosis), or the vessels leaving the heart (patent ductus arteriosus) can increase the workload placed on the heart and can lead to heart failure as the affected pet gets older. If detected early enough, many of these defects can be surgically corrected at a young age, before associated signs become severe. In those that cannot be repaired, treatment is similar to that of other forms of heart disease.

Symptoms of a Failing Heart

Regardless of the inciting cause, the clinical signs associated with a failing heart include coughing (especially at night and after exercise), breathing difficulties, distended abdomen, weight loss, and exercise intolerance. Suffering pets might stand with their front legs spread wide apart and their necks lowered and extended to afford the passage of more air into the lungs. Affected dogs and cats might collapse even after the slightest exertion or excitement.

If the right side of the heart is involved, owners might notice a bulging abdomen. This occurs secondarily to a backup of blood within the abdominal vessels, leading to a fluid buildup within the abdominal cavity.

All of these signs might start off subtly, yet they usually progressively worsen as the disease progresses and failure begins.

Diagnosis

Diagnosis of heart disease or heart failure is made using clinical signs, radiographs, ultrasound, and/or electrocardiogram findings. In addition to the classic clinical signs listed above, many forms of heart disease are accompanied by heart murmurs, which can be detected by a veterinarian on listening to the chest using a stethoscope (Fig. 9.2).

A *heart murmur* is an irregular sound caused by the disruption of normal blood flow within the heart. By far the majority of heart murmurs heard are caused by diseases of the heart valves and the abnormal blood flow through these valves that results. Still other murmurs can originate from the defects in the heart muscle or vessels that alter normal blood flow. Unusually forceful and rapid heart contractions, such as those seen within overly excited animals or in pets suffering from anemia, can even lead to an irregular heart sound. Interestingly, murmurs are not commonly detected in dogs suffering from heartworm disease, even when their hearts are full of the parasites.

Heart murmurs are usually classified according to their intensity as heard through a stethoscope. A trained veterinarian can identify which portion of the heart is affected and arrive at a diagnosis just by

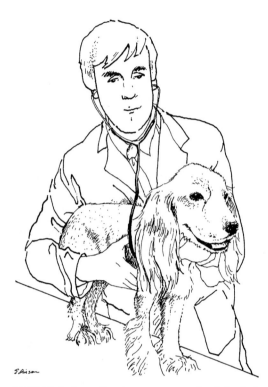

FIGURE 9.2 Heart murmurs can be detected by your veterinarian using a stethoscope.

pinpointing the area on the chest where the murmur is the loudest, and by determining when the murmur occurs, whether it is during the heart's contraction phase, relaxation phase, or both.

OTHER DIAGNOSTIC TESTS

One parameter that cannot be determined from the intensity of a heart murmur is the stage of heart disease or failure the animal is in. For instance, severe mitral insufficiency might not be associated with any murmur whatsoever, whereas a loud one might accompany an early case. This is because in the later stages, the valve might become so diseased and worn that it offers so little resistance to blood flow back through it that a murmur-causing disruption of blood flow might not arise.

Radiographs and/or ultrasonography of the chest are essential for establishing a diagnosis of heart disease. Animals with primary lung disease, including pneumonia, can exhibit clinical signs very similar to those seen in patients with heart failure, and these tests are needed to differentiate the two. Diseased hearts will appear abnormally enlarged on both tests. This enlargement can occur in compensation for the heart having to work harder to pump blood, or it could be due to a thinning and bulging of the heart wall resulting from constant bombardment with high-pressure streams of blood escaping through faulty heart valves. Regardless of the cause, an enlarged heart, combined with clinical signs or murmurs, signifies heart disease. If such a combination exists, the next test most practitioners will perform is an electrocardiogram.

The electrocardiogram (ECG; often phonetically pronounced EKG) is a test used widely to assess the condition of the heart (Fig. 9.3). Remember that a heartbeat is produced when a wave of electrical energy moves through the tissues of the chambers, starting in the atria and moving down to the ventricles. This electrical wave then makes the muscle wall of these chambers contract, pumping out the blood contained within. The ECG helps evaluate the status of this electrical conduction system, and at the same time, can give the veterinarian useful information regarding the size of the heart itself, and indirectly, the condition of the heart as a pump. In addition, with the information gained from an ECG, proper drug treatment dosages can be more easily established.

Treatment

Because most cases of heart disease or failure are nonreversible, the treatment goal for any dog or cat suffering from such a condition is to create an environment that relieves some of the workload on the heart and slows the progression of the disease.

Canines and felines with bad hearts need to be fed special diets that are moderately restricted in sodium to help reduce blood pressure and discourage the accumulation of fluid within the lungs and/or the abdomen. Diets formulated especially for this purpose are available from veterinarians.

Diuretic drugs are also used in heart failure patients to help mobilize and eliminate excessive fluid that might be accumulating within the body. In many instances, this diuretic therapy, combined with a low-sodium diet, might be all that it takes to relieve the coughing and discomfort seen in affected pets. Remember that a dog or cat on diuretic medication will drink lots of water and urinate with greater frequency, so be sure to provide it with plenty of water to drink at all times, and be prepared for plenty of walks outside or frequent trips to the litterbox.

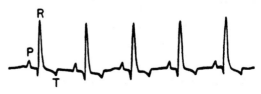

FIGURE 9.3   An electrocardiogram (ECG) measures electrical conduction within the heart.

Medications designed to dilate the blood vessels, making it easier for the diseased heart to pump blood through them, are usually the next in line if the special diet and diuretics don't seem to be enough to correct the problem.

If none of the treatment regimens described above prove effective, the final medicating step often taken to manage the heart failure is to give drugs designed to help slow and strengthen the heart's contraction. Such medications can have many undesirable and serious side effects if a veterinarian does not carefully monitor therapy, but, on average, they will prolong the life of a pet in heart failure for an average of 4 to 6 months.

Arterial Thromboembolism (Cats)

Cats afflicted with cardiomyopathy suffer from impaired circulation, which in turn can lead to a condition known as *arterial thromboembolism*. This disorder is characterized by large blood clots that form within the left side of the heart and pass into circulation, only to lodge within one or more blood vessels within the body, usually at the point where the large aorta divides into two smaller arteries that supply the hindlimbs.

When such a clot restricts blood flow to the back legs, pronounced hindlimb weakness results. The hind paws might feel cold to the touch, and the clear nails might take on a bluish hue. As the muscles of the hind end are deprived of blood and oxygen, they become firm and painful to the touch.

Diagnosis of arterial thromboembolism is based on clinical signs and physical exam findings. Ultrasound can be used to assess the condition of the heart and to identify thrombi still within the organ. A total absence or partial reduction in hind limb pulse is diagnostic of a thromboembolism as well (Fig. 9.4).

Treatment for arterial thromboembolism is difficult at best. Surgery is usually unrewarding, and the existing heart disease in these cats makes them high anesthesia risks. Medical therapy can be somewhat effective if instituted within a few hours of onset. This involves administering drugs designed to dissolve the blood clot, prevent further thrombi from developing, and restore normal blood flow.

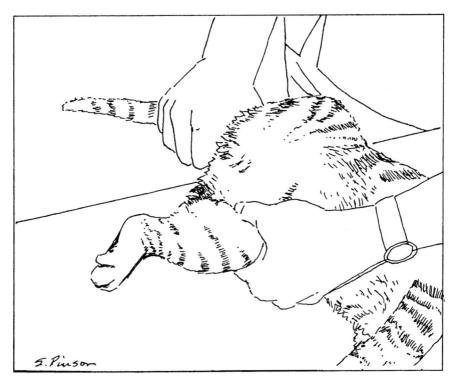

FIGURE 9.4 Cats with thromboemboli often lack a pulse in the hindlimbs.

Prognosis for a full recovery is guarded, simply because of the preexisting heart disease and because of chronic pain and tissue damage caused by the temporary loss of oxygen. However, with physical therapy and attentive nursing care, many cats experience at least partial functional restoration in 1 or 2 months. Obviously, management of the preexisting cardiomyopathy is necessary as well.

Anemia

Anemia is defined as an overall reduction in the number of red blood cells within the bloodstream relative to normal levels within that pet. This reduction can occur from a number of processes, including an increased destruction or decreased production of red blood cells within the body. The overall consequence of anemia is the inability of the blood to supply desired levels of oxygen to the tissues.

Signs seen in an anemic pet include intense lethargy, weakness, increased respiratory and heart rates, and a pallor of the mucous membranes. Depending upon the cause of the anemia, signs related to a blood clotting disorder might be seen as well. Finally, if red blood cells are being destroyed within the body, the skin and mucous membranes might become jaundiced.

A simple blood test performed by a veterinarian can tell you if your dog or cat is anemic. Treatment of anemia depends on the underlying cause. In severe cases, blood transfusions and oxygen therapy might be required to save the pet's life until the cause can be identified and treated. Therapy utilizing special compounds called *colloids* and other oxygen-carrying solutions can be lifesaving as well.

Bleeding Disorders

Whenever an injury or illness compromises a blood vessel and leads to bleeding out of that vessel, a remarkable mechanism or chain reaction begins within the body in an effort to stop the leakage of blood from the damaged vessel and prevent the individual from bleeding to death. This mechanism is known as *hemostasis.*

When a blood vessel is compromised, the first reaction that occurs is constriction of the vessel to help slow blood loss. Following this, special blood cells called *platelets* begin to adhere to the injured vessel wall, forming a temporary plug. At the same time, a coagulation (clotting) pathway is activated within the body, involving a complex interaction of blood and tissue components, as well as calcium and vitamin K. The end result of this pathway is the formation of a more permanent clot at the site of injury.

DID YOU KNOW?

Liver disease can lead to bleeding disorders because many of the components needed for proper blood clotting are manufactured in that organ.

Bleeding disorders can occur whenever any part of the clotting mechanism is interfered with. Diseases or substances such as toxins, drugs, cancers, autoimmune hemolytic anemia, and infectious agents, such as *Ehrlichia canis,* can interfere with platelet numbers or function. In addition, kidney disease and certain inherited defects can also lead to poor platelet function and secondary bleeding.

Any disruptions of the coagulation pathway also spell trouble for hemostasis. For instance, most rodent poisons contain substances that interfere with the vitamin K component of the coagulation pathway. If a dog or cat accidentally ingests these, its coagulation pathway will be effectively disrupted. Also, inherited defects in the coagulation pathway can cause bleeding disorders known as *hemophilia* and *von Willebrand's disease.*

Serious diseases or injuries such as heartworm disease, viral diseases, and massive trauma (such as that caused by a car) can lead to a secondary condition known as *disseminated intravascular coagulation* (DIC). In DIC, tiny blood clots form throughout the body. Not only are these clots detrimental to the health of the animal, but DIC also leads to a depletion of the body's clotting components. This, in turn, predisposes the pet to a bleeding disorder. DIC is invariably fatal to a pet unless rapid supportive treatment is instituted.

Clinical signs of a bleeding disorder usually include noticeable bruising of the skin and mucous membranes. Blood in the urine or feces, nosebleeds, joint pain, abdominal pain, and breathing difficulties might be seen as well. Because of the variety of potential causes, a veterinarian will need to run a series of tests to determine the exact cause and to formulate a proper treatment regimen.

Initial treatment for any bleeding disorder entails blood transfusions until the exact cause is discerned. If rodenticide poisoning is suspected, vitamin K injections, followed by oral vitamin K tablets, will help reverse the effects of certain rodenticides. These tablets should be given daily for a minimum of 4 weeks, since the ingested poison could linger within the body and exert its effects for this length of time.

Finally, for autoimmune clotting defects, steroid therapy can be used to help control the disease and subsequent bleeding.

The Respiratory System

The respiratory system works in conjunction with the circulatory system to provide oxygen to and to remove carbon dioxide from the body tissues. Oxygen is the driving force behind all chemical reactions that occur internally. Obviously, life could not exist without it. As a result, the function of all body systems, including the respiratory system itself, depends first on the ability of this system to deliver its product. In addition to this vital function, the respiratory system also serves as a means of thermoregulation, or body heat exchange, in the dog. Since dogs can't sweat in the conventional way, they rely on heat transfer out of the body through exhaled air. Hence, dogs pant when they get hot.

Anatomy and Physiology

The respiratory system begins with the mouth and nose, which, under the influence of the breathing mechanism, facilitate the passage of air into the trachea. The wall of this cylindrical structure is lined with rings of tough cartilage which prevent it from collapsing during normal breathing activity. The

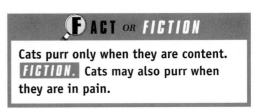

FACT OR **FICTION**

Cats purr only when they are content. **FICTION.** Cats may also purr when they are in pain.

trachea enters the thorax, or chest cavity, and eventually branches into bronchi and smaller bronchioles within the lungs themselves. Thin membranes called *pleura* line the lungs and inner wall of the thorax. *Pleuritis* is the term used to describe inflammation of these membranes, which can make normal respiration difficult and painful.

The smallest unit of the respiratory system is the *alveolus,* located at the terminus of the bronchioles. It is within these alveoli that gas exchange occurs between the lungs and the circulatory system. *Surfactant* (surface-active agent) is a special substance found lining the insides of normal alveoli. It is responsible for preventing alveolar collapse during the breathing cycle.

The major blood supply to the lungs and alveoli comes from the pulmonary artery originating from the right ventricle of the heart. In dogs and cats, heartworms reside in the right side of the heart and can effectively clog this artery and its branches supplying the lungs. The resulting disruption of blood flow and increase in pulmonary blood pressure can have devastating consequences on respiratory function.

The only air within the thorax, or chest cavity, is contained within the lungs. As a result, a negative pressure system exists that facilitates normal breathing. Intake or inspiration of air occurs as the diaphragm, the large muscular band separating the thorax from the abdominal cavity, flattens and lowers itself, and the ribcage expands. The resulting negative pressure caused by the increased thoracic size actively draws air through the trachea and into the lungs. On exhalation, or expiration, the diaphragm and ribcage are returned to their normal size, forcing air out of the lungs. Pneumothorax is a life-threatening condition in which air is allowed into the thoracic cavity, either through a penetrating wound through the skin and ribcage or through a tear in the lung tissue. Either way, the loss of negative pressure within the thorax quickly collapses the lungs, and renders the normal breathing mechanisms inoperable.

Because of its direct exposure to a hostile environment, the respiratory system contains several defense mechanisms to help keep foreign invaders and particulate matter out of the lungs. The sticky substance called *mucus,* produced by cells lining the trachea and bronchi, serves to trap contaminants and foreign debris that might gain external access to the respiratory system.

In addition, tiny, movable, fingerlike projections called *cilia* line the surface of airways and function to mechanically maneuver trapped contaminants in a direction away from the lungs. Any significant buildup of respiratory mucus or irritation to the respiratory lining results in a cough, and (hopefully) the forceful expulsion of any offending substance.

The airways are also lined with surface antibodies that provide a first line of defense against infectious organisms. In dogs, intranasal vaccines against the disease canine cough are designed to stimulate such antibody production. In an unprotected dog, infecting canine cough organisms can destroy the lining of the trachea, predisposing the unfortunate victim to all kinds of secondary infections and to a life of continual coughing.

Rhinitis

Inflammation involving the nasal passages of dogs and cats is termed *rhinitis.* The hallmark clinical signs seen with a case of rhinitis include sneezing and nasal discharge. Causes of rhinitis include bacterial infections, nasal tumors, trauma, and foreign bodies. In addition, the fungal organism *Aspergillus fumigatus* can invade the bones and tissues constituting the nasal passages in dogs and cats, resulting in rhinitis. The fungal organism *Cryptococcus neoformans* infects cats in the same way. The nasal discharges associated with fungal disease, which are usually green and thick in nature, might persist for months at a time. In addition, ulceration involving the outer surface of the nose is sometimes seen. Aspergillosis can occur primarily on its own or secondarily to other conditions that might compromise the immune system.

Nasal Foreign Bodies

Occasionally, foreign bodies can gain entrance into the nasal passageways of dogs and cats via the mouth, causing extreme irritation and rhinitis or sinusitis. The chief culprits in this category seem to be blades of grass, which is not unusual since many dogs and cats love to chew on vegetation.

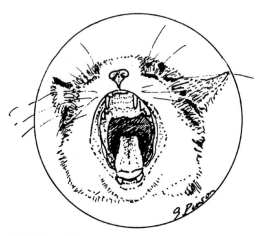

FIGURE 10.1 A veterinary inspection of the mouth and nasal passages may be needed to detect an elusive foreign body in those areas.

Pets with nasal foreign bodies will sneeze and usually have a cloudy or bloody discharge coming from one or both nostrils. Veterinary inspection of the back of the mouth and inner entrances into the nasal passages while the pet is sedated or anesthetized is often enough to identify and extract the culprit. If not, surgery might be required to remove it and to prevent secondary complications associated with bacterial infections (Fig. 10.1).

Nasopharyngeal Polyps (Cats)

Nasopharyngeal polyps are benign, pendulous masses that are associated with chronic ear infections in cats. These polyps normally arise within the throat region and extend into the latter part of the nasal cavity. They may grow to significant sizes and actually interfere with the normal flow of air into the trachea and respiratory airways, causing breathing difficulties.

Clinical signs associated with nasopharyngeal polyps in cats include noisy breathing sounds, sneezing, nasal discharge, and swallowing difficulties. If the polyps arising from the ear canal are large enough, vestibular signs including head tilting, head shaking, incoordination, and falling may also be associated with this condition.

Diagnosis of nasopharyngeal polyps can usually be definitively made on visual examination of the oral cavity of cats suspected of having this disease. Treatment involves surgical removal of the polyps. However, such a procedure is not without its potential complications. Because of the number of nerve fibers that course through the middle ear canal, surgical removal of polyps can lead to localized nerve damage. Such damage can lead to side effects such as paralysis of the muscles of the face and excessive drooling.

Tracheobronchitis (Dogs)

Inflammation occurring within the trachea and bronchi of the respiratory tree is properly termed *tracheobronchitis.* In dogs, the leading cause of tracheobronchitis is canine cough. Other causes can include allergies, foreign bodies, and chemical or gaseous irritants.

Incessant coughing is the hallmark sign of tracheobronchitis. A dry, hacking cough is seen in cases of canine cough, whereas in other cases, such as chemical irritation, the cough might be moist and productive. Treatment of tracheobronchitis depends on the underlying cause.

Collapsed Trachea (Dogs)

Collapsed trachea is a respiratory disease primarily seen in the smaller, toy breeds of dogs, such a toy poodles and Yorkshire terriers. It can occur in dogs of any age, but most cases are seen in dogs over 6 years of age.

A weakening of the muscles that interconnect the band of cartilaginous rings that normally support the trachea causes the syndrome. The end result of this malformation is that instead of the trachea maintaining its normal round shape during respiratory activity, it collapses or flattens out (Fig. 10.2). Depending on which section of the trachea is involved, this collapse might occur on either inspiration or expiration. In some cases, it might be so severe as to become life-threatening.

Obviously, such a situation leads to noticeable

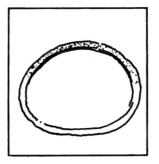
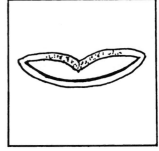

FIGURE 10.2 Top left: diameter of a normal trachea. Bottom right: reduced diameter caused by collapsing trachea.

respiratory distress in affected individuals. In addition, dogs suffering from a collapsing trachea can have a dry, harsh cough with a characteristic "goose honk" sound to it.

Diagnosis is assisted by the type of breed involved and the type of cough heard. Radiographs taken of the trachea are usually diagnostic and will help differentiate this disorder from other diseases of the airways, including tracheitis, bronchitis, and pneumonia. Actual examination of the affected portion of the trachea with an endoscope can be used to help determine the extent and severity of the problem.

Mild cases of collapsing trachea can often be managed through medical means. If an affected dog is overweight, a weight-loss program is a good place to start. Cough suppressants and drugs designed to dilate the airways can help relieve the symptoms. Overexertion and excitement should be discouraged, since the increased respiratory rate resulting from such activities can exacerbate the condition.

Depending on the location of the collapse, surgical correction might afford a more permanent solution to the problem. This involves the implantation of special artificial support rings around the circumference of the trachea for additional support. The postoperative complications associated with such a procedure are usually minimal.

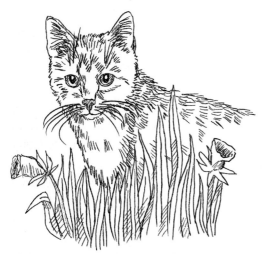

FIGURE 10.3 Pollen and other foreign substances in the air can trigger an attack of feline asthma.

Feline Asthma

Cats can suffer from asthma attacks very similar to those seen in people. They are usually triggered by an allergic reaction to pollens and other allergens that are breathed into the lungs (Fig. 10.3). The reaction caused by the immune system's response can be minor, or it can be quite severe, causing bronchitis and pneumonitis (inflammation of the lungs). This, in turn, can lead to severe breathing difficulties, coughing, and gagging in affected felines. Any cat can suffer from feline asthma, regardless of age.

Along with a good history of occurrence and clinical signs seen, diagnosis of feline asthma is aided by radiographic X rays of the lungs. Longstanding, recurring cases can actually exhibit scarring or fibrosis of the lung tissue.

Treatment of feline asthma involves identifying the source of the allergic reaction and using corticosteroids and other drugs to reduce the allergic response. When looking for the source, some experts recommend starting with the cat litter, especially dusty ones. Often, though, the source of the problem cannot be pinpointed, and symptomatic therapy will be needed each time a flare-up occurs.

Pleural Effusion

Pleural effusion is not really a disease entity in itself; rather, it is a sign of disease. It occurs more frequently in cats than it does in dogs. The *pleural space* is an air-filled space located in the thoracic cavity between the inner thoracic wall and the thoracic organs themselves. *Pleural effusion* is a buildup of fluid—such as blood, pus, or serum— within this pleural space. This effectively interferes with the normal functioning of the heart and lungs.

Some of the potential causes of pleural effusions include infectious diseases (bacterial and fungal infections, FIP, feline leukemia), foreign bodies within the chest, rupture of lymphatic vessels, heart disease, or cancer.

Pets afflicted with a pleural effusion must fight for every breath, often exhibiting open-mouthed breathing with their necks extended forward. In severe instances, they can collapse from lack of oxygen. Emergency treatment is a must.

If pleural effusion is present, treatment will involve drainage of the fluid from the chest. This usually entails placement of a temporary drain tube within the chest to facilitate continued drainage as it is required until the exact cause of the problem can be discerned. The nature of the fluid removed from the pleural space will usually afford the veterinarian enough information to pinpoint the exact cause of the effusion. Treatment is then directed accordingly.

Pneumonia

When inflammation strikes actual tissue within the lungs themselves, a condition of pneumonia is said to exist. *Pneumonia* doesn't necessarily mean that an infection is present; on the contrary, there are a number of noninfectious causes of pneumonia that need to be considered whenever a dog or cat is showing signs of lung disease. For instance, aspiration pneumonia can result from the accidental inhalation of a substance originally destined for the stomach. Dogs and cats suffering from seizures, persistent vomiting, or structural abnormalities, such as megaesophagus or cleft palate, are very susceptible to this type of pneumonia. Pneumonia can also result from inhalation of smoke and certain caustic chemicals. The damage caused by these noninfectious sources is often so severe that the unfortunate victims develop bacterial pneumonia as a secondary problem.

Pets suffering from pneumonia will cough incessantly and often spit up mucus and phlegm. Obvious breathing difficulties are noticed in severe cases, with a reluctance by the pet to move or exert itself. Dogs so affected might stand with their front legs spread wide apart and their necks lowered and extended to afford the passage of more air into the lungs. Fever, lethargy, and loss of appetite are also seen in patients with pneumonia.

Clinical signs combined with abnormal lung sounds detected with a stethoscope can lead a veterinarian to suspect a case of pneumonia (Fig. 10.4). Chest radiographs are needed to confirm such suspicions. If a bacterial or fungal component is thought to exist, a culture of the fluid and mucus within the respiratory tree might be performed as well. Blood work will usually show an elevated white blood cell count.

With infectious pneumonia, high doses of appropriate antibiotics and/or antifungal medications will be required to bring it under control. Drugs designed to expand the airways are helpful in improving airflow into and out of the lungs. Intravenous fluids are also useful to replace important body fluids lost in the increased respiratory secretions and to prevent existing secretions from becoming thickened as a result of dehydration. (*Note:* Medications designed to suppress coughing should not be used in most cases, since this only serves to prevent the removal of mucus and other respiratory secretions from the lungs.)

Cases of aspiration or inhalation pneumonia are treated in a similar fashion, yet these carry a much poorer prognosis. Attempts to suction the foreign material out of the lungs through the trachea are often unsuccessful. Pets that survive are often afflicted with a residual cough for the rest of their lives.

Chronic Obstructive Pulmonary Disease (COPD)

Chronic obstructive pulmonary disease (COPD) is a disorder of the lungs and respiratory tree often linked to aging. It is seen primarily in dogs. COPD is actually a catch-all phrase for all those conditions that affect and restrict normal air move-

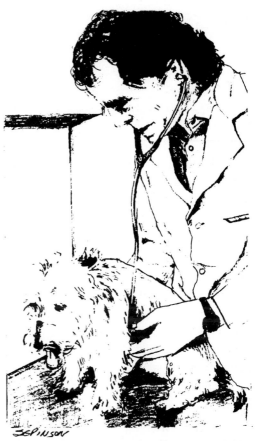

FIGURE 10.4 The lungs sound harsh in dogs suffering from pneumonia.

ment into and within the lungs. Chronic bronchitis and age-related scarring of the actual lung tissue are the two most common causes of COPD in canines.

COPD is characterized by persistent coughing, mucus buildup within the airways, and breathing difficulties. Definitive diagnosis of chronic obstructive pulmonary disease can be made by ruling out other potential causes of clinical signs (pneumonia, canine cough, etc.), evaluating the duration of the clinical signs, and obtaining biopsy samples of lung tissue to determine whether scar tissue is indeed present. Unfortunately, if diagnosed, there is no treatment presently available that can reverse the effects of COPD. However, medications designed to dilate the airway passages can provide some degree of respiratory relief to the affected pet. In addition, anti-inflammatory medications can also be utilized to reduce inflammation and slow scar tissue formation that may be contributing to the COPD.

Metastatic Lung Disease

One characteristic of most highly malignant tumors, regardless of their point of origin, is that they invariably spread to and end up in the lungs if not detected and treated soon enough. Some cancers spread, or metastasize, more readily to the lungs than others. For instance, malignant melanoma of the skin might be present in the lungs even before the actual skin tumor becomes noticeable.

The clinical signs exhibited by pets afflicted with metastatic lung disease can be similar to those seen with pneumonia. Unfortunately, the prognosis for dogs and cats harboring such tumors in their lungs is grave, even with specific cancer treatment.

The Digestive System

The digestive system of the dog and cat is made up of a collective network of organs designed to supply the body with the nutrition it needs for growth, maintenance, and repair. It also functions to rid the body of waste. Because of this, diseases involving the digestive system can have a profound effect not only on the region so afflicted but on the entire body as well.

Anatomy and Physiology

Those organs or regions of the body categorized under the digestive system include the oral cavity (teeth, tongue, salivary glands, etc.), esophagus, stomach, small intestine, large intestine, rectum, anus, pancreas, liver, and gallbladder. In order to understand diseases and their adverse effects, a brief overview of the digestive process is warranted. Keep in mind, however, that the following description is an oversimplification; the actual digestive process is so complex and involved that it warrants the devotion of an entire book in itself!

Once food enters the oral cavity, the process of digestion begins. The teeth mechanically rip, crush, and grind down the food, while the saliva secreted by the salivary glands into the mouth moistens and partially digests carbohydrate portions of the food before it is swallowed. In puppies and kittens, the eruption patterns of these teeth do not start until around 2 to 4 weeks of age. By the time the neonate is 7 weeks of age, it should have a full complement of deciduous (baby) teeth. By 7 months of age, all the permanent teeth should have fully erupted and replaced the deciduous ones.

From the oral cavity, food, water, and saliva are passed back into the esophagus with the aid of the tongue and are swallowed. The walls of the esophagus consist of bands of muscle, which contract in a rhythmic fashion, pushing the food down toward the stomach. This unique muscular action is called *peristalsis.*

From the esophagus, the food passes through a muscular sphincter into the stomach. This sphincter is very important, for it keeps stomach acids and enzymes from entering into and burning the esophageal lining. If it is defective, ulcers and that feeling humans describe as "heartburn" can result.

The stomach is lined with cells that secrete acids and special digestive enzymes, designed to further break down ingested proteins and carbohydrates (Fig. 11.1). The muscular walls of the stomach help gently churn and mix the contents, until such time as they're ready for passage into the small intestine. Again, the food must pass through another sphincter to reach the small intestine. Once the food passes through the sphincter, the stomach acids mixed in the digesta are neutralized and rendered harmless by secretions in the small intestine.

The small intestine is the site where most digestion occurs, and where the resulting nutritional building blocks are absorbed into the body. Bile produced by the liver and stored in the gallbladder is added to the digesta here to break down fats. Enzymes from the pancreas further digest fats, proteins, and carbohydrates until, finally, the nutrients can be absorbed through the intestinal lining and into the body.

The lining of the small intestine consists of millions of small, fingerlike projections called *villi,* designed to increase the absorptive surface area within the intestine. And as if this weren't enough, each of these tiny villi are lined by even tinier projections, called microvilli—again, to further increase the surface area for nutrient absorption. One reason why a parvovirus infection can be so deadly is that the virus

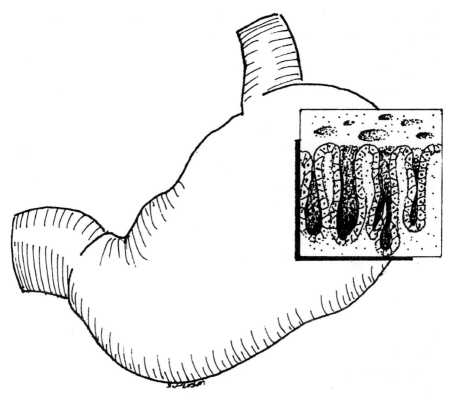

FIGURE 11.1   The stomach is lined with cells that secrete acids and special digestive enzymes.

can effectively destroy these villi lining the small intestine, blocking
absorption of nutrients and "starving" the victim.

As digested nutrients are absorbed, they enter into either the circulatory system or into the lymphatic system. End products of protein
and carbohydrate digestion travel by way of the blood to the liver,
where any toxic by-products are promptly eliminated. Other functions
of the liver include the production of serum proteins, the storage of
vitamins and other nutrients, the destruction and removal of old red
blood cells from the bloodstream, and the secretion and excretion of
bile into the small intestine to aid in the digestive process.

Fatty acids, resulting from fat digestion, travel initially via the
lymphatic vessels and later enter into the bloodstream, where they

are broken down and absorbed into the body tissues. The lymphatic system also plays an important role in immunity.

Digesta and waste that are not absorbed from within the small intestine then pass into the large intestine, which is responsible for removing water and electrolytes from the material and lubricating it for passage out of the body through the rectum and anus.

One special portion of the large intestine is called the *cecum,* which corresponds to the human appendix. In dogs, whipworms inhabit this portion of the large intestine and exert their deleterious effects from within.

Gastrointestinal Response to Disease and Treatment

Considering what they have to go through each day, the stomach and intestines make up a remarkable organ system. In the performance of their daily nutritional functions, they must be on constant guard to protect themselves from autodigestion by digestive acids and enzymes produced and must constantly battle foreign organisms and agents that are inadvertently taken in by mouth.

When the stomach and/or intestines become acutely diseased, three major factors come into play that can quickly turn a sometimes seemingly harmless situation into a life-threatening predicament; these include pain, secondary bacterial invasion, and dehydration (Fig. 11.2).

F ACT OR *FICTION*

A dog that eats grass has an upset stomach **FICTION.** Dogs eat grass because they instinctively crave it. In the wild, when a herbivorous prey is hunted and killed, the stomach and its contents are usually the first to be eaten. The partially digested vegetation found in the stomach provides valuable nutrition for the canine predator. Unfortunately, when domestic pets try to mimic the eating habits of their wild cousins, they often vomit, since the grass has not been predigested for them. If your dog craves grass, boil some vegetables (predigest them!) and offer them as treats. You'll be a hero in its eyes.

Pain

Any inflammation and/or excessive smooth-muscle contractions occurring within the gastrointestinal system can be quite discomforting and painful. In fact, in severe cases of viral enteritis, intestinal obstructions, and intussusceptions, this pain can be so great that the patient goes into life-threatening shock. As a result, the sooner therapeutic measures are undertaken to correct the problem and stifle the pain associated with it, the less chance of complications occurring.

Secondary Bacterial Invasion

The second factor to contend with is secondary bacterial invasion. Normally, the intestines are inhabited

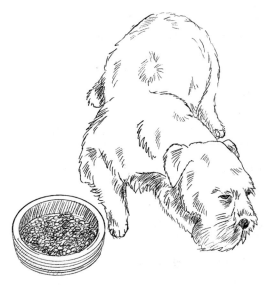

FIGURE 11.2 Pets with gastrointestinal disturbances invariably lose their appetites.

by billions of bacteria that peacefully reside there without causing any problems whatsoever. In fact, the very presence of these non-disease-causing bacteria actually helps prevent the growth of pathogenic, or disease-causing, bacteria within the intestinal setting. However, if disease strikes the small or large intestine, these "friendly" bacteria can be wiped out, allowing pathogenic ones to proliferate and cause disease themselves. If the inflammation persists, or if an intestinal perforation occurs, these and any other bacteria within the intestines can leak out of the gut and even gain entrance into the bloodstream, causing a life-threatening systemic infection and shock.

For these reasons, it is obvious that antibiotics become very important in the treatment of moderate to severe cases of gastroenteritis, even if the original cause is nonbacterial in origin.

Dehydration

The final threatening factor that arises when acute gastroenteritis strikes a pet is dehydration. Pets suffering from vomiting and/or diarrhea can

---

F ACT OR **FICTION**

Force-feeding water can help correct dehydration in a sick pet **FICTION.** Whenever a pet reaches a state of true clinical dehydration, intravenous fluids are required to correct the problem. This is especially true for dehydration caused by vomiting or diarrhea. Most fluids given orally to such animals will pass right through their diseased digestive systems without being absorbed and could actually make the dehydration worse.

---

quickly become dehydrated as a result of water loss through the bowels. Since inflamed bowels cannot regulate water absorption as they do when they are healthy, any fluid intake that indeed occurs will usually pass right out of the body via vomiting and/or diarrhea without being absorbed.

In fact, the disruption of normal motility and distension occurring within the affected bowel can actually attract and draw water right out of the body and into the intestinal lumen. As a result, pets that have become dehydrated or are on the verge of dehydration due to gastroenteritis require intravenous fluids to correct the dehydration occurring within the body's cells, at least until the gut has healed sufficiently to resume these functions once again.

Treatment

Once the gastrointestinal system is on the mend, and all vomiting has been brought under control, a good level of nutrition is required to counteract any malnutrition induced by the disease. Bland diets that are easily digested are prescribed until complete healing of the stomach and/or intestinal linings has taken place. Offering a convalescent pet some type of electrolyte replacement drinks during these first few days can also promote rapid recovery as well. Feeding plain yogurt is also helpful toward repopulating the gastrointestinal tract with non-pathogenic bacteria.

Disorders of the Teeth and Oral Cavity

Diseases and disorders affecting the teeth or oral cavity interfere with a pet's ability to prehense and process food for digestion. In addition, other general signs associated with conditions involving these areas usually include increased salivation, swallowing difficulties, bad breath, gagging, and decreased appetite.

Malocclusion

Malocclusion occurs when the teeth lining the upper jaw fail to line up and fit properly with the teeth of the lower arcade. In the normal bite, the upper canine teeth should rest just behind the lower canines. Disruption of the normal bite pattern can be caused by trauma, improper tooth eruption, and genetics.

Brachygnathism refers to a condition in dogs in which an overbite, or overshot upper jaw, exists. Conversely, *prognathism* is the term referring to the undershot jaw (underbite). Both conditions are inheritable traits, passed from one generation to another. In fact, prognathism is considered normal for certain breeds, such as pugs, boxers, and bulldogs. Although not life-threatening, these anatomic maladies can interfere with normal biting action and eating, and can predispose to dental and jaw problems in affected dogs. As a result, dogs suffering from distinct overbites or underbites (unless normal for the breed) should be surgically neutered to prevent the propagation of these undesirable traits.

Malocclusion can also result from improperly positioned deciduous teeth creating abnormal eruption pathways for the permanent ones. Dental examination of the deciduous teeth performed on puppies and kittens as early as 8 weeks of age can help identify potential problems. In many instances, simply removing the offending deciduous tooth clears the path for the proper eruption of its permanent successor.

Surgical repair or reconstruction of the jaw can be used to repair trauma-induced malocclusions, which is the most common type of malocclusion seen in cats. Orthodontic correction of brachygnathism and prognathism has been utilized in select cases, yet for ethical reasons, such procedures should be performed only for medical purposes, not for cosmetic gains.

Supernumerary Teeth

Supernumerary teeth are extra teeth within the mouth. These can be retained deciduous teeth, or can actually be permanents.

Retained deciduous teeth are commonly seen in small dog breeds, including miniature poodles and Yorkshire terriers. In these dogs, the deciduous canine teeth have the greatest propensity for remaining behind (Fig. 11.3). Such retained teeth can crowd the permanent ones, creating abnormal eruption pathways. In addition, because of their close proximity with their permanent counterparts, these extra teeth can serve as niduses for dental calculus buildup and infection. As long as the eruption pattern for the corresponding permanent tooth is not being interfered with, most veterinarians will postpone removal of the retained tooth (teeth) until another elective procedure, such as neutering or teeth cleaning, is performed. However, if the permanent tooth is being interfered with in any way, immediate removal is recommended.

In rare instances, duplicated permanent teeth, consisting of one or two isolated ones, or an entire arcade, can erupt. Removal of these permanent supernumerary teeth is seldom necessary unless they interfere with the normal biting action of the dog. Because of the genetic predisposition of this condition, affected dogs should not be bred.

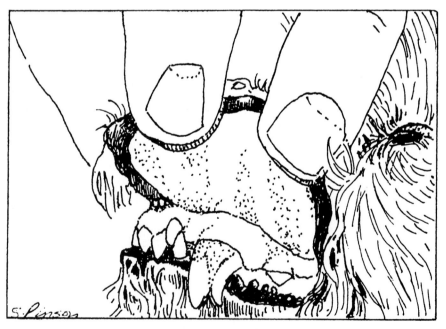

FIGURE 11.3 A retained deciduous upper canine tooth.

Enamel Hypoplasia

This unfortunate condition involves the incomplete development of the hard, protective layer of enamel that normally surrounds the crown of the tooth. Enamel hypoplasia results when the enamel-producing cells within the dental arcade, called *ameloblasts,* are injured or destroyed prior to eruption of either the deciduous or permanent teeth. The canine distemper virus is the most notable culprit causing enamel hypoplasia to occur; other causes can include severe malnutrition and fluorine toxicity.

Teeth that lack enamel have coarse textures (due to exposed dentin) and tend to stain brown. The absence of the protective enamel coating makes these teeth especially susceptible to decay and to traumatic fractures.

For puppies and kittens suffering from enamel hypoplasia on their permanent teeth, enamel restoration procedures (such as crowning) performed by a veterinary dental specialist can add a protective layer to exposed surfaces. Ask a veterinarian for more details regarding these dentistry procedures now available for pets.

Broken Teeth

Occasionally, teeth will break or fracture as a result of trauma or disease (such as in enamel hypoplasia). If the pulp cavity of the tooth is not exposed by the break, treatment measures, aside from filing down any sharp edges, are rarely required. However, if the damage does extend down into the pulp cavity, inflammation, infection, and pain could result.

Endodontic therapy, or root canals, can be performed to salvage teeth with exposed or infected pulp cavities and dentin. The procedure involves the removal of the pulp tissue and infected dentin, thereby alleviating pain and the further progression of disease within the tooth. Cracks and fractures in the tooth can then be filled, completing the restoration procedure.

Discolored Teeth

The administration of certain antibiotics to a pregnant dog or cat can result in yellow-stained dentin within the teeth of her offspring. The same holds true for adolescents administered these drugs prior to eruption of their permanent teeth. Although this staining has no effect on the health of the teeth, it can be unsightly and detrimental in the show ring.

Calculus buildup can certainly discolor teeth so affected. If allowed to persist on a long-term basis, the tooth surface can often take on a yellow hue, even after the calculus has been removed. In these instances, the complete removal of the calculus is far more important than any discoloration left behind.

As mentioned previously, a brownish discoloration to the teeth could be the result of enamel hypoplasia. Enamel restoration procedures can be employed to deal with this problem.

Finally, a bluish-gray discoloration to a tooth is indicative of inflammation within the pulp cavity, warranting endodontic management if the tooth is to be saved.

Dental Caries (Cavities)

Because of uniquely high pH of the saliva, cavities rarely form in the teeth of dogs and cats. When they do, they are often secondary to some trauma that has disrupted the continuity of the dental enamel. Cavities in pets are managed the same way as they are in people, with dental fillings.

Periodontal Disease

Periodontal disease, or tooth and gum disease, is one of the most prevalent health disorders in dogs and cats. Studies have shown that most canines show some signs of this disease by 3 years of age. Early signs can include tender, swollen gums, and, most commonly, bad breath. More importantly, though, if left untreated, periodontal disease can lead to secondary disease conditions that can seriously threaten the health of affected pets (Fig. 11.4).

It all begins with the formation of plaque on tooth surfaces. This plaque is merely a thin film of food particles and bacteria. Over time, however, plaque mineralizes and hardens to form calculus. Owners who lift up their pet's lip and glance at its teeth, especially near the gumline, might notice brownish to yellowish buildup of calculus on the outer surface of the teeth.

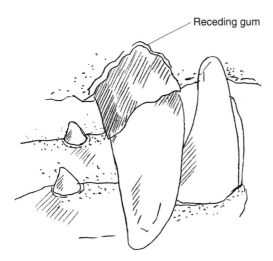

Receding gum

FIGURE 11.4 Receding gums caused by periodontal disease.

Calculus tends to accumulate worse on the outer surface of the large fourth upper premolars and on the inner surfaces of the lower incisors and premolars. This is because canine saliva is conducive to calculus formation, and the ducts from the salivary glands empty into the mouth at these particular sites. Buildup of this substance tends to be worse in smaller breeds of dogs, such as miniature poodles, Yorkshire terriers, Maltese, and schnauzers. In fact, it is not at all unusual for some of these dogs to start losing teeth by 4 to 5 years of age without at-home preventive dental care!

Along with these breed predispositions, diet can play an important role in the development of periodontal disease. For instance, moist foods high in sugar content promote plaque formation much more readily than do the dry varieties. In addition, diets containing too much phosphorus (such as all-meat rations) have been linked to periodontal disease.

Certain underlying disease conditions might also promote periodontal disease as a side effect. For example, hypothyroidism can lead to gingivitis and dental complications associated with it. Periodontal disease can also occur incidentally with tumors involving the gum tissue and/or teeth.

Pets suffering from periodontal disease can exhibit a diverse selection of clinical signs. Early periodontal disease might be marked only by a decreased appetite due to swollen, painful gums. Pet owners often complain of

DID YOU KNOW?

Both feline leukemia and feline AIDS are common causes of periodontal disease in cats.

bad breath in their pets, and might notice signs of gagging or retching as secondary tonsillitis sets in.

As the disease progresses, these signs might worsen, and other symptoms, such as gum recession, gum bleeding, and tooth loss, might arise. Infected teeth that do not fall out can form abscesses, marked by sinus infections, nasal discharges, and/or draining tracts appearing on the face.

But the damage caused by periodontal disease doesn't stop there. Bacteria can gain entrance into the bloodstream by way of the teeth and gums, seeding the body with infectious organisms. In advanced cases, these bacteria can overwhelm the host's immune system and set up housekeeping on the valves of the heart. The resulting valvular endocarditis in turn can lead to heart murmurs and eventual heart failure.

Besides the heart, the bacteria that gain access to the body because of periodontal disease can lodge in the kidney, causing infection, inflammation, and acute damage. Over time, signs related to kidney failure might develop in affected pets.

Early cases of periodontal disease can be treated by a thorough scaling and polishing of the teeth to remove the offending calculus. This scaling needs to be professionally performed under sedation or anesthesia to ensure complete removal of the calculus under the gumline.

Using special instruments to hand-scale a pet's teeth at home without anesthesia is not only dangerous but also highly ineffective at cleaning the teeth where it counts the most, up under the gumline. Furthermore, such scaling, if not followed by polishing, will leave etches in the enamel covering of the teeth that can serve as foci for future plaque and calculus buildup.

Antibiotics will also be prescribed for dogs and cats suffering from moderate to advanced periodontal disease to combat the associated bacterial infection. Teeth that are excessively loose within their sockets serve only to propagate infection, and should be extracted. For infected teeth that are still deemed viable, a root canal can be performed as a salvage procedure. See Chapter 4 for prevention tips to help protect pets against the adverse effects of periodontal disease.

Tonsillitis

The *tonsils* are lymphoid tissues located in the back of the oral cavity near the esophagus. Since they are lymphatic tissues, tonsils have an immune function. *Tonsillitis* refers to the inflammation and/or swelling of these lymphoid structures in response to infections, foreign bodies, and sometimes even noninfectious diseases. For instance, long-term coughing, such as that seen in cases of canine cough, can result in a secondary tonsillar inflammation. Periodontal disease is another common cause of tonsillar swelling. Finally, certain tumors, such as lymphosarcoma and squamous cell carcinoma, can cause the tonsils to swell and should always be kept in mind anytime an older dog or cat develops tonsillitis.

Signs of tonsillitis include gagging, retching, and difficulty swallowing. Affected animals might also go off feed and have a tendency to salivate excessively. Because tonsillitis is usually secondary in nature, other signs of illness related to the primary disease might be present as well.

Diagnosis of tonsillitis is easy when it is based on clinical signs and actual visualization of the swollen tonsils within the oral cavity. Treatment depends on the underlying cause. For example, if the disease is infectious, appropriate antimicrobial therapy will clear up the tonsillitis. If a tumor is suspected, or if a seemingly simple case of tonsillitis is refractory to standard treatment, then the tonsils should be removed and biopsied.

Cleft Palate

The *palate* is a fleshy structure located at the roof of the mouth that separates the oral cavity from the nasal passages. The firm portion located toward the front of the mouth is termed the *hard palate,* whereas the softer, flexible portion toward the back of the mouth is called the *soft palate. Cleft palate* is a disease condition in which the palate fails to fully develop, leaving a communication gap between the mouth and the nasal passages. This condition is hereditary in breeds such as English bulldogs, Boston terriers, and cocker spaniels. It can also be acquired secondary to foreign bodies puncturing the palate, or by burns caused by puppies and kittens chewing on electrical cords.

Puppies and kittens born with cleft palates often die because they are unable to suckle properly. Those that do survive initially can develop nasal infections and aspiration pneumonia if the problem is not surgically corrected in time. The recommended time of surgery for these individuals is around 6 weeks of age. Until then, daily feedings using a tube passed directly into the esophagus are indicated to prevent these secondary complications.

Feline Stomatitis

Feline stomatitis is a condition of the oral cavity in cats characterized by red, friable gums that often grow over and cover the teeth, as well as inflammation of the teeth and bony tissue of the jaw.

Cats affected with this disorder often have difficulty chewing their food, have foul-smelling breath (Fig. 11.5), salivate profusely, and might even have inflamed lips. The inflammation associated with the disease can also spread to the back of the throat, making it difficult to swallow.

The exact cause of this disorder in cats is unknown; however, conceivably any type of chronic inflammation that attracts inflammatory cells to the area could cause such a reaction. Diagnosis of feline stomatitis is made by collecting a biopsy sample of the affected tissue and radiographing the oral cavity to determine the extent of involvement. Treatment consists of surgically removing and/or cauterizing the excess gum tissue, as well as any teeth or bony tissue affected. In especially severe cases, steroid anti-inflammatory medications, antibiotics, and pain relievers may be used as well.

Owners can help slow the recurrence of this disorder by following a strict regimen of dental care for their cats, including the daily treatment of both teeth and gums with a paste, gel, or solution containing chlorhexidine.

Esophageal Disorders

Disorders involving the esophagus will manifest themselves as difficulty in swallowing. Effortless regurgitation of solid food, which must be differentiated from vomiting and its associated abdominal spasms, often tips off the pet owner and veterinary practitioner to an existing problem with the esophagus. Because of the inability to properly swallow food, dogs and cats afflicted with esophageal disease are at high risk of accidentally aspirating food into their lungs, causing serious, life-threatening pneumonia.

Megaesophagus

Megaesophagus is a condition in which a generalized enlargement of the esophagus occurs, making it unable to push food into the stomach. Seen primarily in dogs, this condition might be inherited, or seen secondary to esophageal obstructions or neuromuscular diseases such as myasthenia gravis.

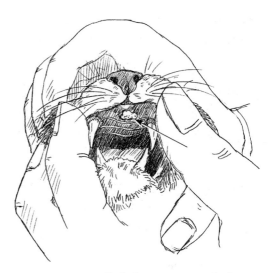

FIGURE 11.5 Oral ulcers can cause foul breath in cats.

Diagnosis of megaesophagus is made by taking radiographs of the esophagus or actually visualizing the enlargement with an endoscope inserted into the esophagus via the mouth. Those dogs diagnosed with this disorder must be fed with their front end elevated on a chair or table to encourage gravity flow of food and water into the stomach. Feeding liquid or semisolid food will also help facilitate this passage into the stomach. Depending on the cause, some individuals do improve with time. In select cases, surgery might be performed to help improve esophageal function.

Esophagitis

Inflammation occurring anywhere along the esophagus is termed *esophagitis.* Esophagitis can be instituted by foreign bodies that injure the organ's lining, by ingestion of caustic substances, and by reflux of stomach contents and acids up into the esophagus. In keeping with the latter cause, chronic, long-term vomiting can also lead to esophagitis.

Regurgitation, loss of appetite, and weight loss are the most frequent signs seen. If left untreated, damage to the lining of the esophagus could occur, causing strictures and secondary megaesophagus.

As with megaesophagus, diagnosis is made using clinical signs, physical exam findings, and endoscopic exam or radiographic X rays of the esophagus using barium as a contrast medium. Treatment of esophagitis consists of treating any primary problems that might be present, and, if stomach acid reflux is to blame, reducing the amount of stomach acid secretions and increasing the rate of stomach emptying.

Esophageal Obstructions

Obstructions can occur secondary to tumors, infections, strictures, and the ingestion of foreign objects (especially bones). As with megaesophagus, obstructions can be diagnosed using radiographs and/or endoscopy (Fig. 11.6). Treatment is aimed at surgical removal of the offending agent.

Gastric Dilatation–Volvulus Complex (Dogs)

Gastric dilatation–volvulus complex (GDV), or "bloat," is a serious, life-threatening disorder that can strike the gastrointestinal systems of dogs, particularly those of large, deep-chested breeds. Great Danes, St. Bernards, Irish setters, standard poodles, boxers, and English sheepdogs are only a few of the many breeds that can be suddenly afflicted with GDV. Although they don't fit the anatomical mold of these other breeds, dachshunds and Pekinese also have a higher incidence of GDV than do other similar-sized breeds. Regardless of the size and age, death can quickly ensue in these dogs if the condition is not recognized and treated with speed.

Rapid ingestion of a large amount of food and water, followed by exercise, is an important predisposing cause for this disorder. As the stomach dilates due to the large food and water content within, and due to the gas formed within the stomach secondary to vigorous exercise, it can rotate or

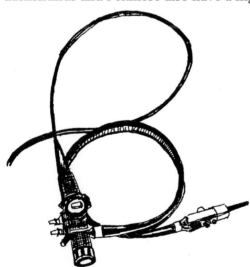

FIGURE 11.6 An endoscope is useful for retrieving foreign objects in the upper airways, esophagus, and stomach.

twist in such as way as to block off all entry into and exit from the stomach. The condition snowballs as the food, water, and gas within are not allowed to escape, and more and more gas and fluid are produced by the churning action and secretions of the distressed stomach. In addition, as the stomach dilates and/or rotates, it can effectively put pressure on the large blood vessels located within the abdomen and seriously reduce blood flow through them. This, in turn, places almost every major organ within the abdomen in serious jeopardy.

Dogs suffering from an acute case of GDV will exhibit signs such as a distended, bloated abdomen, vomiting, excessive salivation, and rapid breathing. In the early stages, the dog will be quite restless because of the pain; as the disease progresses, weakness, recumbency, and shock set in.

A diagnosis of GDV is based on history and clinical signs seen. As mentioned before, treatment must be instituted in earnest to save the life of the pet. The attending veterinarian will try to pass a tube into the stomach to relieve the stomach distension; however, if the stomach is twisted, this passage might be impossible. In these cases, immediate surgical intervention is required. Intravenous fluids, antibiotics, and steroids to combat shock are among the medications used in these patients. The prognosis is guarded with any dog presented with GDV, and recurrence is not uncommon.

If a dog likes to gulp down its food as soon as it is set down, protect it from the dangers of GDV by feeding smaller portions at more frequent intervals throughout the day. In addition, discourage exercise for at least 1 hour after mealtime. For dogs that have recurring bouts with GDV, surgery can be performed as a preventive measure to "tack" the stomach down to the inner abdominal wall, thereby preventing it from twisting if bloating occurs.

Gastrointestinal Ulcers

An ulceration within the stomach or intestines occurs when the protective barrier of mucus covering the inner surfaces of the gastrointestinal tract is lost or destroyed, allowing stomach acids and bile acids to erode the gastrointestinal lining. The same type of heartburn humans can sometimes experience with this problem can affect dogs and cats as well, leading to inappetence, vomiting, and lethargy.

Ulcers actually are indicators of disease rather than distinct disease syndromes in themselves. Sharp foreign bodies or harsh chemicals that are swallowed can scrape, injure, and—in the case of the latter—burn the gastrointestinal lining and cause a primary ulceration.

Ulcers occur secondary to stress, infectious diseases, intestinal parasites, bacteria (including *Helicobacter*), and metabolic diseases such as Cushing's disease and kidney disease. Certain drugs can also have a deleterious effect on the stomach lining when given orally.

Diagnosis of an ulcer relies heavily on clinical signs seen and the history or evidence of an underlying disorder. Radiographs taken after the oral administration of barium can be used to pinpoint the exact location of an ulcer. In addition, direct visualization of the actual stomach or intestinal lining using an endoscope is another means of diagnosing ulcers in a pet.

Obviously, when formulating any treatment regimen for ulcers, any underlying source for the ulceration must be identified and treated. Specific ulcer treatment is aimed at reducing the amount of stomach acid secretion and providing a protective coating over the existing ulcer until it has time to heal. Medications used to treat ulcers in humans are very effective at treating the same in pets.

Hairballs (Cats)

The accumulation of hair within the stomach is the most common cause of vomiting in cats. Because of their self-grooming habits and the roughened nature of their tongues, cats are prone to hairballs. Incidence of this problem increases during the spring and fall months because of increased shedding (Fig. 11.7).

When the hair is swallowed, it can coalesce into a ball within the stomach and act as a gastric foreign body, irritating the stomach lining. Vomiting, often right after eating, and gagging are usually the result when this happens; coughing might also be noticed. Aside from these signs, those cats affected seem otherwise clinically normal.

DID YOU KNOW?

Shorthaired cats can develop hairballs just as readily as their longhaired peers.

Diagnosis of hairballs is based on clinical signs (and the absence of other clinical signs) and physical examination. If the vomiting is continuous or severe, radiographs of the stomach or direct endoscopic examination might be required to rule out other gastric foreign bodies common to cats, such as cloth, strings, and plastic wrap.

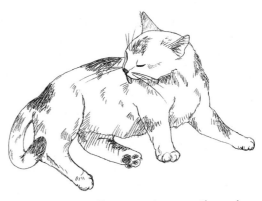

FIGURE 11.7 Because cats groom themselves so efficiently, they are highly prone to hairball formation.

Another way to make a diagnosis of hairballs is to monitor response to treatment. There are numerous "cat laxatives" on the market that can be given to a cat suspected of harboring hairballs. These agents, most of which are merely flavored petroleum jelly, act to lubricate the hairball and facilitate its passage out of the stomach and into the stool. Once this occurs, the clinical signs seen should abate. In severe instances, surgical removal of a prominent hairball might even be required to afford a cure.

Pet owners can do their part to prevent hairballs in their cats. Giving a laxative in a preventive manner once or twice weekly should help keep things moving smoothly through the gastrointestinal tract. One word of caution: Mineral oil should never be used as a hairball laxative, primarily because this substance can be easily aspirated into the lungs. In addition to giving hairball laxative periodically, brushing a cat's haircoat on a daily basis will help reduce the amount of hair available for ingestion.

Hemorrhagic Gastroenteritis (Dogs)

Hemorrhagic gastroenteritis is a life-threatening condition that can be rapidly fatal if not treated promptly. Characterized by an explosive onset of bloody diarrhea, hemorrhagic gastroenteritis can quickly cause dehydration, depression, shock, and toxemia in affected dogs. It is most often seen with dietary indiscretions and/or bouts of pancreatitis. Toxins produced by bacteria within an irritated gut cause such extensive inflammation that overt bleeding within the digestive system results. Toxins and bacteria may then permeate these blood vessels and gain entrance into the body, with serious consequences.

Diagnosis of hemorrhagic gastroenteritis is based on history and clinical signs seen, as well as ruling out other causes of digestive system disturbances. Treatment consists of intravenous fluids to control dehydration, high levels of antibiotics to combat infection, and high dosages of steroid anti-inflammatories and other medications to control shock and to counteract the effects of toxemia.

Intussusception

An *intussusception* is a life-threatening condition involving an abnormal invagination of a portion of a dog or cat's small or large intestine into a dilated portion of bowel situated just ahead of it, causing obstruction to normal flow within the intestine (Fig. 11.8). Peristalsis involving the affected gut segments further aggravates the intussusception, making it worse with time. In especially severe instances, the blood supply to the portion of the intestine involved will be cut off, resulting in the death of that tissue and serious health problems. The site at which an intussusception is most likely to occur in dogs is where the small intestine links up with the large intestine.

The causes of an intussusception can include any type of inflammation within the gut, viral infections,

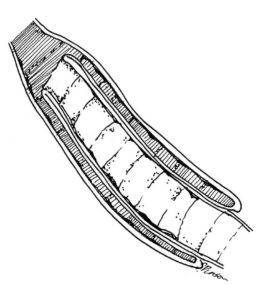

FIGURE 11.8 An intussusception occurs when a portion of the bowel folds over and invaginates on itself.

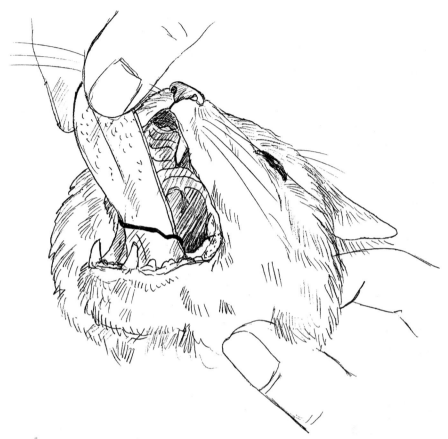

FIGURE 11.9   String foreign bodies commonly become lodged under the tongue.

parasites, tumors, and swallowed foreign objects. Strings (Fig. 11.9) and other linear foreign bodies are often the underlying causes of intussusceptions in cats. Signs seen in pets affected include lethargy, abdominal pain, fever, and vomiting.

Radiographs are the most useful tools in the diagnosis of an intussusception, since it has its own characteristic appearance on a radiograph. If intussusception is suspected or diagnosed, immediate surgery is necessary to correct the invagination and to remove any dead portions of bowel that might be present. Obviously, the underlying problem that initially caused the intussusception must be corrected as well.

Intestinal Obstructions

In addition to intussusception, other items can obstruct normal flow through the gut and result in clinical signs, such as lethargy, vomiting, and black, tarry stools, and abnormal posture (Fig. 11.10). Swallowed foreign bodies (such as bones, rubber balls, and stones), tumors, fungal infections, and herniations are all capable of causing either partial or complete obstructions if large or extensive enough. Unless the obstruction is relieved in a timely fashion, usually through surgical means, loss of blood supply to the affected portion can occur, resulting in the death of that portion of bowel, systemic infection, and shock.

Inflammatory Bowel Disease (IBD)

Inflammatory bowel disease (IBD) is actually a group of chronic digestive disorders characterized by the infiltration of the walls of the bowels with inflammatory cells, leading to abnormal wall thickening and irregularities. IBD has been recognized as a significant cause of chronic vomiting and/or diarrhea in both dogs and cats. As far as the etiology of IBD, research to date has failed to uncover an exact cause. Many veterinarians believe that bacterial and/or dietary proteins may stimulate an autoimmune type of reaction in these pets. This reaction, in turn, manifests as a buildup of immune cells on and within the surfaces coming in contact with these proteins.

The classic clinical sign associated with IBD in cats is chronic vomiting. Often misdiagnosed as hairballs, vomiting induced by IBD usually occurs intermittently over months to years, gradually worsening and increasing in frequency with time. In addition to

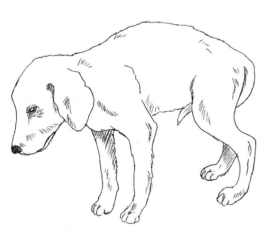

FIGURE 11.10 Characteristic "hunched up" appearance of a dog with an intestinal obstruction.

vomiting, bloody diarrhea and abdominal pain are also clinical signs seen in both dogs and cats suffering from IBD. In cats, lymphosarcoma is not an uncommon sequela to severe cases of IBD that cannot be controlled through medical means.

Diagnosis of IBD is made through the use of a thorough history, physical exam findings, radiographs of the abdomen, and more specifically, biopsy samples from affected portions of bowel. Diagnostic techniques such as these will help differentiate this condition from other disorders that may cause similar clinical signs, including foreign bodies, pancreatitis, tumors, and bowel obstruction.

Treatment for inflammatory bowel disease employs the use of drugs designed to reduce the inflammatory response, as well as medications designed to locally suppress the immune system response within the gut. Administration of these medications may be required on a long-term basis to control this disorder. Since food allergies are thought to be an underlying cause in some instances, most treatment regimens for IBD also employ rations that are hypoallergenic in nature.

Unfortunately, a complete cure for IBD is rarely possible. However, with appropriate treatment, most cases can be managed enough to allow the affected pet to live a relatively normal life otherwise.

Colitis

Problems involving the large intestine of dogs and cats are common in veterinary medicine. *Colitis* refers to the inflammation of the lining of the large intestine, resulting in diarrhea, with the feces often containing an abundance of red blood and mucus. *Tenesmus,* or straining to defecate, is another prevalent sign that is often mistaken for constipation.

Acute colitis refers to a sudden onset of signs that usually lasts only a short period of time with proper treatment. Chronic colitis

DID YOU KNOW?

If bright red blood appears in the stool, it has originated from somewhere along the large intestine. On the contrary, when bleeding originates within the small intestine, the blood that is passed in the stool is often partially digested, giving the stool a black, tarry appearance.

is a long-term, recurring condition that might last for the entire life-time of the pet.

Parasites and bacterial infections are common causes of acute colitis in dogs and cats. Dietary indiscretions and stress-induced situations are two other prevalent sources. Less commonly, fungal infections, foreign bodies, intussusceptions, polyps, food allergies, immune system disorders, and tumors can all result in signs related to a chronic colitis. Because of the variety of potential causes, colitis can strike a pet of any age.

Diagnosis of colitis is made from a predisposing history (such as dietary indiscretion), existing clinical signs, and physical examination. Stool examinations and other laboratory tests should be performed in an attempt to identify the underlying cause of the colitis. Radiographs, including barium contrast studies, are indicated in non-responsive, recurring cases. Biopsies obtained using an endoscope or through exploratory surgery can also prove to be helpful for establishing a definitive diagnosis. In some cases, an exact cause of the inflammation can never be discerned, even with extensive laboratory tests.

Treatment of acute colitis is aimed at eliminating the inciting cause. Parasites should be treated using proper dewormers and antiparasitic medications. Antibiotics can be used to help remove any disease-causing bacteria within the colon, and steroid anti-inflammatories might prove helpful in diminishing clinical signs. If polyps or tumors are present, surgical removal might be necessary to afford a cure.

However, understand that in many cases of chronic colitis, especially those caused by stress or by immune system disorders, a complete cure cannot be achieved. In these pets, treatment goals are aimed at managing flare-ups as they occur and maintaining a good quality of life for the pet. Anti-inflammatories, antibiotics, and local protectants such as kaolin and pectin can help provide relief from these intermittent episodes.

Dietary management is an important component of colitis treatment. Acute cases of colitis caused by dietary indiscretion or some infectious process respond well to feeding a bland, easily digestible diet available from a veterinarian.

Chronic, recurring bouts with colitis might be managed by increasing the fiber content in the diet to normalize the gut motility. Finally, for those cases suspected of being caused by food allergies, a hypoallergenic diet can help eliminate the effects of the allergy.

Megacolon (Cats)

Feline megacolon is a disease condition characterized by a large, distended colon that has lost its ability to contract properly. When this occurs, feces build up within the affected segment and prevent normal flow of ingesta through the intestinal tract.

Megacolon is caused by a disruption of or lack of nerve activity in the muscular walls of the colon. It might occur secondary to spinal cord trauma, other diseases affecting the nervous system, or, as in the case of some Manx cats, be inherited.

The clinical signs associated with feline megacolon can vary. Straining to defecate is certainly the most obvious sign; diarrhea can also be seen alongside firm, hard stools. If the obstruction is severe, vomiting, dehydration, and loss of appetite can be seen as well.

Diagnosis of feline megacolon can be made on physical examination and, for confirmation, from radiographs. Treatment involves removing the fecal impaction using warm-water enemas and by infusing the colon with mineral oil.

Enemas designed for use in humans should not be used in cats, as the components of a human enema solution can cause severe dehydration in cats, Severe cases might require surgical relief of the impaction.

There is no effective cure for this condition; as a result, preventive maintenance therapy should be used to prevent recurrences. Giving an oral hairball laxative on a daily basis will help keep fecal matter moving along nicely. Increasing the amount of fiber in the diet has also been shown to be helpful in preventing relapses.

Anal Sac Disease

The *anal sacs* are special structures located at the eight o'clock and the four o'clock positions just below the anus. These sacs are lined with special cells that secrete an odiferous liquid into the lumen of each sac, where it is stored. As feces pass out of the anus, these sacs are depleted of their stored material via small ducts located just below the anal opening. Some dogs and cats even have the skunklike ability to express these sacs on their own free will! No one knows quite for sure what the purpose of the anal sacs and their secretions is, but many suspect that they serve as a means of communication and identification between strangers!

Anal sac infections and irritation can occur if the material within the sacs isn't emptied on a regular basis. Secretions that are allowed to remain within the sacs for long periods of time often become thick and gritty, making future anal sac emptying that much harder. Any inflammation of the skin caused by allergies, fleas, and other problems can lead to this problem. Changes in frequency or consistency of bowel movements caused by diarrhea, constipation, or dietary changes can also result in improper emptying of the sacs and secondary anal sac disease. Tapeworm segments are notorious for finding their way into the sacs and causing marked irritation. Small breeds of dogs under 15 pounds seem to have more problems with their anal sacs than do larger breeds because the sacs' emptying ducts are smaller as well. Fortunately, cats rarely have problems associated with their anal sacs.

Dogs suffering from anal sac irritation often show obvious signs of discomfort, including constant licking in that region, and "scooting" their hind ends along the floor in an attempt to empty the sacs (Fig. 11.11). In these instances, manual emptying of the sacs often leads to dramatic improvement in the pet's overall disposition.

If one or more anal sacs become infected, actual pus or draining tracts might be observed around the affected region. These dogs are in a great deal of pain and will resist attempts at inspection. The amount of licking activity will also increase.

Infected anal sacs need to be treated with topical antibiotics instilled directly into the affected sac(s) on a daily basis. In extensive cases, oral antibiotics might also be used to quicken the cure.

Anal sac problems can be prevented in a number of ways. Increasing the fiber and bulk content in the diet, and hence in the fecal material, will promote a thorough emptying of the sacs with each bowel movement. If a dog is showing early signs of problems, such as scooting, prompt evacuation of the sacs by a veterinarian can help prevent further progression of the problem.

Routine expression of healthy anal sacs is not advised, since, if done improperly, it could actually inflame these sacs and lead to impaction. Surgical removal of the anal sacs is certainly an option for those dogs that suffer miserably from this affliction. If infection is present, it must be cleared up before this type of surgery is performed.

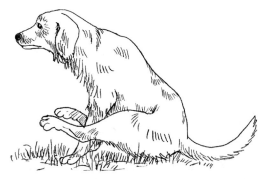

FIGURE 11.11 A dog with impacted anal sacs will "scoot" along the ground in an attempt to empty them.

Pancreatitis

Inflammation of the pancreas, or pancreatitis, is a painful condition characterized by an overproduction of digestive enzymes by the pancreas, which actually begin to damage the pancreatic tissue itself. This disorder can strike both dogs and cats with equal vengeance. In dogs, it is seen most often in middle-aged, overweight females. Dogs and cats that are fed poor-quality, high-calorie diets with or without table scraps are also at high risk of developing pancreatitis. Heredity can also come into play with certain canine breeds, such as schnauzers, which are at greater risk than are some of their counterparts.

Signs of a pancreatitis attack include loss of appetite, excessive salivation, vomiting (Fig. 11.12), diarrhea, depression, and marked pain in the abdominal region on the right side just behind the ribcage. Dogs so afflicted will sometimes assume a "praying" posture, with the front legs bent and the hind end stuck up in the air, in an attempt to alleviate some of the pain.

With severe involvement, shock and death can result if the pain and inflammation are not relieved promptly. Diabetes mellitus can also be an unfortunate consequence with repeated bouts of pancreatitis as digestive enzymes destroy the insulin-producing cells within the pancreas. Because of the similarity of the clinical signs, acute bouts of

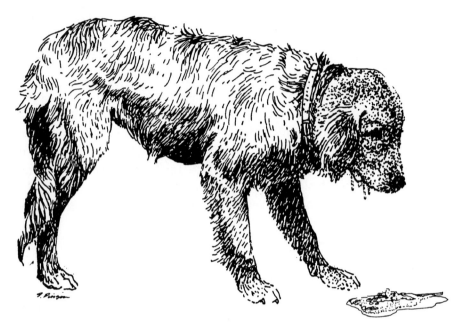

FIGURE 11.12 Pancreatitis causes severe vomiting in dogs so affected.

pancreatitis must be differentiated from other gastrointestinal disorders such as foreign bodies and intestinal obstructions.

Dogs and cats suffering from mild flare-ups of pancreatitis will often recover spontaneously when food and water is withheld. In fact, this is one method of diagnosing this condition. Measuring the blood levels of the pancreatic enzymes amylase and lipase can also be a helpful diagnostic tool, since both tend to be elevated during an acute attack. Radiographs are useful for ruling out other potential causes of the clinical signs, such as intestinal obstructions.

When treating pancreatitis, it is imperative that all food, water, and even oral medication be discontinued for a period of 48 to 72 hours. This will help lower the amounts of digestive enzymes being produced by the pancreas. Intravenous fluids are required to prevent dehydration during this time of fasting.

Pain relievers and medications designed to reduce pancreatic secretions are very important to prevent secondary complications from arising. Since the gastrointestinal tract is involved, antibiotics are indicated as well to prevent secondary bacterial infections.

Pancreatitis is usually a recurring problem that can never be eliminated completely. However, there are certain measures owners can institute at home to protect pets from acute flare-ups and the health problems associated with them.

Dogs and cats with a history of this disorder should be fed low-calorie, easily digestible diets that don't require much pancreatic effort for their breakdown within the intestines. Such a diet, or a recipe for its formulation, is available from veterinarians. All table scraps should cease; even sneaking a small treat from the table could result in a life-threatening pancreatitis attack.

Increasing exercise levels and promoting weight loss will also serve protective functions against recurrence of this disorder.

Hepatitis and Liver Disease

While *pancreatitis* means inflammation involving the pancreas, *hepatitis* involves inflammation of the liver. Contrary to popular belief, not all cases of hepatitis are infectious and contagious in nature. There can be numerous noninfectious causes of liver inflammation as well. Some of these include diabetes mellitus, heart disease, accidental poisonings, starvation, and cancer.

Hepatic lipidosis is a common type of liver dysfunction in cats that has baffled researchers for years. It is characterized by an extensive infiltration of the liver by fatty tissue that, in essence, crowds out the normal liver cells and interferes with normal liver function. It is seen in all ages of cats, and the exact cause of this condition is unknown, yet obesity and/or prolonged periods of food deprivation due to loss of appetite are

FACT OR FICTION

Aspirin, acetaminophen, and other types of oral human pain medications are poisonous to cats. **FACT.** The feline liver, unlike that of most other species, is deficient in a certain enzyme called *glucuronyl transferase*. This enzyme is normally responsible for metabolizing and detoxifying certain therapeutic drugs that reach the liver. This is why cats are so sensitive to drugs such as aspirin and acetaminophen; even small doses can be deadly!

thought to increase the body's utilization of fats for energy, the metabolism of which is carried out in the liver.

As an organ responsible for metabolism of the multitude of nutrients absorbed from the intestines, and detoxification of poisons and drugs circulating in the blood, it is remarkable that the liver is normally very resistant to injury or breakdown resulting from its normal day-to-day functions. Unfortunately, because of this heartiness, clinical signs of liver inflammation seldom appear until serious damage to liver function has already taken place.

Like so many other diseases affecting the gastrointestinal tract, acute flare-ups of hepatitis can cause loss of appetite, vomiting, diar-

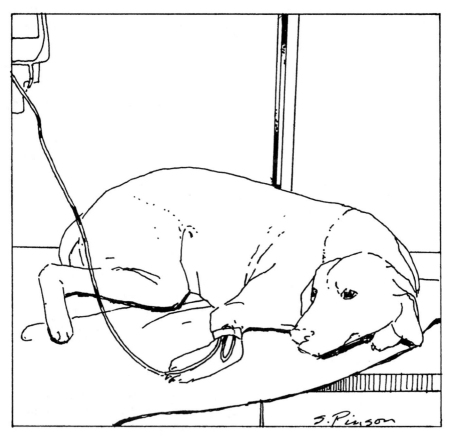

FIGURE 11.13   Acute liver disease requires intense veterinary support.

rhea, and fever in affected dogs and cats. One unique sign often seen with hepatitis, both acute and chronic, is jaundice, or icterus. *Jaundice,* caused by elevated levels of bile pigments in the bloodstream, is characterized by a yellow discoloration of the skin, mucous membranes, and the liquid portion of the blood.

Other clinical signs that can result from chronic, long-term hepatitis and liver disease include a fluid buildup within the abdominal cavity (ascites) due to increased resistance to blood flow through the liver, bleeding tendencies, and anemia. Seizures and other neurologic disorders can also appear with advanced cases as blood levels of ammonia are allowed to build up.

Diagnosis of hepatitis is based on clinical signs, elevated serum levels of liver enzymes, and/or the demonstration of an enlarged liver on radiographs or ultrasonography. For those more subtle cases, special liver function tests and even biopsies might be required to confirm a diagnosis of hepatitis or discover its cause.

Treatment objectives for hepatitis and liver disease are aimed at eliminating the injurious agent and its harmful effect on the liver tissue and at promoting healing of the affected tissue. In cats with hepatic lipidosis, this means force-feeding them if necessary. The liver is one of the few organs within the body that can actually regenerate itself after injury, provided, of course, that the source of the injury is dealt with properly (Fig. 11.13).

If vomiting is a problem, intravenous fluids (Fig. 11.14) might be needed until the stomach settles down enough for oral ingestion of food and water. An easily digestible diet with high biological value (available through veterinarians) is ideal for dogs and cats suffering from a liver disorder. Oral antibiotics designed to eliminate ammonia-forming organisms are useful for those cases exhibiting neurological signs. Ascites can be

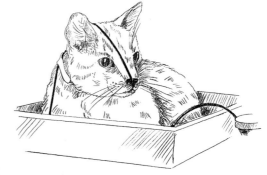

FIGURE 11.14   Sick cats that refuse to eat may require tube feeding. This particular tube passes through the nose, down the esophagus, and into the stomach.

treated with diuretic drugs and by reducing the amount of sodium in the pet's diet.

Finally, in chronic cases of hepatitis, steroids might be warranted to increase appetite and to counteract the loss of protein that can occur with liver disease. In addition, certain drugs for liver disease designed for use in humans are being used in animals with variable success.

The Urinary System

In the normal, day-to-day functioning of the body, lots of waste material is formed as a result of metabolic activity. It is the function of the urinary system to handle and to rid the body of these waste products. In addition, through its ability to dilute or concentrate the urine, it serves to regulate fluid levels within the body.

Anatomy and Physiology

The urinary system of dogs and cats is composed of two kidneys, the ureters, a bladder, and a urethra. The kidneys are composed of cells called *nephrons,* which are responsible for filtering the waste material out of the blood and returning vital fluids and nutrients back into the bloodstream that would otherwise be lost in the urine (Fig. 12.1). Those

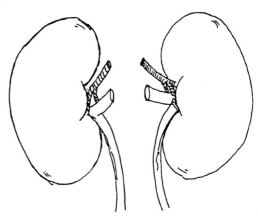

FIGURE 12.1 The kidneys function to filter waste material out of the bloodstream.

solids and fluids not put back into the blood by the nephrons will eventually make up the urine. All the nephrons empty urine into a specific portion of the kidney, which then empties into the ureter for transport to and storage in the bladder.

The bladder wall is composed of smooth muscle and is capable of expanding to enormous sizes. Special muscular sphincters prevent the urine from passing out of the bladder prematurely. Urinary incontinence, characterized by an inability to voluntarily hold urine within the bladder, can result from malfunction of these sphincters. Once the bladder is ready to release its contents, the urine then passes out of the body by way of the urethra.

Because of its vital function, any interference or alteration of urinary system function can quickly lead to serious health consequences. For this reason, prompt and proper diagnosis of urinary tract disorders in dogs and cats is essential. Periodic checkups by a veterinarian can help detect potential problems before they reach such a magnitude as to threaten the health of the pet.

Kidney Disease

The kidneys are responsible for eliminating waste products produced by the body's normal metabolism. If they fail to perform this function adequately, the body will literally poison itself. For this reason, special attention must be directed at keeping these organs healthy, or—if a disease state already exists—at treating to prevent further functional deterioration.

In dogs and cats, kidney (renal) disease is the most common disorder associated with old age. In essence, through normal wear and tear, the kidneys become unable to perform their functions in the same way that they did when they were young. Worn-out kidney cells die and are replaced by scar tissue, which can't filter out toxins from the blood. When enough of these nephrons die and the buildup of toxins in the blood becomes great enough, the pet begins to exhibit signs of kidney failure.

DID YOU KNOW?

It takes a loss of over 75 percent of the functioning capacity of both kidneys to lead to signs of kidney failure in pets.

But don't get the idea that only older pets can suffer from kidney impairment. Young dogs and cats might have been born with inadequate kidney function, or they might suffer from other diseases (such as feline infectious peritonitis or leptospirosis) or toxic agents that kill nephrons and impair renal performance.

For example, systemic infections, heat stroke, heart disease, and autoimmune diseases are only some of the acquired conditions that can lead to kidney disease and kidney failure. Many therapeutic drugs, such as aspirin and certain antibiotics, can be damaging to the kidneys if used indiscriminately. Antifreeze, or ethylene glycol, is deadly to dogs and cats when ingested because of the profound damage it causes to the kidneys. Finally, periodontal disease, with its associated complications, can predispose pets, both young and old, to kidney problems in the future.

The clinical signs associated with kidney disease can be quite variable depending on the extent of damage to the kidneys. Interestingly, dogs and cats rarely show outward signs of kidney disease until at least 75 percent of the function in both kidneys is lost! As a result, when signs do finally become apparent, it is vital that therapeutic measures be taken quickly to prevent loss of the remaining 25 percent.

Sudden, acute kidney failure, the type that can result from the ingestion of a poison such as antifreeze (Fig. 12.2), can lead directly into intense dehydration, shock, unconsciousness, and death without manifesting any other signs.

Chronic, more long-term kidney disease and kidney failure rarely have such a dramatic presentation, yet such conditions can eventually turn into acute kidney failure if measures aren't instituted to prevent this progression. Dogs and cats with chronic renal failure will exhibit an increased thirst and an increased desire to urinate. Depression and loss of appetite might also set in. In addition, since renal disease can cause stomach ulcers, vomiting might occur.

Veterinarians can diagnose kidney disease through

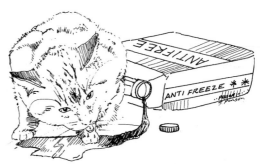

FIGURE 12.2 Antifreeze will destroy the kidneys!

a series of laboratory tests performed on the blood and the urine. Two blood parameters, blood urea nitrogen (BUN) and serum creatinine, will be elevated if the kidneys are failing.

The urine specific gravity is also an important parameter that helps the veterinary practitioner determine the extent of damage to the kidneys. Under normal circumstances, the specific gravity of the urine, which measures how concentrated the urine is, should fluctuate depending on the body's own needs for water. Diseased kidneys, however, are unable to conserve water for the body; hence, the specific gravity of the urine in a pet with advanced kidney disease will be diluted, even if the pet is clinically dehydrated.

Dogs and cats suffering from acute renal failure must be hospitalized and placed on intravenous fluids to correct dehydration. Other medications designed to stimulate kidney function will be given as well. If the pet survives this acute attack, support measures for chronic kidney failure must then be implemented.

Stress reduction is vital in dogs and cats with chronic renal disease and/or failure. Unlimited access to clean, fresh water should be provided at all times, since water deprivation could lead into an acute kidney-failure crisis. Special diets that are low in phosphorus and contain only high-quality protein should be fed to help reduce toxin buildup within the bloodstream. These are available from veterinarians. Vitamin supplementation should also be considered to replace those lost in the increased urine flow.

DID YOU KNOW?

A test is now available from your veterinarian that can detect kidney disease before symptoms even appear!

Since renal disease can alter, among other things, the blood levels of calcium and phosphorus, medications designed to keep levels of these electrolytes constant are used as well. If a pet is having trouble with vomiting, human antiulcer medications can be employed to help settle the stomach.

Finally, since kidney disease places an incredible burden on the affected pet's immune system, all underlying disease processes and disorders (such as periodontal disease) need to be addressed.

Urinary Incontinence

Dogs and cats that are unable to willfully control their urination habits are said to be suffering from incontinence. Pets with urinary incontinence might simply urinate spontaneously without warning, or might drip urine continuously throughout the day. Inappropriate urination while sleeping is another common complaint. Dermatitis in the genital and hind-leg regions can also be seen as a result of incontinence and urine scalding in these areas.

The potential causes of urinary incontinence are numerous; as a result, a proper veterinary workup is essential to obtain a correct diagnosis. Spinal trauma, anatomical changes or irritation caused by inherited defects, infections, tumors, urinary calculi, and metabolic diseases such as diabetes mellitus or diabetes insipidus can all be underlying causes of incontinence. In these instances, treatment is geared toward correcting the underlying cause if possible.

It has been noted that a small number of female dogs that are spayed at an early age can suffer from incontinence when they enter their geriatric years. Although the exact cause of this incontinence is unknown, it can usually be controlled with medications designed to increase sphincter tone within the lower urinary tract.

Puppies and even some adult dogs might urinate spontaneously when they become excited or frightened. Most puppies will "grow out" of this problem as they mature. For these and others, treatment for behavioral incontinence is directed toward minimizing the stimuli that cause the incontinence in the first place. For instance, when dealing with dogs that urinate because of excitement, avoiding eye contact or exaggerated greetings when approaching the pet often help curb excitement and prevent urination. For those dogs that urinate when frightened, easing their fear through behavioral modification is the key to a cure.

Feline Lower Urinary Tract Disease (FLUTD)

Feline lower urinary tract disease [known in the past as *feline urologic syndrome* (FUS)] is a disease syndrome of cats characterized by the

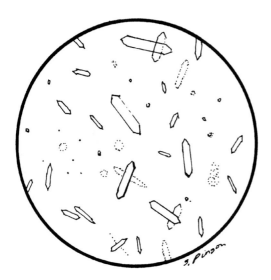

FIGURE 12.3 Urine crystals as seen under a microscope.

formation of crystals (the most common are struvite and calcium oxalate crystals) within the urinary bladder. These crystals, in turn, cause inflammation, urinary bleeding and straining, and sometimes life-threatening obstruction to the normal flow of urine out of the bladder (Fig. 12.3).

No one knows for sure why some cats get FLUTD and others don't. Many potential causes have been hypothesized, including viruses, abnormal urinary retention, obesity, bladder defects, and—the most popular theory to date—improper diet. In reality, one or all of these factors might play a role in the occurrence of FLUTD.

If a cat is prone to this disorder, it will usually show some signs of the disease by the time that it is 3 years of age. Both male and female cats are at risk of developing FLUTD; however, males have a greater likelihood of developing a life-threatening obstruction simply because the male urethra is smaller than that of the female and can become plugged with crystals more easily. If such an obstruction occurs, urine can flow back into the kidneys, causing damage to these organs and also causing toxins to begin building up in the bloodstream.

Early clinical signs of FLUTD result from the irritation that these crystals cause within the bladder itself. These can include inappropriate urination in places other than the litterbox or normal elimination areas, increased licking at the genital region, straining, frequent attempts at urination with crying or vocalization, and blood in the urine (Fig. 12.4). Cats often lose their appetites and become more irritable as well. More seriously, male cats suffering from partial or complete obstruction of the urethra can exhibit vomiting, intense lethargy, and a distended, painful abdomen.

Diagnosis of FLUTD is based on clinical signs, physical examination, and a urinalysis. An enlarged, painful bladder can also be palpated in those cats suffering from some degree of obstruction. If a bladder infection is suspected, then urine cultures might also be performed.

The obstructed cat will usually have high levels of kidney enzymes (BUN, cre-

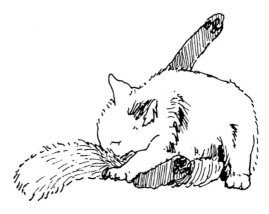

FIGURE 12.4 Cats with urinary tract disease will lick incessantly.

atinine) present in its bloodstream, signifying the toxin buildup and kidney destruction that is occurring. Most veterinary hospitals are equipped to monitor these enzymes.

If an actual obstruction is suspected, then rapid treatment is essential to save the life of the cat. Obstructed cats are immediately placed on intravenous fluids to help dilute the toxin levels within the bloodstream. A catheter is then inserted into the urethra to "unplug" it in order to reestablish urine flow. Once this flow is reestablished, the bladder is flushed repeatedly with sterile saline to remove any crystals that might be remaining within (Fig. 12.5).

The veterinarian must decide whether to keep the urinary catheter in place for a few days. While catheterized, these cats are placed on antibiotics to prevent the occurrence of any secondary bladder infections as a result of the catheter. Intravenous fluids are

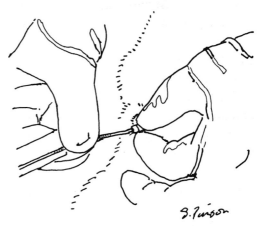

FIGURE 12.5 A urinary catheter may become necessary to relieve an obstruction.

continued in the hospital setting for 2 to 3 days after the obstruction is relieved.

For the cats that are not obstructed but still are showing signs of FLUTD, smooth-muscle relaxants and anti-inflammatory medications can be used to help reduce the discomfort and urge associated with this disease. The use of antibiotics in such patients is still controversial; studies have shown that bacterial infections are present in less than 20 percent of the cases. However, if urine culture confirms the presence of such, antibiotics are, of course, indicated.

If struvite crystals have been diagnosed, altering the pH of the urine in order to dissolve any crystals present within the bladder is another important step in treating this disease in both obstructed and unobstructed felines. Rendering the urine more acidic will help dissolve existing struvite crystals and help prevent the formation of new ones.

> **DID YOU KNOW?**
>
> Special cat litter additives are now available from your veterinarian that can help detect the presence of blood in the urine, allowing for the early detection of FLUTD.

Most veterinary researchers agree that diet plays the foremost role in the creation and in the treatment and prevention of this disease syndrome. Dry diets with high contents of magnesium and ash (mineral) levels are the biggest culprits in promoting FLUTD in cats.

Unfortunately, many of the commercial supermarket brands of cat food contain these excesses. Diets specially formulated for the prevention of FLUTD can be obtained in both moist and dry forms from most veterinary offices and some pet supply stores. Because of its high calcium and mineral content, cow's milk should never be offered to those individuals prone to FLUTD.

Besides feeding a diet that promotes a healthy urine pH and is low in magnesium and ash, providing cats free access to a fresh water supply is a must. Increased water consumption will help increase the number of urinations each day, effectively keeping the bladder flushed out. In fact, most commercial diets formulated for the prevention of FLUTD have an increased salt content to promote increased water consumption. With these increased urinations comes the responsibility of keeping the litterbox cleaned on a regular basis. Many cats refuse to urinate in a dirty litterbox, a practice that encourages urine retention and FLUTD.

Although it might not seem important, regulating the frequency of meals fed can play a direct role in the prevention of FLUTD. After a cat consumes a meal, its urine undergoes a temporary rise in pH. For those cats allowed to eat and nibble all day long (such as those fed dry foods), this might promote relatively constant alkaline urine, and thereby predispose to struvite crystal formation. As a result, in terms of preventing FLUTD, offering one or two meals a day rather than free-choice meals is preferred.

Obese cats are more prone to FLUTD than their slimmer counterparts, so weight control is an important preventive measure to follow as well. Overweight felines, especially those who have exhibited signs of FLUTD in the past, should be placed on a reducing diet prescribed by their veterinarians and have their activity levels increased until the desired weight is reached. Once weight loss is accomplished, they can be switched back over to preventive-type rations.

Without proper dietary management, FLUTD can be expected to recur over 50 percent of the time. In some cats, however, FLUTD recurs over and over again, even with dietary management. In these instances, treating the symptoms when they first appear and continuing with preventive measures will usually prevent such episodes from turning serious.

For those male cats that have had recurring obstruction, a special operation known as a *perineal urethrostomy* might be indicated to reduce the danger of death due to urinary blockage. This surgery involves the removal of the end of the penis and widening the urethral opening, effectively allowing for free passage out of any and all crystals. Keep in mind that such a procedure is not intended to cure the FLUTD; it merely lessens the risk of severe, life-threatening complications associated with it.

Canine Urolithiasis (Urinary Stones)

Urinary tract infections that go unnoticed for a period of time can predispose a dog to urolithiasis. A urolith or stone results from the coalescing of crystals that form within the bladder environment. In dogs, these stones form more readily within the bladder than they do in other portions of the urinary system. Urolithiasis presents itself in dogs in two forms: cystic (bladder) calculi and urethral calculi.

Cystic calculi are found mainly in females and appear when infectious bacteria within the bladder cause a shift in the urine pH, which in turn causes the crystals to form. The two most common types of crystals generated are struvite and calcium oxalate crystals. Stones formed by these crystals are often discoid in shape.

Urethral calculi occur in male dogs and are typically composed of cystine or urate crystals instead of struvite. This type of urolithiasis is seldom caused by infections; rather, an inherent metabolic disorder is responsible for crystal formation. If these stones lodge in the male urethra, they can prevent normal urination, and can seriously threaten the life of the pet.

Straining to urinate, bloody urine, constant licking at the urethral opening, and/or frequent unsuccessful attempts to urinate are all signs of a urinary problem. Stones might or might not be present in a dog exhibiting these signs, but this warrants a professional evaluation. Some dogs, especially females, might carry stones in their bladders for long periods of time without exhibiting any signs at all. This is one good reason for having a veterinarian perform a routine urinalysis on an annual basis.

Diagnosis of urolithiasis is made on the basis of microscopic examination of the urine for crystal formation, abdominal palpation, and radiographs (Fig. 12.6). Most stones will show up readily on regular radiographs; however, those composed of urate or cystine might require special contrast radiographs in order to identify them. In addition, for male dogs sus-

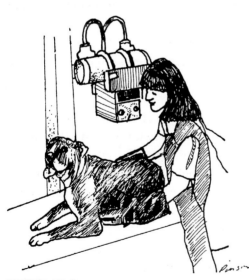

FIGURE 12.6 Radiographs (X rays) can be used to detect many types of bladder stones.

pected of having urethral calculi, inability to pass a urinary catheter is a sure sign that stones are present. In these cases and others, the attending veterinarian will often elect to run blood tests as well to ensure that the kidneys and other organs are functioning properly in the presence of these uroliths.

Treatment of urolithiasis depends on the size and number of the stones present and their location within the urinary tract. Obviously a male dog whose urinary tract is completely plugged by one or more of these stones requires emergency care immediately. Catheterization is performed in an attempt to dislodge the stones, pushing them back into the bladder and freeing up the flow of urine. Most of the time, these stones must then be removed from the bladder surgically.

In those cases uncomplicated by obstruction, the size of the stones involved determines the treatment regimen. Large stones located within the bladder will undoubtedly require surgery for their removal. In contrast, smaller struvite stones or crystals can often be effectively managed only with special diets designed to dissolve the stones.

Typically, this dietary approach to treatment might take anywhere from 1 to 4 months to accomplish the desired results. If a pet is placed on a urolith-dissolving diet, be sure to follow the veterinarian's instructions closely. These diets should not be administered for any term longer than that prescribed by the veterinarian. Once the stones have dissolved, the pet needs to be switched to a different diet.

Of course, whether a surgical or medical approach is used, concurrent antibiotic therapy is also necessary if an infection is underlying the bladder stones.

Because the rate of recurrence of urolithiasis is relatively high even after successful treatment, preventive measures should be instituted to help lower the odds. For urethral calculi, special diets that can help promote a urine pH that is nonconducive to crystal formation are available from veterinarians. These diets are also low in those dietary components that might be incorporated into crystals.

Cystic calculi can be prevented in a similar fashion, using special diets available from veterinarians designed for the prevention of struvite uroliths. In addition, prompt identification and treatment of urinary tract infections will help ensure that crystals and stones won't develop as a consequence.

Urinary Tract Infections

Infections of the urinary tract can occur anywhere along the system pathway, including the kidneys, the ureters, the bladder, the urethra, and the prostate gland. One particular site might be exclusively affected, or multiple sites could be involved at the same time. Most urinary tract infections are caused by bacteria gaining entrance into the body through external urinary orifices and traveling upward into the system (termed *ascending infections*). Other routes of infection can include the blood or the lymphatic system, and through direct penetrating trauma. Urinary tract infections are relatively uncommon in cats unless they occur secondary to FLUTD.

Because of the shorter length of their urethras, female dogs are more prone to urinary tract infections than are males. In all animals, regardless of sex, normal body defense mechanisms are constantly at work preventing the establishment of infections within the tract. Antibodies lining the surfaces of the bladder and urethra provide a first line of defense. Sphincter systems, controlled by contracting smooth muscle, help seal off the different portions of the tract from one another. An acidic pH to the urine is another safeguard against the multiplication of undesirable organisms. Finally, normal, frequent urination is also very effective at eliminating undesirable bacteria from the bladder and other parts of the system. For this reason, any disruption in the normal urination routine (e.g., not taking a dog outside enough, dehydration) can predispose an individual to a bacterial infection.

Clinical signs of urinary tract infection will vary, depending on the region(s) involved. Signs associated with infections of the bladder and urethra include straining when trying to urinate (often mistaken for constipation), passage of only small amounts of urine at a time, and/or bloody urine. In the latter case, blood noted at the beginning of urination often signifies a urethral infection, whereas blood noticed near the end of elimination might indicate that the bladder is involved. In many cases, dogs won't show any other signs of illness or fever.

If the kidneys or ureters are involved, similar clinical signs might be noticed, along with other obvious signs of illness, such as fever, depression, vomiting, abdominal pain, and/or back pain. In cases of upper urinary tract infections, it is vital that treatment be instituted at once to prevent permanent damage to the kidneys.

A urinary tract infection can be associated with other disease processes as well, so its presence can sometimes be overshadowed by clinical signs associated with another primary disease. For instance, diabetes mellitus can predispose to urinary tract infections due to the high sugar content in the urine caused by the disease (sugar can provide an ideal growth medium for bacteria). Disorders of the nervous system can even lead to urinary infections if the nerve supply to the muscles and sphincters of the tract is disrupted, thereby eliminating some of the body's natural means of defense.

One unfortunate sequela that can result from any type of urinary tract infection that is not treated promptly is urolithiasis, or urinary stones. Stones have a propensity to form when an increase in urine pH occurs, often as a result of bacteria acting within the urinary tract to break down urine. When this breakdown occurs, ammonia is released, increasing the pH of the bladder environment.

Diagnosis of a urinary tract infection is based on clinical signs, urinalysis, and urine cultures designed to identify the actual bacteria involved. In addition, a veterinarian might choose to order a blood workup on a pet to rule out any disorders, such as diabetes mellitus, that might be underlying the infection. Furthermore, if crystals are noted on microscopic examination of the urine, radiographs will be needed to rule out the presence of any bladder or kidney stones.

Treatment for a urinary tract infection involves the use of an appropriate antibiotic for a minimum of 10 days. Since bacteria can become resistant to certain antibiotics over time, urine cultures to determine antibiotic sensitivity should be performed if a response to treatment with a particular antibiotic is poor.

Large urinary stones might need to be removed surgically. Smaller stones and crystals can often be dissolved by feeding a special type of diet designed to accomplish this task.

For those dogs that suffer from chronic, recurring flare-ups of urinary tract infections, long-term, low-dose antibiotic therapy might be prescribed by a veterinarian. This involves the administration of a single dosage of antibiotic just before the pet's bedtime. Because of the overnight buildup of urine within the bladder, the antibiotic is allowed to reach high concentrations within the urine, effectively combating any bacteria that might be present. It is important to take a dog outside to eliminate just before bedtime, to ensure that the new urine that is formed will contain high levels of the medication.

Owners can help prevent the occurrence of a urinary tract infection in their dogs by providing plenty of fresh water to drink at all times, and by encouraging frequent urination. Special diets that promote a healthy environment within the urinary tract and help discourage infections are available from veterinarians.

For dogs with long hair, especially females, keep the hair trimmed around the external urinary structures to reduce the chances of bacteria gaining entrance to the urinary system via contamination by this hair.

Finally, because uncomplicated urinary tract infections might not show any outward signs, a routine urinalysis on a pet is encouraged on an annual basis, along with its regular checkup and vaccinations.

The Reproductive System

Diseases and conditions involving the reproductive tract tend to be either infectious or anatomical in nature. Prompt medical attention is warranted in any disorder involving the reproductive tract.

Anatomy and Physiology

The Male Reproductive System

Starting with the male dog and cat, the major parts of the reproductive system include the testicles (with associated epididymis and ductus deferens), the scrotum (containing the testicles), the penis (containing the urethra), and the prostate gland. Tomcats also have two bulbourethral glands, which contribute fluid to the semen.

The testes are the organs responsible for the production of spermatozoa. This production is directly influenced by the hormone testosterone, also produced by the testicles. Aside from regulating sperm production, testosterone is also responsible for normal male sexual behavior, as well as the aggressive, territorial behavior exhibited by some males.

> **FACT OR FICTION**
>
> All calico cats are female. **FICTION.** Ninety-nine percent of all calicos are female, yet the occasional male slips through. When he does, he is sterile.

261

Normally, the testicles should descend into the scrotum shortly after birth, usually no later than 8 weeks of age. If this event fails to occur, the pet is said to be *cryptorchid,* and surgical removal of the testicles is required to prevent medical problems (such as testicular tumors) in the future and to prevent the passage of that undesirable trait to offspring.

From the testicle, sperm is shunted into the *epididymis,* a structure closely attached to each testicle, where it finishes its maturation process. On copulation, the mature sperm is transported from the epididymis through the ductus deferens and to the tubelike urethra coursing within the penis.

The feline penis is covered with tissue "spines" that serve to stimulate ovulation in the female when mating occurs. The canine penis has the uncommon ability to swell near its origin during erection, effecting the unique interlocking "tie" with the female during reproduction. In addition, the dog's penis contains a bony structure called the *os penis,* which is grooved underneath to allow for passage of the urethra. If its support function seems somewhat sedentary, its medical significance is not. Because the penis and urethra are parts of the urinary system as well as the reproductive, this os penis can exacerbate complications associated with certain urinary disorders, including urethral calculi.

The *prostate gland,* considered an accessory sex gland, is located surrounding the urethra near the neck of the bladder. It functions to produce prostatic fluid, which mixes with sperm to form semen, and helps increase the survivability of the sperm within the female reproductive tract. Enlargement or inflammation of this gland can occur as intact male dogs mature. Constipation, discharges from the penis, and painful urination can be clinical signs of a prostatic disorder.

The Female Reproductive System

The major reproductive organs of the female dog and cat include the ovaries, the oviducts, the uterus, the vagina, the vulva, and the mammary glands. The ovaries are responsible for the production and release of eggs destined to be fertilized by the male sperm. In addition, several important reproductive hormones are produced by these structures.

Unfertilized eggs are released, or ovulated, by the ovaries, and pass into the small oviducts. It is within these oviducts that fertilization takes place. The fertilized egg, or embryo, continues its passage down the oviducts on its way to the uterus.

When an embryo reaches the uterus, it attaches itself to the uterine wall and begins its development. If fertilization has not taken place, this attachment won't occur and the body eventually resorbs the egg.

The uterus is separated from the vagina by a ring of muscle known as the *cervix.* Most of the time, this cervix remains open. During pregnancy, however, the cervix will close, preventing outside access to the uterine environment. At time of parturition, the cervix relaxes, allowing the birth to take place.

The external opening of the vagina is termed the *vulva.* As a female dog enters into her heat cycle, the vulva will begin to noticeably swell, tipping off owners to the impending heat.

Dogs and cats typically have a total of 8 to 10 mammary glands (4 to 5 on each side), designed to supply newborn offspring with life-sustaining milk (Fig. 13.1). The size of these glands will fluctuate, depending on the stage of the estrous cycle and the pregnancy status of the female.

The "estrous cycle" is the term used to describe a series of events that occurs within the female reproductive tract between actual heat,

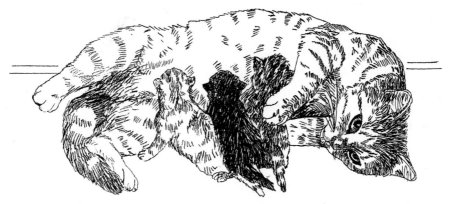

FIGURE 13.1 Newborns receive colostrum from their mother's milk during their first 24 hours of life. This colostrum contains antibodies that help protect the neonates against disease.

or periods of estrus. On the average, this cycle lasts from 6 to 8 months in the female dog (bitch) and in cats (queens), 12 to 20 days. Cats are considered "seasonally polyestrous," meaning that the estrous cycle tends to occur during only certain months of the year (February to October), with anestrus (see the next paragraph) settling in during the fall and early winter. However, cats kept indoors exposed to continuous artificial lighting may not experience anestrus at all.

DID YOU KNOW❓

Queens are induced ovulators; that is, mating stimulates the egg to be ovulated from the ovary, increasing the chances of a successful fertilization.

The four phases of the estrous cycle include anestrus, proestrus, estrus, and metestrus. *Anestrus* is the period of time in which there is no reproductive activity going on in the ovaries. The duration of anestrus is typically 4 to 5 months in the average dog. As mentioned above, the period of anestrus in cats occurs seasonally and is influenced the length of daylight. From anestrus, the reproductive cycle enters the period of *proestrus.* Signs seen during proestrus are related to the ovaries' increased production of the hormone estrogen, and, in dogs, they include vaginal bleeding and a gradual swelling of the vulva. Proestrus can last anywhere from 7 to 14 days in the dog and 3 days in the cat. Normally, females will not stand to be mated until the waning days of this phase.

In dogs, as vaginal bleeding subsides and proestrus ends, estrus, or true heat, begins (the term *estrus* should not be confused with *estrous cycle*). This heat period can last 1 to 2 weeks in both dogs and cats and is characterized by sexual receptivity of the female to the male. Some dog breeds, particularly husky-type breeds and basenjis, can undergo a phenomenon known as "wolf heat." Thought to be a carry-

🔍FACT OR FICTION

Once a female dog starts bleeding from her vagina, she is "in heat." **FICTION.** In reality, such females are beginning their proestrual period and won't enter into true heat until the bleeding stops. Unfortunately, many pet owners trying to guard against accidental pregnancies learn this fact 2 months later when an unexpected litter arrives!

over from their wild ancestors, dogs exhibiting such a pattern might not enter directly into heat after the proestrual period. Instead, the estrous cycle actually comes to a halt for 2 to 3 weeks before starting up again. Another interesting fact about the heat period in the dog is that eggs that are ovulated from the ovaries can mature and be fertilized at different times. As a result, it is possible for mixed litters to occur if the female dog happens to be bred by more than one male.

The last stage in the estrous cycle is *metestrus,* which can last from 2 to 3 months in the dog and 3 to 14 days in the cat. This stage begins when the female refuses to accept the male for further breeding. It is the period of uterine repair or, if fertilization is achieved, the period of pregnancy. False pregnancies appear during this phase as well (see the next section).

Accidental Mating (Mismating)

The question about what to do with the female dog or cat that is accidentally (Fig. 13.2) bred is not an easy one to answer. In the old days, all that a pet owner needed to do was to take her in to the veterinarian for a "mismating" shot or pill. What these treatments consisted of were formulations of the female hormone estrogen, which, if given within the first 36 hours after mating occurred, would effectively terminate a pregnancy.

However, it is now known that significant side effects can occur if such drugs are used. For starters, external sources of estrogens have been demonstrated to actually cause infertility in some female dogs, rendering them unable to conceive at

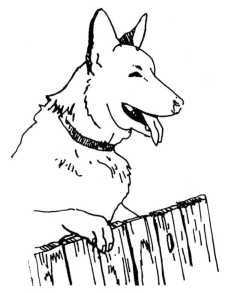

FIGURE 13.2 Be on guard: Male dogs will go to great lengths to be with a female in heat.

later dates. On a more serious note, estrogens can also cause a life-threatening anemia in sensitive cases. And if that weren't enough, they can also predispose a pet to pyometra after administration.

To be safe, use of such estrogen-containing drugs is not an acceptable method for dealing with mismatings in dogs or cats. So what are the options open to pet owners? To begin, valuable breeding females should be allowed to just go ahead and have the litter of puppies or kittens instead of chancing it with mismating medications. If this is not acceptable, then either surgical removal of the fetuses from the uterus at a later stage of development or an actual ovariohysterectomy is warranted.

Remember: All of this is assuming, of course, that a viable mating did indeed take place and that a pregnancy resulted from it! Many mismatings do not result in pregnancy, and cause owners to grieve needlessly. Pregnancy detection tests are available through veterinarians and can be used to confirm whether a pet is indeed pregnant.

False Pregnancy

When the ovaries release eggs to be fertilized, they then start to produce a hormone called *progesterone.* The function of this hormone is to maintain pregnancy if egg fertilization occurs. However, a unique feature seen in dogs is that even if fertilization does not occur, progesterone levels will remain high for up to 10 weeks after heat is over. It is precisely this behavior that is responsible for the condition dog owners know as *pseudopregnancy,* or "false pregnancy." False pregnancies can also occur in cats, yet rarely of the same magnitude as seen in dogs.

All female dogs exhibit some form of pseudopregnancy after they come out of heat. In most, signs associated with it go unnoticed by the owner. However, some dogs do exhibit marked changes as a result of these high progesterone levels, including mammary gland enlargement with or without the production of milk, and behavioral changes that include restlessness, nesting, mothering of inanimate objects, and loss of appetite. In short, they might actually appear to be expectant mothers! Often, there is no way to be sure that they are not, without the use of ultrasound or radiographic X rays. Dogs that undergo marked false pregnancies are also prime candidates for mastitis, a common sequela.

Therapy to control signs associated with pseudopregnancy is seldom needed, unless mastitis becomes a recurring problem, or if marked behavioral changes occur. Hormones prescribed by a veterinarian can provide relief in many cases, yet prolonged use of these agents can have undesirable side effects, especially in females used for breeding. For this reason, unless you have a valuable breeder on your hands, ovariohysterectomy is the safest and most effective way to deal with pseudopregnancy.

Eclampsia

Eclampsia is a serious, sometimes life-threatening disease that can occur in the female either just prior to giving birth or within 3 weeks after parturition has taken place. More common in the smaller, toy breeds, it is characterized by abnormally low levels of blood calcium in their systems. The condition is rarely seen in cats.

In dogs, early signs seen with eclampsia include nervousness, whining, pacing, and trembling. This might progress into incoordination, muscle spasms, and seizurelike activity. If the eclampsia is left untreated, death can result from respiratory difficulties and high fever (Fig. 13.3).

Diagnosis of eclampsia is based on history, clinical signs, and blood calcium levels. Fortunately, treatment consisting of intravenous injections of calcium is highly effective and provides instant relief from the life-threatening signs seen.

After treatment is performed, and clinical signs have abated, owners need to take special precautions to ensure that a relapse does not occur, For starters, puppies should not be allowed to nurse for 24 hours after such an episode. Instead, a commercial milk replacement formula should be fed to them. In fact, periodic supplementation should continue even after the puppies are placed back on their mother's milk to reduce the load on her. In some cases, putting the puppies back on their mother's milk will cause another episode of eclampsia, in which case they should be permanently placed on supplements.

Female dogs that are prone to eclampsia should be placed on oral calcium supplements throughout the nursing period. In fact, if there is

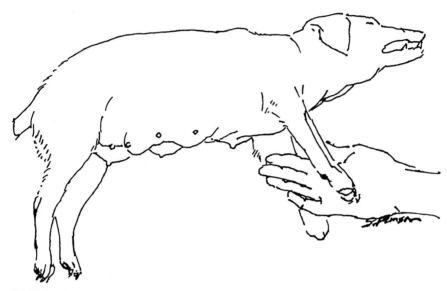

FIGURE 13.3 Eclampsia causes rigid (spastic) convulsions in affected female dogs.

a past history of such a problem, calcium supplementation started during the last 2 weeks of pregnancy and continued throughout lactation can be quite helpful in preventing a recurrence.

Vaginitis and Metritis

Inflammation involving the uterus is termed *metritis*; that involving the vagina is properly termed *vaginitis.* Both vaginitis and metritis can occur independently of each other, or together. Causes of vaginitis and metritis can include venereally transmitted organisms, metabolic diseases like diabetes mellitus, retained fetuses or placentas, and, as mentioned earlier, treatment with estrogen-type drugs.

Female puppies under 1 year of age can suffer from a condition termed *juvenile vaginitis,* characterized by a thick, greenish vaginal discharge. Aside from the discharge, affected puppies generally show no other ill effects, and the condition will, in most instances, spontaneously resolve on its own when the puppy enters into her first heat cycle.

Classic signs of vaginitis or metritis include a thick, yellow-to-green discharge seen coming from the vagina. Owners might notice their pets licking excessively around this area. In especially dire metritis cases, loss of appetite with an increased water intake, fever, and abdominal pain might become apparent. The discharge might also become discernibly blood-tinged. Because of the intimacy of the urinary tract with the reproductive tract in females, bladder infections that occur secondary to the vaginitis or metritis are also common.

The type of treatment used for reproductive tract infections depends on which portions are involved. For instance, in mild cases of vaginitis, including juvenile vaginitis, direct infusion of the vagina with antibiotics or povidone-iodine douches provides effective results. If the vaginitis is severe or if the uterus is involved, high doses of antibiotics given orally or by injection are required. To determine which antibiotics will work the best, a bacterial culture is indicated. Certainly, if there are any puppies nursing on the affected female, they should be removed and placed on formula.

In critical metritis cases, intravenous fluids might even be required for support. Unless the female is a valuable breeding animal, an ovariohysterectomy should be performed on these pets to directly eliminate the source of the problem, and to prevent metritis from recurring at a later date. For those dogs and cats that are considered too valuable to be spayed, special medications called *prostaglandins* can be utilized to help the uterus contract and empty. These, however, must be used with extreme care under the direct supervision of a veterinarian, and even then, only as a last resort.

Cystic Endometrial Hyperplasia (Pyometra)

In older dogs that have experienced numerous heat cycles, *cystic endometrial hyperplasia complex* (CEHC), or *pyometra,* can develop. Because of repeated hormonal stimulation of the uterus year after year, glands lining the inside wall of the uterus become larger and more active with each heat cycle. Large amounts of fluid are secreted into the uterus by these glands, which can then accumulate, causing uterine swelling. Obvious problems can arise if this fluid is not allowed to drain out of the uterus. Unfortunately, this is precisely what happens in many instances. Because of high progesterone levels associated with metestrus, the cervix remains closed, prohibiting drainage from the uterus. At the same time, the trapped fluid provides an ideal medium for bacteria to grow in, leading to bacterial infections and pus formation. As a result, the uterus literally becomes a bag full of pus. And because of the continued buildup of fluid and pus, an infected uterus can reach an enormous size within the dog's abdomen. In advanced cases, actual rupture of the uterine wall might result, often with fatal consequences for the unfortunate dog.

Females afflicted with pyometra usually exhibit the classic signs of metritis, including depression, loss of appetite with a markedly increased thirst, and abdominal pain. As mentioned earlier, a discharge might or might not be associated with pyometra, and the lack thereof might be associated with the more serious form of the disease.

Abdominal enlargement due to uterine filling might also become apparent, with radiographs revealing a huge uterine outline. Blood work performed on these patients will reveal an enormously elevated white blood cell count and mild anemia (due to the long-term nature of the disease). Pyometra has also been shown to induce kidney disease in affected dogs; as a result, increased urination, vomiting, and dehydration might also be present.

Complete ovariohysterectomy is the treatment of choice for pyometra. Those cases involving a grossly enlarged uterus filled with pus and fluid should be regarded as emergencies, and the surgery should be performed as soon as possible.

Spaying nonbreeding females at an early age can prevent pyometra and its associated complications. For those dogs used for breeding purposes, spaying is recommended after their useful breeding life is finished (usually around 8 years of age).

Phimosis and Paraphimosis (Dogs)

Phimosis and paraphimosis are two conditions that occur in male dogs resulting from a preputial opening that is too small.

Phimosis refers to the inability to extrude the penis through the opening, effectively interfering with reproductive activity; *paraphimosis,* is just the opposite: the inability to retract the penis back into the prepuce once extruded. The exposed organ is very susceptible to trauma and lacerations, which can exacerbate the problem even more.

Phimosis can be treated by having the prepucial opening surgically enlarged. In cases of paraphimosis, reducing the penile swelling by soaking it in Epsom salt will usually allow the replacement of the penis back into the prepuce. Antibiotic ointment can then be instilled into the prepuce to speed healing.

Prostate Disorders

The prostate gland in male dogs and cats lies just at the base of the bladder at the origin of the urethra. Its normal function is to produce secretions that make up a portion of the semen. Disorders of this gland in cats are rare, yet can occur in dogs, and can include bacterial infections, benign prostatic enlargement, cysts, and tumors. Signs of prostate disease include straining to urinate, painful urinations, blood in the urine, abdominal pain, and/or hind limb lameness.

Prostate pain or enlargement can be detected on a physical exam using rectal palpation and/or radiographs. If an infection is present, treatment consists of antibiotic therapy. If a tumor or cyst is suspected, surgical treatment is necessary. Neutering should be performed on all dogs that suffer from prostate problems to help prevent recurrences in the future.

CHAPTER 14

The Skin and Haircoat

The *skin,* or *integument,* functions to protect the body from outside foreign invaders and from water loss. It provides a focus for the sense of touch and assists in the regulation of the temperature within the body. In addition, special modifications of the skin, such as claws and pads, provide a means of traction and defense, as well as shock absorbency.

Anatomy and Physiology

The skin is composed of three layers: the epidermis, the dermis, and the hypodermis. The *epidermis* is the outermost layer of the skin. Beneath the epidermis lie the *dermis* and *hypodermis,* which are composed of, among other things, an array of connective and fatty tissue. Sebaceous glands, embedded within these layers, secrete natural oils out onto the skin surface that lubricate and moisturize the skin.

The haircoats of dogs and cats consist of guard hairs, which make up the rougher outer coat, and the wool hairs, which constitute the fine dense undercoat of most breeds. In addition, special hairs called *tactile hairs* (more commonly known as "whiskers") can be found on the head region. These fulfill a sensory function.

A hair cycle exists in dogs and cats that involves the seasonal shedding of old hair and replacement by new hair. This cycle is dependent on light, not on temperature, and increasing or decreasing amounts of daylight trigger it. As a result, peak shedding periods for the dog and cat occur in the springtime, when the days begin to get longer, and in the fall when the days get shorter. Of course, as more pets spend more time indoors with artificial lighting, the hair cycle can be altered, with shedding occurring year-round.

Hair color is dependent on the amount of pigment present within the hair shaft. Large amounts of pigment result in black hair; hairs that lack pigment are white. Different levels of pigmentation that fall between these two extremes result in all other coat colors. Changes in the natural color of the hair can occur with inflammation, trauma, or constant licking of a particular region or regions of the coat. Of course, as a pet enters its senior years, the appearance of gray hairs is not an uncommon sight as well.

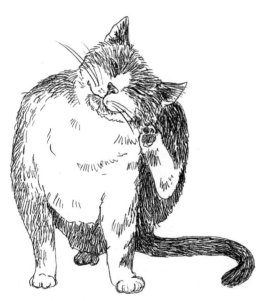

FIGURE 14.1 Fleas and ear mites are two common reasons why cats will scratch their heads.

The Itchy Pet

Many disease conditions can produce itching in the dog and cat. However, only a few disorders result in severe and/or prolonged itching. The primary symptoms of the "itchy pet" are scratching, licking, and/or biting of the skin. Early signs that might be noticed include wet hairs, reddened skin, and hair loss in the areas of biting and scratching. Prolonged itching results in further hair loss, excessive scaling and thickening, and discoloration of the involved skin. Secondary skin infections are common (Fig. 14.1).

Severe and/or prolonged itching is most always a symptom of an underlying skin disorder. As a result, correction of the underlying problem (see list in Table 14.1) is imperative if the symptom of itching is to be successfully controlled.

External Parasites

Refer to specific discussions of external parasites found in this book (Chapter 7).

Inhalant Allergic Dermatitis (Atopic Dermatitis; Atopy)

Table 14.1 Common Causes of Itching and Hair Loss in Cats

Fleas
Food allergy
Inhalant allergies (atopy)
Neurodermatitis
Feline endocrine alopecia
Ringworm
Mange

Inhalant allergic dermatitis represents one of the most common causes of itching in dogs and cats across the United States. Atopy often produces severe itching and is frequently accompanied by skin infection (folliculitis), scaling, hair loss, and discoloration. Atopy parallels human hay fever, except that itching is the primary symptom in the dog and cat rather than the respiratory symptoms exhibited by people. Licking and chewing of the feet, legs, and flank are common symptoms reported by owners, along with generalized scratching.

Atopy is inherited and usually develops between the ages of 6 months and 4 years, following exposure to immune-system-stimulating substances called *allergens.* Although atopy is seasonal, sporadic, and relatively mild in its early stages, it often becomes perennial, and worsens in severity with time. Unfortunately, pets do not outgrow these allergies. Dust (and dust mites), fungal spores, and pollens from trees, shrubs, and grasses can all initiate an allergy in dogs and cats (Table 14.2). Since these substances are present in the air and can be carried hundreds of miles by wind, trying to avoid them by restricting a pet's environment is not possible.

Diagnosis of atopy is based on clinical signs seen, seasonality of such signs, and allergy testing. There are currently two methods of allergy testing available: intradermal skin testing and serum testing.

Intradermal skin testing involves injecting a number of different allergens into the skin of the patient and observing the injection sites

Table 14.2 Wind-Pollinated Plants and Trees That Can Lead to Atopy in Dogs and Cats

Red-root pigweed	Common sagebrush
Meadow fescue	Wild oat
Bermuda grass	Short ragweed
Johnson grass	Kentucky bluegrass
Sweet vernal grass	Redtop
Quackgrass	Smooth brome
Velvetgrass	Broncho grass
Ryegrass	Prairie ragweed
Russian thistle	Cocklebur
Lamb's quarter	Sheep sorrel
Western waterhemp	Annual June grass
Box elder	Oak
Silver maple	White elm

for a corresponding allergic reaction. This type of testing has been used effectively for allergy diagnosis for years and provides the most definitive way to find out what a pet is actually allergic to.

Serum testing is also used to diagnose allergies. These tests involve the evaluation of a serum sample from the allergic pet for antibodies to substances to which it might be allergic. The advantage such testing affords over skin testing is that it is much easier to perform and causes little discomfort to the patient. However, since the accuracy of such tests is still being debated within the veterinary community, intradermal skin testing is still considered by some experts to be the most definitive way to diagnose atopy.

There are four ways to approach treatment for atopy: steroid anti-inflammatory (cortisone-type) drugs, antihistamine/fatty-acid therapy, topical therapy, and allergy shots or hyposensitization.

STEROID ANTI-INFLAMMATORIES (CORTISONE-TYPE DRUGS)

These medications temporarily suppress the itching sensations produced by the allergy. Steroid anti-inflammatories are never curative, yet they can offer effective relief from itching for days to weeks. Increases in water consumption, urination frequency, and appetite are sometimes seen in pets placed on steroid therapy. Unfortunately, prolonged steroid usage over months might produce side effects much more unpleasant than these, including bloating (water retention), muscle atrophy, skin thinning, hair loss, and decreased resistance to infection. In addition, while these steroids are being administered to a pet (especially dogs), its body's ability to produce its own cortisone is suppressed, and might not return even when the steroid therapy is discontinued. If this happens, the pet could go into shock and die. As a result, long-term usage of these drugs for allergic dermatitis should be done only under the close scrutiny of a veterinarian.

> ## FACT OR FICTION
>
> The type of steroid used to treat allergies in dogs is different from those commonly used by people to build muscle and strength. FACT. The steroids used to treat allergies in dogs (glucocorticosteroids) are actually catabolic in nature, meaning that they tend to diminish muscle size and strength with prolonged use. Steroids used to increase muscle size and strength are called anabolic steroids, which, by the way, are sometimes used in veterinary medicine to counteract the effects of aging in older pets.

ANTIHISTAMINE/FATTY-ACID THERAPY

Scientific studies have shown that antihistamine medications alone do little to suppress itching caused by atopic dermatitis. Because antihistamine drugs can cause drowsiness, they can be useful for helping calm down a frustrated pet that can't stop itching and chewing on itself.

Omega-3 fatty acids can be quite beneficial to atopic dogs. It seems that these fatty acids, which are derived from cold-water fish such as salmon, do have the ability in some cases to reduce inflammatory responses and stop itching. Some allergic dogs do fantastic just on these alone. Others require additional medications, such as antihistamines, in order to achieve an acceptable comfort level. Although the effectiveness of this therapy can vary between cases, it does provide a unique alternative to steroid therapy.

TOPICAL THERAPY

Topical treatments by themselves do little to provide lasting relief to the atopic pet. However, when used in combination with other forms of therapy, they can potentiate the effects of these other treatments. One such topical product, a colloidal oatmeal conditioner, can provide effective topical relief for atopic dogs and cats. Along with applying it after bathing, it can also be used as a daily spray (create a 10 to 25% mixture with filtered water and place in a spray bottle) as well. The advantage of using oatmeal conditioners versus shampooing is twofold: (1) A conditioner will help moisturize and soothe the skin with repeated use, whereas shampoos can dry out the skin; and (2) colloidal oatmeal is known to be an effective anti-itch agent and can be applied as many times during the day as necessary to provide relief. Just be sure to brush your pet thoroughly after each application to work the conditioner down to the skin.

ALLERGY SHOTS OR HYPOSENSITIZATION

An alternative approach to treating allergies aside from the ones just mentioned is to hyposensitize the pet using allergen injections. This approach requires allergy testing to be performed, followed by a series of injections of the exact allergens or agents causing the reaction. Although this approach is not effective in all instances, some veterinary dermatology specialists do report at least an 85 to 90 percent success rate; this rate is based on at least 50 percent overall improvement in the allergic pet's condition. However, since inhalant allergens are poor stimulators of immunity, this improvement takes some time. Owners should allow anywhere from 1 to 6 months before making a final judgment as to the effectiveness of the treatment. In most cases, maintenance injections given monthly will be required for the lifetime of the pet.

Hypersensitivity

FLEABITE HYPERSENSITIVITY

Aside from the discomfort caused by the actual bite of a flea, dogs and cats might develop an allergic response to the flea's saliva deposited in the skin during feeding. Moderate to severe itching and hair loss can result, especially along the back near the tail, hips, and hind-leg areas (Fig. 14.2).

Some allergic pets can harbor staphylococcal bacteria not found on the skin of nonallergic pets. Irritation resulting from fleabites can produce a skin infection (fol-

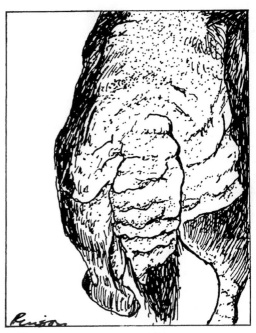

FIGURE 14.2 A flea allergy causes characteristic hair loss from the hips, tail base, and lower portion of the back.

liculitis) on the damaged skin surface and hair follicles. Toxins released from these bacteria might further intensify the itch-scratch cycle. As one might guess, successful treatment of a flea allergy is heavily dependent on the ability to control fleas on the pet and in the environment.

FOOD HYPERSENSITIVITY (FOOD ALLERGIES)

Food allergies are a potential cause of nonseasonal itching in dogs and cats. Other dermatological symptoms might include hives, facial swelling, and chronic ear infections as well. Besides these skin-related problems, food-related allergies have also been implicated in gastrointestinal disorders, such as diarrhea, vomiting, and/or excess gas.

Diagnosis of food hypersensitivity requires the exclusive feeding of a hypoallergenic diet containing a protein source that is not commonly used in commercial pet foods for 8 weeks. Such diets are available through veterinarians.

DID YOU KNOW?

Of all the different types of allergies that can affect pets, food allergies are among the rarest!

If a positive diagnosis is made, the pet will need to remain on the hypoallergenic diet indefinitely. Simply changing food brands or types seldom benefits food allergy cases since most commercial foods contain similar ingredients. Food items such as milk, animal proteins, and vegetable proteins are the most common culprits causing food-induced allergies in pets.

CONTACT HYPERSENSITIVITY (CONTACT ALLERGY)

The haircoat of dogs and cats offers an efficient protective barrier to many substances and agents that could produce an allergic reaction just by coming in contact with the skin. Therefore, those areas relatively devoid of hair such as the chest, abdomen, and feet are more susceptible to contact allergies.

The most common contact-allergy-producing agents include detergents, shampoos, pet sprays, collars, and insecticides, which, in liquid form, can penetrate the normally protective haircoat. In addition, bedding that is moldy or has been chemically treated can cause contact hypersensitivity.

Symptoms of such exposure include redness and swelling of the skin and intense itching. These signs will generally develop within 24 to 72 hours after exposure.

Chemicals that can normally irritate the skin might produce similar symptoms immediately after contact. Such reactions are not to be confused with slower developing hypersensitivity. Treatment of contact allergies requires the removal of the offending agent and administration of topical and/or systemic anti-inflammatory drugs. A thorough history of the pet's exposure to chemicals and exposure to any environment vegetation is imperative in the veterinarian's effort to identify the allergy-producing agent.

Bacterial Infections

Bacterial infections involving the skin are itchy in themselves. As a result, when they occur secondarily to an allergy or parasitic infestation, it can mean sheer misery for a pet. It is for this reason that many treatments for other skin ailments are combined with antibiotic therapy.

Hair Loss (Alopecia)

Loss of hair, either locally or generalized over the coat of a dog or cat, is another type of skin problem that owners may face. As with itching, the causes of hair loss can be quite numerous, and sometimes very complex. A proper diagnosis is essential for restoring a full-bodied haircoat.

Shedding

Although the normal shedding cycles for dogs and cats tend to occur in the spring and fall, some pets, especially those kept indoors, might actually shed year-round. In fact, some of these pets can fill a brush with hair every day! If the dog or cat is otherwise healthy and is on a good nutritional program, this seemingly excessive shedding is of no real consequence. If normal shedding is truly the cause of the hair loss, rarely do raw spots or patches of exposed skin appear. If they do, another cause of the hair loss should be suspected. If the dog or cat is of the type that sheds excessively, be sure to brush it daily to remove the dead hairs and make way for the new ones. Failure to do so can predispose the pet to skin infections.

Any event that is associated with abnormally high amounts of stress can cause increases in shedding activity and, in some cases, overt alopecia. A good example of this is a female dog undergoing pregnancy or lactation. The physiological stress and demands placed her body might lead to an accelerated hair-loss situation. Fortunately, in most instances, the hair will return once the stress abates.

Malnutrition

The hair cycle in dogs and cats is dynamic and active, with new hairs constantly growing in to replace old, dead hairs that are naturally shed. These new hairs require a bounty of protein and other nutrients for their proper formation and development. If these are not supplied, the replacement hairs might not grow in at all, or they might be weak, brittle, and easily broken. As a result, dogs and cats suffering from poor nutrition often have scanty, lackluster haircoats, not to mention unhealthy skin. Since the source of the problem is internal in nature, the distribution of this hair loss tends to be symmetric over the entire body.

Feeding the wrong type of diet is not the only way to cause nutrition-related hair loss. Failure to have a pet checked routinely for internal parasites can also lead to malnutrition secondary to parasitism. Because intestinal parasites can steal vital nutrients, the haircoat can become deprived of essential nutrients and bear the brunt of the consequences.

Obviously, providing quality nutrition and correcting any internal parasite problems that might exist are the two key means of restoring normal hair growth in these cases.

Itching

Virtually all the disorders that cause itching can cause loss of hair as well. This hair loss might be due to self-trauma from licking, chewing, and/or scratching, or it might be secondary to inflammation affecting the hair follicle (e.g., *Demodex*, folliculitis). The distribution of the hair loss can be localized or diffuse, symmetric or asymmetric, depending on the extent of the causative disorder. For instance, if allergies are to blame, the resulting hair loss is often symmetric, affecting both sides equally. On the other hand, hair loss caused by mange or bacterial folliculitis usually appears localized to certain portions of the body at first, although this hair loss can spread to other parts if the disease is left unchecked.

Identifying and correcting the underlying problem are the most important steps to take for restoring the scanty coat (Fig. 14.3). Realize that in many conditions involving inflammation of the hair follicle, the coat might look worse with treatment before it gets better because of treatment-induced shedding of dead or damaged hair. A good plane of nutrition, one that is adequate in protein and fatty acids, will also speed replacement of the lost hair in recovered pets.

Hormonal Imbalance

Symmetric, nonitchy hair loss in middle-aged to older dogs might be the result of hormonal disturbances within the body. Abnormally low amounts of thyroid hormone, deficiencies in insulin, and/or unusually

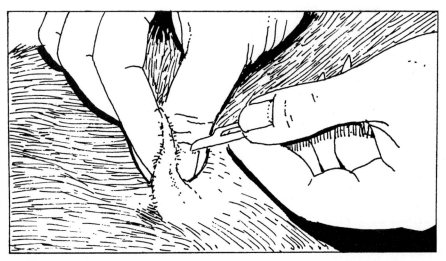

FIGURE 14.3   A special test called a "skin scraping" is needed to definitively diagnose mange in a dog.

high amounts of steroid hormones in circulation can all cause this type of alopecia. Although one would expect to see other signs associated with such disorders, this is not always the case. Regardless of which hormone(s) is (are) involved, stabilization and normalization of their circulating levels within the body are needed to correct the existing alopecia.

Imbalances in circulating amounts of sex hormones (estrogen and testosterone) have also been implicated in some cases of alopecia. *Feline endocrine alopecia* is one example of this in cats. Seen in neutered male and female cats, this condition is characterized by a nonitchy, symmetric hair loss affecting the abdomen, thighs, and posterior region; however, the underlying skin in these areas appears healthy and unaffected. Diagnosis of this disorder is based on ruling out other potential causes of hair loss and on experiencing a positive response to therapy. Treatment using special drugs can sometimes help stimulate hair regrowth in these cats.

Ringworm

Fungal infections involving the skin and hair can cause hair loss without associated itching. Certainly the most prevalent fungal infection affecting the integument of dogs and cats is ringworm. For more information on ringworm, see Chapter 6.

Treatment of Hair Loss

As illustrated, itching and hair loss can be a complex challenge to diagnose and treat. Owners should no longer ignore or simply blame external parasites in all cases of itchy or balding pets. A complete and thorough history provided to a veterinarian, combined with the vet's dermatological examination, are important first steps in all cases of problem itching and/or alopecia.

Seborrhea

The term *seborrhea* refers to an abnormality in the normal turnover of skin cells, which can lead to excessive secretion of sebum by the sebaceous glands in the skin. Dogs and cats afflicted with seborrhea might have dry, flaky skin (seborrhea sicca), or, if the sebaceous glands are active, greasy skin with a rancid odor to it (seborrhea oleosa). Itching and infections can also be unpleasant components of both types.

Seborrhea can be caused by a number of diseases, including allergies, fleas, and, in dogs, poor thyroid function. It can also be a primary disease entity, with no apparent underlying cause. Cocker spaniels and Doberman pinschers are two examples of breeds that can suffer from primary seborrhea.

Diagnosis of a seborrheic condition is not difficult; what can be challenging is determining the underlying problems if they exist. Laboratory tests, including skin biopsies, might be needed to determine whether the seborrhea is primary or secondary. By knowing which it is, the better the chances are that the treatment will be successful.

Successful treatment of seborrhea depends on correcting any underlying sources (secondary seborrhea), and then focusing attention on normalizing the abnormal cell turnover occurring in the skin. Special medicated shampoos containing chlorhexidine, tar and sulfur, and/or selenium disulfide have all been used to clear up infections and remove dead epithelial cells and excessive oils associated with seborrhea.

In cases of dry seborrhea, moisturizing skin rinses and fatty-acid supplements (available from veterinarians) can be helpful. In especially tough cases, prednisolone can be used to lessen the severity of signs and help stop the itching.

Because of its inherent nature, a complete cure will rarely be afforded in those cases of primary seborrhea. However, veterinary researchers are looking with interest at new treatments for primary seborrhea, including retinoid therapy. Although research is still ongoing, the results so far at least look promising.

Acanthosis Nigricans (Dogs)

Acanthosis nigricans is a hormonal condition seen primarily in dachshunds and cocker spaniels, and characterized by hair loss, increased pigmentation, and thickening of the skin. This increased pigmentation usually begins in the armpit region and spreads to the chest and other regions of the body. As the skin thickens, it becomes itchy and inflamed. Seborrhea and secondary bacterial skin infection could also result.

The exact cause of this disease is unknown, but a hormonal imbalance resulting in increases in the melanin pigment is suspect. Hyperthyroidism, although rare in dogs, must be ruled out as the cause of the increased pigmentation; so must allergic skin disorders. Skin biopsies can be used to help confirm or rule out cases of acanthosis nigricans.

Treatment of acanthosis nigricans is nonspecific, using cortico steroids to reduce pain and inflammation, and antibiotics to combat skin infection. Aloe vera gels applied topically can also be used to soothe and comfort irritated regions. Finally, if seborrhea is present, antiseborrheic shampoos should be used on a weekly or twice-weekly basis.

Bacterial Skin Disease

Bacterial skin disease in dogs and cats seldom occurs unless there is some underlying disorder promoting it. Trauma, malnutrition, parasitism, hormonal abnormalities, and immune system malfunctions can all predispose to the proliferation of bacteria on the skin.

Healthy skin has several mechanisms by which it resists infectious organisms. A dry, outer layer of keratin, combined with periodic shedding of dead skin cells, helps discourage population of the skin surface with harmful bacteria. Even sebum, produced by the sebaceous glands of the skin, is antibacterial at normal concentrations. Finally, a normal population of bacteria that resides on the skin surface and in the hair follicles competitively inhibits the growth of disease-causing bacteria.

Problems can start to occur when the integument becomes traumatized, or underlying disease alters the normal integrity of the skin. If the skin's defenses are penetrated in such a way, disease-causing bacteria found naturally in the environment can set up housekeeping.

Superficial bacterial skin disease can take on a number of appearances. These infections are limited to the outermost layers of the skin; however, if left untreated, they can spread to the inner layers, making treatment difficult and lengthy.

DID YOU KNOW ?

Most bacterial skin infections in dogs occur secondary to other underlying disorders.

Acute Moist Dermatitis

Acute moist dermatitis ("hot spots") is characterized by moist, weeping lesions with hair loss and noticeable redness and swelling of the skin. These lesions are quite itchy and painful to the touch, and can spread rapidly over a dog's body if not treated soon enough. Although any breed can be affected, thick-coated breeds such as golden retrievers and chow chows seem to suffer from these the most.

Impetigo

Impetigo, also known as "milk rash," is a bacterial skin disease affecting puppies 6 weeks to 6 months of age. Characterized by small pustule formations, especially in the abdominal region, impetigo is usually an aftereffect of some debilitating disease that stresses the immune system, such as intestinal parasites or viruses. Most puppies seem nonirritated by their presence, and with proper treatment, cases of impetigo clear up very rapidly.

SKIN-FOLD PYODERMAS

Skin-fold pyodermas can strike those breeds with lots of extra skin. This type of infection occurs secondary to moisture, warmth, and friction occurring within prominent folds of skin. Many breeds and breed crosses can be affected by skin-fold pyoderma. For instance, cocker spaniels can have this problem in their lip region; Pekingese and similar flat-nosed breeds, in the facial region; pugs, in the tail region; and bulldogs and shar-peis, just about anywhere on their bodies! Keeping these areas clean and dry can help discourage this problem. In some cases, plastic surgery to remove the skin fold in question is truly the only way to afford a cure.

DEEP PYODERMAS

Deep pyodermas extending into the depths of the skin layers warrant prompt attention. Unless hit hard with treatment, these infections can spread throughout the body. As mentioned above, superficial pyodermas can easily become deep if neglected.

Juvenile pyoderma is a form of deep pyoderma that can strike young dogs less than 6 months of age. Affected dogs have marked swelling, inflammation, and pain in the facial and ear regions. Lymph nodes in the neck region might be noticeably swollen as a result of such infections, and these dogs are noticeably depressed, sometimes running fevers of up to 104 degrees Fahrenheit. Unless juvenile pyoderma is treated promptly and aggressively, permanent scarring and hair loss around the face and head can be an unfortunate side effect.

Cellulitis and *abscesses* are types of deep pyodermas that appear secondary to tissue injury. Cellulitis involves a poorly defined region of inflammation involving the deeper layers of the skin with no apparent rim or border, whereas abscesses do have a well-demarcated line of surrounding inflammatory cells that make them stand out. Both can be characterized by a painful buildup of pus, and usually cause fever and depression. Both can also lead to blood poisoning if not treated. Because of their isolated nature, veterinarians often lance and flush out abscesses to help speed the healing process.

Other types of deep pyoderma are named for the region of the body affected. These include nasal pyoderma, interdigital or foot pyoderma, and elbow callus pyoderma. *Generalized pyoderma* refers to a deep bacterial infection involving all areas of the body.

Folliculitis

Folliculitis is bacterial infection that affects the hair follicles. Because the hair within the follicle suffers from the infection, the coats of dogs and cats with folliculitis often develop a moth-eaten appearance as the damaged hair falls out. In addition, as the inflammation progresses, pustules and small crusty lesions often form over the hair follicles. The amount of itching seen with folliculitis can range from mild to severe. One special type of folliculitis, called *bacterial hypersensitivity,* is a type of allergic reaction to the bacteria residing on the skin. Dogs affected with bacterial hypersensitivity exhibit severe itching and hair loss. In fact, because the hair loss is usually in a circular pattern, bacterial hypersensitivity is often mistaken for a case of ringworm.

Treatment of Bacterial Skin Disease

Prompt treatment of bacterial skin disease is a smart idea to prevent unnecessary complications. For all types, both superficial and deep, there are certain principles that should be followed when treating such diseases.

If there is an underlying cause for the infection, it *must* be identified and corrected first. For instance, if fleas seem to be the source, insecticidal treatment is warranted. If this problem is not controlled, the infection will recur after other treatments are stopped.

Skin lesions should be kept clean and dry at all times. This is especially true for cases of acute moist dermatitis. Astringents (drying agents) should be applied daily to assist in healing and prevent further spread. Many of the ear cleansers available have excellent drying properties and can be used topically for such a purpose. Creams and ointments should not be used on moist skin lesions, since such vehicles are counterproductive to drying efforts. Ideally, bacterial skin lesions should be allowed direct access to surrounding air, which means that the hair in the affected region(s) should be shaved and bandages avoided.

High doses of antibiotics used for extended durations are the mainstay of treatment for bacterial skin infections. Mild, superficial infections might require only 10 to 14 days of medication to afford a cure; severe, deep infections might require antibiotic therapy that can last as long as 8 weeks!

Bacterial resistance to the effects of certain antibiotics has become an unfortunate reality. As a result, do not be surprised if a veterinarian elects to perform a bacterial culture or sensitivity study to determine the exact antibiotics that are effective against that particular infection. If a pet is placed on oral antibiotic therapy for a skin infection, it is imperative that owners complete the entire prescription as directed, even if the skin clears up after only a few days of medication.

Topical therapy for bacterial skin infections is an important adjunct to any treatment regimen. Many medicated shampoos are available that can be used to help speed healing. Those shampoos containing chlorhexidine are preferred, since this substance has excellent antibacterial properties. In some cases, these medicated shampoos should be used daily until the infection is brought under control. For best results, medicated shampoos should be allowed to remain in contact with skin in the affected area(s) for at least 15 minutes before rinsing. Remember to follow all veterinary recommendations concerning the frequency and duration of this type of topical therapy.

Pets should be shampooed and rinsed thoroughly, then dried off completely. This last step is vital because moisture will only serve to promote the infection. If needed, a handheld blow dryer set on low heat can assist in this task.

Medicated creams and ointments are also popular therapeutic additions for pets with skin infections. Triple antibiotic formulations available over the counter or by prescription are preferred, and should be applied three to four times a day to the lesions. As mentioned before, use these products only on lesions that have been properly dried; do not use on moist lesions.

When using a medicated cream or ointment, avoid those preparations containing hydrocortisone or other steroid anti-inflammatories unless specifically prescribed or recommended by veterinarians. Indiscriminate use of such products could actually delay healing and allow the infection to worsen.

Miliary Dermatitis (Cats)

Miliary dermatitis refers to a specific way in which feline skin responds to inflammation and/or irritation. Such a skin reaction is characterized by the formation of tiny, seedlike crusts that frequent the head, neck, and tail regions of the body. In extensive cases, the entire body might be involved. Furthermore, the miliary reaction is quite itchy, and leads to scratching, rubbing, and licking of the affected skin. Hair loss often results as a result of these activities. Often the irritation that miliary dermatitis causes is so great that the affected cat becomes easily agitated and twitches its skin when disturbed or touched.

The potential causes of miliary dermatitis are numerous. Irritation caused by external parasites is the most common cause of localized miliary reactions. Allergies, including food, inhalant, and contact allergies, are other potential causes. In addition, adverse reactions to medications and drugs and fatty-acid deficiencies in the diet have also been implicated as inciting feline miliary dermatitis.

Treatment for feline miliary dermatitis is aimed at correcting the underlying cause of the disorder, if this is known. For those cases in which an underlying cause cannot be identified, treatment with corticosteroids can provide relief from the clinical signs. Antibiotics are rarely necessary, since bacterial infection is rarely a component of this disorder.

Eosinophilic Granuloma Complex (Cats)

This dermatopathy of cats is characterized by the unexplained appearance of red to yellow-brown ulcerated lesions with associated hair loss occurring at various locations around the body. On the average, it tends to strike female cats that are under 6 years of age.

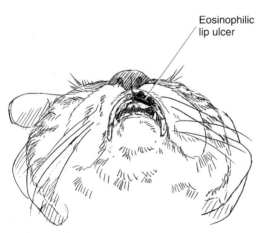

Eosinophilic lip ulcer

When the raised, well-demarcated reddish ulcers appear on the lips of affected felines, they are termed *eosinophilic ulcers* or "rodent ulcers" (Fig. 14.4). Linear granulomas are eosinophilic granulomas that can occur anywhere on the body, but usually on the

FIGURE 14.4 Eosinophilic lip ulcers appear as red, angry lesions.

back portion of the hind legs. These ulcerations are yellowish to pink in appearance, and, as the name implies, they tend to run in a straight line down the affected portion of skin.

With both eosinophilic ulcers and linear granulomas, pain and itching do not appear to be significant factors. However, prompt treatment is still important, since some of these lesions, especially eosinophilic ulcers, can evolve to skin cancer if left alone.

Eosinophilic plaques are types of eosinophilic granuloma that are associated with intense itching. These well-demarcated, raised ulcers are often bright red in appearance and show up primarily on the abdomen and on the upper, inside portions of the back legs. Cats so affected will often lick constantly at the lesions because of the irritation and itching that they cause.

Diagnosis of eosinophilic granuloma complex in cats is routinely made on physical exam and on microscopic examination of cells or tissues from the lesions. Treatment employs corticosteroids given orally or by injection for 3 to 4 weeks. In cases that don't respond to standard treatment, alternate therapy such as radiation therapy may be used in an effort to bring the lesions under control. As with miliary dermatitis, antibiotics are rarely necessary to afford a cure unless a secondary infection is present.

Feline Acne

Superficial bacterial skin disease in cats can take on a number of appearances. Feline acne is perhaps the most common type seen in veterinary circles. This disease is characterized by infection of the hair follicles and the appearance of blackheads and/or pustules on the chins of affected cats. Although the exact cause of this disorder remains unknown, many researchers feel that it is due to the cat's inability to adequately groom this area.

Treatment for feline acne consists of clipping the hair away from the chin and scrubbing the chin daily with a mild antibacterial solution containing benzoyl peroxide or chlorhexidine. Afterward, a drying agent such as alcohol or ear-cleansing solution should be applied to the chin. In severe instances, systemic antibiotics might be required to completely clear up an infection.

As far as other superficial skin infections are concerned, any at-home treatment that uses topical antibacterial creams or ointments should be first approved by a veterinarian. Avoid those preparations containing hydrocortisone or other steroid compounds. In cases where the infection is spreading or is not responding to topical medications, then oral antibiotics will be required.

Neurodermatitis (Cats)

Feline neurodermatitis results in hair loss and/or skin irritation due to nervous licking and chewing. The highly emotional breeds of cats, such as Siamese and Himalayan, are more prone to this disease than others.

This nervous licking and chewing can be triggered by any disruption or stress in the cat's normal daily routine, such as moving into a new home or introducing a new addition to the family. The lesions caused by this abnormal grooming activity can resemble eosinophilic ulcers, or it might present itself as a "stripe" of hair loss on the back or sides of the body (Fig. 14.5). Often the hair loss resembles that seen with ringworm.

A diagnosis of neurodermatitis is made after carefully examining the history of occurrence, plus ruling out other causes of similar dermatological signs. If possible, eliminating or correcting the inciting cause is the best way to treat neurodermatitis. In difficult cases, therapy using antianxiety or mood-altering drugs might be necessary to calm the nervous feline and prevent self-trauma to the skin and coat.

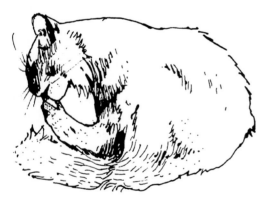

FIGURE 14.5 Cats suffering from neurodermatitis harbor characteristic lesions.

Solar Dermatitis

Initiated by the ultraviolet rays of the sun, solar dermatitis can occur in cats and dogs with insufficient skin pigmentation to block the harmful effects of sunlight. Cats with white haircoats (or those with white ears and/or white faces) and dogs with pink noses that live in hot, sunny climates are most prone to this dermatopathy.

In cats, lesions usually begin at the tips and margins of the ears, yet they can also appear on the eyelids, nose, and/or lips. Hair loss, scabs, and ulcerations characterize these lesions. If left unattended, the affected skin can eventually become cancerous, and metastasize to other parts of the body.

Diagnosis of solar dermatitis is confirmed through surgically obtaining a biopsy sample of the affected areas. Treatment is geared toward reducing exposure to the sun's rays via indoor confinement and through the use of commercial sunscreen products. Corticosteroids applied topically can also help reduce any associated inflammation. For those lesions suspect of becoming cancerous, surgical removal (if possible) and/or radiation therapy is needed to prevent its spread.

Skin Lumps and Masses

Whenever a lump or mass appears on/or beneath the skin of a dog or cat, five possibilities exist as to its source:

1. An abscess

2. A hematoma or seroma

3. A cyst

4. A granuloma

5. A tumor

Obviously, because the cause can vary, owners will need to employ the help of a veterinarian for identification of the mass. A fine-needle aspirate of the mass or an actual biopsy sample will assist the vet in a diagnosis (Fig. 14.6).

Abscesses

Abscesses are usually painful to the touch and are often associated with other signs, such as fever, depression, and loss of appetite. They also

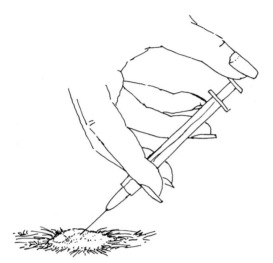

FIGURE 14.6 Cell and fluid samples taken from an unidentified lump can be used to assist in a definitive diagnosis.

tend to be fluctuant when direct pressure is applied to them. Abscesses are seen in cats more often than dogs.

Hematomas and Seromas

Hematomas and seromas result from leakage of blood or serum, respectively, from damaged blood vessels. Traumatic blows to the skin can result in hematoma or seroma formation beneath the affected area of skin. The swellings caused by these lesions are also fluctuant, and because of the traumatic nature of their occurrence, they can be painful as well.

In most cases, the swellings caused by hematomas and seromas will resolve on their own with time, assuming that infection does not occur in the meantime.

Cysts

A *cyst* is simply a well-defined pocket filled with fluid, secretion, or inflammatory debris. Unlike abscesses, cysts are seldom painful to the touch.

Sebaceous cysts or epidermoid cysts develop within the skin of dogs when the sebum normally formed within sebaceous glands is not allowed to escape. There does seem to be a breed predisposition for this problem, with cocker spaniels, springer spaniels, terriers, and shepherds most commonly affected.

Sebaceous cysts can arise in multiple locations over the body of these dogs, and can constantly recur throughout the life of the pet. Although they pose no specific danger to the health of a dog, extra large cysts should be surgically excised.

Granulomas

Granulomas are firm, raised masses consisting chiefly of inflammatory cells sent to the particular area by the body in response to skin penetration by a foreign substance or infectious agent. In essence, the body attempts to quickly surround and wall off the foreign invader before it can spread to other parts of the body. Thorns, insect stingers, vaccines, fungal organisms, and certain bacteria are only a few of the things that can trigger granuloma formation.

If a pet develops one of these growths, an attempt should be made to determine the cause of its appearance. If an infectious agent is suspected, appropriate antimicrobial therapy is warranted to prevent further development of the granuloma.

Granulomas might recede with time, depending on the cause. In some cases, surgical removal of the mass gets rid of the unsightly lump and its cause all at the same time.

Tumors

Skin tumors or cancers can appear in a variety of types, sizes, and shapes. Common tumors that might appear as a lump or mass on or beneath the skin include sebaceous adenomas, lipomas, carcinomas, fibrosarcomas, and mast cell tumors. It is imperative that a biopsy is performed in all instances to determine whether the tumor is malignant.

Sebaceous gland tumors are among the most prevalent of all skin tumors in dogs. These wartlike growths are especially common in cocker spaniels and poodles. They can appear anywhere on the body, including the eyelids. The vast majority of these growths are benign and cause no problems whatsoever, unless they become traumatized as a result of sheer size. Excision of these tumors is curative locally, but others often appear elsewhere with time.

Lipomas are benign, soft, fatty tumors that often form beneath the skin of dogs and cause noticeable lumps. They occur with greater frequency in older dogs that have weight problems. Although a diagnosis of lipoma might seem obvious, a fine-needle aspirate should always be performed to rule out the presence of its less common malignant counterpart, liposarcoma.

Lipomas can be surgically removed, yet because they can infiltrate into the muscle bundles and surrounding tissue, this removal might be unknowingly incomplete and the tumor might recur. As a result, many practitioners will choose to remove only those lipomas that are extralarge or those diagnosed as malignant.

Fibrosarcomas in cats have been known to occur infrequently after certain vaccines are administered. As a result, any lump that appears 2 to 6 weeks following vaccination should be brought to the attention of a veterinarian.

Mammary tumors are relatively common in intact dogs. Treatment involves surgical removal of the affected gland(s). For extensive tumors, chemotherapy might also be employed.

It is imperative that a biopsy be performed on all firm lumps to determine whether or not a tumor exists. For more information on cancer and its treatment, see Chapter 43.

The Eyes and Ears

THE EYES

The visual acuity of the average dog (see anatomy of the canine eye in Fig. 15.1) has been compared to that of a human at sunset. Most see only generalized forms rather than distinct images or features. Exceptions to this rule include the sight hounds (greyhounds, afghans), which indeed have keen eyesight.

Contrary to popular belief, dogs might not be as colorblind as people think. In fact, the canine eye possesses all of those structures necessary to perceive their world in color. Now, whether they take full advantage of this is still a matter of speculation. It seems, however, that since the sense of sight is not as vital to most dogs as, let's say, the sense of smell, there might be no real need for color perception.

The sense of vision is important to nocturnal hunters such as the cat, more so than their canine counterparts. Unique adaptations of the feline eye allow for this greater visual acuity. For instance, the unique slit-shaped design of the feline pupil allows it to dilate exceptionally wide in dimly lit surroundings. In addition, the ability to focus in on objects and to detect even the slightest of movements is highly refined.

Certainly such visual characteristics account for the effectiveness of the feline as a hunter. As do dogs' eyes, cats' eyes also posses those structures necessary to perceive the world in color. As far as visual

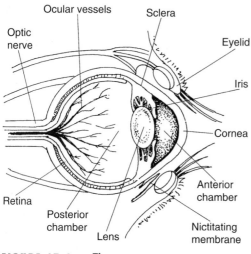

Ocular vessels   Sclera
Optic nerve
Eyelid
Iris
Cornea
Anterior chamber
Retina
Posterior chamber
Nictitating membrane
Lens

FIGURE 15.1   The eye.

DID YOU KNOW⁇

Color receptors in the eyes of cats and dogs enable them to see their world in greens and blues, and any combinations thereof.

---

capabilities are concerned, one interesting breed to take note of is the Siamese cat. Although anatomically their eyes differ little if at all from those of their brethren, research has revealed that they might perceive their world a little bit differently. While binocular vision (visualizing one scene with both eyes) is the standard for humans and most animals, Siamese cats might actually visualize two different presentations for the same scene—one for each eye. Confusing? Imagine a set of keys sitting on a countertop. That is what a person would see, a set of keys. A Siamese cat, on the other hand, might visualize two sets of keys because each eye is focusing in on the set separately. Because of this apparent lack of binocular vision, depth perception is not as refined in this breed as with others. Could all this explain the unique behavior exhibited by this fanciful breed?

Anatomy and Physiology

Each eye is housed within a bony socket of the skull, and is surrounded by an upper eyelid and a lower eyelid. In addition, a nictitating membrane, or third eyelid, is located on the inside corner of each eye. Serving a protective function similar to that of the conventional lids, this third eyelid will passively extrude over the eye in the event of injury or illness. Special glands lining the inside portion of this lid also bear significance in the disease condition in dogs known as "cherry eye."

The conjunctiva is the delicate membrane seen lining the pink inner portion of the eyelid and a substantial portion of the eyeball itself. *Conjunctivitis* is the term applied to inflammation involving this membrane. It often results in red, weeping eyes.

The white portion of the eyeball is properly termed the *sclera.* Changes in the color of the sclera can be indicative of underlying disease. For instance, a sclera that is yellow-tinged could reflect a serious underlying liver or bleeding disorder.

The *cornea* is the clear, transparent structure at the front of the eye through which the colored iris and black pupil can be seen. When light passes through the cornea, it enters into the fluid-filled anterior chamber of the eye, which is located between the cornea and the iris.

Monitoring the pressure maintained within the eyes by this fluid is a valuable diagnostic tool for the veterinarian trying to diagnose eye disorders in pets. For instance, *glaucoma,* or increased pressure within the eye, is a serious disease that can lead to blindness if not treated promptly. It can originate as a result of increased amounts of this anterior chamber fluid. On the contrary, a decreased pressure reading signifies active inflammation within the eye itself (uveitis), prompting appropriate treatment measures.

The *iris* is the structure that contains the pigment that gives the eye its characteristic color. In dogs, brown is by far the dominant eye color seen, with a few blue eyes interspersed here and there.

The *pupil* is a hole formed by the iris. The size of the pupil is determined by the contraction and expansion of the iris in response to varying degrees of light. Thus, the iris serves to regulate the amount of light that is actually allowed into the eye. Injury or illness can affect pupil size. For example, poisonings caused by organophosphate insecticides can cause the pupils to be pinpoint in size. Furthermore, pupils that are unequal in size can be indicators of a primary neurological disease, including disorders of the middle ear.

Once through the pupil, light enters into the posterior chamber of the eye, containing the lens and the retina.

FACT or FICTION

Night vision in cats is far superior to that of humans **FACT**. This assumes, however, that the moon is up. In pitch darkness, cats can see no better than we do!

The lens serves to gather incoming light and then focus it in on the retina, which lines the back surface of the eye. Special fibers attaching to the lens allow it to change sizes to accommodate for distances.

The *retina* contains a multitude of nerve endings that, when stimulated by light, send nervous impulses which feed into the optic disk and then into the brain. The end result is a visualized, perceived image. The appearance of the retina can be altered by a variety of disease states, offering valuable diagnostic insight to the veterinarian attempting to pinpoint the source of an illness.

The *tapetum* is a specially pigmented structure that lines the back surface of the eye along with the retina. The tapetum serves as a light-gathering, reflective device that improves night vision in the dog and cat. It is responsible for the characteristic green color seen when light from approaching automobile headlights or other sources reflect off of it.

Corneal Ulcers

The transparent cornea enclosing the front portion of the eye is a remarkable organ in itself. Responsible for gathering light and directing it into the eye, healthy corneas are essential for proper vision. It stands to reason, then, that ulcerations (loss of surface epithelium) or scratches involving one or more corneal surfaces can seriously threaten eyesight if not managed promptly.

Corneal ulcerations in dogs and cats can occur secondary to poor tear production, entropion or ectropion, dust and foreign debris in the eye(s), nail scratches and other direct trauma, and infections.

Some of the most common sources of corneal ulceration seen by veterinarians are soap or shampoo burns caused by inadequate eye protection when bathing. Pet owners should always apply a sterile ophthalmic ointment to their pet's eyes prior to any procedure that involves potentially caustic substances around the eyes. Since corneas are so sensitive, even shampoos with touted "no tears" formulations should never be used without applying this protection first.

Clinical signs of a corneal ulcer include squinting and aversion to light, ocular discharge, and obvious discomfort, often signified by pawing at or rubbing the affected eye. A change in the normal color or transparency of the corneal surface is also an indicator that something is wrong.

Definitive diagnosis of a corneal ulcer is made by veterinarians using special fluorescein dyes to stain the corneal surfaces. Dead, diseased corneal tissue will readily take up such stains whereas healthy tissue will not.

Fortunately, the cornea is one organ that will heal quite rapidly if treatment is administered quickly and vigorously (Fig. 15.2). For ulcers involving only the superficial layers of the cornea, topical antibiotic ointments or solutions designed for use in the eyes and applied three to six times daily will help speed healing.

Of course, if an underlying cause, such as foreign debris, still exists in the eye, it must be removed before proper healing can take place. Superficial ulcers can heal in 36 to 48 hours with proper treatment applied.

Deep Corneal Ulcerations

Deep corneal ulcerations are treated the same way that superficial ulcerations are, yet these require close observation for progression or worsening of the ulcer. Bacterial cultures of such ulcers are necessary to be certain that the antibiotics being used are effective against any organisms involved.

For deep ulcers that worsen or fail to respond to conventional treatment, additional procedures might be necessary to speed healing or to prevent the cornea from actually rupturing. A favorite procedure among veterinarians consists of surgically freeing and extending a portion of the thin conjunctiva over the ulcer and actually tacking it down against the ulcer using suture material (conjunctival

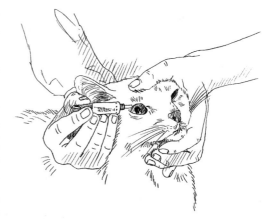

FIGURE 15.2   Whenever applying eye ointment, keep the tip of the tube parallel to the eye to prevent accidental injury if your cat moves.

flap). The flap of conjunctiva provides nutrition and speeds healing to the ulcer, and also allows any medications applied directly to the eye(s) to reach the ulcer without hindrance. Once healing has been accomplished, the flap is released, and excess conjunctival tissue is trimmed away from the healed surface.

Special contact lenses and/or corneal tissue adhesives can also be applied over the damaged surface of the cornea. These serve to protect it from further degradation and help promote rapid healing. For difficult ulcers, actual grafts using fresh or frozen corneal tissue may be required.

Conjunctivitis

Inflammation of the thin, transparent mucous membrane lining the inner portion of the eyelids and front part of the sclera is termed *conjunctivitis.* Conjunctivitis is the most common cause of "red eyes" in dogs and cats. Other signs seen with conjunctivitis include discharge, swelling, and pain.

The type of discharge present can sometimes give a clue as to the underlying cause of the conjunctivitis. For instance, a watery discharge can indicate irritation from an allergy, virus (canine distemper or feline rhinotracheitis), or contact with dirt or dust; a mucuslike discharge often links the problem to abnormal tear formation ("dry eye") or to a bacterial infection, either primary or secondary to any of the causes previously mentioned.

Because conjunctivitis can be secondary to other problems, diagnostic tests performed by veterinarians should be directed at identifying any underlying causes. Corneal staining using a fluorescent stain is usually performed to determine whether the cornea is affected. In dogs, if a mucuslike discharge is present, a tear flow test should be performed to rule out "dry eye" as the cause of the conjunctivitis.

In cases of conjunctivitis that don't respond to conventional therapy, a bacterial culture or sensitivity test should be performed to be sure treatment measures being used are correct.

Treatment of conjunctivitis is aimed at treating or eliminating any inciting causes, and at controlling the localized inflammation. If dust or pollens are the source of the conjunctivitis, daily flushing of the eyes with a sterile saline solution designed for use in the eyes or daily application of a sterile ophthalmic lubricant can help reduce the irritation caused by these offenders.

Ophthalmic drops or ointments containing antibiotics are necessary if a bacterial infection is present (Fig. 15.3). In addition, ophthalmic preparations containing steroids can be used to reduce the inflammation present, provided the surface of the cornea is intact. Preparations containing both antibiotics and steroid compounds for use in the eyes are readily available for pets through a prescription from a veterinarian.

Glaucoma

Glaucoma is a condition characterized by an increase in fluid pressure from the aqueous humor within the eye(s). In the normal eye, pressure and aqueous levels are maintained at a constant plateau by the continual drainage of excess aqueous humor out of the eye through tiny ports (drainage angles) located where the edge of the iris meets the cornea. If this drainage is obstructed or altered in any way, a rise in pressure within the eye can result. Unfortunately, even short-term rises in this pressure can lead to irreversible damage if not detected and treated in a timely fashion.

Conditions such as a buildup of inflammatory material within the eye, luxation of the lens due to trauma or cataracts, and *synechia,* where the iris "sticks" to the lens or cornea, can all effectively prevent the normal drainage of the aqueous humor from the eye.

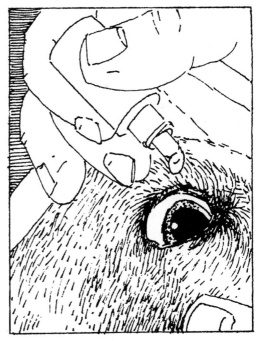

FIGURE 15.3   Antibiotic drops can be used to combat conjunctivitis.

Heredity is also thought to play a role in some cases of glaucoma in dogs, with basset hounds, beagles, and cocker spaniels having a higher incidence of the disease due to improper development of the drainage angles. In addition, a predisposition for lens luxation has been identified along family lines for many of the terrier breeds, predisposing them to glaucoma. Finally, allergies and overactive immune system responses are also thought to be important precursors to glaucoma in dogs and cats.

Clinical signs of a glaucomatous eye include a marked redness affecting both the conjunctival tissue and the sclera; a blue, hazy cornea; a dilated, unresponsive pupil; and apparent blindness due to the pressure the fluid is placing on the optic nerve. In instances where the glaucoma has been present for quite some time, enlargement of the affected eyeball might become noticeable, and actual rupture of the cornea could occur.

Diagnosis of glaucoma can be easily confirmed by a veterinarian through the use of an instrument called a *tonometer*. This instrument, when placed directly on the surface of the cornea, measures the exact pressure within the eye (Fig. 15.4). If the pressure reading is indeed elevated, then treatment should be instituted immediately to prevent lasting damage to the eye.

Treatment for glaucoma is aimed at decreasing the pressure within the eye to an acceptable level as quickly as possible, and then stabilizing this pressure to prevent future increases.

Drugs designed to quickly draw fluid out of the eye and into the bloodstream will initially be used to reduce the pressure within a pet's eye(s). Other drugs that act by decreasing the production of aqueous humor and by increasing the size of the drainage angles are then prescribed for the long-term management and prevention of recurrence. At the same time, anti-inflammatory medications can be used topically on the eye to clear up any primary or secondary inflammation that might be aggravating the glaucoma.

In instances where a luxated lens is causing the increase in pressure, surgical removal of the offending lens should always be performed. Cryotherapy (freezing) can be used as well. This involves surgically inserting a special needle within the eye and freezing the cells within the eye responsible for the production of aqueous humor. With this technique, aqueous production can be reduced by up to 30 percent in some patients.

Cataracts

An opacity involving the lens of the eye that prevents light from reaching the retina is termed a *cataract.* Cataracts can be inherited (juvenile cataracts) or might develop secondary to eye trauma, infections, or metabolic disease, such as diabetes mellitus. As lens opacity increases, the amount of light allowed to reach the retina is diminished, and partial blindness ensues.

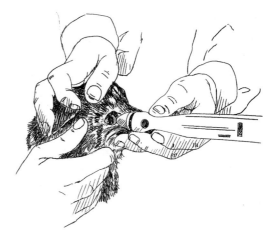

FIGURE 15.4   Testing for glaucoma.

Cataracts can also predispose to rotation or luxation of the lens. Such lens movement can disrupt normal fluid flow within the eye and lead to secondary glaucoma.

True cataracts must be differentiated from lenticular sclerosis seen in older pets. *Lenticular sclerosis* is a lens opacity caused by a normal hardening of the lens material due to age. It is a normal aging change seen in some dogs, and rarely leads to loss of sight as can occur with cataracts. As a result, no specific treatment is required for most cases of lenticular sclerosis. Lenticular sclerosis and cataracts can be differentiated with an ophthalmologic examination performed by a veterinarian.

Treatment for cataracts usually involves surgical removal of the offending lens. A less invasive surgical technique for cataract removal is called *phacofragmentation.* This procedure employs the use of ultrasound to break up the lens material into small pieces, which can then be drawn or sucked out of the eye using special instrumentation. Once cataracts are removed, vision is effectively restored in the affected pet.

Keratoconjunctivitis Sicca (Dry Eye)

Seen primarily in dogs, *keratoconjunctivitis sicca* (KCS), or "dry eye," is a condition affecting the cornea and conjunctiva of the eye resulting from inadequate tear production. Actually, only the water portion of the tear film is deficient; the mucus portion is still produced in adequate quantities. This leads to the characteristic green, mucoid buildup in and around eyes affected with KCS. The lack of adequate tear moisture also predisposes the cornea to damage and ulcers. Long-term sequelae include pigmentation of the corneal surface and blindness.

KCS can have a number of underlying causes. In many breeds— such as Yorkshire terriers, schnauzers, cocker spaniels, bulldogs, and beagles—KCS can be an inherited trait. Other potential causes include canine distemper, certain medications (such as sulfa drugs), hypothyroidism, diabetes mellitus, and autoimmune disease.

Diagnosis of KCS is made using tear flow tests to determine the amount of tear production (Fig. 15.5). Treatment of KCS involves the use of tear replacement drops, followed by an application of a tear replacement ointment to seal in the drops. These replacements must be applied every 3 to 4 hours to be truly effective. If infection or inflammation is present, antibiotics and anti-inflammatory medications should be instilled into the eyes as well.

Medications designed to stimulate more tear production have been used for treatment in the past with varying success. Also, the drug cyclosporine can be quite effective at stimulating renewed tear production in some dogs with KCS. For more information on cyclosporine, owners should contact their pets' veterinarians.

In especially advanced cases of KCS, surgical intervention might become necessary. The standard surgical treatment used, called *parotid duct transposition,* involves repositioning a duct from a salivary gland to the corner of the affected eye(s), thereby providing a constant source of moisture (saliva) to the eye.

Retinal Degeneration and Disease

Retinal degeneration and disease can be a cause of blindness in dogs and cats. For instance, *progressive retinal atrophy* (PRA) is a hereditary condition that can strike middle-aged to older dogs and produce blindness over a period of several months to years. Breeds that are predisposed to this condition include Gordon setters, Irish setters, poodles, Norwegian elkhounds, Labrador retrievers, collies, cocker spaniels, and malamutes. Characterized by a slow degeneration of the receptor cells composing the retina, PRA in its early stages often leads to nightblindness in affected dogs. These dogs tend to fear or shy away from poorly lit areas. As PRA progresses, it eventually causes the pupils to remain dilated and fail to respond to light, causing complete blindness.

Retinal function may also be partially or completely lost due to underlying disease or injury. For example, glaucoma affecting an eye can place so much pressure on the

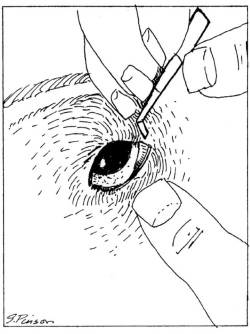

FIGURE 15.5   Special test strips can be used to check for tear production in suspected cases of "dry eye."

blood vessels supplying the retina of that eye that secondary retinal degeneration results. *Sudden acquired retinal degeneration* (SARD) is another nonhereditary condition that can cause blindness in dogs, yet its exact cause remains a mystery. Interestingly, this disease is often accompanied by an increase in thirst and in appetite in those dogs so affected. Infectious diseases, such as ehrlichiosis and Rocky Mountain spotted fever, and fungi can also adversely affect the region of the retina where the optic nerve exits, leading to inflammation and subsequent loss of vision. In addition, neoplasms such as lymphosarcoma can infiltrate the retinas of dogs and cats and inhibit retinal function. Finally, trauma, immune-mediated diseases, and certain toxins can cause retinal injury and lead to blindness.

Diagnosis of retinal disease and degeneration is made using history, physical exam findings, and information obtained from an ophthalmic examination of the retinas themselves. In addition, an *electroretinogram,* which measures the electrical activity taking place within the retinas, will provide a definitive diagnosis of retinal degeneration and retinal blindness. If a disease condition such as glaucoma, infection, neoplasia, or toxicity is suspected, other diagnostic testing procedures specific to these conditions may be required as well to confirm a diagnosis.

Unfortunately, there are presently no known treatments for PRA and SARD, and the prognosis remains grave for the restoration of sight in affected dogs. Other diseases involving the retina may respond favorably to treatments specific for the particular disorder; however, it must be remembered that the longer such treatments are delayed or neglected, the greater the chances are of permanent loss of vision.

Prolapse of the Third-Eyelid Gland (Cherry Eye)

The third eyelid of dogs contains a gland that might occasionally become inflamed and protrude over the edge of the third eyelid, producing a classic "cherry eye" appearance. Certain breeds—such as the cocker spaniel, Lhasa apso, Pekingese, and beagle—seem to be more predisposed to this condition than others.

In the past, treatment for a prolapsed gland of the third eyelid involved complete surgical removal of the gland. However, researchers agree that the gland might play an important role in tear production; hence, complete removal of the gland might predispose a pet to keratoconjunctivitis sicca. As a result, newer surgical procedures involve removal of only a portion of the gland, or actually tacking down the prolapsed portion of the gland to the inner surface of the third eyelid.

Entropion

Entropion is an ophthalmic condition in which the eyelids roll inward, allowing lashes and hair to irritate the surface of the eyes. The condition is inheritable, or it can occur secondary to other types of eye irritation (spastic entropion) or eyelid injury. Congenital entropion has a high incidence in chow chows, shar-peis, English bulldogs, poodles, and rottweilers.

Signs of entropion include excessive tearing, squinting, constant rubbing of the affected eye(s), excessive redness to the eye(s), and a noticeable inward roll to the eyelid, especially the lower lid.

If a pet is suffering from entropion, surgical treatment might be essential to prevent lasting damage to the surface of the eye(s). Some puppies afflicted with this disorder might outgrow it as they mature; hence, surgery is usually delayed in these young animals until they are at least 6 months old, unless the damage to the eye is severe.

In the meantime, topical lubricants designed to protect the corneas can be used on a daily basis in these patients. In some pups, especially shar-peis, temporary eversion of the offending lids with sutures implanted in the skin of the lids can also help prevent complications until they outgrow the entropion or are old enough for the surgery.

Entropion surgery involves the removal of a flap of skin just beneath (lower lid) or above (upper lid) the inverted lid. Suturing close the resulting gap of skin will then provide enough tension to roll the lid back out. In many instances, more than one surgery is necessary to achieve just the right amount of eversion.

After surgery is performed, care must be taken to prevent the dog from irritating the incision line and causing swelling. Hospitalization for a few days after the procedure is performed will help reduce this occurrence.

Because of the inheritable nature of this disorder, all dogs affected with entropion should be neutered to prevent its passing to future generations. When selecting a new pet, especially one that falls into the high-risk category, owners should examine the pup's parents closely for any signs of entropion or for evidence that surgical correction has been previously performed.

Ectropion

Ectropion is the exact opposite of entropion; it is the outward rolling of the eyelid(s), which exposes the pink conjunctival lining within. As with entropion, this condition is inheritable, with cocker spaniels, St. Bernards, and bloodhounds having a high incidence. Facial nerve paralysis, such as that seen secondary to otitis media, can also result in ectropic lids.

Mild cases of ectropion usually cause no problems whatsoever in affected individuals. Moderate to severe cases are often accompanied by conjunctivitis, excessive lacrimation, and eye discharges.

Keeping the eye(s) clean and free of discharge on a daily basis using saline solution or medicated drops or ointments will help keep minor cases of ectropion under control. For more extensive involvement, surgical correction designed to release the tension placed on the skin of the eyelid, allowing it to roll back to its correct position, might be required.

Masses Involving the Eyelids

The integrity of the eyelids is vital to protect the eyes from environmental hazards. Any disruption or alteration in the normal lid anatomy can place vision in jeopardy. And certain masses involving the lids can do just that if they become large enough.

Chalazions are masses involving the eyelid that originate from the small meibomian glands that line the edge of the lid. They result from a buildup of secretion within the glands due to blockage of the ducts leading from the gland. Chalazions appear as yellow to white swellings beneath the conjunctiva on the inner lid margin. Puncturing or incising these to remove the trapped contents will afford a cure.

Hordeolums are pus-filled masses caused by infections within the meibomian glands or hair follicles lining the lid margin. As with chalazions, these can be punctured and expressed to help speed healing. Topical or systemic antibiotics are also used to eliminate infection.

Tumors that affect the eyelid can be very serious due to the inability to remove them surgically without disrupting the integrity of the lid. Sebaceous gland adenomas are common lid tumors, especially in older dogs. Others include adenocarcinomas, papillomas, and melanomas. As an alternative or adjunct to surgical removal, radiation therapy, chemotherapy, or cryotherapy (freezing) can be used as well, depending upon which type of tumor is involved.

THE EARS

The sense of hearing in the average dog and cat (see anatomy of the ear in Fig. 15.6) is much more fine-tuned than that of a human, allowing it to detect much higher sound pitches. The upper range of hearing is thought to be around 50,000 kilohertz for dogs and 60,000 kilohertz for cats, well above the 20,000-kilohertz norm for people.

Silent dog whistles were invented on the basis of this principle, and the pitch emitted was just above human hearing range but well within that of the dog being summoned. Unfortunately, the high pitch emitted by many of the new electronic flea collars available on the market often falls within the dog and cat's hearing range, raising serious questions as to their safe use.

Anatomy and Physiology

The canine and feline hearing apparatus can be divided into three portions: the inner ear, the middle ear, and the external ear canal and associated structures.

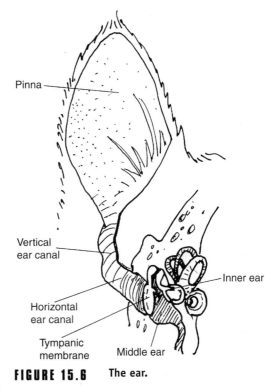

FIGURE 15.6   **The ear.**

The *inner ear* is that portion containing the nerve endings responsible for the sensation of hearing. It also plays a leading role in maintaining balance and equilibrium in your pet (dogs and cats get carsick, too!). The inner ear apparatus lies protected within the bony confines of the skull. The nerves and associated structures within the inner ear are very sensitive and can be damaged through continued exposure to loud, high-pitched noises, infections, and/or toxic medications.

The *middle ear* communicates directly with the inner ear and is contained within a pear-shaped bony cavity originating from the skull called the *tympanic bulla*. This middle-ear cavity is normally filled with air and contains blood vessels and nerves that supply the face and the rest of the head. Inflammation involving the middle ear can adversely affect these nerves, leading to paralysis of the muscles of the face.

The *eardrum,* or *tympanic membrane,* separates the middle ear from the external ear canal. This external canal directly communicates to the outside world, but not without first going through some significant anatomical changes along the way. A horizontal portion of the canal courses a short distance directly away from the eardrum before angling sharply upward (especially in dogs) to form a long vertical portion. This distinct bend has medical significance in that it can lead to the entrapment of wax, hair, and debris deep within the ear, predisposing to inflammation and infection. These substances can be removed by application of a liquid cleansing agent (Fig. 15.7).

The vertical external ear canal—and to a lesser extent, the horizontal ear canal—are lined with special glands that produce ear wax, or cerumen. In the past, cerumen was thought to exert some beneficial antibacterial effects in the ear. Yet research has disproved this and has shown that too much of a waxy buildup can actually promote bacterial growth and infections. In the healthy ear with normal amounts of cerumen produced, this doesn't present much of a problem. Yet when an ear becomes inflamed, wax production increases, and can predispose to infectious complications.

Surrounding the opening of the external ear canals is the earflap, or pinna, which, in dogs, comes in all sorts of sizes and shapes, both natural and synthetic. Each pinna is supported by a sturdy band of cartilage that courses from the vertical ear canal to the tip of each flap. Long droopy earflaps that hang down over the ear openings can effectively cut off proper air circulation within the ear canal (Fig. 15.8); this can potentially lead to ear problems in these dogs unless preventive measures are instituted on a routine basis. Thus, dogs with shorter, more erect pinnae are less likely to develop this condition (Fig. 15.9).

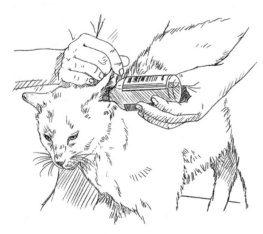

FIGURE 15.7   Commercial ear cleansers can help you keep you pet's ears in tiptop shape.

Otitis Externa

Inflammation involving the external ear canal is called *otitis externa*. It is estimated that up to 20 percent of the dog population in the United States alone suffers from some form of otitis externa. Anatomical features that predispose certain breeds to ear disorders include long, pendulous ears (cocker spaniels), long, narrow ear canals (poodles), and excessive hair within the ear canal which entraps wax and restricts air circulation (poodles). Dogs that spend a lot of time in the water, such as hunting retrievers and

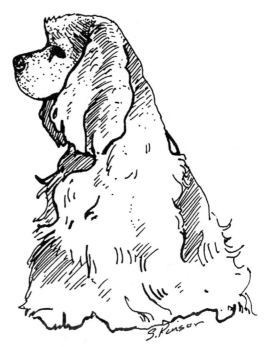

FIGURE 15.8 Long, floppy pinnae can reduce air circulation within the ear canal and predispose the dog to infections.

spaniels, are also prone to otitis externa. Otitis externa is relatively rare in cats, unless it occurs secondary to trauma or to ear mites.

Since the external canals are nothing more than inward extensions of the skin, conceivably anything that can cause skin inflammation can cause otitis externa. This can include allergies, metabolic diseases (hypothyroidism, seborrhea), trauma, foreign bodies such as grass awns and twigs, and parasites such as ticks and mites. Anal sac disease has even been implicated in cases of otitis externa, even though the exact mechanism of involvement is not completely understood.

Signs of otitis externa involving one or both ears include head shaking, itching, painful ears, personality changes, and/or odiferous discharges coming from the ear canal(s). Hair loss might be noticed around the

DID YOU KNOW?

Many chronic ear infections in dogs are caused by allergies.

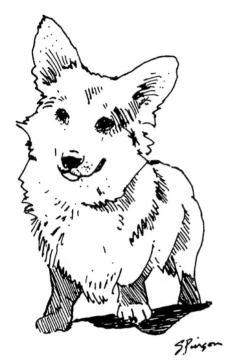

pinnae due to scratching. Aural hematomas might also develop in the wake of such self-trauma.

Diagnosis of otitis externa is based on clinical signs, physical exam, and selected laboratory tests if needed to determine the underlying cause of the inflammation. An otoscopic (ear) exam performed by a veterinarian will help rule out foreign bodies and parasites. This exam is also needed to assess the health of the eardrums. Since many medications cannot be used if the eardrum is torn or ruptured, never attempt to treat otitis externa at home without first having a veterinarian perform this otoscopic exam.

FIGURE 15.9   Dogs with erect ears are less prone to ear problems than are dogs with droopy ears.

The type of medications prescribed by a veterinarian for the treatment of otitis externa will vary, depending on the nature and extent of the causative agent or condition. See Chapter 4 for proper techniques for instilling medications into the ears.

Yeast Infections

Malassezia pachydermatis is the yeast organism most commonly involved in otitis externa. This is not surprising, since *Malassezia* is normally found within the ear canals of healthy dogs and cats, causing no problems whatsoever. However, if inflammation strikes for whatever reason, the yeast takes advantage of a good situation and begins to proliferate. When this growth reaches a certain level, it too can promote inflammation. A characteristic brownish discharge is seen with a buildup of yeast within the ears.

Ear ointments or solutions containing miconazole, thiabendazole, or nystatin can be used to effectively treat yeast infections in the ear. Treating the ears twice daily for 10 to 14 days will clear up most infections.

Because *Malassezia* is considered an opportunist, it is important that the underlying source of the inflammation that led to the yeast infection be identified and treated concurrently.

Bacterial Infections

Failure to detect and treat inflammation within the external ear canal early enough can lead to the establishment of a bacterial infection within the ear. Often, these infections result when the harmless bacteria that normally inhabit the ear are overwhelmed by the inflammation, allowing their not-so-peaceful counterparts to proliferate and take over.

A creamy brown to yellow discharge carrying a foul odor is characteristic of a bacterial disorder within the ear. Bacterial infections can even be found together with yeast infections within the same ear(s), leading to a discharge having characteristics of both types.

If not treated promptly and vigorously, bacterial infections can become firmly entrenched within the ear canal, making a complete cure difficult. For this reason, veterinary practitioners rely heavily on bacterial cultures and sensitivity tests to tell them which bacteria are involved and which antibiotics will be most effective.

Otic preparations containing appropriate antibiotics, often combined with anti-inflammatory medications, are used to combat cases of bacterial otitis externa. Bacteria within the ear have been effectively treated with 5% vinegar (acetic acid) solutions.

If a ruptured eardrum is suspected, selection of treatment agents must be done carefully. For example, antibiotics belonging to the class known as *aminoglycosides* (examples include gentamycin and neomycin) should not be used in the ear directly, since they can cause nerve deafness if exposed to the inner ear. The same holds true for astringent preparations and acetic acid solutions. In addition, if a ruptured eardrum is suspected, only water-soluble treatment solutions should be used. Ointments should be avoided, as they can become entrapped within the middle ear.

In especially severe cases of bacterial otitis, oral antibiotics might be given concurrently with topical ear medications to afford faster results. In chronic longstanding infections that can't be cleared up with antibiotics, a surgical procedure known as a *lateral ear resection* might be necessary to increase the treatment effectiveness. This involves the surgical reconstruction of the external ear canal to eliminate the vertical portion, allowing easy, direct access to the horizontal portion and the eardrum. Although the results might not be the most cosmetic, a lateral ear resection can mean the difference between a life of misery or comfort for a dog afflicted with chronic otitis externa.

Ear Mites

Otodectes cynotis is the mite that most commonly inhabits the ear canals of dogs and cats. These tiny parasites, which are transmitted by close contact with other infected animals, live on the skin surface within the ear and feed on body fluids. Their presence irritates the glands lining the ear canal, leading to an increased cerumen production. Secondary infections with the *Malassezia* yeast are not uncommon, leading to the brown, crusty discharge so often seen with ear mite infestations. In isolated cases, intense allergic reactions to ear mites can occur, causing severe inflammation and secondary infection.

Diagnosis of an ear mite infestation is confirmed by identification of the mites directly on otoscopic exam or through a microscopic examination of an ear swab. Treatment involves the use of medications containing antiparasitic compounds, such as pyrethrins, rotenone, ivermectin, or thiabendazole. Mineral oil has also been employed as a home remedy for killing mites by suffocation. Since secondary yeast infections are commonly found with ear mite infestations, an antiyeast medication should be used concurrently with antimite preparations.

Ear mites can be difficult pests to eliminate (Fig. 15.10). Depending on the

> ## Dr. P's Vet Tip
>
> To help prevent treatment failures and recurrences when treating ear mites in cats, apply a pyrethrin spray to the haircoat at least once a week during the course of treatment. This will kill those industrious mites that may have evacuated the ears prior to or during treatment and are "hiding out" in the haircoat.

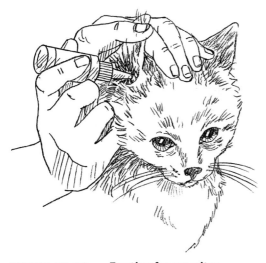

FIGURE 15.10 Treating for ear mites.

medication used, daily treatment for 3 to 4 weeks might be needed to ensure a complete kill. All animals in the household, regardless of whether they are exhibiting signs of infestation, should be treated at the same time. In addition, to prevent reinfestation from the haircoat, an insecticidal spray or shampoo should be used at least twice during the treatment period.

Otitis Media and Interna

Otitis media, infection involving the middle ear, usually results from a chronic, untreated or recurring otitis externa. In such cases, the eardrum might become so diseased as to tear or rupture completely, allowing direct access of infectious organisms into the middle-ear chamber.

The clinical signs of otitis media are essentially the same as those for otitis externa, with a few notable additions. Pets so afflicted will usually exhibit a head tilt toward the side of the affected ear.

In severe cases, paralysis of the facial muscles on the side of the lesion might be seen as the nerves passing through the middle ear become involved. This can result in a characteristic drooping of the eyelids, cheeks, and lips. In addition, a decreased tear production, pinpoint pupil, and protrusion of the third eyelid might be noted in the eye on the affected side.

If the infection extends from the middle ear into the inner-ear apparatus, the signs become even more pronounced. Since the inner ear functions in maintaining balance and equilibrium as well as hearing, pets suffering from otitis interna tend to become very uncoordinated and might fall down frequently or move in circles toward the affected side. A characteristic twitching of the eyeball, called *nystagmus,* also becomes more noticeable.

Although the clinical signs seen are often diagnostic, radiographs of the skull are quite helpful at confirming a diagnosis of otitis media or interna and determining the extent of the disorder.

Therapy for otitis media or interna must be instituted promptly to prevent permanent damage to the hearing apparatus. Oral antibiotics should be started immediately. In cases of otitis interna, continued treatment with antibiotics might be required for up to 30 days to afford a complete cure. In select cases, anti-inflammatory medications have been used to reduce signs associated with inflammation. If not already ruptured, the eardrum on the affected side is usually punctured to allow for thorough drainage of the middle-ear cavity and for the direct infusion of medications. Of course, such treatment steps must be carried out in a veterinary hospital under heavy sedation or anesthesia. In tough, refractory cases, surgical placement of a drain in the bony tympanic bulla affords excellent exposure to the middle- and inner-ear spaces.

Ruptured Eardrums

Eardrums can tear or rupture as the result of direct trauma from a foreign body (a twig, cotton-tip applicator, etc.), sudden pressure changes, or, most commonly, as a secondary complication due to otitis externa. Although a serious and painful condition, a torn eardrum will heal quite quickly provided the underlying cause of the perforation is eliminated.

Medications designed for use in the ears must be used with caution if a dog or cat suffers from a ruptured eardrum. Not only can their application be painful, but also, as mentioned previously, certain antibiotics and solutions, if allowed direct access into the middle- and inner-ear chambers, can cause damage to the auditory nerve endings, resulting in deafness. As a result, be certain to follow a veterinarian's recommendations closely.

Deafness

Veterinarians are often confronted by frustrated pet owners claiming that their pet is going deaf! Now, whether this is a valid claim or rather an actual ploy conceived by a defiant subject will not be known until a thorough ear examination is performed. A pet's apparent inability to perceive sounds can result for a number of reasons.

First, there might be impedance to the sound waves traveling through the ear. An external ear canal clogged with wax and debris can certainly be the culprit, as can constrictive swelling of the ear canal caused by otitis externa. Torn or ruptured eardrums can also diminish the effective transmission of sound waves to the middle and inner ears.

Interestingly, some researchers feel that a dog's eardrums are not altogether necessary for efficient conduction of sound waves; rather, sound waves permeating the bony, air-filled tympanic bullae directly fulfill a major portion of this conductive function. Regardless, researchers do know that sound waves must pass through the middle-ear cavity before reaching the inner ear, and that fluid or inflammation secondary to otitis media can lead to diminished hearing.

Besides interference with the transmission of sound waves, deafness in dogs and cats can also be caused by developmental defects or damage involving the actual nerve endings within the inner ear. Congenital nerve deafness has been reported in some breeds, including dalmatians, collies, and rottweilers. Nerve deafness can also be inherited in some cats. This type of induced deafness is seen primarily in white cats with blue eyes.

Certain drugs, such as the aminoglycoside antibiotics, are well known for their adverse effects on the hearing function in dogs and cats. Chronic, untreated bacterial and fungal infections within the middle and inner ears can undoubtedly lead to nerve deafness, as can certain viral organisms.

Diagnosis of nerve deafness is based on history and special hearing tests. One such test, the brainstem auditory evoked response test (BAER), measures the brain's response to auditory stimuli and is quite helpful in the detection of hearing defects, determining the extent of any defect, and pinpointing its location.

Unfortunately, no known treatment exists for true nerve deafness. Hearing aids designed especially for dogs are now commercially available, and may help improve hearing in select instances. Most deaf pets will adapt to their condition with time. However, because of inherent dangers associated with environmental hazards, deaf dogs and cats should not be allowed outdoors unless closely supervised or maintained on a leash and harness.

Aural Hematomas

Fractures or trauma to the cartilage supporting the pinna of the ear can lead to the accumulation of blood and serum within the affected flap. These aural hematomas cause the pinna to swell, sometimes to enormous sizes. In the majority of cases, the fluid accumulation occurs on the inside portion of the earflap.

Researchers don't know what precipitates many cases of aural hematomas, but they do have a few suspicions. Since these hematomas are often accompanied by otitis externa, many feel that the trauma induced by scratching and shaking the head predisposes to aural hematomas, especially in those dogs with pendulous ears. Still others suspect that an overactive host immune system is the culprit behind this disorder. Regardless of the cause, aural hematomas are painful and irritating, and need to be surgically drained as soon as possible after initial appearance.

The Musculoskeletal System

The musculoskeletal system in mammals is responsible for locomotion, plus support and protection of vital internal organs. The components of this system include muscles, bones, and a variety of supportive structures, including ligaments, tendons, and cartilage. Disorders of the musculoskeletal system can be quite debilitating to a dog or cat and be accompanied by a lot of pain.

Anatomy and Physiology

The type of muscle involved in skeletal locomotion is termed *striated muscle.* This type of muscle is in contrast to the cardiac muscle found in the heart, and the smooth muscle found in many of the internal organs, both of which are under involuntary control by the nervous system. Striated muscle consists of interlocking bands of cells capable of contracting with great force, thereby achieving movement. Tendons are those tough, fibrous bands that anchor the striated muscle to bone and allow this movement to occur. A strain is said to have occurred on injury to a muscle or a tendon.

The axial skeleton of the dog and cat consists of the skull, the vertebrae, and the ribcage. The appendicular skeleton consists of the bones making up the front and hind limbs, as well as the pelvis.

Each type is made up of a hard mineralized matrix with bone cells interspersed within. The centers of most bones are hollow and filled with soft bone marrow. This substance is an important component of the host immune system as the location for white blood cell production. Red blood cells and platelets, those structures involved in the blood-clotting scheme, are also produced exclusively within the bone marrow.

Bone is a dynamic tissue, constantly being reabsorbed and regenerated throughout the life of the individual. Long bones grow in length by means of a special structure called an *epiphyseal plate,* located at the ends of the bones. It is interesting to note that overall health and growth patterns of bony tissue are very dependent on proper nutrition; malnutrition and vitamin or mineral deficiencies can wreak havoc on the development and/or integrity of the skeletal system.

A *ligament* is different from a tendon in that it connects bone to bone, not muscle to bone. Injuries involving ligaments are properly termed *sprains.*

A *joint* is the site at which two bones meet. Not all joints are movable, such as those making up the skull. However, for purposes of discussion, the types of joints referred to most often are called *synovial joints.* These joints, found throughout the body, allow for free movement between bones and also serve a shock-absorbing capacity. Each synovial joint consists of ligaments, cartilage on which the ends of the bones move or articulate, joint fluid designed to lubricate the joint and provide nutrition to the articular cartilage, and a tough, fibrous capsule surrounding it all. In addition, some synovial joints contain special pads of cartilage, called *menisci,* which act as super shock absorbers. The knee joint, or *stifle,* is a good example of such a joint.

Arthritis and Degenerative Joint Disease

Arthritis is the term used in both human and veterinary medicine to describe any type of joint inflammation. *Polyarthritis* describes inflammation involving multiple joints throughout the body. This inflammation might be accompanied by loss of cartilage or bony changes within the joint(s) in question. Causes of arthritis in dogs and cats include infections, autoimmune diseases, and trauma. Even certain drugs, such as sulfa antibiotics, can promote joint inflammation if used indiscriminately.

Osteoarthrosis, or degenerative joint disease, describes the condition in which a cartilage defect or cartilage erosion occurs within a given joint. Although not considered a true inflammatory condition, many people use the term interchangeably with *arthritis.* Osteoarthrosis often occurs as a result of a hereditary defect that may show up at any age. For instance, hip dysplasia is one of the more infamous forms of inheritable degenerative joint disease, and it's one that most dog owners have heard of. But osteoarthrosis doesn't always have to be inherited; it can also occur secondary to joint injury, or it can even be a part of the normal aging process in older pets.

Regardless of the cause, the clinical signs associated with joint disease are basically the same. Stiffness or lameness involving one or more limbs is often the most obvious sign of a joint problem. In many instances, cold weather and/or exercise aggravate this lameness.

Affected pets might be reluctant to play or jump, and they might become more irritable because of pain. If the hips are involved, inability to rise after lying down is a common clinical complaint. Joints can be swollen and painful to the touch, especially with infectious or autoimmune etiologies. Depression, fever, and loss of appetite could become apparent with the latter as well.

Diagnosis of a joint disorder is based on physical palpation of the joint(s) in question, observing the abnormal gait or movement associated with the disorder, and obtaining radiographs.

Treatment approaches for arthritis and osteoarthrosis depend on the cause and severity of the condition. In recent years, new medications and innovative surgical techniques have been introduced which show promise in the treatment of joint disease and alleviation of the pain associated with it.

Infectious Arthritis

As mentioned above, joint inflammation can be secondary to an infectious process. Bacteria that gain entrance into the body's bloodstream can circulate to one or more joints of the body, setting up house-

DID YOU KNOW ?

The onset of hip lameness in an older dog may not necessarily be due to arthritis. Vertebral spondylosis also causes similar signs. Radiographs should be used to differentiate the two conditions since treatment modalities are different for each.

keeping within the joint fluid. Bacterial endocarditis caused by periodontal disease can be an important source of these organisms.

Arthritis can also be a prominent sign in ehrlichiosis, Rocky Mountain spotted fever, and Lyme disease. If the arthritis is left untreated, permanent damage to the cartilage and other joint structures can result.

Fever, depression, and painful, swollen joints are prominent clinical signs seen in most cases of infectious arthritis. Laboratory testing, including cultures of the fluid within the joint, may be needed to positively identify the offender. Once this identification is accomplished, specific treatment, usually involving high doses of antibiotics, can be instituted.

Arthritis Due to Autoimmune Disease

Sometimes, an overactive immune system can lead to an arthritic condition. In these instances, immune complexes consisting of antibodies coalesce within the joints of the body, causing inflammation. The resultant polyarthritis can be very painful and debilitating. Fever and a generalized depression are also features of these diseases.

Dogs can get rheumatoid arthritis just as people can. In dogs, this autoimmunity-related disease is seen more frequently in the toy breeds than in any others. Another autoimmune disease in dogs that can cause arthritis is called *systemic lupus.* In contrast to rheumatoid arthritis, systemic lupus usually favors the larger breeds of dog, such as German shepherds and St. Bernards.

Many cats that suffer from immunity-related polyarthritis are also infected with the feline leukemia virus. As a result, other symptoms not related to the arthritis might be seen. Fever and a generalized depression are two of these that are seen quite consistently.

Special blood tests and/or tests on joint fluid are used to diagnose autoimmune disorders in pets. Treatment usually consists of high dosages of steroid anti-inflammatory medications designed to curb the body's overactive immune response.

Hip Dysplasia

Hip dysplasia refers to an inherited arthritic condition involving one or both hip joints of affected dogs. It presents itself as a partial dislocation, or in severe cases, a complete dislocation of the hip joints. With time, the cartilage lining the joint surfaces wears down as a result of the abnormal stress and strain placed on the joint, and arthritis results (Fig. 16.1).

Although hip dysplasia can be a problem in any breed, it is seen most often in larger purebred dogs, such as German shepherds, golden retrievers, Labrador retrievers, and St. Bernards. In German shepherds alone, the incidence is thought to be as high as 80 percent!

Because of its inherited nature, signs associated with hip dysplasia may appear as early as 4 weeks of age, although as a rule, most cases show up around 8 to 12 months of age. These clinical signs consist of posterior pain, unsteadiness on the hind limbs, difficulty in rising from a prone position, and a reluctance to move or exercise. Manipulation of the hip joints will reveal obvious pain. In less severe cases, signs might appear only after intense activity and exercise.

Diagnosis of hip dysplasia is achieved by radiographing (X raying) suspected joints and from a history of this disorder in the dog's genetic bloodline. Several registries aimed at controlling genetic diseases in

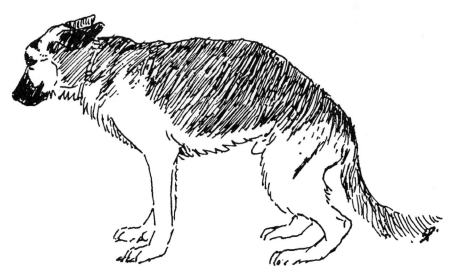

FIGURE 16.1   Hip dysplasia is a crippling and painful genetic disease.

dogs have developed guidelines and testing procedures for veterinarians in an effort to detect this disease in puppies and young dogs before clinical signs even appear.

In otherwise healthy dogs exhibiting marked lameness due to dysplasia, a number of different surgical techniques can be employed to help relieve pain and lameness caused by the disease, and/or to actually reconstruct the hip joint(s). Total hip joint replacements using prosthetic devices can be performed as well in certain cases to afford a permanent cure. As a rule, the smaller the dog involved, the better the results achieved through surgical intervention.

In dogs that are poor surgical candidates, anti-inflammatory medications can be used to temporarily decrease pain and discomfort associated with hip dysplasia. A program of regular exercise and weight loss can also benefit these patients. Also, disease-modifying osteoarthritis drugs (DMOADs) such as the polysulfated glycosaminoglycans, glucosamine, chondroitin sulfate, and hyaluronic acid have been used with great success to stimulate repair of damaged cartilage within diseased joints, instead of just masking the pain caused by the arthritis.

Osteochondrosis

Osteochondrosis describes a condition characterized by abnormal development and growth of joint cartilage. It is seen in young dogs and usually strikes larger breeds. Thought to be caused by trauma and overfeeding, osteochondrosis can precipitate painful joint inflammation and lameness in these pets. The shoulder, elbow, knee, and hock joints are the regions most commonly affected.

Radiographic X rays are used to definitively diagnose osteochondrosis in a dog. In many of these dogs, healing will occur spontaneously over 4 to 6 weeks with strict cage rest. If the cartilage defect is extensive, or if pieces of cartilage have broken off and are floating freely within the joint, surgical intervention might be necessary to remove any dead cartilage and to stimulate healing.

Anti-inflammatory medications can be used to temporarily decrease pain and discomfort associated with this condition. Disease-modifying osteoarthritis drugs such as the polysulfated glycosaminoglycans, glucosamine, chondroitin sulfate, and hyaluronic acid can be employed in the conservative treatment of osteochondrosis in dogs. As in hip dysplasia, these agents appear to satisfactorily set the stage for healing to take place within the defective cartilage.

Legg-Perthes Disease

Legg-Perthes disease, or *ischemic femoral head necrosis,* is an orthopedic condition involving the hips of smaller breeds of dogs, such as Yorkshire terriers and miniature poodles. This condition is characterized by a degeneration of the head of the femur bone—that portion which fits into the socket of the pelvis to form the hip joint (Fig. 16.2). Hereditary in nature, Legg-Perthes disease usually appears around 3 to 9 months of age. Clinical signs associated with this disease include lameness and painful hips.

On radiographic diagnosis, treatment for Legg-Perthes disease involves surgical removal of the head of the affected femur(s). Most dogs, because of their light weight, can return to normal locomotion and activity within a matter of days to weeks after such a surgery.

Patellar Luxation (Dogs)

Patellar luxation is an orthopedic condition in which the patella, or kneecap, "slips" to one side of the knee joint, causing pain and loss of the joint function (Fig. 16.3). *Medial patellar luxation,* in which the patella slips to the inside surface of the joint, is most often seen in the toy breeds, such as Yorkshire terriers, poodles, and Pomeranians. Lateral patellar luxation, where the kneecap migrates to the outer surface of the

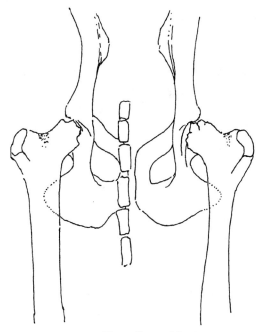

FIGURE 16.2 The radiographic appearance of ischemic femoral head necrosis.

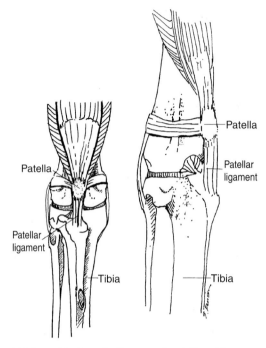

Patella

Patellar ligament

Tibia

Patella

Patellar ligament

Tibia

FIGURE 16.3 Left: normal patellar alignment. Right: a luxated patella.

knee joint, shows no true breed disposition, with larger dogs sometimes affected. Regardless of the type, patellar luxation can occur secondary to direct trauma to the joint, or can be caused by an abnormal anatomic development of the bones comprising the knee joint.

Signs of this problem can occur as early as 6 months of age in affected dogs. Milder cases often go unnoticed for years until arthritis of the affected knee sets in. Symptoms associated with patellar luxation include intermittent lameness, with the dog often reluctant to put the affected hind leg on the ground. Dogs affected with this problem might seem fine one minute, and then suddenly let out a yelp and come up overtly lame. Many times, the patella will slip back into place by itself and the dog will seem fine again. However, if this condition continues for a long time, arthritis of the knee joint eventually occurs, and the lameness signs will fail to disappear.

An easily displaced patella found on physical examination will confirm a diagnosis of patellar luxation. Radiographs are helpful as well to determine the extent of arthritis involvement, if any at all.

Surgical correction of patellar luxation is the treatment of choice in these pets. This involves altering the anatomy of the tibia (the shinbone that makes up the lower portion of the knee joint) in such a way that the patella is not allowed to slip to either side. The prognosis after surgery is good to excellent for complete remission of signs. In those dogs that have problems with both knee joints, surgical repair of both legs may be necessary.

Torn Knee Ligaments (Cruciate Injuries)

The knee joints of dogs and cats (and of people) are held together by a fibrous joint capsule and a number of ligaments; the most prominent of these are the cruciate ligaments. Because of their configuration, the range of motion allowed the knee joint is limited to simple flexion and extension. If an abnormal force is placed on the joint from trauma or from planting the leg wrong on the ground, these ligaments could tear or rupture, leading to instability and pain within the affected knee joint. This instability, if not corrected in a timely fashion, will lead to arthritic changes and permanent pain within the joint (Fig. 16.4).

As with humans, cruciate injuries seemingly affect active, athletic canines more than others do, but older, obese dogs and cats also have their fair share of this type of problem. Ruptured cruciates can also occur secondary to patellar luxation in toy dog breeds. Acute ruptures or tears involving the cruciate ligaments usually result in a sudden, non-weight-bearing lameness in pets so affected. Over time, a gradual return to function can occur even if the condition is not treated, but the lameness will undoubtedly return as the activity level of the pet increases or as arthritis strikes the joint.

A diagnosis of torn knee ligaments is made if a veterinarian can demonstrate an obvious laxity within the affected knee joint. Because of the pain involved with such a diagnostic procedure, sedation might be necessary in order to obtain an accurate assessment. Radiographs might be helpful, depending on the duration of the problem.

Treatment of this condition involves surgical repair and reconstruction of the

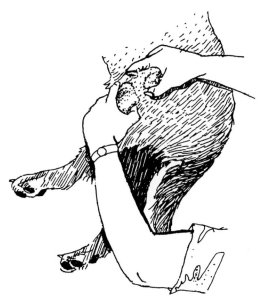

FIGURE 16.4 Cruciate injuries lead to knee joint instability.

torn ligaments in an effort to restore normal knee joint stability. Many techniques for such repair are available for use, depending on the extent of the injury and other circumstances involved. In general, cats and smaller dogs that do not have to carry as much weight around on their knee joints as do larger dogs have the most satisfactory postsurgical results.

Following surgical repair, disease-modifying osteoarthritis drugs (DMOADs) can be used to speed the healing of any cartilage damaged as a result of the injury.

Hip Luxation

One common sequela to car accidents and other types of trauma involving dogs and cats is dislocation, or luxation, of one or both hip joints. These pets usually have a non-weight-bearing lameness on the affected leg, and it is quite painful. Diagnosis can be made with a physical examination and radiographic X rays of the hips and pelvis.

Treatment usually involves surgical stabilization of the hip joint to restore function and to prevent recurrence. In cats and small dogs, the head of the femur may actually be removed to allow a false joint to form at the site.

Fractures

Most bone fractures in dogs and cats are trauma-related. In isolated instances, metabolic diseases, such as nutritional osteodystrophy and bone cancers, can also be underlying causes. A fracture will present itself as a non-weight-bearing lameness, with noticeable swelling and pain in the region of the affected bone. *Crepitus,* or the grinding feel made by broken ends of bone rubbing together, and an anatomical distortion of the site, such as a shortening of an affected limb, might be seen as well.

Diagnosis of a fracture is based on physical exam findings and radiographic X rays. Treatment depends on the type of fracture and the region involved, and it consists of any combination of cage rest, bandaging or splinting, and surgery to reduce and stabilize the fracture.

Minor fractures involving the pelvis will often heal nicely with cage rest alone, whereas displaced fractures of one or more limbs might require surgical fixation using orthopedic pins, screws, and/or bone plates. In general, uncomplicated fractures usually heal quite readily in dogs and cats.

Osteomyelitis

Infections involving bony tissue within the body are termed *osteomyelitis.* Bacterial osteomyelitis in dogs and cats can occur secondary to a deep bite wound or some other type of penetrating trauma. Open fractures can also predispose to bone infections. Furthermore, fungal organisms, such as histoplasmosis and blastomycosis, can also spread from other areas of the body via the blood and infect bony tissue in pets.

Dogs and cats with osteomyelitis are lame and feverish, and usually feel considerable pain at the affected site. These signs, combined with the localized swelling that often occurs, can easily be mistaken for a fracture and must be differentiated from one. To do this, radiographic X rays should be taken of the suspected skeletal region. In addition, bone biopsies might be necessary to differentiate some cases of osteomyelitis from bone tumors, and to collect samples for bacterial or fungal cultures.

Because infections that become embedded in bone can be difficult to clear up with antibiotics alone, surgery is usually needed to actually remove those portions of bone severely affected. Drain tubes are placed as well to allow for postsurgical drainage and flushing of the site with medicated solutions. Following surgery, antibiotic therapy might be required for 1 to 2 months. If a fungal organism is involved, medications might need to be given for 4 to 6 months.

Spondylosis Deformans (Dogs)

Spondylosis deformans is a degenerative bone condition that seems to be related to the aging process in some dogs, especially the larger breeds. It is characterized by the development of bony spurs that originate from intervertebral disks and grow to bridge the gap between adjacent vertebrae. These spurs are evident on radiographic X rays. Most dogs afflicted with this disorder show no clinical signs whatsoever. However, in some dogs, pressure and pain originating from these bony growths can cause prominent hind-end weakness and reluctance to move.

Unfortunately, there is no cure for spondylosis deformans. Discomfort associated with the condition can be temporarily relieved with anti-inflammatory medication.

Metabolic Bone Disease

Metabolic bone diseases are characterized by a thinning and loss of bony mass, predisposing the bone to fractures and growth deformities. The most common metabolic bone disease seen in dogs and cats is *hyperparathyroidism.* This condition is characterized by a calcium deficiency within the body that leads to abnormal bone growth and bone resorption as the body tries to correct the low calcium levels in the bloodstream. Hyperparathyroidism can result from feeding pets all-meat diets (which are naturally low in calcium), or it can result secondary to kidney disease.

Dogs and cats afflicted with metabolic bone diseases exhibit lameness, weakness, bone and joint deformities, and spontaneous fractures. Diagnosis is based on radiographic X-ray findings and on blood calcium measurements. Treatment for nutritionally related bone disease obviously involves changes in the diet and calcium supplementation. Treatment for kidney-related hyperparathyroidism is geared toward counteracting the kidney disease itself.

Another type of metabolic bone disease that can affect cats is called *hypervitaminosis A.* This condition is seen in those cats fed an exclusive diet of liver, which contain high levels of vitamin A. Musculoskeletal changes seen in cats experiencing chronic vitamin A toxicity include bony deformities, outgrowths, and fusion involving the vertebral column, especially in the region of the neck, and bony fusion of the joints of the limbs, resulting in pain and immobility.

A history of an all-liver diet, combined with clinical signs and radiographic analysis of the spine and limbs, can reveal conclusive evidence of hypervitaminosis A. If detected early in its development, this condition can often be reversed by switching the cat to a balanced diet. However, in advanced cases, the bony changes that occur are usually permanent, and anti-inflammatory medications are usually required for the remaining life of the cat to help ease the pain associated with the disease.

Mucopolysaccharidosis (Cats)

Mucopolysaccharidosis is an inherited disorder that has been documented in Siamese cats. It results from an enzyme deficiency that allows polysaccharide carbohydrates to accumulate within the cells of the body.

The skeletal system is particularly affected, with stricken cats suffering from bony spurs on the vertebrae, arthritis and abnormal formation of the joints, and a generalized osteoporosis, or thinning of the bones themselves. These cats also have a characteristic "flattening" of the face, resulting from a widening of the facial structure, and, at an early age, can suffer from opacities or cloudiness involving the corneas of both eyes.

Diagnosis of mucopolysaccharidosis is made by physical examination, blood tests, and radiographic X rays of the skeletal system. A special test that detects mucopolysaccharides in the urine can also be employed in diagnosing this disorder.

Unfortunately, because of the inherited nature of this disease, there is no known treatment. Future generations should be protected by neutering those pets affected to prevent passage of the trait.

Myositis and Myopathies

Myositis is inflammation of muscle tissue that results in pain, weakness, and muscle atrophy (shrinking). Dogs and cats suffering from severe bouts of myositis are reluctant to move and can actually appear as if they are paralyzed as a result of the inflammatory effects on the muscles.

Myositis can be caused by a number of different disease entities, including toxoplasmosis, leptospirosis, bacterial infections (abscesses), low blood potassium (see text below), and autoimmune disease. One special type of myositis, called *masticatory myositis,* affects the facial muscles of affected dogs, causing atrophy and the inability to chew normally. This autoimmune disease is seen most frequently in German shepherds.

Myositis is diagnosed using clinical signs and blood tests designed to detect increased levels in muscle enzymes within the blood. In especially elusive cases, biopsy samples taken from suspected muscle tissue can help veterinarians obtain a definitive diagnosis.

Treatment for myositis is aimed at the underlying cause. If infections are to blame, appropriate antimicrobial or antiparasitic therapy will help relieve the myositis. Anti-inflammatory medications can also be used to relieve the pain and discomfort associated with the inflammation until the underlying cause is treated.

Autoimmune myositis, such as masticatory myositis, is treated with high levels of glucocorticosteroids (such as prednisolone) in an effort to suppress the immune response causing the inflammation in the first place. The prognosis for complete recovery with autoimmune myositis is poor, yet with medications, the signs associated with the disorder can be kept under control.

The term *myopathy* refers to abnormal anatomy and/or function of skeletal muscle tissue within the body. Most myopathies in dogs are inherited. Chow chows, golden retrievers, and Irish terriers are examples of breeds that can suffer from inherited myopathies. Dogs suffering from myopathies exhibit abnormal postures, stiff gaits, and generalized shrinking or atrophy of the muscles. Because of the inherited nature of these diseases, the onset of clinical signs usually occurs within a year of age. Unfortunately, there is no effective treatment to stop the progression of these myopathies.

Hypokalemic Myopathy (Potassium Depletion) in Cats

As an electrolyte, potassium serves a variety of functions within the body, including maintaining proper fluid volume and pH. Potassium is also necessary for normal muscle contraction. Many illnesses in cats can also produce deficiencies in this electrolyte, or hypokalemia, within their bodies. This is especially true for those cats suffering from kidney disease, liver disease, or diabetes mellitus (Fig. 16.5).

Actual signs of hypokalemia can include weight loss, loss of appetite, constipation (due to poor motility of the muscles lining the

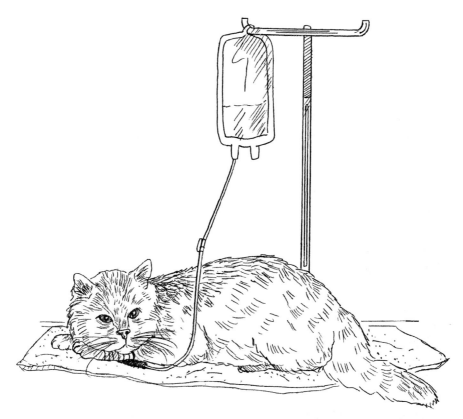

FIGURE 16.5 Critically ill cats require supportive care to prevent secondary potassium depletion.

gastrointestinal tract), muscle weakness, muscle pain, and incoordination. As the condition progresses and respiratory muscles become affected, breathing difficulties might be noted. In severe cases, death from respiratory paralysis could result.

Diagnosis of hypokalemia in a sick cat is based on a history, clinical signs, and measurements of blood potassium levels. If hypokalemia is diagnosed, treatment consists of intravenous injections of a potassium supplement to correct the immediate deficit, followed by oral supplementation as long as deemed necessary. Prognosis for recovery is good if treatment begins early on.

Hernias

A hernia results from a tear or defect in a muscular wall, allowing the contents contained behind the wall to protrude through the opening in the muscle. In dogs, the four most prevalent types of hernias include umbilical hernias, inguinal hernias, perineal hernias, and diaphragmatic hernias. In cats, diaphragmatic hernias are the types most commonly seen.

Umbilical hernias occur on the midline of the dog's stomach at the location of the umbilicus, or the belly button. These usually result from trauma to the muscle wall in this area that occurs when the bitch severs the umbilical cord after birth. Umbilical hernias pose no real health problems, since fatty tissue is usually the only item that ever protrudes through the opening. These hernias can be sutured and repaired at the time of other elective surgeries.

Inguinal hernias occur in the inguinal region of the abdomen, or that region where the abdominal musculature meets that of the hind legs. They are seen as birth defects or secondary to trauma. These hernias are more serious than umbilical hernias, since the herniated material often includes intestines. As a result, normal digestive processes can be disrupted. Treatment involves surgical replacement of the herniated material back inside the abdomen and suturing the defective muscle.

Perineal hernias result from a weakening of the musculature in the region located beneath the tail on either side of the anus. Seen primarily in older male dogs that have not been neutered, perineal hernias can involve portions of the colon and cause impactions and elimination problems if not surgically corrected. Because the hormone testosterone seems to play a role in the development of these hernias, neutering these dogs is also recommended to prevent a recurrence.

By far the most serious type of hernia is the diaphragmatic hernia. The diaphragm is the thick wall of muscle that separates the thorax or chest cavity from the abdominal contents. Tears or ruptures occurring in this band of muscle, resulting either from inherited defects or from traumatic incidents, can allow liver, intestines, and/or other abdominal contents to herniate into the chest cavity. When this happens, the pressure applied to the crowded lungs and heart results in, among other things, breathing difficulties, weakness, and/or gastrointestinal disturbances.

Definitive diagnosis of a diaphragmatic hernia can be made by coupling history, clinical signs, and a physical examination with radiographic X-ray findings. Surgical repair of the torn diaphragm will alleviate the signs and usually result in a complete recovery.

The Nervous System

The nervous system involves a complex interaction between special elements designed to originate or carry unique electrochemical charges to and from the various organs within the body. Like its endocrine counterpart, the nervous system initiates and regulates bodily functions and ensures its owner of an awareness to the surrounding environment.

Anatomy and Physiology

The smallest component of the nervous system is the neuron. There are over 10 billion of these dynamic cells in the body, and they have the ability to originate and propagate nerve impulses. These result from changes in electrolyte ratios, namely, those of sodium and potassium, occurring across the cell membrane of the neuron. For this reason, abnormalities in the amounts of sodium and potassium within the body can have devastating effects on nervous system function.

Generated impulses are transmitted to their respective targets along special cellular projections, originating from the cell body, called *nerve fibers*. Speeds of transmission along these nerve fibers can reach over 110 meters per second. Groups or bundles of fibers coursing together are what are referred to as *nerves*.

Within the nervous system, neurons can link together to form a continuous chain to allow for the uninterrupted passage of a nerve impulse to its desired destination. A *synapse* is described as this connection between two nerve cells. Special chemical transmitters located at synapses (neurotransmitters) transfer the impulses from the end of one neuron to the receptive end of another, allowing the impulse to continue in its travels. Neurotransmitters are also found at the junctions between nerve fibers and their target muscles or organs. In dogs and cats, organophosphate insecticide poisoning exerts its deadly effects by interfering with the normal breakdown of acetylcholine, one of these neurotransmitters.

The brain is the control center for the entire nervous system. Internally, it is composed of gray matter, which is a collection of neuron cell bodies and synapses between nerve cells, and white matter, made up of nerve fibers originating from the neuron cell bodies.

The mammalian brain is divided into three divisions: the cerebrum, the cerebellum, and the brainstem. The largest of the three, the cerebrum, is responsible for memory, sensory awareness, learning, and muscular movement. The cerebellum, located in back of and just beneath the cerebrum, functions to coordinate muscular activity and movement, and control body posture. The final division of the brain, the brainstem, serves a variety of functions. It acts as an important intermediary by relaying messages between the cerebrum, cerebellum, and the spinal cord, and influencing activities such as heartbeat, breathing, vision, and hearing. A special portion of the brainstem, called the *hypothalamus,* provides an important link between the nervous system and the endocrine system.

The spinal cord is the major highway of activity for the transmission of nerve impulses between the brain and the rest of the body. It runs along the course of the back within the spinal canal formed by the vertebral column. Like the brain, the spinal cord also contains gray matter and white matter. Large spinal nerves containing numerous smaller nerve fibers branch off from the main cord along its course and travel to respective target muscles and organs. The spinal cord can also serve as coordinating center for certain reflex activities involving the muscles of the limbs without first requiring a nerve impulse to be sent to the brain. Clinicians can often assess the extent of damage to a spinal cord by evaluating these spinal reflex arcs.

Spinal nerves branching off from the spinal cord contain two main types of nerve fibers: *somatic nerve fibers,* which carry information to and from skeletal muscle, skin, joints, and appendages (effects such as muscle contraction, produced by somatic fibers, are said to be under conscious or voluntary control from the brain), and *autonomic nerve fibers,* which innervate glands and internal organs throughout the body. Unlike somatic nerves, autonomic nerves act mainly on reflex, with little voluntary control. Blood pressure, cardiac output, breathing, gastrointestinal motility, body temperature, and hormone secretion are only some of the many vital life functions under the influence of this unique system.

Three thin layers of tissue called *meninges* cover both the brain and the spinal cord. Between these layers is found a special type of fluid, called *cerebrospinal fluid.* Meninges with their accompanying cerebrospinal fluid serve to protect, support, and nourish the underlying nervous tissue. Abnormal increases in the amount of cerebrospinal fluid can cause serious damage to the spinal cord and brain. Hydrocephalus is the term used to describe such a condition affecting the brain.

Seizures

Those who own a pet that has suffered from seizures know firsthand how scary these episodes can be. A *seizure* is defined as uncontrollable behavior or muscle activity caused by an abnormal increase in the brain's nervous activities. *Epilepsy* is a term used to describe recurring seizures.

Seizural activity in dogs and cats can be quite obvious or quite subtle. In essence, seizures should be suspected anytime that a pet undergoes sporadic, unexplained behavioral changes.

What causes seizures in dogs and cats? Potential causes are numerous and include viral infections (e.g., distemper, FIP), toxoplasmosis, fungal infections (e.g., cryptococcosis), epilepsy, hydrocephalus, brain tumor, intestinal parasites, low blood sugar, low blood calcium, insecticide poisoning, and heat stroke. Sometimes the cause cannot be determined; if so, seizure episodes are termed "idiopathic."

Because causes of seizures are so numerous, a thorough examination and blood workup by a veterinarian is warranted whenever a pet exhibits seizures. In some cases, managing or eliminating an underlying cause will eliminate the seizures. In others, such as with idiopathic epilepsy, there is no known cause, yet by ruling out the other potential causes (e.g., hydrocephalus; see Fig. 17.1) and establishing a pattern of occurrence, most cases can be effectively managed with anticonvulsant medications. With idiopathic epilepsy, seizures can begin at any stage in life, yet, for the most part, they begin around 1 to 3 years of age. While the cause of idiopathic epilepsy is unknown, it has been shown to be inheritable in some dog breeds, including beagles and dachshunds.

Seizures themselves are rarely life-threatening, unless some physical harm comes to the pet as a result of the fit. The typical seizure or epileptic fit has three stages, or phases. The first of these, the *preictal phase,* is marked by anxiety and restlessness on the part of the pet. The actual period of the seizure activity, *ictus,* follows next. Its duration might be for only a few seconds or it might be minutes. Certainly the longer the seizure lasts, the more dangerous it is to the health of the pet. The *postictal phase* following the seizure is characterized by an overall depression or confusion. Postictal pets can appear to be blind, running into walls and objects, or they might just sleep a lot. This phase can last for a few hours or for days, with the pet returning to its normal state after its conclusion.

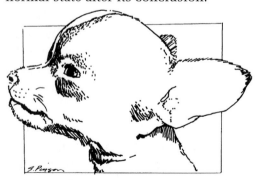

FIGURE 17.1 Hydrocephalus, or "water on the brain," can cause seizures in affected pets.

There is one seizural presentation called *status epilepticus* that can prove fatal to a pet. This condition is characterized by a cluster of seizure events occurring in quick succession. Unless appropriate emergency medication is administered intravenously to stop the seizures, these dogs and cats can lapse into a coma and die. As a result, prompt recognition and action on the part of the pet owner is essential.

When attempting to diagnose the cause of seizural activity, veterinarians will first look at the age and the type of pet involved. For example, seizures occurring in pets under 1 year of age commonly result from birth defects or from infectious diseases, such as canine distemper or intestinal parasites, whereas seizures occurring in a very old dog or cat often indicate kidney failure or cancer. In smaller, toy puppies and in active hunting dogs, low blood sugar brought on by illness, stress, or overexertion can be an important inciting cause. Seizures occurring in a pregnant dog or cat or one that has just given birth are usually caused by "milk fever," or low blood calcium. Finally, as mentioned above, certain breeds are prone to idiopathic epilepsy.

A good history is also vital to help determine the cause of the seizures. Does the pet have access to any type of poison? Has the pet ever suffered any type of physical trauma, such as being hit by a car? Has the intensity of the seizures gradually been getting worse or increasing in frequency? The answers to these and other questions can help a veterinarian narrow the choices.

A complete blood profile and urinalysis should be performed to help rule out the metabolic and infectious causes of seizures. Radiographs and ultrasound can prove to be helpful in certain instances as well. If no underlying cause can be found, and the history supports it, a diagnosis of idiopathic epilepsy is made and treatment is started on this premise.

For cases other than idiopathic epilepsy, treatment is geared toward correcting or managing the underlying problem, whether it is kidney failure, poisoning, low blood sugar, or another condition. In instances in which idiopathic epilepsy is suspect, anticonvulsant medications can be used to control or even eliminate the seizural activity.

Determining the exact dosages of anticonvulsant medications might require frequent adjustments at the start in order to accommodate the pet's individual needs. Pets on anticonvulsant medication may need liver function tests performed annually, since some of these medications can damage the liver over the long term.

Paralysis

Paralysis can be defined as a disruption of the nervous system leading to an impairment of motor function and/or feeling to a particular region or regions of the body. This impairment can be in the form of a spasticity of the muscles in the involved region, or these muscles may become completely limp. In either case, the muscles involved are unable to function in the manner in which they were intended.

Paralysis involving the sensory portion of the nervous system can result in an increased sensitivity to pain or in a complete absence of it. Finally, paralysis resulting in the inefficient function of certain internal organs can occur as well if the nerves supplying these structures are disrupted in any way.

Any disease or disorder that traumatizes the brain, spinal cord, and nerves has the potential to cause paralysis. In dogs and cats, some of the more common causes seen by veterinarians include infectious diseases and parasites, being hit by a car, ruptured disks, and in the case of facial muscle paralysis, ear infections.

Treatment of paralysis is geared toward identifying and treating the underlying cause. If it has been caused by trauma, anti-inflammatory agents combined with drugs designed to draw fluid out of the central nervous system might help reverse signs of paralysis, yet their usefulness is dependent on the extent of the nervous injury and how quickly therapy is instituted.

Pets that have sensory paralysis in a limb might require limb amputation to prevent self-mutilation of the leg. In instances where an irreversible paralysis involves more than one limb, or involves the malfunction of internal organs, pet owners must seriously consider not only their pet's quality of life as a paralytic but their own as well, before prolonged therapeutic or rehabilitative measures are undertaken.

Degenerative Disk Disease (DDD)

Coursing along the length of the back, the spinal cord travels protected within the bony vertebral column. Separating each vertebra, and located beneath the spinal cord itself, are structures called *interverte-*

bral disks, which serve as cushions between each individual vertebra, absorbing shock and forming joints that allow the vertebral column to bend. Each circular disk is composed of an outer band of tough, fibrous tissue called the *annulus fibrosus* surrounding an inner gelatinous center called the *nucleus pulposus.* This latter structure is responsible for absorbing any shock placed on the disk.

Degenerative disk disease (DDD) is characterized by the slow degeneration of the nucleus pulposus within one or more intervertebral disks. As these continue to degenerate, they become less resilient and can even calcify, leaving the intervertebral disk without its shock-absorbing unit. As a result, the disks so affected become very susceptible to compression damage, even from normal day-to-day activity. In pets so affected, continued stress or sudden trauma to the disk or vertebral column can lead to an overt tearing or rupture of the annulus fibrosus, and extrusion of the degenerating nucleus pulposus. Unfortunately, since the top portion of the annulus is much narrower than the bottom portion, this extrusion usually occurs upward directly into the spinal canal, damaging the spinal cord and associated nerves (Fig. 17.2).

Overt disk ruptures may be classified as partial or complete. In *partial ruptures,* the annulus can either be stretched or displaced into the spinal canal, or it can partially rupture, allowing a small amount of the nucleus within to escape and pressure the spinal cord. With *complete ruptures,* the entire nucleus content is allowed to escape into the spinal canal. Obviously, the consequences of such a rupture versus a partial one are much more severe.

The region of the vertebral column most susceptible to rupture is that portion extending from the last rib to the pelvis. The neck region is another area that can be affected. In a pet suffering from DDD, even the slightest wrong move, such as jumping off the couch or running too fast, can cause an affected disk to rupture.

Dogs are the species primarily afflicted with DDD. Although any dog can suffer from DDD, there do seem to be some breed dispositions. The dachshund breed certainly leads the list in the number of cases reported (Fig. 17.3). Other breeds commonly afflicted with degenerative disk disease include poodles, Pekingese, and Lhasa apsos. Beagles and cocker spaniels also have a notable incidence of DDD in their neck region.

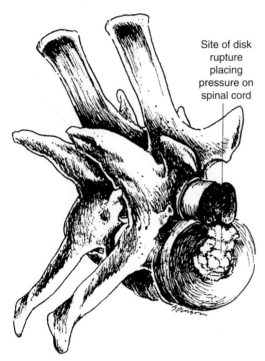

Site of disk
rupture
placing
pressure on
spinal cord

FIGURE 17.2 **Cross section of a ruptured intervertebral disk.**

Problems with DDD can show up in smaller breeds as early as 3 years of age. In larger dogs, the onset of signs might not occur until they are 6 to 7 years old. Overweight dogs are at an especially high risk of developing complications associated with intervertebral disk disease.

The clinical signs seen with degenerative disk disease and/or disk rupture depend on the location of the lesion and the amount, if any, of the rupture that has taken place. In fact, the extent of pressure or damage to the spinal cord can be estimated according to the signs seen.

Dogs with early or mild cases of disk disease causing slight pressure upon the cord will be quite painful and reluctant to move. Many will cry or yelp when picked up. If the neck is involved, any manipulations attempted will be met with vigorous protests. These pets often prefer not to be bothered, and have the tendency to isolate themselves. Appetites are usually reduced as well. Since nerve fibers responsible for coordinated muscle movement run within the outer layers of the spinal cord, owners may also notice weakness and/or incoordination when their pet attempts to walk.

With more severe disk ruptures, damage to the deeper portions of the spinal cord can become a serious factor. When this occurs, partial or complete paralysis of one or more limbs might result, depending on the location of the rupture. If the entire depth of the spinal cord is involved, these animals will also lose all pain sensation to one or all four limbs, again depending on the areas of the spinal cord involved.

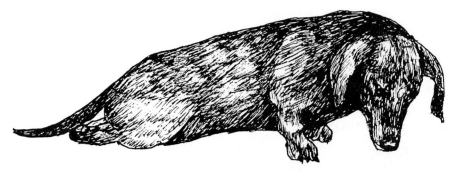

FIGURE 17.3   Degenerative disk disease is a common cause of paralysis in dachshunds.

Such severe cases carry a very grave prognosis, since treatment at this stage is rarely successful.

In most cases, confirmation of a ruptured disk is made via a thorough examination, clinical signs, and with radiographs of the vertebral column. If the exact location of the spinal lesion cannot be pinpointed with regular radiographs, a special test, called a *myelogram,* is performed. This test involves injecting a dye directly into the spinal canal. The dye, which can be identified on a radiograph, helps outline the cord lesion and demonstrate the extent of the disk rupture.

The type of treatment instituted for disk disease and/or rupture depends on the extent of the damage done by the disk to the spinal cord.

For those dogs showing only pain with some mild incoordination, *a strict 2-week confinement* period, either at home or in a hospital setting, is a must! Afterward, short 10- to 15-minute physical therapy sessions, including swimming, can be performed twice daily to help speed recovery and return to normal function.

For cases in which the affected dog is having great

DID YOU KNOW?

Although aspirin and other anti-inflammatory agents can be used to reduce the swelling and pain associated with bone, joint, or back injuries, many veterinarians will choose to forgo them altogether. The reason for this is that any pain experienced by the pet serves to discourage excessive movement and mobility, which, in turn, prevents further damage to the affected site and promotes faster healing.

difficulty walking, strict cage confinement combined with anti-inflammatory therapy and other specific treatment is indicated. If the disease is such that the dog is unable to support weight on the limbs at all, even after medical therapy, then surgery is required to reduce the pressure placed on the spinal cord by the ruptured disk.

This surgery, called a *laminectomy* or *hemilaminectomy,* works best if performed within the first 24 hours of the injury. It involves the removal of part of the vertebra over the affected cord segment. By eliminating the enclosed space through which the spinal cord runs, the pressure on the cord caused by the inflammation is allowed to dissipate. At the same time, surgeons often elect to perform intervertebral disk fenestrations, aimed at removing the offending nucleus pulposus from the disk in question and from adjacent disks as well.

The prognosis is poor for those pets that are unable to walk and have lost deep pain sensation in their legs as a result of a ruptured disk. The loss of deep pain indicates that the entire depth of the spinal cord is invariably involved, and surgical salvage procedures are rarely successful.

In those instances where surgery is unsuccessful, or in which paralysis is permanent, euthanasia is not always the only option left to the owner. Special "wheelchairs" for dogs have been developed for dogs paralyzed by a ruptured disk or other neurological accidents. Although not suitable for every patient, these carts can help afford mobility to select patients willing to wear the apparatus and an alternative for those owners willing to devote much time and care to their paralyzed pet. If you think that such a device could be applicable to your own pet's situation, ask your veterinarian for more details regarding this and other management options available.

There are specific measures that pet owners can take to help protect their dog from a ruptured disk. The first and most important is to prevent obesity. Overweight dogs are prime candidates for such complications; hence, they should be placed on a strict diet to reduce this risk factor.

Jumping should be discouraged in dogs predisposed to intervertebral disk disease. Many ruptured disks result from pets jumping off and on furniture. Pets so inclined should be assisted up or down whenever possible. Even better, a small chair or ramp can be placed in front of the dog's favorite piece of furniture to allow easier access.

Whenever lifting a dog with back problems, be sure to firmly support both the front and hind ends, keeping the back as straight as possible. This stabilizes the position of the spine and affords the handler with better and safer control should the pet struggle (Fig. 17.4).

Surgical intervertebral disk fenestration is often used as a preventive measure in dogs that have previously suffered from bouts of intervertebral disk disease. As mentioned before, this involves the penetration and removal of the nucleus pulposus from one or more intervertebral disks suspected of causing current or future problems. If this is done, the danger associated with later disk rupture is removed with the nucleus.

Vertebral Instability (Canine Wobbler Syndrome)

Seen primarily in Great Danes and Doberman pinschers, vertebral instability is characterized by instability and deformities in the vertebra of the neck region, leading to pressure on the spinal cord in that region. The condition in these breeds is hereditary in nature; however, trauma can predispose any dog to canine wobbler syndrome. Signs associated with vertebral instability include incoordination, weakness, and paralysis. Pain is rarely a feature of this disease. Diagnosis of vertebral instability is made with radiographic X rays. Treatment involves the use of anti-inflammatory medication to reduce the spinal cord inflammation. Surgical decompression of the spinal cord is also warranted in severe cases.

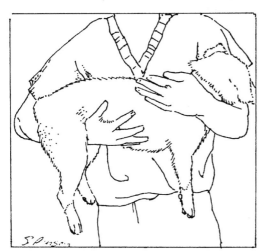

FIGURE 17.4 Whenever handling a dog with a degenerative disk disease, always keep the back straight and well supported.

Myelopathies

Myelopathies are degenerative diseases that strike the spinal cord and nerve fibers coursing throughout the body. These diseases involve the gradual loss of the outer, conductive coating that surrounds certain nerve fibers, called *myelin.* This loss impairs the fiber's ability to transmit nerve impulses. Seen primarily in older, larger breeds of dogs, especially German shepherds, myelopathies are characterized by muscular incoordination, weakness, and atrophy. As the nerves innervating the hindlegs are affected, a turning under or dragging of the hind feet may result. In fact, the hind limb weakness exhibited by some dogs with degenerative myelopathy is often mistaken for arthritis of the hips or spondylosis deformans of the spine. However, pain is rarely a factor in this disease.

A myelopathy is tentatively diagnosed using historical findings, clinical signs, and reflex testing. Dogs afflicted with this condition will exhibit weak to absent reflex activity in their limbs. Electromyograms (EMGs) may be performed as well to evaluate electrical activity associated with the muscle tissue of the body.

Unfortunately, because an exact cause of most myelopathies, other than genetics, remains a mystery, there is no effective treatment to date. Vitamin therapy has been used in some instances to slow the progression of the disease, yet motor incapacitation is inevitable.

Vestibular Disease

The *vestibular system* is a specialized portion of the nervous system found within the inner ear, brain, and spinal cord. Its duty is to maintain a state of equilibrium and balance. By communicating with the nerves supplying the eyes, limbs, and trunk, the body is able to coordinate the position and activity of these regions with movements of the head.

Peripheral vestibular dysfunction (PVD) is a disease that affects the nerves of the vestibular apparatus in the ears. PVD is characterized by a sudden onset of incoordination and loss of balance, which is often accompanied by a head tilt, involuntary twitching of the eyeballs, and in many cases, vomiting. The causes of this disorder can include trauma to the ears, skull infections, and tumors involving the middle or inner ear. Diagnosis of PVD is achieved using clinical signs and various laboratory tests to rule out other potential causes of the symptoms. Radiographs of the skull may be helpful in the detection of any masses or infections that may involve the inner portions of the ears. Treatment, of course, depends on the underlying cause and usually includes high doses of corticosteroid medications designed to reduce inflammation involving the vestibular apparatus.

Vestibular ataxia syndrome is seen in kittens born of queens stricken with feline parvovirus during pregnancy. Owners often

> ## 🔍 **F**ACT *OR* *FICTION*
>
> **When falling from heights, all cats have the natural ability to "right" themselves and land feet first. 🔍F**ACT**. But only if the cat has healthy ears! The vestibular portion of the nervous system, normally responsible for this remarkable reflex, can be disrupted by, among other things, ear infections and nasopharyngeal polyps. As a result, any cat harboring a severe ear mite infestation should think twice before leaping!**

are alerted to a problem when these kittens seem to have trouble in attempting to walk. The condition will not improve as these kittens mature, nor will it usually worsen.

Congenital vestibular syndrome is seen in Siamese and Burmese cats, with signs appearing anywhere from 2 to 4 weeks of age. Many of the Siamese cats affected are deaf as well. The prognosis for Siamese cats with congenital vestibular syndrome is good, with clinical signs usually abating by the time the cat is 6 months of age. In Burmese cats, however, the prognosis is not as good, and the poor quality of life for most of these individuals will usually warrant euthanasia.

Feline Hyperesthesia Syndrome

Feline hyperesthesia syndrome ("twitchy skin syndrome") is a condition characterized by some unique clinical signs. Affected cats exhibit a rippling of the skin on their backs, especially when petted in the lower back region. They might chew or lick at their tail incessantly, and appear to be "spaced out," spontaneously darting throughout a room or house and attacking objects and owners without provocation.

The exact cause of this condition remains unknown. Some researchers feel that it is a form of epilepsy. Because "emotional" breeds such as Siamese, Persians, and Himalayans seem to be most often affected, other researchers believe that it is actually a behavioral disorder brought about by an upsetting experience or circumstance. Even food preservatives used in cat foods have been accused of causing feline hyperesthesia syndrome.

Medical therapy for this disorder consists of the use of antianxiety medications or sedatives in an attempt to modify the cat's behavior. Identifying and correcting any environmental upsets (including any dietary changes) that might have a possible link to the problem are needed as well.

Ischemic Encephalopathy (Cats)

Feline ischemic encephalopathy (FIE) is a neurologic condition that has been known to strike cats. FIE is caused by a sudden disruption of blood supply to the brain, similar to a stroke in humans. Although a definitive cause has yet to be determined, cardiomyopathy, neoplasia metastasis, and even feline heartworms are suspect. Affected cats exhibit marked depression, incoordination, circling behavior, and/or seizure activity. The pupils of the eyes may become dilated, and blindness may be apparent. Acute clinical signs usually resolve within 7 to 10 days; however, residual neurologic deficits of varying degrees often remain indefinitely.

Diagnosis of feline ischemic encephalopathy is based on history and clinical signs seen, as well as ruling out other causes of similar symptoms, such as vestibular disease, feline leukemia, and poisonings. Treatment of this neurologic disorder involves the administration of high doses of anti-inflammatory medications. In addition, medications designed to dilate the brain's blood vessels and thin the blood may be employed in an effort to improve overall circulation to the affected regions of the brain.

The prognosis for survival in cats with FIE is guarded during the first 48 hours following onset of clinical signs. After 48 hours, the prognosis for survival is good, since FIE is a nonprogressive disorder.

The Endocrine System

Within the bodies of all mammals, a complex network of glands (the endocrine system) is responsible for the production and secretion of special proteins and lipids (fats) called *hormones.* In turn, these hormones serve to regulate many vital functions within the body, from growth and development to digestion and utilization of nutrients. Like the nervous system, the endocrine system assumes a regulatory role within the body, and its proper function is essential to the overall health of the animal. Without the endocrine glands and their hormones, a state of chaos would quickly ensue within the body, as the functional harmony existing between the various organ systems would cease to exist.

Anatomy and Physiology

Hormones can be protein in nature, or they can be fashioned from special fatty components, known as *steroids.* "Steroid" is one of the most misused and widely misunderstood terms in today's society.

Corticosteroids are a special group of steroids produced by the adrenal glands that are vital to many everyday functions within the body. Synthetic derivatives of this steroid group are commonly used, among other things, to reduce pain and inflammation resulting from musculoskeletal injuries.

Androgens (i.e., testosterone) and *estrogens,* the sex hormones that influence reproductive activity and secondary sexual characteristics, are also types of steroid hormones produced naturally within the body.

Anabolic steroids, probably the most notorious members of the steroid family, are actually synthetic derivatives of the male androgenic steroid hormones. This is the group that has been largely exploited by athletes for increased muscular strength and size.

Although all the different classes of steroids mentioned above, whether natural or synthetic, share a similar structural design, it is easy to see that their functions and effects differ greatly between each class.

Both protein and steroid-type hormones are secreted directly into the bloodstream from the glands or organs that produce them, and circulate to their specific target cells or organs, where they exert their effect. The amount of hormone required to exert its particular effect is precise. If present in too great a quantity, or if supplies are deficient, abnormal function of its target cells or organs result. As a result, hormonal activities within the body are governed by complex negative feedback mechanisms, which ensure proper blood levels at all times. Unfortunately, certain disease conditions involving the endocrine glands and organs can disrupt this delicate balance, which can pose serious health problems.

The *hypothalamus,* located at the bottom portion of the brainstem, functions as an integration center between the nervous system and the endocrine system. Nervous system functions of the hypothalamus include regulation of body temperature, emotional behavior and sleep, and control of food and water intake. As an endocrine organ, the hypothalamus secretes the hormone ADH (antidiuretic hormone), which controls the water balance within the body; oxytocin, which stimulates lactation and uterine contractions; and a variety of other hormones that exert control over the pituitary gland.

The pituitary gland produces hormones that have effects on other endocrine glands, such as the thyroid and adrenal glands. In addition, pituitary hormones also influence growth and reproductive patterns. In dogs, *Cushing's disease,* a condition characterized by an oversecretion of adrenal gland hormones, is most commonly caused by a tumor of the pituitary gland.

Hormones produced by the thyroid gland control the rate of growth and metabolism within the body, as well as decrease calcium levels within the bloodstream. Closely associated with the thyroid gland are the parathyroid glands, which produce a hormone that counteracts the action of a certain thyroid hormone by increasing blood calcium levels. This balance between the thyroid and parathyroid glands helps maintain proper blood levels of calcium at all time. Too much parathyroid hormone can result in excess resorption of bony tissue, resulting in metabolic bone disease.

The adrenal glands produce a variety of hormones, each exerting unique effects within the body. Among other things, adrenal hormones influence carbohydrate and protein metabolism and storage (cortisol, cortisone), help the kidneys regulate sodium and potassium levels (aldosterone), and control blood pressure and heart rate (epinephrine and norepinephrine). Certain organs can double as endocrine glands. The pancreas is not just responsible for producing digestive enzymes; it secretes two hormones, insulin and glucagon, both involved in carbohydrate (sugar) metabolism within the body. Insulin functions to lower blood sugar by increasing its uptake and utilization by the body organs. Counteracting the effects of insulin, glucagon increases blood sugar levels by decreasing its uptake into the liver and fatty tissue. Diabetes mellitus is a disease in which not enough insulin is produced by the pancreas, prohibiting cells and organs from extracting carbohydrates out of the bloodstream.

Other organs exhibiting endocrine functions include the stomach, which produces hormones that regulate digestion; the ovaries and testicles, which, together with the adrenal gland and placenta (in pregnant females), produce the sex hormones; the kidneys, which secrete hormones that influence blood flow and filtration within the kidneys themselves; and the thymus gland, with hormonal activity that influences the cells of the immune system.

Hypothyroidism (Dogs)

The thyroid gland, through production of thyroid hormones, functions to influence nutrient and oxygen utilization within the body, hence affecting overall metabolism. As a result, deficiencies in thyroid hormone or interference with its function can have profound effects on the body. In dogs, immune system malfunctions, iodine deficiencies, incomplete thyroid gland development, and pituitary gland malfunctions can all lead to a condition of hypothyroidism. Predisposed breeds include cocker spaniels, Dobermans, dachshunds, beagles, and golden retrievers.

Clinical signs associated with this disorder are varied, owing to the tremendous scope of thyroid hormone function. Dogs with hypothyroidism tend to be lethargic, sleeping a lot and tiring easily after exercise. Some exhibit a profound intolerance to cold floors or cool environmental temperatures. Puppies so affected might seem to be slow learners when it comes to training. As the skin around the face of these dogs often thickens as a result of the disease, a dog's voice might change to a lower pitch, and facial features might appear droopy or sad.

In addition, hypothyroid dogs may also have poor appetites, yet still gain weight. Over 50 percent of dogs afflicted with hypothyroidism will exhibit changes to the skin and haircoat. A loss of the undercoat occurs, resulting in a thinned, poor-looking coat. Skin thickening occurs, and secondary seborrhea is not uncommon. Finally, eye problems, neurologic disorders, reproductive infertility, arthritis, and aggressive behavior could all have their roots in a thyroid disorder.

A veterinarian can evaluate your pet's thyroid function right at the office. A simple blood test can be used to screen thyroid hormone levels within the body (Fig. 18.1). If a problem is found, then more extensive thyroid function tests may be ordered to help determine the extent of the problem. If a dog is taking corticosteroid hormones for other problems at the time of the testing, the results could come back falsely low. As a rule, however, if clinical signs correlate with blood test results, then it is safe to assume that a condition of true hypothyroidism exists.

Regardless of the underlying cause, treatment of hypothyroidism in dogs involves daily supplementation with synthetic thyroid hormone tablets. Thyroid hormone levels will need to be monitored during the initial stages of treatment to ensure that the proper dosage is being met. For the most part, this is a medication that affected dogs will need to stay on for the rest of their lives. Clinical response to medicating is usually seen within 2 weeks after initiation, with resolution of signs occurring soon after.

Hyperthyroidism (Cats)

A condition of hyperthyroidism in cats is caused by an increase in circulat-

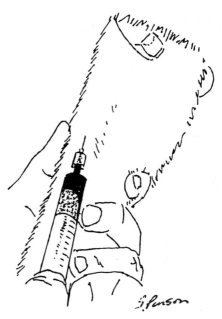

FIGURE 18.1 A simple blood test can be used to assess the thyroid status of a dog.

ing levels of thyroid hormones, namely, thyroxine (T3) and triiodothyronine (T4). When it occurs, hyperthyroidism is most commonly seen in cats greater than 8 years of age, usually as a result of a tumor involving the thyroid gland. Because thyroid hormone helps regulate the body's metabolism, the clinical signs seen with hyperthyroidism can be directly related to the exaggerated increase in the cat's metabolic rate. These symptoms may be mild to severe depending on the amount of excess hormone being secreted. Signs typically include noticeable weight loss in the presence of a voracious appetite (Fig. 18.2), nervousness and hyperactive behavior, and a rough, unkempt haircoat. Other less common signs seen include increased water consumption, regurgitation (due to rapid overeating), panting, and breathing difficulties, especially if the thyroid glands are grossly enlarged. In addition, many cats with elevated thyroid levels also suffer from inflammatory bowel disease (IBD). As a result, vomiting and/or diarrhea related to this may be seen in the hyperthyroid feline as well.

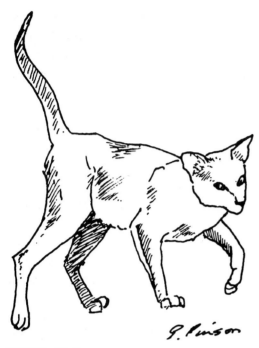

FIGURE 18.2 Hyperthyroidism causes emaciation in the presence of a ravenous appetite!

Diagnosis of hyperthyroidism is made through the evaluation of clinical signs, physical exam findings, and special laboratory tests. On physical examination, nodules can usually be palpated in the neck region because of glandular enlargement. In addition, a rapid heart rate and pulse are often detected because of the effects of the thyroid hormones on the heart. This cardiac affect can be especially dangerous in cats suffering from concurrent cardiomyopathy. A diagnosis of hyperthyroidism can also be verified through the use of special tests designed to detect levels of thyroid hormone in the blood.

If this condition is definitively diagnosed, a number of treatment options exist. The type of treatment chosen will depend on the severity of the thyroid hormone elevation and other underlying disease factors (such as the presence of heart disease or kidney disease). Medical treatment for hyperthyroidism involves the administration of special drugs designed to inhibit production of thyroid hormone by the thyroid gland, thereby controlling clinical signs. Side effects from giving such drugs can include anemia, immune cell suppression, decreased appetite, vomiting, weakness, and itching. Since most cats must stay on this medication for the remainder of their lives, close monitoring by and periodic communication with a veterinarian is essential.

Yet another form of medical therapy that yields successive results in hyperthyroid felines is called *radioactive iodine therapy.* This type of therapy selectively destroys malfunctioning thyroid cells using radiation.

Most cats suffering from hyperthyroidism will respond favorably to medical therapy. However, if drug therapy fails to resolve the disorder and radioactive iodine therapy is unavailable, surgical removal of the thyroid gland (partial or complete thyroidectomy) must be performed. If extensive tumor involvement necessitates the removal of the thyroid, then daily thyroid hormone supplementation will be required for the remainder of the cat's life. Felines placed on such supplementation should have blood thyroid levels checked every 6 to 8 months to ensure that adequate levels are being given.

An inherent risk associated with the surgical removal of the thyroid gland in cats is a complication known as *hypoparathyroidism.* This condition, characterized by low blood calcium levels, is caused by the inadvertent removal of the parathyroid gland (tightly adhered to the thyroid gland) when the thyroid tissue is removed. Signs of low blood calcium, which normally arise within 3 days of parathyroid gland removal, include profound weakness, muscle tremors and spasms, and in some cases, seizures. Felines suffering from this postsurgical complication require prompt treatment with calcium supplements. These supplements, as well as vitamin D tablets, will be required for life to help maintain proper calcium levels within the body.

Hyperadrenocorticism (Cushing's Disease)

Steroid hormones, specifically the class known as *glucocorticosteroids* produced by the adrenal glands, serve over 50 vital functions within the body. Some of the more important ones have to deal with carbohydrate, protein, and fat utilization and with maintaining water and electrolyte balance within the body. Veterinarians fighting allergic reactions or inflammation in dogs and cats rely on glucocorticosteroids for their anti-inflammatory effects when given at low dosages. Similarly, since high doses of glucocorticosteroids can suppress the immune system, they are quite useful in treatment against autoimmune diseases in pets, including *pemphigus,* a disease that causes severe skin lesions in affected dogs.

Unfortunately, since steroid hormones help maintain a delicate balance within the body, an overproduction of these hormones within the body can upset this balance. This is precisely what happens in

Cushing's disease. An overproduction of glucocorticosteroids from the adrenal glands occurs within the body, usually as the result of a tumor affecting one or both glands, or, more commonly, a tumor affecting the pituitary gland. The disease is most common in dogs over 8 years of age. Furthermore, poodles, boxers, and dachshunds seem to be afflicted with a greater frequency than other breeds. Fortunately, the condition is rarely seen in cats.

Some of the clinical signs seen in dogs with Cushing's disease include a marked increase in water and food consumption, an increase in elimination activity, lethargy and exercise intolerance, and a generalized reduction in muscle size and tone, which, when it affects the muscles of the abdominal wall, leads to a characteristic pot-bellied appearance (Fig. 18.3).

The skin and coat changes that occur in a dog with Cushing's disease might be the first clues as to the existence of the problem. A generalized thinning of the haircoat and skin will be seen, with flakiness, pigmentation, and secondary infections. Eye problems are common in these dogs, too, with recurring ulcers affecting the cornea. Because high levels of steroids have a suppressing influence on the immune system, secondary infections, especially bladder infections, are often seen in these dogs as well. Finally, if a tumor is present in the pituitary gland at the base of the brain, neurological problems might occur as pressure is increased on the brain.

These signs can lead a clinician to suspect Cushing's disease, but more extensive blood testing and radiographic X rays are usually required to confirm a diagnosis. Measuring actual blood levels of steroids within the bloodstream is one way to test for Cushing's disease; other methods include injecting small amounts of special synthetic hormones, designed to alter the production of steroids within the body, into the dog and measuring

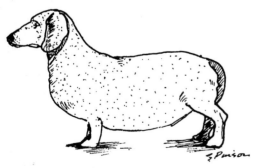

FIGURE 18.3 Hair loss and a pot-bellied appearance are both frequent signs seen with Cushing's disease.

the body's response to them. If these hormones cannot alter the steroid production, then a diagnosis can be made.

Once a dog is diagnosed with Cushing's disease, therapy may be instituted in a number of ways. Surgical removal of the tumor in either the adrenal glands and/or pituitary gland can be attempted, but this is a very difficult procedure associated with many postoperative complications.

Chemotherapy can be employed to target the adrenal glands and reduce the amount of steroids being produced by them. Used correctly, this treatment can reduce or eliminate the clinical signs seen and greatly improve a dog's quality of life. Close veterinary monitoring for the appearance of side effects during the initial treatment stage is recommended. Therapy is usually required for life.

Because of the intense management required with these modes of therapy, some pet owners prefer to stick to conservative treatment when dealing with this disease in their dogs. In these cases, dogs should be placed on high-protein diets to counteract protein loss caused by the disease. In addition, treating secondary problems as they arise—such as skin infections, bladder infections, and corneal ulceration—is necessary. Because the tumors responsible for Cushing's disease are usually slow-growing, most dogs can live for up to 2 years with this treatment approach alone.

Hypoadrenocorticism (Addison's Disease)

While Cushing's disease is caused by too many corticosteroids circulating within the body, Addison's disease is caused by the exact opposite: inadequate amounts of circulating corticosteroids. This includes not only the glucocorticosteroids produced by the adrenal glands but the mineralocorticoids as well. Because the latter are so vital at maintaining a fluid and electrolyte balance within the body, Addison's disease can be acutely life-threatening in the affected individual. Like Cushing's disease, Addison's disease is primarily a disease of dogs; it is rare in cats.

Causes of this disease in dogs can include tumors, infections, autoimmune diseases, and toxins. It can also occur secondarily to overtreatment with corticosteroids.

The clinical signs seen resemble those exhibited by pets afflicted with viral or parasitic gastroenteritis—namely vomiting, diarrhea, and dehydration. Loss of appetite and weight loss accompany these signs as well, yet there might be an increase in water consumption. Because the levels of sodium and potassium, two electrolytes vital to proper muscle contraction, are disrupted, profound muscle weakness, including a slowing of the rate at which the heart muscle contracts, are also observed. In severe cases, collapse of the entire circulatory system, with shock and then death, has been documented.

Diagnosis of Addison's disease can made based on the history (i.e., long-term corticosteroid therapy), clinical signs seen, and determining the ratio of sodium to potassium in the bloodstream. Marked increases in potassium and decreases in sodium are indicative of primary Addison's disease. Physical examination and electrocardiograms will reveal abnormal heart activity in these patients as well.

If Addison's disease is diagnosed or suspected, treatment should be instituted immediately. Dehydration is combated with intravenous fluids, and injections of mineralocorticoids are administered to stabilize fluid and electrolyte levels.

For cases of primary Addison's disease, periodic injections with mineralocorticoids will be required throughout the dog's life to prevent relapses from occurring. If the condition was caused by the sudden cessation of glucocorticosteroid therapy, such therapy is reinstituted and then gradually tapered off over weeks to months.

Hyperparathyroidism

The parathyroid glands, which are closely associated with the thyroid glands in dogs and cats, produce a hormone that is responsible for increasing calcium levels in the blood by drawing stores of this mineral from bone and other regions of the body. *Hyperparathyroidism* is a condition initiated by a deficiency of calcium within the bloodstream. This can result from diet regimens that are high in phosphorus (nutritional hyperparathyroidism), such as all-meat diets, or, more commonly in older pets, from increased phosphorus levels in the body caused by kidney disease. When such a calcium deficiency occurs, the parathyroid glands respond by secreting large amounts of hormone, which draws calcium out of bone in an attempt to normalize blood calcium levels. Over time, these bones become weakened and prone to stress injury.

Diabetes Mellitus

Diabetes mellitus is one of the more common endocrine diseases affecting both dogs and cats. The condition is caused by a deficiency in (or in some cases, a resistance to) the hormone called *insulin,* which is created by special cells within the pancreas. Insulin is responsible for regulating the uptake of blood sugar, or glucose, into cells and tissues of the body for use as energy. Any disease involving the pancreas, including chronic pancreatitis, can cause deficiencies in this hormone. In addition, autoimmune disease, in which the pet's body creates antibodies against its own insulin, has also been known to occur. Overweight pets, especially obese cats, are at high risk for diabetes mellitus. Finally, there is evidence that, in dogs, a risk for diabetes can be inherited. Middle-aged female dogs seem to be more at greater risk.

When a deficiency in insulin does occur, the transfer of glucose from the bloodstream to the tissues does not occur; hence, blood glucose levels become elevated. At the same time, the cells, tissues, and organs of the body don't receive the proper nutrition needed to maintain their function, and they start to look for other sources of energy in the body, namely, proteins and fats. And this is where the problems start.

Dogs and cats with this disease will exhibit an increase in water consumption and, consequently, urination. As the body calls on these alternate sources of energy, pronounced weight loss results. In addition, as body fat stores are called on and metabolized for energy, an excess of ketone bodies, by-products of fatty breakdown, accumulate within the body. In large amounts, these ketone bodies have the ability to damage the liver and to depress the nervous system, leading to depression and coma. Over time, the increased glucose levels within the blood can lead to cataracts and blindness.

Diabetic pets have a decreased resistance to infection; as a result, they often suffer from chronic skin and bladder infections. Damage to small capillaries within the body caused by diabetes mellitus can lead to secondary kidney disease, blindness, and gangrene of the skin and extremities.

The clinical signs associated with diabetes mellitus are similar to those in conditions such as Cushing's disease, kidney disease, and diabetes insipidus; therefore, a thorough laboratory workup is needed to ensure a correct diagnosis. Blood tests on pets with diabetes mellitus will consistently reveal elevated glucose levels, and evaluation of urine samples will reveal the same. In addition, levels of the blood protein known as *fructosamine* will be elevated as well, even if blood glucose levels are borderline. Such findings, along with the exclusion of other potential causes of the clinical signs, can lead to a definitive diagnosis of diabetes mellitus.

Diabetes mellitus can be classified as uncomplicated or complicated. Uncomplicated cases might exhibit mild to moderate signs of the disease, yet none are truly life-threatening. In contrast, pets diagnosed with the disease and exhibiting marked depression, vomiting, diarrhea, heavy breathing, and/or severe weight loss should all be considered complicated cases and should always be considered medical emergencies. In most of these cases, the high levels of ketone acids produced as a result of increased fat metabolism lower the pH of the blood sufficiently to cause the harmful effects represented by the clinical signs. These pets usually become severely dehydrated at the same time.

Treatment consists of immediate hospitalization with intravenous infusion of replacement fluids, medications designed to increase the pH of the blood (if indeed the pH is too low), and insulin. The levels of insulin given and corresponding blood glucose must be monitored closely, since too much insulin is even worse than not having enough. If excess insulin is given, the pet could quickly become hypoglycemic and go into convulsions. Good monitoring and careful planning on the part of a veterinarian will help prevent this.

Often, dogs and cats are presented with complicated cases of diabetes mellitus because of some underlying disorder adding to the problem. For instance, many of these pets suffer from coexisting disorders such as obesity, pancreatitis, kidney disease, and heart disease. In order to increase the chances of recovery from a complicated case of diabetes mellitus, these disorders must be addressed at the same time.

When a pet finally comes home, it will be the owner's job to ensure that the proper insulin dosage (as prescribed by the veterinarian) is given each day and that proper adjustments are made (per veterinary instruction) as needed.

Keep in mind that it is better to give a diabetic pet too little insulin than to give too much. Adjustments to insulin dosages need to be made slowly and carefully in these uncomplicated cases. Giving too much insulin can cause insulin shock (hypoglycemia), which can be fatal. Signs of this can include trembling, weakness, incoordination, and—if it is not rapidly corrected—seizures. Owners of diabetic pets should always keep a bottle of pancake syrup or honey around in case of insulin shock. Two tablespoons or more given orally should be used if such a reaction is suspected.

Owners must keep accurate records each day as to their pet's urine glucose readings, insulin dosage, overall attitude and/or clinical signs that day, and appetite. These will not only be useful in regulating insulin levels, but such records can provide a veterinarian with valuable information should a question or problem ever arise. Periodic blood tests by a veterinarian will also be needed to determine the efficacy of treatment.

A large number of uncomplicated cases of diabetes mellitus in cats are non-insulin-dependent and do not require specific insulin therapy. In these instances, feeding high-protein, low-carbohydrate diets and administering oral medications designed to either stimulate insulin release from the pancreas, decrease insulin resistance, and/or slow glucose absorption from the intestines are indicated. However, if ketosis occurs at any time during treatment, insulin therapy will be needed.

Strict feeding schedules for pets with diabetes mellitus must be followed. Rations high in fiber and protein with restricted fat and special carbohydrate sources are ideal for maintaining the diabetic pet.

Diabetic dogs should be kept on a consistent exercise program, since fluctuations in the amount of exercise performed from one day to the next can affect blood glucose levels and make proper insulin dosing difficult. If a dog or cat is obese to start with, it will need to be placed on a weight reduction program.

Finally, intact females that are diabetic should be spayed. By eliminating female hormonal influences

> **DID YOU KNOW?**
>
> Approximately 50 percent of all diabetic cats are non-insulin-dependent.

on glucose levels in the body, achieving and maintaining proper insulin levels will be greatly enhanced.

Diabetes Insipidus

This type of diabetes should not be confused with *diabetes mellitus,* which involves abnormal glucose metabolism. Diabetes insipidus involves abnormal water metabolism, and it occurs when there is a lack of the antidiuretic hormone (ADH). ADH is normally produced by the hypothalamus of the brain, yet it exerts its effects on the kidneys, causing water to be recaptured from the kidney tubules rather than being lost in the urine. As a result, the delicate water balance within the body is maintained with this hormone's influence.

Too little ADH may be produced by the hypothalamus as the result of an inherited defect or due to head trauma that damages the hypothalamus. In addition, defects present in the kidneys at birth or acquired later in life can make the kidneys unresponsive or only partially responsive to the effects of ADH. If any of these conditions occur, then diabetes insipidus results.

Pets with diabetes insipidus exhibit increased urinations, incontinence (especially at night), and an increased water consumption. Routine laboratory work usually reveals nothing too significant except for very low urine specific gravity (dilute urine). However, a laboratory workup will help rule out other potential causes of the clinical signs seen, such as diabetes mellitus, Cushing's disease, and kidney disease. If these are ruled out, then a tentative diagnosis of diabetes insipidus becomes more likely. To obtain a definitive diagnosis, special laboratory tests, such as water deprivation tests, plasma ADH determinations, and ADH trials, are required.

Diabetes insipidus caused by poor ADH production from the hypothalamus can be treated by administering a natural or synthetic ADH supplement. These can be administered by injection or drops applied directly into the eyes. Such treatment will be required on a daily basis to control the clinical signs. Therapy is usually for life.

Diabetes insipidus caused by kidneys that are nonresponsive to ADH is more difficult to control. Special drugs can be utilized to slow water loss and reduce thirst in pets so affected.

Providing free access to water at all times is the most important therapeutic measure for all pets suffering from diabetes insipidus. Doing so will help prevent dehydration and its undesirable effects from setting in as a result of the excess water loss through the kidneys. The prognosis for most pets with diabetes insipidus is good to excellent, assuming that medical therapy and free access to water are provided. Because these pets are prone to dehydration, any signs of illness such as loss of appetite, vomiting, or diarrhea warrant prompt veterinary attention.

PART II

BIRDS

Just a few short years ago, when one thought of a household pet, a dog or cat came to mind. Not so anymore. As a substitute for these furry companion animals, birds are increasing in popularity. In fact, the pet bird population in the United States now numbers in the tens of millions and is growing every year.

Birds certainly have their place in history, where they undoubtedly served as an important food source for early humans. As human appreciation for their beauty and unique personalities grew, birds were eventually tamed as pets and, as in the case of raptors, hunters in the households of Egyptian, Grecian, and Roman elite. Ever since Christopher Columbus introduced the first parrot to the European community from one of his many voyages to the New World, their popularity as companions has been on the increase.

What accounts for the popularity of birds as pets in our day and age? For starters, they are fascinating creatures to be around. Most people fail to realize how much personality and affection a pet bird can exhibit toward its owner. And when was the last time you carried on a conversation with your dog, and it talked back to you!

Still another reason sparking the popularity of birds as pets is the increase in the number of people who live in apartments and condominiums. Space and lease restrictions against dogs and cats in many of these locations have left potential pet owners seeking options. And pet birds seem to be the perfect choice!

Many books and articles promote the virtue of birds as being fairly maintenance-free pets. Granted, maintaining a pair of finches might not require much expenditure of energy on your part, but keep in mind that husbandry for the average pet bird requires at least as much effort as that for cats and dogs. For instance, cleanliness is a key factor in bird husbandry, and daily attention to it must be given. Also, many birds, such as cockatoos and hand-raised birds, require a definite daily time commitment to satisfy their need for social interaction. Failure to do so can lead to great emotional stress, upsetting behavioral problems, and even disease.

The bottom line is this: Don't purchase a bird with the idea of a low-maintenance pet in mind. Like a dog or a cat, it will require both time and effort on your part to ensure that your relationship with your bird is a happy and healthy one.

Choosing the Right Bird for You

hen purchasing or selecting a bird, there are a number of factors to consider. The first obviously is what variety of bird you want. You have many to choose from. Be sure to visit the library, local bookstore, or the Internet to thoroughly research the variety of bird you are most drawn to prior to becoming an actual owner.

Factors to Consider

The more popular pet birds come from two categories, or orders, of avians: Psittaciformes (psittacines) and Passeriformes (passerines). Psittacines include budgerigars, cockatiels, cockatoos, lovebirds, lories, lorikeets, conures, the large parrots, and macaws. The passerine group includes finches, canaries, and the softbilled mynahs. Another popular pet, the toucan, belongs to the order Piciformes.

DID YOU KNOW?

One way to differentiate psittacines from passerines is to observe their feet when they are at perch. Psittacines will perch with two toes pointing forward and two pointing backward. Passerines, on the other hand, perch with three toes pointing forward and one pointing back.

Varieties

BUDGERIGARS

Budgerigars, or "budgies," are by far the most fancied bird in America, accounting for almost 45 percent of all pet birds purchased (Fig. 19.1). They are referred to by most people as *parakeets,* yet in reality, the word *parakeet* pertains to any long-tailed parrot, including budgies, lorikeets, rosellas, and those birds belonging to the genus *Brotogeris.*

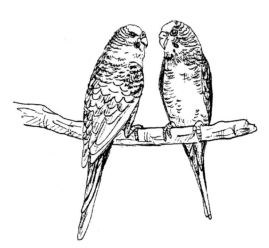

Budgerigars are hardy birds that, for the most part, have gentle dispositions. Their popularity also rests on the fact that they are inexpensive to purchase, require little space, and maintain a relatively low noise level.

Budgerigars have the capability to live 15 to 18 years in captivity. Unfortunately, because of poor husbandry practices on the part of many budgie owners, few of these birds live past 6 years of age. As far as talking is concerned, male budgerigars have the ability to learn a broad vocabulary, and can actually vocalize entire phrases and sentences at a time. Females, on the other hand, won't talk as much as will the opposite sex!

FIGURE 19.1 Budgerigars are by far the most popular of all pet birds.

COCKATIELS

The second most popular companion bird is the cockatiel. In fact, many experts feel that as a first bird for beginners, cockatiels rank among the best. Known for their affection toward their owners and their insatiable curiosity, these birds are relatively easy to maintain and can live as long as 20 years. Compared to budgies, their vocabulary is somewhat limited, yet they (especially males) can be taught to talk. In addition, the female cockatiel tends to have a more laid-back personality than do her male counterparts.

FINCHES AND CANARIES

Finches are small, lively birds. They make excellent pets, and just watching their busy activity can provide hours of enjoyment. The two most popular finch varieties for beginners include "zebra" finches and "society" finches. Because of their gregarious nature, finches should be kept in pairs.

> **FACT or FICTION**
>
> Green budgerigars and gray cockatiels tend to live longer and healthier lives than do their different colored counterparts within the same species.
> **FACT.** Green and gray are the normal colors found in wild budgies and wild cockatiels, respectively, whereas other colors are the result of mutations. Because other genetic mutations often accompany these color mutations, the longevity of these "off-colored" birds tends to be reduced.

Canaries, on the other hand, may be kept as singles and are easier to tame than finches. Another desired feature of canaries is that males have the ability to produce beautiful music and song, much to the delight of their owners. Finches can live anywhere from 6 to 10 years, and canaries even longer.

LOVEBIRDS

Lovebirds make up only a small portion of the pet bird population. These dwarf parrots originate from Africa and are tough to tame, requiring regular interaction with people to maintain any established trust between bird and owner. The peachface lovebird seems to be the most popular among the species available. Energetic and active, lovebirds have a captive life span of 5 to 10 years.

LORIES AND LORIKEETS

Having roots in Australia and the South Pacific, lories and lorikeets are known for their striking colors and playfulness. Although they are visually appealing to novice bird owners, lories and lorikeets can be considered high maintenance and are not good selections for beginners. Since they eat nectars, fruits, and vegetables, their droppings tend to be quite liquid and messy. This necessitates frequent cleanings of the cage and the contents therein. Food must be kept fresh at all times. Lories and lorikeets love to take baths, so frequent opportunities to do so should be offered. Cared for properly, these affectionate birds can live 8 to 15 years in captivity.

CONURES

Conures are a smaller variety of parrot that can make excellent starter pets for the novice. Most have outgoing pleasant personalities and can be quite affectionate. The half-moon conure from Mexico is among the most popular. Be forewarned, however, that these birds like to screech and can be quite loud at times, much to the dismay of neighbors. The average life span of a captive conure ranges from 15 to 30 years.

LARGE PARROTS

The African Grey parrot is the most popular of the larger psittacines. Fancied in ancient Rome for their outgoing personalities and impressive talking abilities, African Greys have proved to be faithful companions of humans throughout history. When raised domestically and hand-fed when young, these birds enjoy and actively seek out the attention and affection of their owners.

One unique feature of African Greys is the vocal growl they won't hesitate to exhibit when surprised or stressed. The average life span of the African Grey in the wild is 50+ years, or 18 years in captivity. Their cost is usually not quite as high as the Amazon parrot, yet many factors, including whether the bird was hand-fed and tamed when young, can influence purchase prices.

Like their African cousins, Amazon parrots are popular choices among bird fanciers, primarily because of their ready availability and to their social attraction to humans. They tend to be more expensive than the smaller psittacines and even the African Grey, with hand-reared birds bringing the highest prices. Amazon parrots can live 80+ years in the wild, yet rarely live past 20 years in captivity.

Within the Amazon parrot family, there are varieties from which to choose, including the popular double yellowhead, yellow nape, and blue-fronted Amazons. The yellowhead Amazon is a popular talker, yet is also known for its somewhat temperamental disposition. The blue-fronted Amazon parrot exhibits talking abilities that rival those of their yellowhead counterparts. Lilac-crowned Amazon parrots are a common species smuggled into the United States from Mexico. Potential purchasers of yellowhead Amazons, especially from a "shady" source, should be on the lookout, since the heads of the inexpensive lilac-crowned parrots are sometimes dyed yellow to fool potential buyers into thinking they are buying a more expensive bird.

Because of the long life span of Amazon parrots, purchasers of these birds are truly accepting a lifelong responsibility. However, most owners will agree that the companionship and joy that these entertaining talkers offer is well worth the commitment.

Because of the danger of the disease psittacosis (see Chap. 44) in birds that are illegally smuggled into the United States, potential buyers of Amazon parrots should buy their pets only from reputable sources.

COCKATOOS

Cockatoos are magnificent birds and are among the most intelligent and emotional members of the entire parrot family. Consequently, they demand more social attention from their owners than do other psittacines.

Cockatoos that feel neglected can become quite destructive and noisy, and can begin to pick at their feathers as a result of emotional stress. However, as current cockatoo owners would agree, the high intelligence level and outgoing personalities of cockatoos rank them among the most entertaining and devoted of all psittacine pets. The average life span of these beautiful birds in the wild is 50 to 80 years, yet only 15 to 20 years in captivity.

MACAWS

Macaws are the largest of the psittacines and among the most beautiful. Highly intelligent birds, they, too, enjoy interaction with people. Common types include blue and gold macaws, scarlet macaws, greenwing macaws, and military macaws. A fifth type, the hyacinth macaw, is the largest of all parrots (Fig. 19.2).

Because of their size, macaws do have large space requirements. This factor, along with their high cost and high maintenance requirements, make them inappropriate choices for first-time bird owners. The incredible power of this bird's beak can quickly wreak havoc on

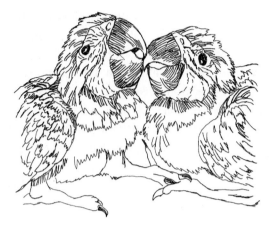

FIGURE 19.2 Baby macaws.

DID YOU KNOW?

A large psittacine can inflict serious physical trauma on any dog or cat.

household furnishings if allowed free access to them. Cages must be sturdy! Inexperienced handlers may also learn the hard way that macaws must be approached and handled with gentleness and care. The loud shrill of these magnificent psittacines and its potential effects on one's neighbors is another factor that must be taken into account by prospective buyers of these birds. Macaws can live 50+ years in the wild, yet rarely live past 15 years in captivity.

MYNAHS AND TOUCANS

Mynahs and toucans belong to a special group of birds known as "softbills" that eat only fruits and other soft foods. Mynahs are probably the most prolific and expert talkers of all birds. Toucans, on the other hand, won't say a word. Both require fruit in their diets, which can make daily cleanup much more arduous than with parrots.

Aside from cleanup, softbills require less social attention than do most conventional psittacines, which can make them excellent choices for those owners who just enjoy having a bird in the house.

Purchase Price

Cost of ownership undoubtedly comes into play when deciding which variety of bird to buy. Purchase prices can range from less than $20 for finches and budgies to over $10,000 for some hand-raised, domestic macaws. One can expect to pay more in food, housing, and veterinary care for the larger parrots and macaws, and for a much longer period of time. Also, birds that are domestically hand-raised and hand-fed by breeders when young command higher prices than do wilder imports, simply because they generally make tamer, more desirable pets. As a result, beginners should plan on paying a little extra for such a bird.

Beware of "special deals" and abnormally low prices advertised for some psittacines. These birds could have undesirable personalities or health problems, which may account for their low price. For example, psittacines that are smuggled into the United States can often be purchased at exceptionally low prices, yet these birds are often quite wild and can be carriers of *psittacosis,* a disease that can threaten human health as well as that of the bird. As a result, always be knowledgeable of the current price trends for the variety of bird you want, and always purchase your bird from a reputable breeder or pet store.

Time

Before you purchase a bird, you should consider how much time you are willing to invest in its care. Realize that acquiring a larger parrot or macaw may constitute a lifetime commitment on your part. If you have doubts about taking on such a responsibility, stick to the smaller varieties of birds with shorter life spans, such as budgerigars or cockatiels. Even with these birds, however, realize that you are still making a 10- to 15-year commitment!

The time you need to devote daily to a pet bird will increase with the size of the bird, with the exception of the cockatoo, which seems to require the most attention of all psittacines. Failure to devote daily attention and time to these birds can lead to many serious behavioral and health problems in the future (Fig. 19.3).

Also remember that owning a pet bird may restrict or interfere with your ability to travel or vacation. Transport-

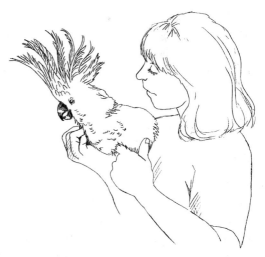

FIGURE 19.3 Many birds require lots of attention from their owners and could exhibit serious behavioral disorders if neglected.

ing your bird between temporary travel destinations is not recommended because of the high level of stress it would ultimately generate, putting your pet's health at risk. The best solution is to hire a pet sitter to care for your bird while you are gone.

Housing

Housing and space requirements should also be figured into your purchase decision. Birdcages need to be roomy enough to provide for safe, adequate movement and exercise within. In addition, realize that most pet birds will require time outside their cages, which can inevitably lead to abuses within your house or apartment. This is especially true with the larger parrots and macaws. Finally, conures, large parrots, and macaws can be quite noisy, which could pose a problem with your neighbors and/or landlord. You must also take this noise factor into account if you run an office from your home.

Age

Consider the age of the bird you are going to buy. As a rule, younger birds are more desirable than older ones simply because they are easier to tame and train, and are less likely to have difficult personality quirks. They are also more likely to develop into good talkers. If possible, purchase budgerigars and cockatiels before they are 3 months of age and larger psittacines before they are 1 year of age.

Eye color can be used as an age estimator for African Grey parrots, cockatoos, and macaws. Young birds tend to have darker eyes that turn grayish around 1 year of age, and then turn white to yellow around 3 to 4 years of age. The iris color of Amazon parrots turns from brown in young birds to a red-orange color as the bird matures.

Sex

The sex of a bird often determines its personality For example, male psittacines tend to be better talkers than do females of the same species, yet the latter are often less aggressive and more content in captivity.

Male budgies can be differentiated from females by the color of their ceres (or nostrils) and legs. The male budgie has a dark blue to lavender cere and a blue hue to his legs; the female will have a tan, pink, or light blue cere and pink legs. Male cockatiels can be identified by yellow and orange markings on the head, in contrast to the grayish coloration of the female. Most cockatoos can be sexed according to their eye color; males have black-colored eyes and females have a red-brown tint to theirs. Male zebra finches can be identified apart from the female by the red-orange patches on their cheeks and sides. On the contrary, male and female society finches and canaries are indistinguishable in terms of color. Male canaries, however, can be identified according to their ability to sing.

For conures, macaws, and the larger parrots, methods other than coloration and behavior must be used to determine sex. One of the most common methods used today is fiber-optic endoscopy to surgically sex these birds. If you wish to breed your bird at some point in the future, have this procedure performed prior to purchase, as part of the prepurchase screening, just so you can be sure of the sex and reproductive health status of your new feathered friend.

Taming and Training Your Pet Bird

Because of their highly intelligent nature, training a pet bird is not as difficult a task as it might seem. The first hurdle you must overcome, however, is the taming process. If you purchased a bird that was hand-reared, this taming no doubt has already been done for you. Your only job is to make friends with your new companion (Fig. 19.4).

Depending on the previous socialization your bird has received, it might take some time for it to become comfortable with you, so be patient. Perform this routine over and over each day. Keep each session short and positive. Remember: This relationship is based on mutual trust (Fig. 19.5).

When trying to win your way into your new friend's heart, go by way of the stomach! Use food, especially seed or pound cake, to entice your bird out of its cage and onto your hand or arm (Fig. 19.6). If you haven't already done so, get your bird's feathers clipped to prevent it from flying away while you are trying to tame it.

Once tamed, birds can be taught to do a variety of tricks using food as a reward. Be careful not to be overzealous when doling out these rewards. You don't want your pet to get fat during the training process!

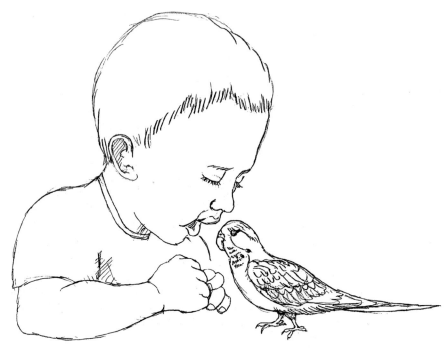

FIGURE 19.4 When properly socialized, pet birds can be fun for the entire family!

Talking

Most psittacines have the uncanny ability to mimic what they hear, a skill that is instinctive. Some species are more talkative than others. Pet birds listed from most talkative to least talkative include African Grey parrots, Amazon parrots, budgerigars, cockatoos, cockatiels, conures, lovebirds, and macaws. In addition, males birds tend to exhibit a greater ability to mimic than do females.

If you want to teach your bird certain words, names, or phrases, *repetition* is the key. Although young birds are the easiest to teach, all birds can learn to speak. Practice with your bird daily, rewarding it with food for a desired response. When you are not there, a tape recording of the word or phrase repeated over and over again is an effective training tool you can leave with your bird. Just be sure you don't leave it on during the night, disturbing your bird's rest. With enough repetition and practice, you will soon find your bird talking like a pro!

Proper Nutrition

There is no doubt that, aside from good sanitation, nutrition leads the list as the most important factor in keeping pet birds healthy. Birds should be allowed access to a high-quality diet twice a day, early morning and late evening, to better satisfy the instinctive food gathering rituals that they exhibit in the wild.

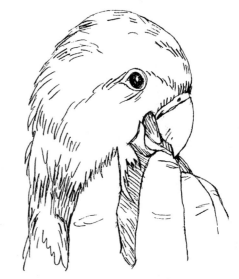

FIGURE 19.5   As part of its training program, don't allow your bird to bite you, even in play.

The most common misconception held among novice owners regarding avian nutrition is that perching birds can be sustained on a diet of seeds alone. Granted, seeds add to the nutritional requirements of birds, yet an all-seed diet or even one where seeds are simply offered as treats is inadequate for captive birds and will eventually lead to serious health problems.

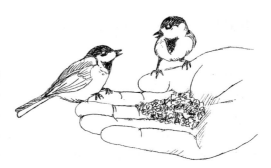

FIGURE 19.6   Food is one of the most effective training aids for birds.

Seeds are high in fat and carbohydrates, yet relatively low in protein and certain essential amino acids. Many obese birds became that way because of too much seed, and consequently, too much fat, in their diets. Seeds alone are also deficient in certain vitamins, including vitamins A, D_3, and B_{12}. The hulls of seeds, which are rich in B vitamins, are often removed prior to consumption, thereby further reducing the seed's nutritional value.

As far as essential minerals are concerned, seeds are deficient in iodine, calcium, and other trace minerals, yet high in phosphorus. For birds fed seed-only diets, this high level of phosphorus can lead to musculoskeletal disease. Old, moldy seed can also cause aspergillosis.

The Best Dietary Choices

A number of high-quality formulated feed mixtures suitable for your particular variety of bird are now available commercially, and are the diets of choice for pet birds. Ask your veterinarian to recommend the mixture best suited for your bird. Because of the wide variety of high-quality bird rations available on the market today, formulating your own mixtures at home is no longer recommended. Limited amounts of green vegetables (such as bell peppers, collards and mustard greens, broccoli, and alfalfa sprouts), yellow vegetables (such as squash and carrots), and fruit (including apples, grapes, and bananas) can still be offered as treats to birds being fed a high-quality formulation. As a rule, these should not exceed 15 percent of your bird's total daily food intake. All foods offered to your bird should be as fresh as possible (Fig. 19.7).

(*Note:* Softbills, lories, and lorikeets require special fruit and nectar diets. Be sure to discuss these dietary needs with your veterinarian.)

Supplements

All birds should also be fed a vitamin supplement containing vitamin D_3, and a mineral supplement that provides extra calcium to the diet. Cuttlebone, mineral blocks, or crushed oyster shells can be used as sources for calcium. As for vitamin supplements, these are readily available from pet stores and can be added directly to food or water. If added to the water, remember to change the water daily to prevent bacterial growth.

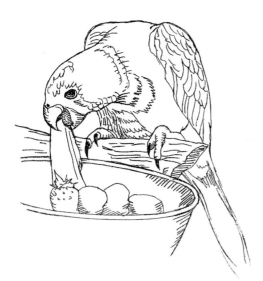

FIGURE 19.7 Fruits and vegetables are important parts of your psittacine's diet.

The Finicky Eater

What happens if your bird appears to be hooked on seeds and refuses to eat its high-quality ration? The first thing to remember is that birds can become malnourished because of food refusal following abrupt changes in diet. For example, finches, which consume about one-third of their body weight per day in food, can die within 48 hours if they choose to go on a hunger strike! Since taste and smell are poorly developed in birds, sight recognition plays an important role in food desirability. Your bird might not like what it sees.

DR. P's VET TIP

A useful tool for coaxing a finicky bird to eat food other than seeds is pound cake. Most birds will readily accept this tasty treat, which, when used to camouflage or cover up new types of foods, can be used to entice the bird into eating them. Over the next few days, gradually reduce the amount of pound cake offered. Pound cake is also useful as a vehicle for giving oral medications to birds!

DID YOU KNOW?

Seed-only diets can lead to malnutrition and liver disease in birds.

Any radical changes to your bird's diet should take place gradually over a 7- to 10-day period. If your bird is addicted to seeds, try to wean it off of them by offering a formulated diet with no seeds in the mornings, and then offering a small amount of seed in the evenings. Leave this seed in the cage for only a few hours, then remove it. Keep repeating this exercise, gradually reducing the amount of seeds and increasing the formulated diet that you are offering.

Other Nutritional Requirements

Grit is often offered to pet birds as an aid to digestion. Commercial grit usually consists of crushed shells and/or limestone. This substance does its work in the bird's gizzard, helping to crush and grind food, making it acceptable for digestion. Not much is actually needed for this purpose—only a few pieces over a week's time. In fact, allowing access to too much grit at one time can actually cause serious health problems, especially in birds that are already ill.

The need for grit in captive birds is still controversial among veterinarians, with many feeling that it is not necessary for those birds fed a well-formulated diet. Ask your veterinarian to decide whether grit is necessary for your particular bird.

Twigs from apple, maple, oak, elm, or cherry trees should also be offered to pet birds. Chewing on these will not only help keep their beaks in fine shape but also contribute essential trace minerals to the diet.

Finally, fresh water should be offered at all times. Smaller birds consume anywhere from a teaspoon to tablespoon of water per day; larger birds, up to 1 ounce (30 milliliters) per day. Filtered or purified water is ideal, and considering the small amount of water the average bird drinks in one day, offering such water is worth the extra cost.

Housing Your Pet Bird

Cages

The cage you select for your bird should be large enough to enable your bird to fully extend its wings and flap them without the tips touching the sides (Fig. 19.8). In addition, your bird must be able to perch without its tail feathers touching the floor or sides of the cage. The larger the cage the better, for a large cage will allow your bird more opportunity for exercise. Many experts recommend birdcages with flat tops versus those with domed tops, since the latter have been implicated in toe and beak injuries from those regions on top where the metal bars converge. If you plan on using an antique or custom-made cage, be certain there is no chance of exposure to lead-based paint and/or solder that might have been used in its construction.

Regardless of the type of cage you choose, the metal bars of the cage should not be spaced sufficiently wide apart to allow your pet to escape or, worse yet, cause injury if it attempts to squeeze through them. For smaller birds, this usually means spacing no greater than $7/16$ inch and for larger parrots, no greater than 1 inch.

For safety, the door leading into the cage should open in an outward direction away from the cage, instead of opening inward or sliding up and down. Also, if the door has a spring action, remove the spring and allow the door to swing freely.

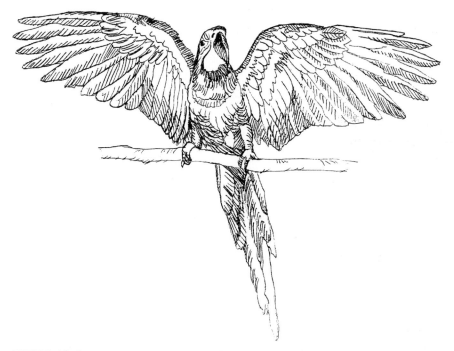

FIGURE 19.8 Your bird's cage should be large enough to allow it to fully extend its wings without touching the sides.

Finally, make sure that the cage you choose is constructed in such a way that it is easy to access and clean. Having to clean an entire cage through the small entry door can be difficult and tedious, and could lead to dereliction of duty!

CAGE LINING

Paper towels or commercial cage pads can be used to cover the bottom of the cage. Newspaper should not be used, since news ink, if ingested, can be harmful to birds. This lining should be cleaned daily to maintain good sanitation. However, always take note of the number and characteristics of the droppings on the liner before throwing it away. As will be pointed out later, these droppings can be useful indicators of your bird's health status (see Chap. 21).

PERCHES

Every pet bird needs a perch to sit on, and choosing the right type will help prevent foot problems from developing later on. Ideally, more

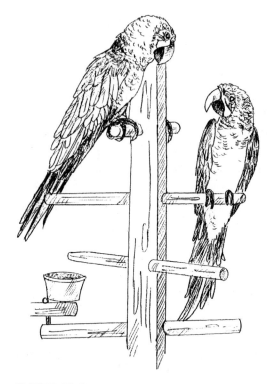

FIGURE 19.9 Be sure to provide your bird with multiple perches of differing diameters.

than one perch should be provided, each of a different diameter and hardness to provide variety for the bird's feet (Fig. 19.9).

The best perches you can offer are simple tree branches of varying widths from northern hardwood, citrus, or eucalyptus trees. Be sure to wash, disinfect, and dry these before placing them in the cage for the first time. Perches shaped like tree branches and made of nontoxic plastic are also available commercially. If you plan to use a painted perch, make certain that a lead-free paint was used. Avoid perches designed with a sandpaper covering (supposedly designed to keep the nails in shape) or those covered with ridges. These are hard on the feet, and can lead to foot problems, including bumblefoot (see Chap. 22).

For sanitary purposes, be sure to position the perches within the cage away from food and water dishes. Like anything else, perches will need to be periodically cleaned and sanitized when they get dirty. Be sure to keep a few spares on hand to minimize the time you must spend on cage cleaning.

CAGE COVERS

Pet birds need at least 12 hours of darkness per day during which to rest and sleep. As a result, a cage cover will be needed to help ensure that your bird gets the beauty sleep it needs. For greatest effectiveness, the cover itself should be made out of a dark fabric. One word of caution: Be sure your bird is at perch before putting on the cage cover. If it is not, it could have difficulty finding the perch in the dark—many a bird has suffered injuries trying to do so.

Toys and Accessories

Toys and accessories for your bird can include small branches, pinecones, rawhide chews, corncobs, and other nontoxic items. Glass mirrors are not recommended for any bird, especially large ones, since the reflection can frighten or anger the bird and lead to a self-sustained injury. In addition, watch out for lead, copper, or zinc contained in some toys. These can be an innocent source of metal poisoning in birds. Finally, food and water dishes should be durably constructed to withstand abuse!

Sanitation

Impeccable sanitation is another key to effective bird husbandry. Cages should be thoroughly cleaned from top to bottom and perches cleaned and rotated at least once a week. Food dishes and water dishes should be cleaned and disinfected on a daily basis. Toys should also be either cleaned or rotated on a daily basis.

Use nontoxic soap and water for cleaning, and afterward, apply a disinfectant. Quaternary ammonium disinfectants, available from most cleaning-supply stores, work well for this purpose. You can use household bleach, diluted $1/4$ cup per gallon of water, as an alternative. Just be sure to rinse all items and surfaces thoroughly with tap water to remove all disinfectant residues.

Avian Anatomy and Physiology

In order to understand the behavior that our pet birds exhibit, and the diseases and disorders that they may encounter, we need to touch on a brief overview of avian anatomy and physiology.

Birds possess some unique features, both externally and internally, that set them apart from the rest of the animal kingdom. For the most part, these variations are geared toward making the bird's primary mode of transportation, flight, easier and more efficient (Fig. 20.1).

The Digestive System

Birds have a short, efficient digestive system. The beak is actually a lightweight substitute for the mammalian cheek, teeth, and lips. It can be used as an effective weapon; the strength contained in the jaws of the larger parrots and macaws is enormous and can lead to serious injuries if the inexperienced handler is not careful.

The tongue of birds, as in mammals, helps manipulate food to the back of the throat, where it can enter the esophagus. As food passes down the esophagus, it enters the *crop*. The crop represents an outpouching of esophagus at the point just before it enters the chest cavity. It serves as a temporary storage place for food. Canaries have no crop.

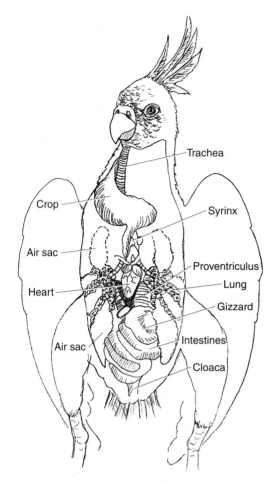

From the crop, food then passes into the *proventriculus,* or *glandular stomach,* and then into the *ventriculus,* or "gizzard." Within the gizzard of the bird, strong muscular contractions, combined with ingested grit, serve to grind up food. Digesta leaves the ventriculus and enters the small intestine, where most of the nutrient absorption takes place. Afterward, it passes into the large intestine. The terminal portion of the large intestine is termed the *cloaca.* It is here that fecal matter is mixed with urates and urine from the urinary system, all of which then pass out through the external opening of the cloaca, called the *vent.*

As far as accessory digestive organs are concerned, the liver, pancreas,

FIGURE 20.1 The internal organs.

and gallbladder (when present) serve similar functions in birds as they do in mammals.

The Respiratory System

The unique respiratory system of the bird begins with the nares, which are two small slits located in the upper portion of the beak. These mark the external entrances into the nasal cavity The trachea extends from the back portion of the mouth down toward the chest cavity and splits off into two branches as it nears its destination. At this bifurcation is located the *syrinx.* This organ corresponds to our vocal cords and is responsible for a bird's singing and talking abilities.

From the syrinx, tubelike bronchi enter into the lungs. Birds have no functional diaphragm that separates the chest and abdominal

cavities; as a result, they rely on the active movement of the ribcage for expansion and contraction of the lungs. This is one reason why gentle restraint is a must when handling pet birds.

Finally, attached to and surrounding the lungs are unique structures called air sacs. Serving as large storage areas for air during respiratory activity, air sacs contribute to the aerodynamics of flight. Interestingly, some of these sacs actually communicate with the cavities inside certain bones, filling them with air. This is why a fractured bone can lead to inflammation of the air sacs, called *airsacculitis.*

The Urogenital System

The kidneys and ureters of birds function in essentially the same way as those of mammals. Birds have no urinary bladder, which would only serve to weigh them down in flight. Instead, the ureters empty their contents directly into the cloaca, which, as mentioned previously, communicates to the outside through the vent.

The reproductive system of the male bird, or cock, consists of testicles and associated structures, *ductus deferens,* and a copulatory apparatus. Female birds, or hens, have two ovaries, yet the left ovary is usually the only one active. When the egg, or yolk, is ovulated from the ovary, it enters the oviduct. In most birds, the left oviduct is the only one that is functional. Within the oviduct, the *albumen,* or "whites" of the final egg are added to the yolk. From the oviduct, the unfinished egg enters into the uterus. It is within the uterus that the hard shell is added. From here, the egg is transferred through the vagina to the cloaca, and from there is laid through the vent. Females lay eggs in groups known as *clutches,* the size of which depends on the species involved.

"Sexing" Your Bird

Certainly the first item on a successful breeding agenda is to be sure you know the sex of your bird(s). This might sound funny, but for many birds, especially the larger psittacines, the sex can't be reliably determined by physical appearance.

Most small psittacines, finches, and canaries can be sexed using physical appearances and/or characteristic behavior. For instance, male budgies can be differentiated from females by the color of their ceres. The male budgie has a dark blue to lavender cere, whereas the female will have a pink or tan cere.

Similarly, male cockatiels can usually be identified by yellow and orange markings on the head, in contrast to the grayish coloration of the female. Cockatoos can often be sexed according to the color of their eyes; males have black eyes and females have red-brown eyes. Male zebra finches can be identified by characteristic red-orange patches on their cheeks and sides.

Not all finches can be differentiated sexually by their coloration. For instance, both male and female society finches look similar. However, behavior can be used to identify male society finches, which will often sing and dance in the presence of a female. The same holds true for male canaries, which can be distinguished by their unprecedented singing ability when spring is in the air.

For larger psittacines such as conures, macaws, African Grey parrots, and Amazon parrots, special lab tests and/or surgical procedures are required to accurately determine the sex of these birds. One such test veterinarians can use is called a *fecal steroid analysis,* which tests for sex specific hormones within the bird's feces. This test is noninvasive, easy to perform, and fairly accurate.

Another sexing method that is popular and can be used to actually view and identify the reproductive organs within the bird's abdomen is called *endoscopy.* With this method, a bird is placed under light anesthesia and a tiny incision is made in the bird's side, into which a fiber-optic device can be inserted. Once inside, the endoscope can be used to visualize the ovaries or testes. One big advantage endoscopy has over other methods of sexing psittacines is that while the endoscope is inside the abdomen, the veterinarian can also assess the overall internal health and breeding condition of the bird in question. For example, endoscopy can be used to detect excessive fat within the abdomen, abnormally developed reproductive organs, and infections, all of which can affect breeding performance. The disadvantage of this procedure, of course, is the risk associated with using anesthetics, although this risk is generally quite low in the hands of an experienced veterinarian. It is up to each individual bird owner to weigh the benefits and risks of having an endoscopic procedure performed. Also, it is a good idea for potential bird owners who are purchasing birds specifically for breeding purposes to arrange with the seller to have the procedure performed as part of the prepurchase exam, if it has not already been done.

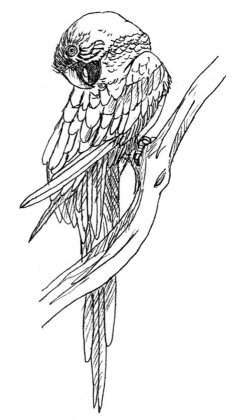

FIGURE 20.2 Preening is a natural way for birds to keep their feathers in top shape.

The Endocrine, Circulatory, and Nervous Systems

These three organ systems are very similar to those in dogs and cats. Heart rates in birds can range anywhere from 175 beats per minute for large macaws to over 1000 beats per minute for small finches and canaries. Birds do have lymphatic channels within their bodies that serve an immune capacity, yet they lack actual lymph nodes.

The Musculoskeletal System

As you might suspect, the muscles and bones of birds are geared toward efficient flight. The skeleton of the typical bird is very lightweight, making flying easier. As mentioned earlier, some of the bones are actually air-filled, communicating directly with air sacs.

The muscles making up the breast of the bird, which are responsible for wing motion, are not surprisingly the largest and strongest in the body. Wasting of these muscles secondary to disease will cause the large *keel bone* or breast bone to protrude and become easily palpable.

The Integumentary System

In contrast to most mammals, the skin of birds is very thin and has minimal blood and nerve supply. In addition, this skin contains no glands per se, except for a special one located near the base of the tail called the *uropygial gland.* The oils produced by this gland are used by the bird during self-grooming, or *preening,* to lubricate and smooth the feathers (Fig. 20.2). Contrary to popular belief, these oils do not waterproof the bird.

The legs and feet of birds are covered in scales. The beak, which corresponds to teeth, cheeks, and lips seen in dogs and cats, is made up of a tough, horny material. The *cere is* a soft tissue structure located at the top portion of the beak. Often used to sex smaller psittacines, overgrowth of this structure could signify nutritional imbalances or parasitic infestations.

The feathers of birds are not only necessary for flight but also play an important role in the regulation of body temperature and in courtship displays. In addition, the overall structure and overlap of feathers helps waterproof the bird and protect it from the elements.

Two Types of Feathers

Contour feathers make up the majority of feathers seen on the head, wings, body, and tail of a bird. The flight feathers are contour feathers, and can be further broken down into the *remiges,* which include the primary and secondary flight feathers of the wings, and the *rectrices,* or those flight feathers making up the tail. *Semiplumes* are smaller contour feathers that blend in with the second main type of feathers,

the *down feathers,* the small, soft feathers found beneath the contour feathers. These serve as effective insulators against environmental temperature fluctuations. In addition, some species, such as cockatiels and cockatoos, have special down feathers called *powder down feathers.* These give off a fine powder that the bird uses in preening.

Molting

Birds go through a molting period one or more times a year in which feathers are lost and then replaced (similar to shedding in dogs and cats). Molting usually occurs seasonally, depending on species. Signs of an impending molt include an increase in preening activity, not to mention the increased number of feathers that will be seen lying at the bottom of the cage. Molting birds may become noticeably lethargic, as the process uses up lots of calories! Some birds will lose most of their feathers all at once; others will lose them more gradually. The entire process usually takes 4 to 6 weeks to complete.

The new feathers that grow in after a molt are encased within feather sheaths, which are eventually shed once eruption is complete. These new feathers also have a rich blood supply that will disappear when the feather reaches its mature length. If a growing feather is accidentally injured and begins to bleed, the entire feather should be plucked from its shaft. This will stop the bleeding, and allow for a new feather to replace the damaged one. On the other hand, mature feathers that are plucked will not be replaced until the next molt.

As indicated above, the molting period for birds is very stressful. Otherwise talkative birds might choose to remain silent during this time, and songbirds might stop singing. It is important that you take appropriate husbandry actions to ensure that other sources of potential stress are avoided. Be sure to provide extra privacy and warmth during this time. Also, increasing the protein, fat, and calcium in diets offered to birds in molt will help ensure that the molt is a successful one and that the new feathers are bright, shiny, and healthy.

Abnormal molting can result in new feathers that are ragged or incomplete, or ones that contain abnormal markings or streaks caused by improper feather development (stress bars). If you suspect that your bird has had an abnormal molt, contact your veterinarian right away.

Vision and Hearing

Eyes

The bird's sense of vision is generally sharper and more acute than that of their furry household counterparts. This is to be expected, considering the maneuverability required for flight and the keen visual perception necessary for safe takeoffs and landings. For example, the eyesight of birds of prey is so acute that they can pick up even the slightest movements on the ground from hundreds of feet up in the air! Researchers also believe that certain species of birds even have the ability to perceive and differentiate colors in their environment.

Anatomically, the eyes and ocular components of birds and those of cats and dogs are essentially the same. There are, however, some unique features of the avian eye worth mentioning.

For starters, the muscles that control eye movement in birds are somewhat small and underdeveloped. As a result, birds must cock, tilt, and turn their heads when trying to focus in on a subject. The iris of the bird eye is also unique in that the bird can, at any time, voluntarily control the size of its pupil. This could account for the exceptional visual acuity displayed by birds, especially birds of prey while in flight. Finally, unlike the eyes of other companion animals, birds have small bones situated within the sclera of the eyes, giving the bird's eye its characteristic shape.

Ears

The structure of the avian ear is also similar to that of dogs and cats, except that it lacks a pinna and has a much shorter ear canal. Located just behind and below the eyes, the ears are rarely a source of health problems in birds. However, because of the ear's importance in maintaining balance and equilibrium, infections or injuries can seriously impair a bird's ability to fly and should be suspected if flight difficulties arise.

Preventive Health Care

As with dogs and cats, the best treatment for any avian disease or injury is prevention (Fig. 21.1). With birds, this takes on a special importance when you consider that they have the ability to hide signs of disease quite effectively, and when evidence of illness does appear, subsequent treatment efforts are often futile. As a result, bird owners can and should play an active role in preventing disease in their pets. Listed below are 11 effective ways to do so:

1. Avoid overcrowding. Housing too many birds in a cage that is too small will not only lead to sanitation problems but also increase the chances of physical trauma and injury.

2. Clean food and water bowls on a daily basis.

3. Keep fresh food and water in the bowls at all times. This might mean replacing the food and water more than once a day. Use filtered or purified water if possible.

4. Provide adequate ventilation in and around your bird's living quarters. Environmental temperatures should be kept between 60 and 85 degrees Fahrenheit, and cages should be placed clear of any drafts in the room. If there are smokers in the household, be sure that such smoke is kept away from your bird.

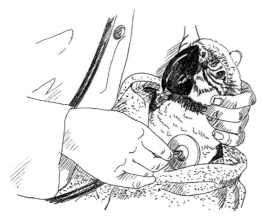

FIGURE 21.1 All birds should receive regular veterinary checkups as part of a complete preventive health care program.

5. Be sure your bird is getting adequate amounts of sleep. Keep bedtimes constant and predictable.

6. Feed a well-balanced diet. What more can be said?

7. Don't let your bird mingle with its wild peers. Wild birds can transmit infectious diseases such as avian pox and internal parasites.

8. Quarantine new birds brought into the household for 6 to 8 weeks before introducing them to an existing bird in the house. A new-bird checkup by your veterinarian is also warranted to help detect any diseases or parasitism already present.

9. Minimize other sources of stress as much as possible. Avoid moving your bird's cage to a different location unless absolutely necessary. Keep the cage free from drafts, as these can quickly lead to stress and respiratory problems in exposed birds. Remember that dogs and cats in the household can place a great deal of stress on some birds, so it makes sense to keep them separated. Also, other sources of stress such as loud noises and blaring music should be kept to a minimum.

10. Vaccines do exist against some of the more common diseases seen in pet birds. For instance, vaccines against avian pox, polyomavirus, and Pacheco's disease are available, and might be effective in preventing the spread of disease within

FACT OR **FICTION**

You shouldn't kiss your bird. **FACT.** Pet birds can develop serious bacterial infections from contact with human saliva.

aviaries, or in those instances in which access to wild birds cannot be controlled. Ask your veterinarian for details.

11. Unnecessary and close physical contact between humans and birds could expose the bird to various infections; avoid such contact if possible.

Preventing Injury or Accidental Poisoning

Aside from the aforementioned tips for preventing disease in pet birds, there are also steps bird owners can take to minimize the chances of injury or accidental poisoning involving their feathered pet within the home.

> **DID YOU KNOW?**
>
> One common source of poisoning in birds during the holiday season is ornamental dough, used to make Christmas tree decorations. This dough contains high levels of salt, which, if consumed by an unsuspecting bird, can cause rapid dehydration, diarrhea, and neurologic signs.

Flying Hazards

To prevent your bird from embarking on an unexpected trip outdoors, get into the habit of keeping all doors and windows closed. In addition, place conspicuous stickers on clear glass doors, windows with the curtains or shades drawn, and mirrors to help prevent midair collisions.

Feather-clipping should also be performed periodically, especially after molting, to help limit your bird's ability to fly freely within the house.

Other Household Hazards

Other hazards that the average house can pose for pet birds include exposed lightbulbs, ceiling fans, and hot stove burners or ovens. Poisonous substances that your pet bird could encounter inside your home include toxic plants, alcohol, pesticides, crayons, pencils, mothballs, chocolate, cedar, redwood, and tobacco. Toilet bowl cleaners that are hung within the tank can pose a special hazard to the innocent bird that sees the open toilet lid and decides it is time to take a bath.

Noxious fumes emitted from paint, cleaners, cigarettes, and even from the nonstick coating of certain types of cookware (when heated) can quickly overcome a bird if adequate ventilation is not available. Jewelry and other small metal items may be eaten by a curious bird, with unfortunate consequences. You must also guard against and eliminate potential sources of lead poisoning, such as lead-based paint, caulking, ceramic glazing, linoleum, and curtain weights. Even excess lead in the water supply (caused by lead-lined pipes) can lead to lead toxicity in a pet bird if levels are high enough.

DID YOU KNOW?

Many perfumes and colognes can be toxic to birds.

The clinical signs of lead poisoning can vary, depending on the amount consumed. General signs include lethargy, vomiting, diarrhea, and increased urination. Also, neurologic signs, such as seizures, apparent blindness, tremors, excitability, and lack of coordination, are usually a tipoff to lead poisoning in birds.

Diagnosis of lead toxicity can be made using radiographic X rays, and actually seeing the lead particles within the gastrointestinal tract. Prompt therapy using the antidote EDTA (ethylenediaminetetraacetic acid) can help relieve the clinical signs in these birds. Surgical removal of the remaining lead particles may also be necessary.

Restraint

When it comes to physical restraint of a bird, the ultimate goal is to cause the least amount of stress to your bird as possible. As a result, knowing how to safely restrain your bird is a must!

There are three important principles regarding bird restraint that owners must be aware of:

1. Birds have no muscular diaphragm to help them breathe, so they rely on active movements of the ribcage to draw and expel air to and from the lungs. Grasping a bird too tightly can severely restrict its breathing ability, and could lead to death through suffocation.

2. Birds, especially overweight budgerigars, can experience a phenomenon known as *cardiac racing* if they are extremely stressed

or frightened. The heart rate in these birds can increase to such a high level that the heart itself can't pump blood properly, and death can result. As a result, certain measures should be taken to ease excitement as much as possible.

3. Birds that are exhibiting signs of illness are poor candidates for any kind of restraint, except when needed for treatment. These birds are already so stressed out that even the slightest anxiety attack could lead to death.

Proper Procedure for Restraint

Before reaching into a cage or carrier to capture a bird, be sure that all toys, perches, and bowls have been removed. Also, make certain all doors and windows in the room are closed. For smaller birds, dimming the room lights can help immensely in their capture, since most are reluctant to fly in the dark.

Camouflage your hand when capturing a bird to prevent it from becoming hand-shy in the future. A towel, or for larger birds, a pair of welders gloves works just fine. Reach into the cage slowly and intently, waiting until the bird grasps the cage bars with its beak as it tries to avoid your approach. Then grasp the bird's head between your thumb and forefinger (Fig. 21.2). Let the bird chew on the towel if it chooses. Remember: The key to capturing and handling pet birds is to gain control of the head right from the start.

For small birds, gently cradle the body with your remaining fingers and the palm of your hand. For large birds, wrap them up completely in a towel, leaving their head exposed, yet under the control of your hand. Keeping the birds in an upright position will facilitate their breathing (Fig. 21.3).

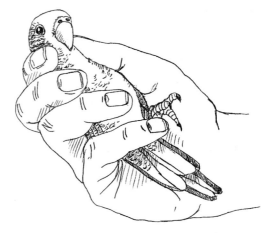

FIGURE 21.2 Restraining a budgerigar.

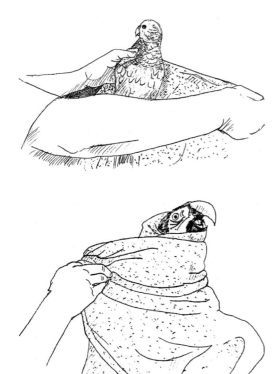

FIGURE 21.3   Using a towel to restrain a large parrot.

At-Home Physical Exam

The physical exam is a useful tool that you can use to assess the overall health of your bird. It can be performed prior to purchase, and thereafter at periodic intervals, preferably at least four times per year. In addition, your bird should receive a complete professional checkup by your veterinarian at least twice a year.

At-home or prepurchase physical exams are easy to do and take little time. Owners should be cautioned, however, that if their pet is showing obvious signs of illness, veterinary attention is warranted at once. Here is the reason why. As mentioned previously, birds have an incredible ability to mask signs of illness to protect them against predators looking for sick and wounded prey on which to feast. However, such a tendency presents a problem in that birds kept as pets will also exhibit the same type of instinctive behavior, and illnesses might brew for months before a bird owner has any indication that something is wrong. Unfortunately, by the time the sickness overwhelms the bird's ability to mask its signs, subsequent treatment efforts often are unrewarding. Therefore, as an owner of one of these extremely stoic creatures, you must be constantly on the lookout for early, subtle clinical signs that can alert you to an illness. Performing periodic at-home physical examinations on your bird will assist you in these efforts. This same examination technique can also be used for your prepurchase screening, and can alert you to any health problems before any cash changes hands.

If possible, these exams should be performed without physical restraint, in the comfort of your bird's own surroundings. For a closer look, see if your bird won't stay perched on your hand or arm while you perform the exam, or, in the case of a prepurchase exam, on the seller's arm. However, if the subject simply refuses to cooperate, physical restraint might need to be employed.

Examine Droppings

Every examination should start with a good look at your bird's droppings in the cage. Have they changed in color or consistency? Normal bird droppings consist of three fractions:

1. A formed fecal fraction, which will appear green if the bird is eating seed; brown if eating pellets
2. A white, creamy urate fraction
3. A liquid urine portion

Again, the consistency and color of the droppings can vary with the type of diet the bird is on, so learn what is normal for your particular bird. Abnormal droppings are characterized by changes in frequency, volume, color, and consistency. Birds can have anywhere from 20 to 40 droppings per day. A decrease in the frequency of elimination or in the volume of the fecal portion is a good indicator of a decrease in food consumption, which could be secondary to disease and stress. Keep in mind that birds can't go without food for more than 2 to 3 days at a time without suffering serious health consequences.

Gastroenteritis usually causes the fecal portion to be liquid, whereas pancreatic disease can cause the feces to be bulky and gray in color, due to inadequate digestion of food. On the other hand, undigested seed and/or grit in the feces points to a potential problem in the gizzard region of the digestive tract. Pea-green stools are often seen with psittacosis or other serious infections. Finally, overt blood in the feces could signify a tumor or an ulcer somewhere within the digestive tract.

Changes in the urate and urine fractions of the droppings can also result from underlying disease. Urates having a yellow-green tinge often reveal the presence of an underlying liver disorder. Also, increases in the amount of urate or urine produced can be caused by, among other things, kidney disease and diabetes mellitus. Finally, lead poisoning should be suspected if blood is noted in the urine.

Observe Your Bird

Observe the way your bird carries itself. Does it seem uncomfortable on the perch? Is it shifting its weight back and forth? If so, it could have sore feet or it could be acting restless because of an underlying illness. Are there any signs of lameness? Certainly musculoskeletal injuries and gout are two leading causes of lameness in birds. In addition, internal tumors can cause paralysis in one or both legs, resulting in apparent lameness.

How about your bird's posture? Is it upright and attentive? Is it active? Birds that are ill often appear sleepy and exhibit unsteadiness at perch. A decrease in singing or vocalization could also indicate problems.

WEIGHT

How is your bird's weight? For small birds, weight can be monitored using a small postal scale or food scale. Excessive weight gain is as undesirable and unhealthy in pet birds as it is in dogs and cats. Obesity tends to be a problem in budgerigars more than in other species of birds. What is thought to be weight gain must be differentiated from internal masses or swellings. Have your veterinarian check it out. On the other hand, apparent weight loss could mean that your bird's appetite is off or it could mean dehydration, both signifying disease.

One key indicator of disease is the status of the large breast muscles. Disease often produces a wasting of these muscles, which results in a protruding keel (breast) bone that is easily palpable.

DID YOU KNOW?

Weight gain in birds can be caused by tumors, reproductive challenges, and liver disease, while noticeable weight loss results from chronic infections and metabolic diseases.

EYES

The eyes should be bright, shiny, and sharp. Look for signs of irritation and/or swelling. Green discharges coming from the eyes or crusty material surrounding the eye are indicators of infections. Clear discharges could indicate an allergy problem or a foreign body in the eye. Cataracts, which are common in older psittacines, will appear as a cloudy space within the pupil of one or both eyes. Are the eyelids droopy? This could be the result of a former eye infection, especially in cockatiels.

FACIAL AREA

The beak, nares, and cere should be smooth and free of growths and discharges. Discharges from the nares could indicate an active *airsacculitis*. Sneezing could be a sign of an early respiratory infection. Does the beak seem to be wearing evenly? Does it close properly? How about its length? Overgrown beaks can be a sign of liver disease in birds. A scaly, flaky beak could be infected. The mite *Knemidokoptes* should also be suspected if the beak appears crusty and scaly.

BREATHING

The respirations of a bird should be barely noticeable. Also, healthy birds breathe with their mouths closed. Labored respirations with or without open-mouth breathing signify serious respiratory distress. A wheezing or clicking sound is also indicative of respiratory disease in birds, as is tail bobbing when at perch.

WINGS AND PLUMAGE

Observe the wings and plumage. A droopy wing might be injured or held that way because of sheer weakness. The feathers of a healthy bird should appear crisp, sleek, and bright and should lie smoothly against the body. Ruffled feathers could indicate cool environmental temperatures or worse, illness. Are any feathers missing or broken? Broken tail feathers might mean that your bird's cage is too small. Missing or misshapen feathers can result from an abnormal molt or from feather picking.

Look at the feathers around the vent. Pasting of the feathers with fecal material should alert you to a potential gastrointestinal disorder. At the same time, observe the head feathers and those around the mouth for signs of matting and pasting. This could indicate regurgitation and/or vomiting.

FEET AND LEGS

Check the feet and legs for signs of irritation, inflammation, or tissue proliferation. The feet should be smooth. Keep in mind that poor perch selection and maintenance are the most common causes of foot problems in pet birds.

Overgrown nails can also adversely affect perching, and can pose a danger to the bird's health if they get caught in the cage. Also, leg bands on confined birds can do more harm than good and should be removed.

If your physical examination reveals any abnormalities, seek the advice of your veterinarian. Avoid further handling of your bird until you get it to your veterinarian, since unwarranted handling could kill a seriously ill bird. Transport your bird to the veterinary hospital in its cage (very important!). Don't clean the cage before you go, as your veterinarian will want to observe the character of your bird's droppings and all toys, food, and medicine that have been offered. However, you should empty water dishes and remove grit and perches from the cage prior to transport. Cover the cage for warmth and to minimize stress. If it is cold outside, warm your car up first before loading your bird.

Nail Trimming

The nails of your bird should be kept at a proper length, since overgrowth can cause nail breakage and predispose the legs and feet to injuries. Most of the time, the nails stay worn down by themselves as a result of normal perching activities. However, disease can sometimes cause overgrowth to occur. If your bird is otherwise healthy, yet suffering from nail overgrowth, take a close look at the perches in the cage. Soft, narrow perches can contribute to this problem.

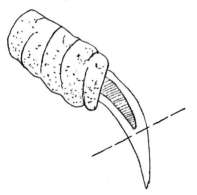

FIGURE 21.4 The dashed line indicates where to cut a bird's nail.

You can trim the nails of your bird using a pair of dog or cat toenail clippers.

For smaller birds, use a set of human nail trimmers. Before performing this procedure, always have clotting powder on hand in case you cut a nail too short. This is readily available from your veterinarian or a local pet supplier.

Simply capture and restrain your bird (assuming it is not ill), then snip off the sharp ends to the nails (Fig. 21.4). If one or more of the nails start to bleed, apply clotting powder to the bleeding tips. Keep the bird restrained for a minute or two before putting it back in its cage to be certain the bleeding has stopped.

Beak Care

Healthy birds will keep their beaks in shape through normal eating habits and by chewing on soft wood and toys within their cages. The absence of such items within the cage, as well as injuries, various diseases, and poor nutrition, can all lead to uneven beak wear and/or overgrowth. Budgerigars seem to be the pet birds that are most in need of periodic beak trims (Fig. 21.5).

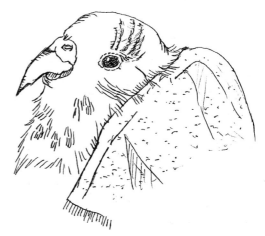

FIGURE 21.5 A budgie suffering from an overgrown beak.

Beak trimming should be performed only by a qualified avian veterinarian. At the same time, your veterinarian can show you how to perform minor touchups at home to keep your bird's beak looking nice.

Feather Clipping

Feather clipping is a procedure performed on pet birds to limit their flight capabilities. This not only prevents inadvertent escape out of an open window or door but also protects the birds from hazards associated with flight within the house (such as ceiling fans).

To minimize stress and possible harm to your bird, have your veterinarian perform this procedure. If you are determined to do it on your own, you should at least receive hands-on training from your veterinarian, who can show you several methods of doing so. The first method involves starting from the tip of the wing, skipping the first two or three primary feathers, and then using scissors to cut the remaining primaries down to the level of the covert feathers. Secondary flight feathers may be left intact. Scissors are then used to clip the very outer edges of the remaining flight feathers to prevent their adherence to one another (Fig. 21.6). An alternate method of deflighting pet birds is to strip every other flight feather bare, leaving only a shaft. This effectively eliminates adherence between the feathers, making it difficult to fly.

Evaluate your bird's flight capabilities after the clipping. If it is still able to fly well, secondary feathers may need clipping. In some instances, the opposite wing will need to be clipped as well. In general, the smaller the bird, the harder it is to keep them from flying.

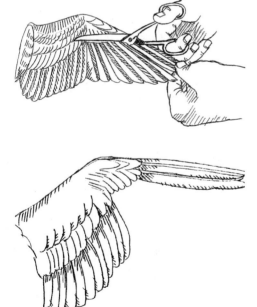

FIGURE 21.6 One method of feather clipping to prevent flight.

Feather clipping must usually be repeated every 6 to 8 months, or 6 to 8 weeks after the start of a new molt. If clipping is to be performed soon after molting, use caution to avoid the new blood feathers that have come in. If one of these is accidentally clipped and begins to bleed, the feather should be plucked from its shaft and temporary pressure applied to the follicle to stop the blood flow. A new feather should replace it in 6 to 8 weeks.

Permanent flight-restraint procedures that can be surgically performed by your veterinarian include pinioning, which involves amputation of a portion of the wing, and tenotomy, a procedure in which the tendon of the main extension muscle of the wing is severed, rendering the wing nonfunctional.

Bathing

Most birds enjoy periodic water baths, so provide them with the opportunity. A shallow bowl filled with water can be placed in the cage for this purpose. Some birds would rather use the kitchen sink containing a small amount of water for their bath once allowed out of their cage. Other birds find toilet water attractive, which is fine as long as no detergents or automatic cleaners are present within the water (these can be highly toxic to the unsuspecting bird).

Many owners choose to use a spray bottle filled with water to give their bird a daily mist bath. If you do so, be sure the spray bottle you use did not previously contain any chemicals or residues that could harm your bird.

Finally, some birds enjoy showering with their owners. If this is the case, the temperature within the shower should not exceed 98 degrees Fahrenheit. To be safe, leave the bathroom door opened slightly to allow your bird an easy exit if the need arises.

Avian Diseases and Disorders

This chapter covers some of the more common afflictions seen in pet birds. General signs of illness in birds include the following:

Decreased appetite or water consumption

Weakness

Fluffed-up feathers

Broken, bent, or lost feathers

Labored breathing

Reluctance or inability to perch

Loss of muscle mass on breast

Shifting leg lameness

Abnormal lumps, bumps, or swellings

Change in color or character of droppings

Vomiting or regurgitation of food

Overgrown beak and/or nails

Discharges from eyes or nares

Prolonged molting period

As mentioned previously, the appearance of one or more of these symptoms warrants a consultation with your veterinarian.

Most of the diseases discussed in this chapter are grouped according to major organ systems affected. However, it is important to note that many of them, especially the infectious diseases, can affect multiple tissues and organs at a time, resulting in a potpourri of clinical signs. For this reason, the infectious diseases are presented in their own section within this chapter and are not listed under the respective organ systems that they affect.

Respiratory Tract Diseases

Refer to Chap. 20 for details regarding the anatomy and physiology of the avian respiratory system. Respiratory tract disease is undoubtedly the number 1 health disorder seen in birds. The causes are numerous, and can include viral, bacterial, and/or fungal etiologies.

Regardless of cause, clinical signs that indicate a respiratory problem in a bird include an increased breathing rate, tail bobbing, labored or open-mouthed breathing and abnormal respiratory sounds, nasal or eye discharge, and loss of voice. Other nonspecific signs, such as ruffled feathers, reluctance to fly, and a depressed, sleepy attitude, could also accompany these signs.

If respiratory disease is suspected, rapid diagnosis and treatment of the underlying cause are imperative for a happy ending. Supportive care designed to reduce stress, combined with appropriate antibiotic therapy and, if needed, oxygen therapy, are the benchmarks for treating respiratory disease in birds. For increased effectiveness, antibiotic therapy can be delivered using a *nebulizer,* a device that converts medications into a fine mist that can then be inhaled directly into the respiratory tract.

Aspergillosis

Aspergillosis is caused by a fungal organism that is normally found in the bird's environment. Because of this ubiquitous nature, disease caused by this organism is usually seen only in those birds that become highly stressed because of poor sanitation and/or poor nutrition. Old, moldy seeds and foods are major sources of this organism.

The disease caused by aspergillosis is primarily respiratory in origin, with infected birds exhibiting clinical signs such as sneezing, nasal discharge, and breathing difficulties. Occasionally, the organism will spread to other organs within the body, leading to a wide variety of clinical signs.

Diagnosis of aspergillosis is based on history (e.g., poor husbandry), clinical signs seen, and physical examination. Radiographic X rays can be used to confirm lung and/or air sac involvement, and cultures of respiratory secretions can help isolate and identify the causative organism.

Treatment of aspergillosis is often successful if the disease is caught in its early stages. Antifungal medications can be employed to combat such an infection. Certainly changes in nutrition, sanitation, and other husbandry practices are warranted at the same time.

Airsacculitis

The term *airsacculitis* refers to inflammation and functional impairment of the air sacs. The most frequent culprits causing airsacculitis include infectious diseases (bacteria, fungi, and viruses), parasites such as air sac mites, and traumatic rupture of the sacs themselves. Diagnosis can be made using radiographic X-ray findings. Nebulization of antibiotics can be an effective mode of treatment for airsacculitis.

> ### DID YOU KNOW?
>
> The air sacs are not only important for aerodynamics but also function to help deliver oxygen to the tissues and to dissipate the tremendous amount of body heat generated by the act of flying.

Gapeworms

The "gapeworm," *Syngamus trachea,* is a parasite that can inhabit the wall of the trachea in finches and canaries. Its colloquial name is derived from the clinical sign it causes in affected birds, namely, an open-mouthed "gape" due to interference with normal airflow down the trachea.

The parasite gains entrance into the body through infected soil or, in some cases, via ingested earthworms and insects harboring the worm larvae. From the gastrointestinal tract, the larvae migrate to the trachea. These migrating larvae can also cause pneumonia along the way. A variety of medicines can be used to treat gapeworms. In fact, in larger birds, manual removal of the worms by a veterinarian can often be accomplished. Because of the damage and distress gapeworms cause in birds, early treatment is a must.

Digestive System Diseases

See Chapter 20 for details on the anatomy and physiology of the digestive system in birds.

Specific signs of gastrointestinal disease usually include regurgitation, vomiting, diarrhea, and/or weight loss. Some of the more prevalent diseases affecting this system in birds include those discussed below.

Candidiasis

Candidiasis is not a primary disease syndrome, but rather a disease seen secondarily to long-term antibiotic therapy, malnutrition, and/or poor husbandry. This yeast organism causes lesions and ulcers in the mouth, esophagus, crop, or even the proventriculus. A characteristic white film, or plaque, usually covers the ulcerated areas.

Birds afflicted with candidiasis often regurgitate food due to the irritation caused by the lesions. Others may exhibit only nonspecific signs of illness, such as depression, ruffled feathers, and decreased appetite. Candidiasis is a serious disease in baby cockatiels, as it can quickly lead to death.

Diagnosis of this disease can be made by your veterinarian by identifying the characteristic plaques within the mouth or throat, and by examining swabs taken from the mouth and other affected areas, and demonstrating the yeast organisms under the microscope. Once this condition is diagnosed, specific antifungal treatments can then be instituted. Correcting husbandry shortcomings is also a must to prevent recurrences.

Sour Crop

Diseases affecting the crop invariably lead to one clinical sign common to all birds affected: regurgitation. One of the more prevalent conditions affecting this region is known as "sour crop," which occurs when the crop becomes inflamed and ulcerated, usually secondary to bacterial or fungal overgrowth within. Birds affected with sour crop will regurgitate foul-smelling food that has been sitting and fermenting within the irritated crop. Spoiled or moldy feed is thought to play a role in the development of this condition. Continual tube feeding can also predispose the crop to infection.

Treatment involves removing the crop contents using a feeding tube, and then repeatedly flushing out the crop using a special mixture of baking soda (1 teaspoon) plus kaolin and pectin ($1/2$ teaspoon mixed into 8 ounces of water).

Appropriate therapy for bacterial and/or fungal infections that may be present is also necessary. Feeding should be resumed in small increments several times a day until the crop heals. Sour crop can be prevented by observing good hygiene when tube feeding pet birds, by not overfeeding, and by feeding only fresh rations.

Crop and Gizzard Impaction

Impaction of the crop is another problem that can occur in pet birds. It can result when birds are allowed to engorge themselves on seed or grit, causing a grossly overdistended crop. Impaction can also occur secondary to infections, tumors, foreign bodies, and enlarged thyroid glands, all of which can affect the crop's contractility and ability to empty.

Palpation of the crop region will confirm a diagnosis of impaction. If this condition is diagnosed, treatment is aimed at emptying the crop of its contents and treating any underlying disease condition present. In severe cases, surgical removal of the crop contents and/or partial removal of the crop itself might become necessary.

Like crop impactions, impactions of the gizzard can be seen in birds that overfeed on grit or seeds. For instance, sick birds have a tendency to engorge themselves on grit. As a result, all grit should be removed from the cage of an ill bird.

Signs of a gizzard impaction include scant, bloody droppings that may have undigested seeds in them. Radiographic X rays can be used to reveal grit buildup within the gizzard. As mentioned above, surgery might be required to alleviate the impaction.

Macaw Wasting Disease

Probably the most infamous psittacine diseases affecting the gastrointestinal tract of birds is termed *macaw wasting disease* (MWD). As the name implies, this condition, which is characterized by an abnormal distension of the proventriculus, is seen mostly in macaws, although other psittacines can be affected. The exact cause of this disease syndrome is still unknown, but a virus is suspect. Researchers do know that it is a disorder characterized by poor nerve supply to the proventriculus and other organs, leading to muscular degeneration and weak contractions.

Once signs appear, the course of the disease is usually short. Sick birds will exhibit weight loss and muscle wasting, especially along the breast. Regurgitation can occur as the crop becomes affected, and as other normal digestive processes are disrupted, diarrhea containing undigested seed is seen. Birds severely afflicted exhibit incoordination and other nervous system signs. A radiographic X ray that reveals a distended proventriculus is diagnostic for MWD.

Unfortunately, there is no treatment available. As a supportive measure, these birds should be put on a liquid diet to promote normal passage of nutrients through the gastrointestinal tract.

Gastrointestinal Parasites

The most prevalent worm seen in the intestinal tract of psittacines is the roundworm, or *ascarid.* Affected birds often exhibit signs of unthriftiness, poor growth, weight loss, and sometimes diarrhea. Birds pick up infestations through contact with infected fecal material. In some cases, earthworms can act as intermediate carriers for the parasite.

Diagnosis can be difficult, and repeated examinations of stool specimens under a microscope might be necessary to identify the characteristic eggs. Once infestation is diagnosed, treatment using a dewormer is usually effective. Thoroughly steam-cleaning the cage a few days after treatment will help prevent reinfestation originating from the bird's own droppings.

THREADWORMS

If ascarids are the most common internal parasite seen in birds, *Capillaria* (the threadworm) runs a close second! These hairlike worms live in the small intestines. In canaries and finches they can inhabit the esophagus and crop as well. Transmitted between birds through contact with infected soil or with earthworms, threadworms cause loss of appetite, weight loss, and profuse diarrhea—often bloody—in affected birds.

Microscopic examination of fluid from the crop or of a stool specimen can lead a veterinarian to a diagnosis of threadworms in a pet bird. Again, treatment for this parasite is similar to that for ascarids.

OTHER INTESTINAL PARASITES

Other worms that can affect pet birds include tapeworms and stomach worms. Both have the ability to cause diarrhea and generalized unthriftiness in birds.

Tapeworms can be easily treated with special dewormers once identified in the stools. Stomach worms burrow into the lining of the proventriculus and gizzard, and can actually cause perforations if allowed to persist. As a result, expedient diagnosis and deworming can be lifesaving.

Other intestinal parasites that can adversely affect the health of pet birds include flagellates (*Trichomonas*), coccidia, and *Giardia*. The

> **DID YOU KNOW?**
>
> *Giardia* is the most common human intestinal parasite worldwide.

Giardia organism can cause high mortality rates in baby budgerigars and cockatiels affected with the organism, and has been implicated as the cause of cockatiel feather syndrome.

All three of these latter parasites can cause pronounced unthriftiness, lethargy, and gastroenteritis. *Trichomonas* can also infect the throat, causing oral exudates and breathing difficulties (*frounce*). Microscopic examination of a fecal sample can help your veterinarian establish a definite diagnosis and institute a proper treatment regimen.

Other Intestinal Diseases

While infectious and parasitic diseases can play major roles in gastrointestinal disease, poisonings, such as lead poisoning or plant toxicity, can also cause their share of intestinal upset, and usually lead to profound diarrhea. A good history combined with microscopic examination of droppings can often reveal the cause of the problem, or at least rule some out. Once a diagnosis has been established, appropriate treatment measures can be instituted.

Constipation can be a problem in dehydrated birds, overweight birds, or in those birds that eat too much grit. It can also affect females getting ready to lay eggs, due to pressure placed on the rectum from the maturing egg. Treatment consists of administering mineral oil or adding more fruit to the diet, and correcting any underlying problems.

Prolapse of the cloaca out of the vent can occur secondarily to egg laying and to straining, as seen with persistent diarrhea or constipation. Mild prolapses can often be replaced with minimal effort; more extensive ones might require surgery.

Liver Disease

Liver impairment in birds can present itself as a variety of clinical signs, including weight loss, seizures, abdominal enlargement, diarrhea, regurgitation, and blindness. Various infectious diseases, such as psittacosis, Pacheco's disease, and salmonellosis, can all adversely affect the liver. In addition, ingestion of toxic substances can also impair liver function.

DID YOU KNOW?

Overgrown toenails can be indicative of liver disease in birds.

Demonstrating elevated levels of liver enzymes in a blood sample is indicative of a liver disorder. Treatment is generally aimed at the underlying cause.

Neurologic Disorders

Disorders of the nervous system in birds can manifest themselves in the following clinical signs: seizures, weakness, paralysis, incoordination and inability to perch, weight loss, vomiting, and abnormal posturing. Conditions that can induce such signs in pet birds include trauma, malnutrition (especially vitamin deficiencies), infectious diseases (such as Pacheco's disease, psittacosis, exotic Newcastle disease), liver disease, proventricular wasting syndrome, parasites, and toxic substances such as lead or insecticides. Budgerigars suffering from tumors of the kidneys or pituitary gland can also exhibit neurological signs.

Seizures caused by epilepsy have been diagnosed in budgerigars and certain Amazon parrots. During an epileptic fit, these birds may fall off the perch, shiver, rock back and forth, and appear to be in a trancelike state. Some birds may even exhibit abnormal aggressive tendencies. Anticonvulsant medications, similar to those used in cats and dogs, can be administered to control the seizures.

Because of the wide variety of potential causes, a proper diagnosis by a veterinarian is essential for establishing an exact source of a seizure. Once this has been done, an appropriate treatment, if available, can be instituted.

Cardiovascular Diseases

Fortunately, noninfectious diseases affecting the heart are not seen much in pet birds. Certainly older birds can suffer from the wear-and-tear effects of aging;

> **DID YOU KNOW?**
> Older birds on fatty diets can develop atherosclerosis of the blood vessels just as humans do!

chronic heart disease is one such effect. The two clinical signs seen most in these birds suffering from heart disease include exercise intolerance and breathing difficulties.

Parasites

Interestingly, parasites that inhabit the bloodstream are common in birds. Types include microfilaria, trypanosomes, *Hemoproteus, Plasmodium,* and *Leukocy-*

> **DID YOU KNOW?**
> Up to 50 percent of otherwise healthy caged birds harbor some type of bloodborne organism!

tozoon. Fortunately, most of the blood parasites seen in birds are harmless to their hosts, except when those birds are ill or highly stressed. In these individuals, bloodborne parasites can cause clinical disease, usually in the form of anemia or impaired blood circulation, and will require specific treatment.

Endocrine Malfunctions

Endocrine malfunctions resulting in diabetes mellitus, adrenal gland insufficiency, and hypothyroidism have been known to occur in pet birds. Because of their systemic nature, clinical signs associated with these disorders can be quite variable and originate from multiple organ systems. Diagnosis can be achieved through the use of laboratory blood testing.

Eye Disorders

Eye disorders can afflict birds of all ages. Traumatic eye injuries resulting from flight injuries, fighting, foreign objects, and burns can disrupt the outer corneal surface of the eye, leading to corneal ulcerations and abrasions. Corneas so affected usually appear cloudy and opaque, with the bird reluctant to keep its eye open. Certainly such a condition can seriously threaten eyesight if not managed promptly with ophthalmic antibiotics and other medications.

Conjunctivitis is another type of eye problem seen in pet birds. Swelling and inflammation of one or both conjunctival membranes are most often associated with respiratory infections in birds. In addition, cockatiels have been known to suffer from bacterial conjunctivitis, which can cause ocular discharge and swollen, protruding conjunctival membranes. Such infections usually respond to antibiotic eyedrops.

Inflammation of the internal structures of the eye, called *uveitis,* can be seen secondary to any generalized disease. If allowed to continue untreated, a cataract in the affected eye could result. A *cataract* is an opacity of the lens within the eye that does not allow light to penetrate to the retina, ultimately resulting in vision loss. Not all cataracts are caused by inflammation or infections. They can be inherited as well, especially in canaries.

The avian poxvirus causes serious eye disease in birds. The eyelids of these birds become scabbed shut, and corneal ulcers, conjunctivitis, and uveitis can result. Manual removal of these scabs can lead to intense scarring around the eyes and lids if the bird survives. Treatment is aimed at combating secondary infection with antibiotic ointments for the eyes, and at preventing the lids from becoming scabbed shut using daily warm-water lid washes. Vitamin A supplementation is thought to also be of some help in these birds.

Finally, parasites known as *conjunctival worms* can set up house-keeping within the eyelids and conjunctival sacs of unfortunate cock-atoos and macaws. Affected birds are seen constantly rubbing and scratching at their eyes. Antiparasitic drugs can be used to get rid of these pesky parasites. However, if treatment is not prompt, these worms could actually penetrate the eye itself, making removal all the more difficult and threatening vision in the affected eye(s).

Ear Problems

The ears are rarely a source of health problems in birds. However, because of the ear's importance in maintaining balance and equilibrium, infections or injuries can seriously impair a bird's ability to fly and should be suspect in such cases.

Disorders of the Skin and Feathers

Diseases of the skin and feathers are major concerns for most bird owners, not only for the health of their pets but for cosmetic reasons as well. Disorders involving the integument and feathers are among the most frequent seen by veterinarians and can be among the most challenging to treat. Feather loss and skin involvement might signify a primary disorder, or they might occur incidentally to an unrelated disease process. The goal is to find out which it is!

External Parasites

Dogs and cats are not the only species that can suffer from external parasites. Pet birds can have their share as well.

Knemidokoptic mange is a skin and feather disease caused by a mite that burrows into the skin and feather follicles. In parrots and other psittacines, these parasites manifest disease as deformities and overgrowth of the beak, and deformities of the legs, feet, and nails (Fig. 22.1). In fact, severe infestations can actually lead to sloughing of the toes and nails!

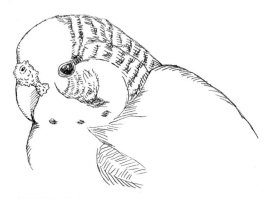

FIGURE 22.1 Abnormal growth on the cere caused by mite infestation.

Canaries and finches can also be infested with this parasite, yet their legs and feet are affected more often than are their beaks. Lesions caused by this mite have been known to take on a characteristic "honeycomb" appearance. Itching is usually not seen with this disease.

Your veterinarian can diagnose this condition by taking skin scrapings of affected skin and examining them under the microscope for the presence of mange mites. Treatment using topical insecticides should be applied to the affected regions every 3 days for five treatments total, then repeated weekly until the lesions have cleared. Systemic antiparasitic drugs, given orally or injected, have also been shown to be even more effective in eliminating these mites. During the treatment process, loosened scabs should be removed and the beak, if affected, should be kept trimmed.

Other mites that pester pet birds less frequently include red mites, feather mites, *Myialges,* and *Ornithonsyssus,* the northern mite. The tracheal mite, *Sternostoma tracheacolum,* can inhabit the upper airways of birds and can cause loss of voice and some breathing difficulties. Air sac mites can also cause breathing difficulties and coughing in affected birds. A characteristic "smacking" sound emitted from these birds should alert owners to a potential problem involving these mites. Systemic drugs administered by your veterinarian are the best treatment for these mites as well.

Feather Picking

Feather picking is one of the most frustrating syndromes affecting pet birds (Fig. 22.2). Characterized by a loss of or damage to the feathers below the neck, this condition can exert devastating cosmetic effects on a prized pet. It is important to realize that feather picking is a sign of some other underlying problem, which must be addressed before the disfiguring habit can be stopped.

Medical illnesses can certainly play a role in the development of feather picking. Diseases that need to be ruled out as causes are numerous, and include the following:

Endocrine diseases (such as hypothyroidism)

Infectious diseases (poxvirus, psittacosis)

Poor nutrition

Food allergies (especially to seeds)

Contrary to popular belief, external parasites such as feather mites are rarely a cause of feather picking in pet birds. However, internal parasites such as roundworms and tapeworms must be ruled out as potential causes. *Giardia* infections have also been implicated as a cause of feather picking in cockatiels and budgerigars.

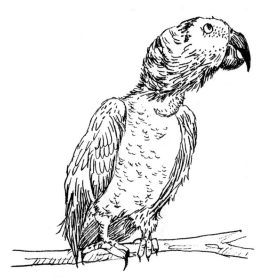

Another reason why a bird might pick at its feathers is stress due to emotional upset. Birds that have moved into a new home or those that are being handled excessively and unwillingly have been

FIGURE 22.2 Feather picking can have devastating effects.

known to start feather picking. Often, a new addition to the family will trigger an emotional episode, resulting in feather loss. Finally, if a bird does not receive enough attention on a daily basis, it might turn to feather picking to relieve its frustration.

Treatment for feather picking is directed at the underlying cause. If a medical reason exists, appropriate medications can be used to clear up both problems at the same time. Improved nutrition and husbandry are a must in all instances. In some birds, feather picking might lead to secondary bacterial infections of the feather follicles. As a result,

> ## Dr. P's Vet Tip
>
> For the emotional bird prone to feather picking, try leaving a radio or television on while you're not at home. Just hearing a familiar, consistent noise is often enough to thwart the nervous anxiety that can lead to this bad habit.

antibiotic therapy might be needed to treat this secondary problem.

For those cases that are psychologically induced, owners can take a number of measures to curb their bird's anxiety. Sometimes simply moving the cage to a different location with more privacy is all that is necessary to calm an upset bird. Providing a larger cage with lots of safe toys and more room to move around also helps in some instances.

If lack of attention is the suspected cause, the obvious solution is to increase the amount of time you devote to your bird each day. If you haven't done so already, get your bird on a regular schedule of feeding, exercise, and sleep. This will help reduce its stress level.

Finally, if you are having difficulties fulfilling your time commitments to your bird, you might want to even go so far as to purchase your bird a feathered companion with which it can play and interact in your absence.

In especially tough feather-picking cases that are psychologically induced, your veterinarian may prescribe tranquilizers for your bird. Special collars designed to prevent the bird's access to its feathers can also be used to temporarily spare the remaining feathers from a similar fate while the underlying problem is being worked on. Please note that these collars should be used only for temporary relief and should not be relied on on a long-term basis. Because birds wearing these collars cannot preen themselves, owners must be sure to remove the sheaths from any new feathers that grow in. Any feathers that have been traumatized and broken should be pulled out to allow the new ones to grow in.

Psittacine Beak and Feather Disease

This disease, first identified in cockatoos years ago and subsequently in other parrot species, is caused by the psittacine circovirus (Fig. 22.3).

Affected birds suffer from feather loss and deformities in new feathers attempting to replace those lost. The beaks and nails of these birds are also affected and often chip, split, or fall off as a result of the disease.

Diagnosis of psittacine beak and feather disease is made by obtaining biopsy samples and performing microscopic examinations of deformed feathers and affected follicles. Unfortunately, an effective treatment for this disease is not available. Affected birds eventually die as a result of secondary complications and infections associated with this disease.

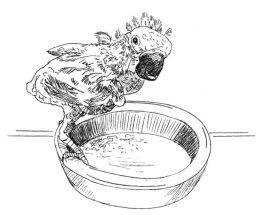

FIGURE 22.3 Psittacine beak and feather disease.

French Molt

Seen in budgerigars and other smaller psittacines, this condition is characterized by the abnormal development or overt absence of tail and flight feathers. The exact cause is unknown, although a genetic viral etiology is suspected. Unfortunately, as with the previous disease, there is no effective treatment.

Feather Cysts

Bulging nodules under the skin that contain abnormal feather shafts are characteristic of feather cysts. Their exact cause is unknown, but they have been shown to be genetic in nature in canaries. Feather cysts must be differentiated from other lumps and bumps that can arise on the skin of a bird, such as abscesses, tumors, and cysts affecting the feather follicles themselves. Once a feather cyst is diagnosed, treatment consists of surgical lancing or removal of the cysts as they occur.

Hormone-Induced Feather Loss

Feather loss can occur secondary to hormonal influences. In male canaries and budgies, a testosterone deficiency can cause such a loss.

Accordingly, administration of testosterone hormone for 4 to 6 weeks will usually prevent further feather loss.

Deficiencies in thyroid hormone (*hypothyroidism*) due to iodine deficiencies or inflammation of the thyroid gland can, among other things, lead to feather loss. Treatment consisting of daily administration of a thyroid hormone supplement in the bird's water is usually quite rewarding.

Overgrown Beak and Cere Changes

In a year's time, the beak of a healthy budgerigar should grow 2 to 3 inches; that of a larger psittacine should grow 1 to 1½ inches. The normal length of the beak is usually well maintained by the normal wear and tear from eating and from chewing on wood and other hard objects in the bird's cage. As a result, when beak overgrowth occurs, it is usually a sign of underlying disease. Genetic deformities can predispose a bird to beak overgrowth, as can other diseases such as malnutrition, bacterial and fungal infections, trauma, tumors, and liver disease.

MITES

The *Knemidokoptes* mite is a common instigator of beak overgrowth in budgerigars. Characteristically, this mite causes proliferation and crusting not only of the beak but also of the cere, face, neck, and legs. Fortunately, these mites can be treated effectively with miticides.

BROWN HYPERTROPHY

Unexpected changes in the color of the cere can be caused by a condition known as *brown hypertrophy* of the cere. This condition is seen primarily in budgerigars and is characterized by a brown, crusty thickening of the cere region, often becoming unicornlike in appearance. The exact cause of brown hypertrophy is unknown. Removal of the crusts and application of a skin-softening cream or lanolin to the region might help cosmetically, but you should count on the condition to recur.

INTERNAL TUMORS

Internal tumors can also cause a brownish discoloration of the cere in budgerigars. However, in most of these instances, there are other clinical signs, such as weight loss and neurologic defects, and an apparent abdominal mass will be seen as well.

Tumors of the Integument

Lipomas and papillomas are the two most common types of tumors affecting the integument of pet birds.

Lipomas are fatty tumors that can appear on the breast, abdomen, wings, and neck of pet birds, especially budgerigars. These tumors can get so large that they interfere with flying, walking, and perching. *Hypothyroidism* is thought to be one of the predisposing causes of lipomas. Diet might also play a role in their development. Feeding white millet on a regular basis has been shown to reduce the size of lipomas in select instances. Large and encumbering lipomas will need to be removed surgically.

Papillomas are warty proliferations that can affect many species of pet birds. The neck, toes, lower beak, and uropygial region are commonly affected. These pink-to-white growths are often covered with dry, brown crusts that can be easily removed. As far as the papilloma is concerned, surgical removal will ensure a cure.

Oiled Feathers

We have all seen and heard of the devastating effects spilled oil can have on a bird. The harmful effects of oil are numerous. The bird's insulating mechanisms are lost, and the oral cavity and vent become clogged with the substance, creating breathing and eating difficulties. Oil is also toxic to birds and can quickly lead to dehydration, gout, and organ failure in affected birds. See Chapter 23 for management of birds exposed to oil and other petroleum products.

Musculoskeletal Disorders

Lameness, the primary clinical sign seen with musculoskeletal disease, can be caused by a wide variety of illnesses and syndromes. Certainly one prevalent cause of lameness is sore feet due to poor perches. Perches that are too large or are covered with ridges or sandpaper are the major culprits.

Nutritional deficiencies, such as vitamin A deficiencies, can also lead to unhealthy skin on the bottom of the feet and, eventually, to lameness. Filthy living conditions and perches can cause bacterial infections of the feet. Other causes of lameness can include arthritis, gout, *Knemidokoptes,* tight-fitting leg bands, abdominal tumors, bone tumors, and bone fractures.

Gout

Gout, a condition causing lameness in pet birds, is characterized by a disposition to uric acid in the tissues and joints. Diets high in protein, dehydration, kidney disease, and vitamin A deficiencies have all been implicated in causing gout. Besides obvious lameness, joint swellings, and flight difficulties, gout can also lead to weight loss, diarrhea, and breathing difficulties as other organs within the body become affected.

Diagnosis of gout is based on clinical signs seen and on laboratory detection of abnormal levels of uric acid within the tissues. Treatment consists of lowering protein levels and increasing vitamin A levels in the diet; providing low, soft perches; and adding allopurinol to the drinking water daily. Analgesics such as aspirin can be added to the drinking water to reduce the discomfort. Unfortunately, not much can be done with the uric acid deposits that already exist within the tissues; therefore, the overall prognosis for recovery is poor.

Broken Bones

Broken wings and legs often result when birds fly into sliding glass doors, windows, and mirrors that are not properly marked. Ceiling fans can also cause broken bones in pet birds. Obviously, one of the best ways to protect your bird from such injuries is to keep its wings clipped to impair its flying abilities.

Poorly designed cages can also be implicated in many cases of broken bones. Cages that are too small or those that have narrow bar spacings or convergences in which a nail or wing could be trapped pose the biggest hazards.

Birds with broken wings will droop the affected wing or allow it to drag the ground when walking. If a break is suspected, immobilize the wing by pinning it against the bird's body using gauze wrap or a small towel. Be sure not to wrap it so tightly that you impair your bird's breathing. Transport your bird immediately to the veterinarian. For leg fractures, a toothpick or pencil can be used as a temporary splint while you transport your bird to the veterinarian.

Reproductive Disorders

Refer to Chapter 20 for information about the reproductive system in pet birds.

Egg Binding

Egg binding is the most prevalent challenge seen involving the reproductive organ system. Failure or inability of a maturing egg to be expelled from the reproductive tract characterizes this condition. It occurs more frequently in small birds, such as budgerigars, canaries, and finches. Predisposing factors to egg binding include obesity (especially in budgerigars), exhaustion from repeat layings, and the presence of any underlying disease process. Also, calcium deficiency in the diet can lead to the formation of soft, thin-shelled eggs that can easily become bound.

Clinical signs of egg binding include tail wagging, swaying and unsteadiness while at perch, abdominal swelling, and a penguinlike stance, with the bird resting its weight on its tail with its legs spread apart. Some of these birds might show signs of leg paralysis due to the pressure the egg is placing on the nerve supply to one or both legs.

Egg binding can be diagnosed using clinical signs, physical examination, and radiographic X rays. Treatment involves calcium injections and/or removing the contents of the egg with needle and syringe prior to manual extraction. In some cases, actual surgical removal might be required.

Specific medical therapy can be instituted to help prevent future egg-binding episodes in pet birds. Ask your veterinarian for details.

Tumors

Occasionally birds, especially budgerigars, can suffer from tumors affecting the structures of the reproductive tract. Signs associated with such growths include inability to fly, abdominal enlargement, breathing difficulties, and, characteristically, leg paralysis. Unfortunately, once clinical signs are manifested, surgical treatment is generally unrewarding.

Infectious Diseases

Infectious agents account for many of the disease conditions seen in pet birds. These agents can occur as primary disease entities, or they can occur secondary to stress, poor nutrition, and/or poor sanitation. Regardless of the organism involved, infectious diseases can be quite deadly to pet birds.

Psittacosis

Psittacosis, or *chlamydiosis,* is a serious disease in birds that must be considered whenever a bird becomes ill. Not only can it become life-threatening if it remains undetected, but it also can pose a health threat to an owner. It is caused by the organism *Chlamydia psittaci,* which is transmitted from bird to bird (and from bird to man) via dried feces and nasal discharges. Ingestion or inhalation of infected particles directly exposes birds.

Many birds, especially cockatoos, can become carriers of the disease, not showing any outward signs until stressed. Psittacines that are smuggled into the United States from Mexico and other countries without passing through a quarantine station are important sources of this zoonotic disease. Because of this, when purchasing a bird, always do so from a reputable source. If you do, the birds you choose will usually have already been tested for psittacosis, and should pose no health threat to your family.

Psittacosis has been known to cause severe and sometimes fatal flu-like illness in people. The disease can be transmitted by both exotic birds and pigeons, and can be caught by humans breathing infective aerosols from dried bird droppings.

The history of a bird affected with psittacosis usually involves recent exposure to other birds and to some stressful situation. Many will suffer from chronic, intermittent, low-grade illnesses and fail to fully regain their health.

The clinical signs of psittacosis include depression, muscle wasting, poor feathering, regurgitation, sneezing, nasal and eye discharges, and breathing difficulties. Psittacine birds will usually exhibit a classic sign: lime-green diarrhea. In addition, the urate portion of the droppings often takes on a yellow hue, signifying liver inflammation. Heart disease can also occur secondary to infection with the psittacosis organism.

Your veterinarian can diagnose psittacosis using laboratory tests. Increases in the number of white cells in the blood, evidence of anemia, and elevated liver enzymes in the blood can all point toward psittacosis. Specific diagnostic tests, including fecal cultures, selected antibody screens, and tissue stains, are also useful in the diagnosis of this disease.

Treatment of this disease involves the use of special antibiotics that are added to the bird's feed or water. Treatment might be necessary for 30 to 45 days or, in some birds, for an entire lifetime. During their convalescence, sick birds must be isolated from others to prevent transmission of the disease and to reduce stress.

Because of its zoonotic potential, owners should always practice good hygiene when caring for a bird with psittacosis. Cages and utensils should be thoroughly disinfected on a daily basis, using a quaternary ammonium compound or a dilution of bleach (1/4 cup of bleach per gallon of water).

Owners can prevent unwelcome surprises by having all new psittacines examined and tested for psittacosis prior to bringing them into the household. This is especially true for birds with questionable origins. If you have other birds in your household, it is a good idea to keep new birds away from these existing pets for 2 to 3 weeks before introducing them to the others. This will protect your existing birds not only from the threat of psittacosis but also from the threat of other diseases.

Exotic Newcastle's Disease (Avian Distemper)

Exotic Newcastle's disease (END) has been effectively eradicated from the United States, but it bears mentioning, since not all new birds entering the country pass through quarantine stations as they should. This viral disease is spread by ingestion or inhalation of the infective virus in food, in water, or on the hands of a handler. Among the psittacines, cockatoos and cockatiels are especially susceptible to END.

Clinical signs of the disease in affected birds include depression, loss of appetite and weight, breathing difficulties, nasal and eye discharges, diarrhea, and nervous system signs, such as incoordination, weakness, and paralysis.

If END is suspected in a pet bird from history and clinical signs, the United States Department of Agriculture is notified immediately, and the bird is placed in quarantine at a USDA facility. Unfortunately, there is no effective treatment for this disease.

Pox (Avian Diphtheria)

Avian pox is a viral disease characterized by severe respiratory and skin disease. Almost all birds can be infected with a poxvirus; the most likely candidates are canaries, finches, parrots, and pigeons. Cockatoos and cockatiels are relatively resistant to the disease. Exposure to the pox organism occurs via inhalation or by skin penetration, usually secondary to trauma. Insects, especially mosquitoes, can even spread the disease between susceptible birds. Pox seems to be a nagging problem in exotic bird quarantine stations.

The clinical signs associated with a pox infection include sneezing, breathing difficulties, discharges from the eyes and nose, and ulcers or scabs in the mouth, on the face, or on the extremities. The eyes of affected birds are often inflamed and painful. With severe involvement, death can ensue 1 to 7 days after clinical signs appear.

Diagnosis of a pox infection is based on clinical signs seen and microscopic examination of infected tissues and fluids. Unfortunately, not much can be done for treatment. Preventing secondary infections with antibiotics and treating any eye involvement are certainly warranted.

A vaccine can be used to help protect canaries against the ravages of canary pox. In addition, owners can help reduce chances of transmission by preventing their pets' access to wild birds (or vice versa), by controlling mosquitoes, and by quarantining all new birds before introducing them into the household.

Polyoma Papovavirus Infection (Budgie Fledgling Disease)

The *polyoma papovavirus* has been implicated as the cause of budgie fledgling disease, a highly fatal syndrome that affects young birds less than 4 weeks of age. The disease is transmitted through contact with infected droppings and other body fluids. Mother-to-egg transfer has also been documented. Fledglings stricken with this disease suffer from a severe gastroenteritis with accompanying diarrhea. The heart, liver, and kidneys become additional targets for the virus as well.

Because of the disease's intensity and the lack of an effective treatment, these young birds usually die within 1 to 2 days after the onset of signs. Those rare birds that do survive often experience stunted growth and feather development.

Pacheco's Disease (Inclusion Body Hepatitis)

Pacheco's disease is caused by the psittacine herpes virus, which causes severe illness in affected birds. It is seen most often in newly imported and illegally smuggled birds. Transmission between birds occurs through contact with infected feces, usually from contaminated food and water bowls. Some birds can become carriers of this disease, with stress playing an important role in the appearance of clinical signs.

The clinical signs seen with Pacheco's disease are the result of liver, spleen, gastrointestinal, and respiratory involvement. Bright yellow diarrhea, yellow-green urates, vomiting, breathing difficulties, nasal discharges, depression, and a generalized wasting are all signs that can be seen with this disease. Incoordination and head tilting can also occur if the nervous system becomes involved. In severe instances, sudden death might occur.

Diagnosis of Pacheco's disease is made using history and clinical signs. Fecal cultures for the herpes virus can be performed as well. Unfortunately, definitive diagnosis is often made only after the bird has died.

There is currently no effective treatment for Pacheco's disease, although the effectiveness of certain human antiviral drugs against this disease agent is being tested in the laboratory.

A vaccine for Pacheco's disease does now exist and is available through veterinarians. As with psittacosis, new birds should be quarantined and screened for Pacheco's before introduction into the household.

Bacterial Infections

The bacterial organism *Salmonella* and others can cause significant disease in pet birds, particularly those stressed because of poor husbandry and nutrition. Pigeons are effective carriers of salmonellosis, yet rarely show any signs of infection. In contrast, pet birds that become infected can suffer from severe clinical signs and syndromes, some of which include depression, diarrhea, breathing difficulties, arthritis, and bone infections. Salmonellosis and other bacterial infections are spread from bird to bird via contact with infected fecal material. Rodents and certain insects such as cockroaches can also play an active role in the spread of these diseases.

General Treatment of Sick Birds

Keep in mind that a sick bird is fragile, and requires lots of attention and care to ensure that a proper recovery takes place. Because of the importance of minimizing stress, many veterinarians encourage convalescence at home in the environment in which the bird is most comfortable. As a result, owners should know how to best care for a sick or injured bird during that all-important convalescent period.

Care for Sick Birds

The cornerstone of any treatment regimen for birds is to reduce stress as much as possible. For starters, this means that handling should be kept to a minimum at all times during the recovery period (Fig. 23.1).

If applicable, remove other birds from the cage. It is essential to keep the cage environment between 85 and 90 degrees Fahrenheit and adequately humidified (Fig. 23.2). A heating pad set on low may be placed beneath (not *in*) the cage. Be sure that a towel or blanket separates the pad from the metal of the cage and clear the

> **DR. P'S VET TIP**
>
> Ill birds have a tendency to overindulge in grit. As a result, if your bird is sick, remove all grit from its cage.

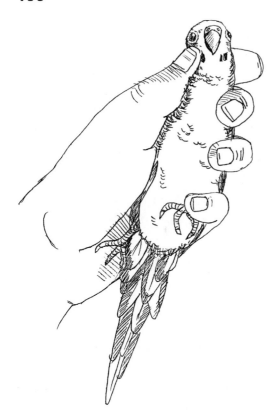

cage of grit. Always use a thermometer to monitor cage temperature.

An incandescent light-bulb can also be installed overhead to provide extra warmth. Avoid using white bulbs because the bright light they emit will inter-fere with sleep. Instead, use a 40- to 60-watt green bulb. It can provide a source of heat, while at the same time respecting your bird's seclusion.

A cage cover can be used for the convalescing bird to help provide additional seclusion and warmth. It should cover three-fourths of the cage during the day and the entire cage at night. It is vital that convalescing birds receive at least 12 hours of undisturbed rest per day.

FIGURE 23.1 Unless administering a treatment, keep handling of sick birds to an absolute minimum.

Also, lower perches to make access easier and to reduce the chances of injury from falling. Place food and water within the bird's easy reach.

Tube Feeding

If a bird refuses to eat or drink on its own, tube feeding might be necessary. Before doing this, however, try to hand-feed your bird.

Warmed baby food or oatmeal may be sufficiently enticing to stimu-late an appetite. To encourage drinking, add sugar or honey to your bird's water, and offer it with a dropper or small syringe. This is espe-cially helpful if medications are to be administered in the water. (If you decide to add sugar or honey to the water, be sure to change the water

2. Attach the feeding syringe filled with the desired amount of formula to the tube, and expel any air present within the tube. With the bird held upright, insert the speculum into its mouth. Pass the feeding tube through the speculum starting from the left side of the bird's mouth and progressing toward the right side of the throat. As you pass the tube, feel for the tube in the esophagus as it passes down. This will help ensure that the tube is in the correct place and not in the airways. Insert the tube the premeasured distance (Fig. 23.3).

3. Slowly administer the desired amount of food. Palpate the crop for fullness. It should not feel tight, but rather still slightly fluctuant to the touch. Once finished, withdraw the tube. If the bird regurgitates food at any time during the feeding, withdraw the tube immediately. Be sure to clean and disinfect the equipment after each feeding and put leftover formula back into the refrigerator. Discard any unused commercial formula after 48 hours.

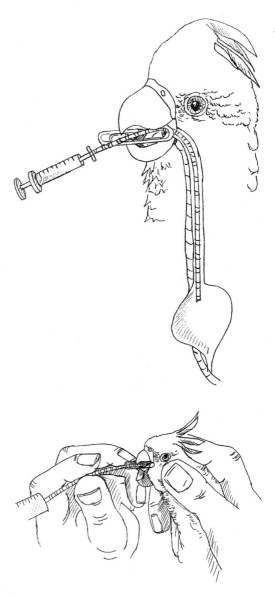

FIGURE 23.3 Prior to passing a feeding tube, measure the approximate length of tubing it will take to pass from the bird's mouth to its crop. The crop will be situated near the forwardmost tip of the breastbone (keel bone). (Refer to Fig. 20.1.) Mark the proper length directly on the tube using tape or a permanent-ink marker.

Hand-Raising Baby Birds

At some time you might be faced with hand-raising a baby bird, perhaps because the mother bird has abandoned the baby or was abusive toward it. Many bird breeders choose to hand-raise new offspring in order to stimulate the parents to produce more eggs. Birds that are hand-raised as babies are also tamer and generally make better pets.

Hand-reared baby birds must be kept warm, and a good way to do this is to either place a heating pad (low setting) under the portion of the box in which the baby is being kept, or by using a 75-watt lightbulb clamped overhead. Always use a thermometer to monitor environmental temperatures. For the first 10 days of the baby bird's life, the environmental temperature should be kept between 90 and 95 degrees Fahrenheit. Afterward, it can be dropped to about 85 degrees Fahrenheit for the next 30 days. Once the bird is feathered, maintaining an environmental temperature of around 75 degrees Fahrenheit is ideal.

The floor of the box should be kept spotless at all times. Paper towels or soft facial tissue can be used as floor covering. Wood shavings are not recommended, since birds may eat them.

Feedings need to be performed at regular intervals, depending on the age of the bird. Just-hatched birds will receive nourishment from the yolk sac for up to 12 hours and seldom require feeding during this time. Once feeding is to commence, an eyedropper or syringe can be used to deliver the food mixture. Commercial formulas should be used. However, if one is not readily available, then the following formula can be substituted:

Baby food, including
High-protein cereal	1 cup
Vegetable (any type)	1 teaspoon
Fruit (any type)	1 teaspoon
Lowfat milk (powder)	1/4 cup

This formula should be blended with warm water to form a mixture that can easily be fed using a syringe or dropper. The water used to prepare the feeding formula should not be soft water because of its high salt content. Purified or filtered water is the best. Additionally, a vitamin-mineral supplement can be added to the mixture, dosing according to the supplement's label instructions. Keep the formula refrigerated when not in use. Discard unused homemade formula on a daily basis.

Warm your bird's food up to 100 degrees Fahrenheit before feeding. When administering food into your bird's mouth, have the bird facing you and slowly squirt the food into the mouth aiming from your right to your left. This will help guide the food down the esophagus instead of the trachea. Give just enough food to lightly distend the crop; don't overfill! The idea is to have the crop three-quarters empty by the time the next feeding rolls around. If a meal sits in the crop too long, it can predispose to crop infection. If you find that the crop is not emptying properly, try cutting back on the amount you are feeding, or add more water to the formula. Also, recheck the temperature of the food. If the formula is too cold, crop emptying can be delayed. Do not force-feed a bird that is reluctant to eat. If its appetite remains depressed, call your veterinarian for instructions.

Feed birds 1 to 7 days of age every 2 hours (feed only once or twice during the night to avoid totally interrupting your bird's sleep). When the bird is 7 to 21 days old, feed it every 4 hours; at 3 to 6 weeks of age, feed three times daily. When the bird is 6 to 8 weeks of age, feed it twice daily. Birds over 8 weeks of age should not require more than one hand-fed meal, given at bedtime. At this age, they will usually start eating and drinking on their own.

Emergency and First Aid Procedures in Birds

Because any injury or illness in a bird can lead to serious complications and even death, you must be prepared in the event of an emergency involving your pet (Fig. 23.4). Some of the more common emergency situations that might arise include bleeding, broken bones, respiratory distress, and poisonings. As far as first aid is concerned, minor injuries such as bleeding toenails or minor lacerations

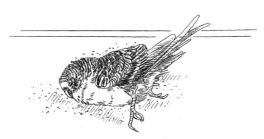

FIGURE 23.4 Any injury or apparent illness in a bird should be treated as a medical emergency.

can be effectively doctored at home. On the other hand, those first aid procedures related to more serious injuries or illnesses are only palliative, and must be followed up immediately with a visit to your veterinarian. Remember: The life of an injured or ill bird is fragile and could easily be lost unless prompt action is taken.

Ideally, transport your bird to the veterinary hospital in its original cage. Remove all perches and empty all water containers prior to moving. Also, place a cover over the cage for seclusion and warmth. If your bird is so debilitated that it cannot stand or balance itself, gently wrap it in a towel large enough to prevent movement. Keep the temperature within the car above 85 degrees Fahrenheit to minimize stress.

First Aid for Birds

BLEEDING (HEMORRHAGE), CUTS, AND WOUNDS

Apply direct, firm pressure over the area for a minimum of 5 minutes using a cloth, towel, or article of clothing. Be aware of how you are restraining your pet; don't grasp it so tightly that breathing is impaired.

After applying pressure for 5 minutes, remove the covering and observe for further bleeding. Reapply pressure if necessary or apply a clotting cream or powder (if a toenail is involved). Do not use clotting powders or creams on other open wounds. Instead, gently wash the wound with soap and water, and rinse thoroughly. Apply an antibiotic ointment to the wound. In addition, if the wound is large, cover it with a sterile dressing. If the wound and/or bleeding is severe, wrap your bird in a towel and transport it to your veterinarian.

BREATHING DIFFICULTIES AND NASAL DISCHARGE

These two clinical symptoms indicate respiratory disease or heart disease, both of which can be rapidly fatal if not treated promptly. Do not try to treat these symptoms at home. Take your bird to your veterinarian immediately.

DIARRHEA AND CONSTIPATION

Bird owners should not attempt to treat diarrhea in birds at home, because of the high probability of an underlying infectious disease.

The longer you postpone professional treatment, the greater the chances are for your bird's condition to worsen.

For the constipated bird, try adding mineral oil or more fruit to the diet. If the problem persists for more than 2 days or if the bird shows other signs of illness, immediate veterinary attention is indicated.

CLOACAL PROLAPSE

If such a prolapse occurs, gently clean the prolapse with warm water and soap, and rinse well. Coat and lubricate the prolapsed region with lubricating jelly and attempt to gently push it back in. Then take your bird to your veterinarian. If it won't go back in easily, discontinue your attempts and enlist the help of your veterinarian. Prolapsed birds should be placed on antibiotics to prevent secondary infections from developing.

EGG BINDING

There is no specific treatment that you can do at home for an egg-bound bird. This condition requires immediate veterinary attention.

OILED BIRDS

Loosely tape your bird's mouth shut to prevent ingestion of the oil. Flush the eyes, nose, and mouth to remove any oil that may be present. Using mild dishwashing liquid, wash the feathers thoroughly and

Dr. P's Vet Tip

Nontoxic mechanic's waterless hand cleanser can be an effective tool for removing oil and dirt from the feathers of birds. Just be sure to dry the feathers thoroughly after use.

rinse well. Repeat as necessary. Blot the feathers dry using a towel, and take your bird to your veterinarian for further treatment.

POISONINGS

If the poison was ingested, rush both bird and poison container to your veterinarian as soon as possible. If the poison contacts the skin and feathers, rinse the bird well with copious amounts of warm water and blot dry with a towel. Transport to your veterinarian at once, being sure to take the poison container with you.

SEIZURES

Wrap a seizuring bird gently in a towel to prevent self-injury. Transport immediately to a veterinarian.

EYE INJURIES AND DISORDERS

If a noxious substance gets in the eye, gently flush the eye liberally with an ophthalmic solution or tap water. Use a tissue or soft cloth to wipe away any discharge or foreign matter from the skin surrounding the eye. Transport to your veterinarian.

HEAT STROKE AND SMOKE INHALATION

Quickly remove the bird from the offending environment and provide free access to fresh air. Fan the bird to increase air circulation. For heat stroke, wrap the bird in a cool (not cold) moistened towel and transport it immediately to your veterinarian.

FRACTURES AND BROKEN BONES

For broken wings, immobilize the wing by pinning it against the bird's body using gauze wrap or a small towel. Be sure not to wrap so tightly as to impair your bird's breathing. Transport it immediately to your veterinarian. For leg fractures, toothpicks, pens, or pencils can be used as temporary splints while you transport your bird to the veterinarian.

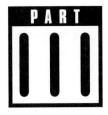

PART

III

EXOTIC PETS

For the purpose of this book, any creature that doesn't bark, meow, or fly falls into the category of "exotic pet." In reality, most of these pets are not truly "exotic" or unconventional, owing to their ever-increasing popularity and numbers in households across the country. As American lifestyles change, it appears that pet preferences may be changing as well!

Popular exotic pets include rabbits, guinea pigs, small rodents (gerbils, hamsters, mice, and rats), chinchillas, sugar gliders, prairie dogs, hedgehogs, ferrets, pot-bellied pigs, reptiles, amphibians, invertebrates, and fish. Each one of these pets has special husbandry, nutritional, and preventive health care requirements that are essential for its health and happiness. It is vital that prospective owners do their research *before, not after,* obtaining such a pet. Veterinarians are becoming more specialized in exotic medicine, and can serve as excellent information resources for first-time owners.

Keeping an exotic pet healthy and happy is not difficult and can be loads of fun. The following chapters are designed to touch on the main points of husbandry and health care of the more popular exotic species seen today. If more in-depth information is needed, consult your veterinarian or pet health care professional.

Rabbits

The domestic rabbit that we are all familiar with, *Oryctolagus cuniculus*, is actually a descendant of the European wild rabbit. Rabbits have been used for centuries for food and pelts, yet their importance and popularity as delightful house pets are rapidly increasing. Well over 50 breeds exist from which to choose, depending on aesthetic preference. Common breeds kept as pets include several varieties of angora, lop-eared, and dwarf rabbits. Many of the popular lop-eared rabbits have ears that hang all the way down to the floor! In addition, rabbits come in three basic sizes: large, medium, and small, with the larger rabbits weighing in as much as 15 pounds! Docile and easy to handle, rabbits are relatively easy to care for. Many can be trained to perform tricks and even walk on a leash! As with other pets, the key to disease prevention and control in these creatures is good husbandry. Well maintained, the average rabbit can live to be 5 to 10 years old.

Restraint

When handling a rabbit, grasp the loose skin over the shoulder and neck region with one hand, and support

DID YOU KNOW?

Lagomorphs (rabbits) and rodents can be differentiated by their teeth. Lagomorphs have four upper incisor teeth, whereas rodents have only two.

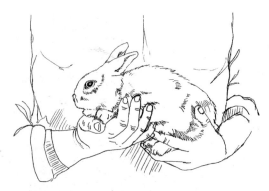

FIGURE 24.1 When holding a rabbit, always maintain support of its powerful hind legs to prevent injury.

the hind legs against your chest with the other (Fig. 24.1). Not only will this keep you from being bitten or scratched, but it is also necessary to prevent accidental injury to the back and spine of the rabbit. A rabbit that is restrained with its rear legs unsupported can kick and thrust with such force as to actually fracture its spine in the struggle!

Housing

Rabbits can be allowed free access to the house and can be readily litter-trained. If a litterbox is to be supplied, use only pelleted paper or non-toxic organic litter in the box. Standard clay or gravel can be harmful if ingested by your rabbit. With rabbits that are allowed to roam freely, realize that they can be quite destructive with their teeth and nails. Rabbitproof your home as you would for any new puppy or kitten.

If your rabbit is to be kept in a cage, be sure it provides plenty of room in which to move around. Metal cages can be purchased commercially or can be constructed out of wire mesh (Fig. 24.2). This wire mesh should be 1 × 2 inches on the sides and no more than $1/2$ × 1 inch on the floor.

Because wire mesh is hard on the feet of rabbits, supply a plastic or metal resting board to place over a portion of the cage floor. This will provide your rabbit with both a space for resting and a space for activity. Cover this portion of flooring with straw or aspen shavings. Just remember to remove all feces and urine that may accumulate on a daily basis. To ensure utmost sanitation, a tray filled with cat litter or other absorbent material can be placed beneath the open flooring to capture urine and fecal material that passes through the wire mesh. Many cage setups have sunken flooring beneath the wire mesh that slides out and makes cleanup much easier (Fig. 24.3).

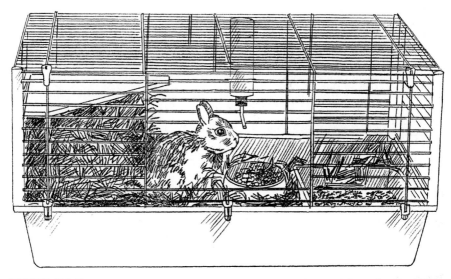

FIGURE 24.2 One example of a housing setup that can be used for a dwarf rabbit.

Cages should be placed in well-ventilated areas to prevent buildups of ammonia fumes emitted from urine. If kept outdoors, they should also provide protection against the wind and other elements. Rabbits enjoy environmental temperatures that range between 65 and 80 degrees Fahrenheit. Temperatures exceeding 85 degrees are not well tolerated.

Sipper bottles suspended from the sides of the cage should be used in place of water bowls, since sippers prevent fecal contamination of the water supply and also reduce the chances of sore hock and other moisture-related diseases. Cages, food bowls, and water dispensers should be cleaned

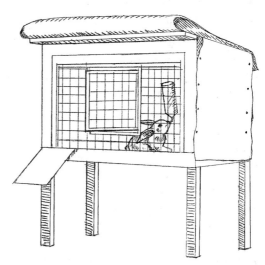

FIGURE 24.3 A classic outdoor rabbit hutch with plastic sheeting on the side to protect against the wind.

and disinfected at least twice weekly. Chlorhexidine or a quaternary ammonium compound diluted in a 1:10 solution (1 part ammonium to 10 parts water) can be used as the disinfectant. Be sure to rinse well after application. For cages located outdoors, waste material should be removed at least every other day to keep it from attracting flies and other insects.

Nutrition

Commercial rabbit pellets can be purchased for your rabbit, along with unlimited amounts of hay. All food offered should be as fresh as possible and be free of mold. The daily allotment should be offered free-choice for consumption throughout the day. In addition to pellets, small portions of dark green or yellow vegetables (e.g., broccoli, brussels sprouts, alfalfa sprouts, carrots, squash) and fruit (e.g., apples, melon, strawberries) should be offered daily. (*Note:* To prevent digestive upset, green, leafy vegetables should not be offered to young rabbits under 6 months of age.)

As always, provide plenty of clean, fresh water delivered through a water sipper that hangs from the side of the cage. Both food (uneaten) and water should be changed daily.

Because a rabbit's teeth are in a constant growth mode, provide a hardwood chew block and/or tree branches (e.g., elm, maple, birch, apple, pear, peach) to help keep the teeth worn down properly and to satisfy its desire to chew (Fig. 24.4). Avoid branches from trees such as cedar, redwood, cherry, and oleander, as these can be poisonous.

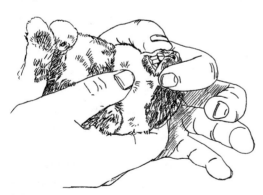

FIGURE 24.4 A rabbit's incisor teeth are constantly on the grow and need to be worn down through normal chewing activity. As a result, rabbits should be provided with plenty of hardwood chew blocks and/or tree branches to help keep the teeth in top shape.

One behavior of rabbits that might surprise new owners is *coprophagy,* or the consumption of their own fecal material. This usually occurs during the morning hours. This practice shouldn't be frowned on, as it actually increases nutrient utilization and absorption within the rabbit's body.

DID YOU KNOW?

When a rabbit rubs its chin on an item, it is claiming it as its personal property!

Reproduction

Justifiably, the rabbit has been accused of being one of the most prolific breeders of all time. One reason for this fecundity is that the female rabbit, or doe, is *polyestrous,* that is, continually in heat. Rabbits are also induced ovulators, which means that an egg is released from the ovary only on copulation.

Three weeks after breeding, a hay-filled nesting box should be introduced into the cage for the doe to make final preparations for birth. It must be large enough for the doe to easily stand in and be equipped with a doorway to allow for the doe and her babies to come and go as they please. Pregnancy in does lasts 28 to 34 days.

The number of offspring to be expected is around three to nine. Baby rabbits, or pups, are born in the nest naked, blind, and helpless, yet are usually well cared for by the doe. Eyes will open up at around 10 days of age.

After the birth, the doe's food allowance should be increased gradually over a week's time to compensate for lactation. Do not increase it suddenly, as this can lead to serious gastrointestinal problems. In 3 weeks, the nest can be removed from the cage. Weaning will occur 3 to 4 weeks after its removal. Young rabbits reach puberty at 4 to 10 months of age.

Orphaned pups or those that have not been fed properly during the first 2 days of life can be raised on commercial milk replacements intended for puppies and kittens. Feedings should be offered every 8 to 12 hours, up to a daily amount of 10 to 20 milliliters of formula. Pups should be stimulated to urinate and defecate after feeding by massaging their anal regions with a cotton ball soaked in warm water. Most young rabbits can be weaned onto commercial

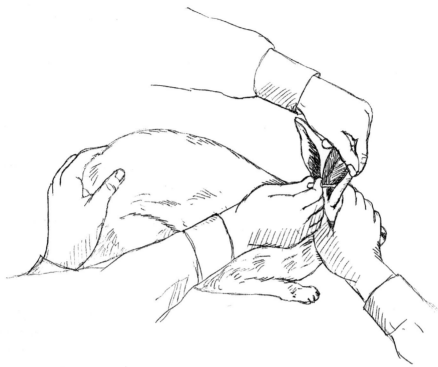

FIGURE 24.5 Treat ear mites in a rabbit as you would in a cat.

pellets as early as 3 weeks of age. As always, warmth, sanitation, and tender loving care are vital whenever raising orphans.

Preventive Health Care

Routine vaccinations are not required for rabbits, but annual veterinary checkups and stool checks are highly recommended. The nails should be trimmed monthly (or more frequently if needed), and the haircoat should be brushed at least twice weekly (longhair varieties more frequently). Rabbits will shed their haircoats every 3 to 4 months. Feline hairball laxative should be administered weekly to prevent hairball formation. While administering this medication, take note of the teeth for any apparent overgrowth. If detected, contact your veterinarian. Fleas and ear mites can be controlled using safe topical products designed for puppies and kittens (Fig. 24.5).

Adult does can be spayed to prevent further pregnancies and to reduce the incidence of uterine cancer as they grow older. Similarly, bucks can be neutered when they are 8 to 12 months of age. Ask your veterinarian for more details.

Strict sanitation, environmental control, and high-quality rations must be given top priority in order to prevent disease. Keep a close eye on your pet's behavior, eating habits, elimination habits, and physical characteristics. Notify your veterinarian of any changes. Care should be taken to prevent obesity, which can have the same deleterious effects in rabbits as it does in humans. And don't forget to offer a liberal dose of attention to your pet each day to help fulfill its mental and emotional needs.

Diseases and Disorders of Rabbits

Table 24.1 lists some selected diseases and disorders seen in rabbits. Remember that others do exist, which is why a definitive diagnosis should be made by a qualified veterinarian. Identifying and treating diseases in their early stages is the key to successful treatment and cure.

Table 24.1 Diseases and Disorders of Rabbits

Disease or disorder	Clinical signs	Treatment and comments
Respiratory disease		
Bacterial rhinitis/ pneumonia (snuffles; pasteurellosis)	Sneezing; nasal and eye discharge; breathing difficulties; head shaking	Common in stressed rabbits; treat with antibiotics
Gastrointestinal diseases		
Malocclusion of teeth ("slobbers")	Excessive salivation; inability to eat; weight loss; lip lacerations	Trim incisor teeth every 2 weeks

Table 24.1 Diseases and Disorders of Rabbits (*Continued*)

Disease or disorder	Clinical signs	Treatment and comments
Hairballs	Loss of appetite; abdominal pain	Treat using laxatives; surgical removal sometimes needed; prevent with brushing, hairball laxative weekly
Mucoid-enteropathy	Abdominal pain and distension; diarrhea; arched back; dehydration	Highly fatal in young rabbits; exact cause unknown; treat with antibiotics to prevent secondary infection; replace fluids; high-fiber diet might help
Coccidiosis	Abdominal pain and distension; loss of appetite; diarrhea; jaundice; weight loss	Associated with poor sanitary conditions; treat with sulfa drugs
Bacterial enteritis	Diarrhea; weight loss; jaundice	Associated with poor sanitary conditions; also can be associated with improper antibiotic therapy; treat using a select group of antimicrobial agents
Skin and coat diseases		
"Sore hocks" (bacterial dermatitis)	Moist, ulcerated skin lesions on hind feet	Caused by trauma from wire floors, environmental filth; treat with antibiotics; change environmental conditions
Ringworm	Hair loss; crusts on head, ears	Treat with antifungal medications
Ear mites	Head shaking; scratching at ears; crusts and scabs in ears; hair loss on head and neck	Very common problem in pet rabbits; treat with ear mite medication; ivermectin for tough cases

Table 24.1 Diseases and Disorders of Rabbits (*Continued*)

Disease or disorder	Clinical signs	Treatment and comments
Mange (*Sarcoptes*)	Intense itching; hair loss on face, ears, genitalia	Very contagious to other rabbits; treat with safe insecticidal shampoo; ivermectin for tough cases
Fleas, ticks	Itching; hair loss; anemia	Treatment same as that for cats
Pox viruses	Wartlike growths on face, legs, and feet; swollen eyelids; eye discharge; subcutaneous lumps	Transmitted by biting insects; no treatment; wartlike growths usually regress on their own
Reproductive system diseases		
Pregnancy toxemia	Loss of appetite; depression; seizures in pregnant or lactating does	Cause unknown; high mortality; support with antibiotics
Uterine adenocarcinoma	Infertility; weight loss; loss of appetite; vaginal discharge	Common in older females; spay if not metastasized
Urinary system diseases		
Normal urine	Urine cloudy, thick; often orange or brown in color	
Nephroma	Loss of appetite, depression; variable signs (associated with kidney disease)	Usually benign, yet affects kidney function

Table 24.1 Diseases and Disorders of Rabbits (*Continued*)

Disease or disorder	Clinical signs	Treatment and comments
Neurological diseases		
Parasitic encephalitis	Tremors; convulsions; incoordination	Can be caused by exposure to raccoon, roundworms, or other infected rabbits; *Cuterebra* larvae can also cause similar signs
Musculoskeletal diseases		
Splayleg	Inability to walk, support weight; one or all legs can be affected	Can be genetic or traumatic in origin; treatment generally unrewarding
Spinal fractures	Paralysis of hind end and hind legs	Caused by improper handling or trauma; treatment generally unrewarding

Guinea Pigs

avia porcellus, the guinea pig, is a native of the south American continent, where it was raised by the Incas for food and for religious sacrifice. Introduced into Europe centuries ago, the guinea pig became popular as a laboratory animal, then as a pet. In the United States, the same functions hold true today. As pets, there are a number of popular breeds from which to choose, including the *English,* characterized by smooth, short hair; *Peruvians,* which have long, silky hair; *Abyssinians,* which sport short, coarse hair arranged in multiple whorls; *crested,* which are similar to English guinea pigs but with a white crest on the head; and *Teddys,* characterized by coarse, kinky hair. Guinea pigs also come in a variety of colors, such as solids, agouti, Himalayan, and tortoise shell.

Like hamsters, guinea pigs have no tails. Good-natured, they rarely bite, yet will emit a loud squeal when frightened or handled. They are easy to maintain, and require minimal preventive health care. They do require periodic brushing and nail trims. In addition, their front teeth may require trimming if overgrowth occurs. Guinea pigs average about 1 to 2 pounds in weight when fully grown, and can live up to 8 years when well cared for.

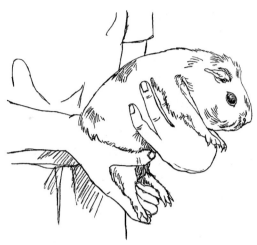

FIGURE 25.1 Use two hands when lifting your guinea pig.

Restraint

Restraint of the guinea pig is similar to that of rats. The shoulder and chest regions can be encircled with one hand and the hind end supported with the other hand as you lift. Be sure to control the guinea pig's hind feet and rump to prevent it from scratching you (Fig. 25.1).

Housing

Male guinea pigs can be housed with females, yet two males living together will fight. Housing for guinea pigs should consist of a wire cage or aquarium at least 12 inches high and providing at least 2 square feet of space for each pig. The smooth flooring of the cage can be lined with aspen shavings (avoid cedar shavings), commercial rodent bedding, or hay. Bedding should be spot-cleaned daily and changed completely every week. Most guinea pigs appreciate a hiding box or enclosure made of plastic, ceramic, or wood in which to crawl and hide when the feeling arises (Fig. 25.2). Also, guinea pigs like to climb. Providing multilevel shelving within the cage would make your pet extremely happy!

Water delivery systems should be kept up off of the cage floor for sanitary purposes. Since some pigs might actually regurgitate food back up into the water sipper, be sure to check and maintain the patency of such devices on a daily basis. A sturdy, chew-resistant food bowl is a must. The entire cage and its contents should be thoroughly cleaned and sanitized weekly using soap and water.

Guinea pigs do not tolerate heat and humidity very well. Ideal environmental temperature for them is around 70 degrees Fahrenheit. Temperatures exceeding 80 degrees Fahrenheit can quickly lead to heat stroke.

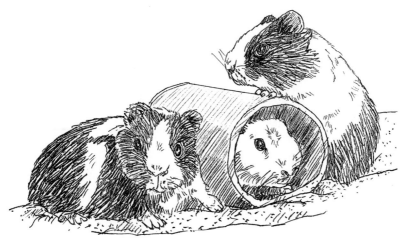

FIGURE 25.2 Provide your guinea pigs with lots of places in which to hide!

Nutrition

Guinea pigs must have adequate amounts of vitamin C in their diets, since their bodies are not capable of synthesizing the vitamin internally. Commercial guinea pig rations, in pellet form, can more than satisfy this requirement if the pellets purchased are fresh. However, to be safe, offer fresh fruits (e.g., one-quarter of an orange or apple) and vegetables (e.g., collard greens, parsley, kale) along with the regular pelleted rations to ensure adequate amounts of vitamin C in the diet. Like rabbits, guinea pigs also enjoy gnawing on carrot sticks.

Because a guinea pig's teeth are in a constant growth mode, provide a hardwood chew block and/or tree branches (e.g., elm, maple, birch, apple, pear, peach) to help keep the teeth worn down properly and to satisfy its desire to chew. Avoid branches from trees such as cedar, redwood, cherry, and oleander, as these can be poisonous.

Clean food bowls (these should be ceramic to discourage chewing) daily, as some guinea pigs enjoy defecating therein. Also, provide plenty of clean, fresh water delivered through a water sipper that hangs from the side of the cage (Fig. 25.3).

Reproduction

Female guinea pigs cycle every 16 days and, if mated, will carry the developing offspring for an average of 68 days. Females that are not bred

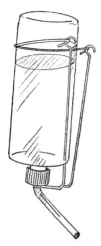

FIGURE 25.3 A water bottle that hangs from the side of the cage is the most sanitary method for delivering water to your guinea pig.

until after 6 months of age have a higher incidence of birthing complications than do those bred earlier in life. If a pig is not bred before this time, its pelvis might fuse together, making passage through the birth canal difficult. As a result, a C-section operation might be necessary to deliver the litter. Also, pregnant guinea pigs are especially susceptible to heat stroke if environmental temperatures are not kept well regulated.

Litter sizes usually range from one to eight cavies. Baby guinea pigs are born with eyes open and with hair. This enables them to be weaned almost immediately if the situation warrants it. However, survival rates are better if babies are weaned around 3 weeks of age (Fig. 25.4). Sexual maturity in guinea pigs is reached at 3 months of age.

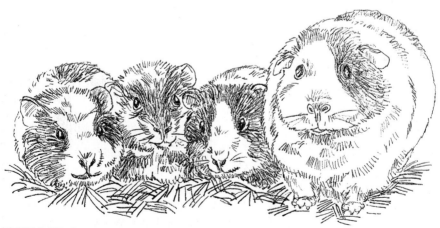

FIGURE 25.4 Young guinea pigs are weaned at 3 to 4 weeks of age.

Preventive Health Care

Routine vaccinations are not required for guinea pigs, but an annual veterinary checkup is highly recommended. The nails of guinea pigs should be trimmed monthly (or more frequently if needed), and the haircoat should be brushed at least twice weekly (longhair varieties more frequently). Monitor your pet's teeth monthly for any apparent overgrowth. If detected, contact your veterinarian. Fleas can be controlled by spot-treating with safe, topical products designed for puppies and kittens.

Guinea pigs can be prolific breeders, so many owners opt to have their pets neutered to prevent their households from becoming overpopulated with these cute creatures!

Strict sanitation, environmental control, and high-quality rations, including vitamin C supplements, must be given top priority in order to prevent disease in guinea pigs. Always keep a close eye on your pet's behavior, eating habits, elimination habits, and physical characteristics. Notify your veterinarian of any changes. Care should be taken to prevent obesity, which can have the same deleterious effects in guinea pigs as it does in humans. And be sure to offer your pet a liberal dose of attention each day to cater to its mental and emotional health.

> **FACT OR FICTION**
>
> A guinea pig that rubs its rump on the ground has worms. **FICTION.** In reality, it is just marking its territory!

Diseases and Disorders

Table 25.1 shows selected diseases and disorders seen in guinea pigs. Stress, overcrowding, improper nutrition, and poor sanitation all play important roles in the development of many diseases, especially the infectious ones.

> **DID YOU KNOW?**
>
> The same *Bordetella* organism that causes kennel cough in dogs can cause life-threatening disease in guinea pigs. As a result, it is always a good idea to have a *Bordetella* vaccine administered to any dog or cat living in the same house as a guinea pig.

Table 25.1 Diseases and Disorders of Guinea Pigs

Disease or disorder	Clinical signs	Treatment and comments
	Infectious diseases	
Salmonellosis	Weight loss; conjunctivitis, diarrhea	Often transmitted via contaminated food (greens); treat with antibiotics; good sanitation; wash greens prior to feeding
Streptococcosis	Enlarged lymph nodes ("lumps"); variable signs and organ involvement; breathing difficulties	Treat with antibiotics
Bordetella bronchiseptica	Nasal discharge; breathing difficulties	Same organism that causes canine cough; treat with antibiotics
Lymphocytic choriomeningitis virus	Poor growth; eye discharge; locomotion difficulties; seizures; breathing difficulties	Transmitted by wild rodents; no treatment available; zoonotic disease
Adenovirus	Breathing difficulties; nasal discharge; weight loss	No treatment available
Inclusion conjunctivitis	Eye crusting, discharge in young guinea pigs; swollen eyelids	Treat with topical eye ointments; will usually clear up without intervention
	Digestive system diseases	
Malocclusion of teeth ("slobbers")	Excessive salivation; inability to eat; weight loss	Usually involves premolars and molars; causes include nutritional deficiencies, genetics; file down overgrown teeth—repeat every 3 weeks

Table 25.1 Diseases and Disorders of Guinea Pigs (*Continued*)

Disease or disorder	Clinical signs	Treatment and comments
Hairballs	Loss of appetite; abdominal pain; palpable mass within abdomen	Surgical removal necessary
Coccidiosis	Abdominal pain and distension; loss of appetite; diarrhea; weight loss	Associated with poor sanitary conditions; treat with sulfa drugs
Bacterial enteritis	Diarrhea; weight loss; abdominal pain	Associated with poor sanitary conditions; also can be associated with improper antibiotic therapy; treat using a select group of antimicrobial agents
Hemorrhagic syndrome	Jaundice; diarrhea; blood clotting problems	Seen in pregnant pigs; caused by uterus disrupting liver function; treat by C-section;* vitamin K therapy
Skin diseases		
Pododermatitis	Moist, ulcerated skin lesions on feet	Caused by trauma from wire floors, environmental filth; treat with antibiotics; change environmental conditions
Hair loss	Can occur anywhere on the body	Causes can include skin parasites, chewing ("barbering"), fighting, pregnancy, ringworm
Ringworm	Hair loss; crusts on head, ears, back	Treat with antifungal medications

Table 25.1 Diseases and Disorders of Guinea Pigs (*Continued*)

Disease or disorder	Clinical signs	Treatment and comments
Mange (mites)	Intense itching; hair loss on face, ears; seizures	Very contagious to other pigs; treat with safe insecticidal shampoo or dip
Fleas, ticks, lice	Itching; hair loss; anemia	Treatment with pyrethrin spray
Reproductive diseases		
Pregnancy toxemia	Loss of appetite; depression; seizures; breathing difficulties in pregnant or lactating pigs	Obesity, genetics, stress, fasting can play a role; treat with dextrose
Urinary diseases		
Urethral obstruction	Inability to urinate; painful abdomen; irritable behavior; blood-tinged urine	Seen in older males; obstruction must be manually removed
Kidney disease	Weight loss; loss of appetite; variable clinical signs	Common in older pigs; treatment generally unrewarding
Nervous system diseases		
Hind-end paralysis	Inability to walk and support weight on hind legs	Often due to spinal fracture or spinal cord damage secondary to pregnancy, vitamin C deficiency, arthritis; treatment depends on severity

Table 25.1 Diseases and Disorders of Guinea Pigs (*Continued*)

Disease or disorder	Clinical signs	Treatment and comments
Musculoskeletal diseases		
Hind-leg fractures	Inability to bear weight on hind leg; dragging leg	Caused by foot getting caught in flooring of wire cage, other trauma; treatment depends on severity
Myopathy	Reluctance to move; depression	Due to vitamin E deficiency; treat with vitamin E supplements
"Stiff wrist" syndrome	Bone deformities; muscular stiffness; abnormal posture	Due to magnesium deficiency; treat by correcting ration

*Cesarean section.

If your guinea pig shows signs of illness, do not give it any medications unless prescribed by your veterinarian. For instance, antibiotic preparations containing penicillin or erythromycin can be deadly if given to guinea pigs.

Remember that with the appearance of any clinical signs, a definitive diagnosis should be made by a qualified veterinarian. Identifying and treating diseases in their early stages are the keys to successful treatment and cure. Sick guinea pigs are fragile creatures, and require prompt veterinary attention.

Hamsters and Gerbils

The most popular species of pet hamster is by far the golden (Syrian) hamster (*Mesocricetus auratus*). Its smaller cousin, the Chinese (striped-back) hamster (*Cricetus griseus*), is probably next in popularity. Hamsters are native to both the European and Asian continents. They are larger than gerbils and lack tails. Depending on the variety, hamsters can sport either a long or a short haircoat, and come in variety of colors, including brown, cinnamon, white, and blends thereof.

Hamsters can be fun and loving pets, providing hours of enjoyment and fascination just watching their busy activity. Notorious escape artists, hamsters are most active at night (sometimes to the dismay of their owners!) and like to sleep during the day. The average life span of a hamster in captivity is approximately 2 years.

Gerbils can be differentiated from hamsters by their smaller size and by the presence of a hairy tail. The presence of hair on the tail can also be used to differentiate gerbils from mice, which have hairless tails. The Mongolian gerbil, *Meriones unguiculatus,* is by far the most popular type. It is native to the deserts of Mongolia and China. Because of their origin, gerbils possess many unique features, including a very low daily water requirement. Like camels, gerbils can

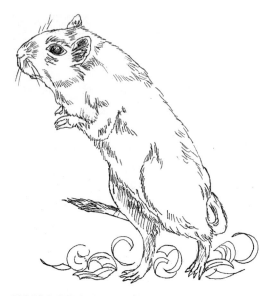

FIGURE 26.1 One unique feature of the gerbil is that it has a very low daily water requirement.

regulate water reserves within their bodies quite efficiently, and can go for days without water (Fig. 26.1)! Gerbils tend to be friendlier than hamsters, rarely biting the hand that feeds them. They are curious creatures, yet rarely try to escape. Unlike hamsters, they enjoy daytime as well as nighttime activity. Gerbils that are well cared for can live 4 years or more in captivity.

Restraint

When handling or restraining hamsters, use caution because some may have a tendency to bite. Grasp the skin over the shoulder and neck region with the thumb and first two fingers of one hand and support the body with the other hand. For restraining hamsters that are known biters (this includes sick hamsters), be sure to grasp as much skin as you can.

Gerbils are much easier to handle than hamsters because of their friendly and gentle dispositions. Most will climb right into an open hand; others might need to be restrained similar to mice (see Fig. 26.2). Never pick up a gerbil by its tail. If you do, the skin covering the tail could come off in your hand, leaving your rodent friend in an unhealthy predicament!

DID YOU KNOW ?

During winter months, hamsters might become lethargic and appear ill (or even dead) if environmental temperatures drop to below 50 degrees Fahrenheit. But don't fret! These hamsters are only thinking about hibernating, and a little warmth and rousing will soon bring them back to life!

Housing

Hamsters, especially females, should be housed individually, owing to their somewhat belligerent behavior toward cagemates. Adult gerbils placed in a cage together for the first time may fight as well. However, gerbils that were raised together for the first 2 months of life will coexist quite comfortably within the same enclosure (Fig. 26.3).

Housing accommodations for hamsters and gerbils can be readily purchased from a local pet store or pet supplier. Well-ventilated wire or plastic cages with solid flooring are preferred. For hamsters, setups containing divided compartments connected with tunnels work well also. Cages with wire mesh flooring should be avoided because they can be hard on the feet and, in the case of gerbils, be a source of tail injuries. Finally, hamsters are notorious escape artists, so be certain that all cage outlets are secured at all times!

Aspen shavings or commercial rodent bedding can be used to line the bottom

(F)ACT or *FICTION*

Hamsters are more likely to bite their owners during daylight hours.

(F)ACT. Hamsters get most of their sleep during the day and tired or sleepy hamsters can easily become cranky when handled.

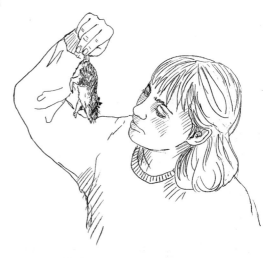

FIGURE 26.2 When picking up a gerbil by the tail, be sure to grasp it at the base—instead of the end—of the tail.

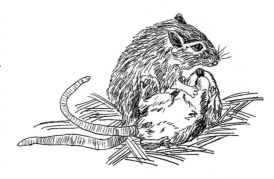

FIGURE 26.3 Gerbils are happiest when kept in pairs.

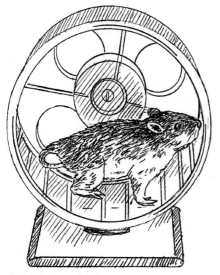

FIGURE 26.4 All small rodents should be provided with an exercise wheel to help keep them fit and trim!

of the cage and help absorb waste material. This bedding should be changed at least twice weekly. Cedar shavings should not be used, as the oils contained in cedar can be irritating to the skin and mucous membranes of rodents. Be sure to also provide nesting material consisting of shredded tissue or cotton.

Exercise wheels, toys, and makeshift huts or sleeping quarters should be installed for your pet's enjoyment (Fig. 26.4). When choosing a wheel for gerbils, select one constructed of plastic. Avoid metal wheels with spokes, since these can cause serious injuries to tails if they become intertwined in them.

Both hamsters and gerbils should be provided with 12 hours of light and 12 hours of darkness each day. Environmental temperatures should be kept around 70 degrees Fahrenheit for maximum comfort. Humidity should not exceed 50 percent.

Nutrition

Rations for a hamster or gerbil should consist of commercial rodent pellets with a few treats such as sprouts, fruits (avoid oranges) such as raisins, or nuts thrown in for good measure. Seeds can be offered as treats as well, but only in limited quantities. Some pets will prefer to eat the seeds over their regular ration, leading to nutritional imbalances and obesity. At the same time, be careful not to overfeed regular rations. Obesity causes the same ill effects in these small animals as it does in larger ones. Hamsters are notorious for gathering and storing food, which may trick you into thinking that you aren't feeding enough.

Ceramic food dispensers can be attached directly to the side of the cage. This method of food delivery is much more sanitary than simply placing a food bowl on the floor of the cage. Water sippers can also be attached to the side of the cage. Just be sure that both food and water are within easy reach and that the delivery end of the water sipper remains patent. Many hamsters and gerbils die each year because food and water sources are innocently placed out of reach or are inefficient at delivering their products!

Natural wood blocks or sticks for chewing should be placed in the enclosure as well to help keep the incisors worn down and healthy.

Reproduction

Male hamsters can be differentiated from females by the presence of two dark, pigmented spots on the hip regions. These identify the location of hip glands used for marking territory and attracting females.

Female hamsters experience a heat cycle every 4 days. Toward the end of their heat period, a white discharge might be seen coming from the vagina. This is normal and should not be mistaken for an infection. Male hamsters should be introduced into the cage at this time.

Because it could take a few days for the female to become adjusted to the male, watch for aggressiveness on her part, and remove the male immediately if it occurs. Reintroduce him the next day, following the same precautions.

Once breeding takes place, the gestation period is approximately 18 days. Litter size normally ranges from 6 to 10 pups. They are born hairless and blind. Although not common, cannibalism of offspring by young females has been known to occur if the new mother becomes disturbed during the first week after giving birth. This can be aggravated by owners handling the young during the first week of life, improper nesting material, cage cleanings, and difficult access to food and water. As a result, be sure to leave mom alone and undisturbed with her pups for the first week, except, of course, to provide her with food and water. Hamster pups reach weaning age in 3 to 4 weeks and should be removed to their own housing at that time. Puberty is achieved at 8 weeks of age.

The breeding habits of gerbils are similar to those of hamsters. Interestingly, male and female breeding pairs form strong bonds that can last a lifetime. Male gerbils can be differentiated from females by the distance between the anal opening and the genital opening; the distance for the male is much longer.

Females undergo a heat period every 4 to 5 days, and once bred, they experience a gestation period of approximately 24 days. Litter sizes usually range from four to five pups, which, like hamsters, are born hairless, blind, and helpless. A full coat of hair is usually in place by day 10, and the eyes open around day 18.

Cannibalism is not as serious a problem in gerbils as in hamsters. However, it can occur if the female becomes stressed or ill. Pups are weaned at 21 to 24 days, and will reach sexual maturity themselves at about 12 weeks of age.

Preventive Health Care

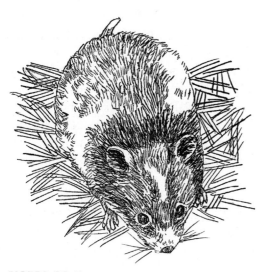

FIGURE 26.5 Stress, improper nutrition, and poor sanitation play important roles in the development of disease in hamsters and gerbils.

Strict sanitation, environmental control, and high-quality rations must be given top priority in order to prevent disease (Fig. 26.5). Keep a close eye on your pet's behavior, and its eating habits, elimination habits, and physical characteristics. The teeth should be examined monthly for overgrowth. Also, the appearance of an unkempt haircoat should alert you to a potential health problem. Notify your veterinarian of this or any other noticeable changes. (*Note:* Remember that hamsters kept in cold temperatures might undergo behavioral changes and appear lethargic or lifeless. Increasing the environmental temperature will restore these hamsters to normal behavior and activity.)

Diseases and Disorders

Tables 26.1 and 26.2 list some selected diseases and disorders seen in hamsters and gerbils. Sick hamsters are generally very irritable and can bite! Stress, improper nutrition, and poor sanitation play important roles in the development of many diseases, especially infectious diseases. Remember that with the appearance of any clinical signs, a definitive diagnosis should be made by a qualified veterinarian. Identifying and treating diseases in their early stages are the keys to successful treatment and cure.

> **DID YOU KNOW?**
>
> Gerbils that are frightened or stressed might exhibit spontaneous epileptic seizures. This tendency for seizure is an inherited trait seen in some strains of gerbils, but don't be alarmed if this happens to your pet. The convulsions will subside on their own, and they require no specific management.

Table 26.1 Diseases and Disorders of Hamsters

Disease or disorder	Clinical signs	Treatment and comments
Digestive system diseases		
Malocclusion of incisor teeth	Excessive salivation; inability to eat; weight loss; nasal discharge	Trim incisors every 8–12 weeks as needed
Salmonellosis	Weight loss; diarrhea; variable signs and organ involvement	Often transmitted via contaminated food (greens); treatment rarely helpful
"Wet tail"	Weight loss; diarrhea; ruffled fur; dehydration; rectal prolapse	Can be rapidly fatal; treat with antibiotics and fluids to correct dehydration
Antibiotic-induced colitis	Severe diarrhea, dehydration, death	Bacterial overgrowth in intestines caused by improper selection of antibiotic
Tapeworms	Weight loss; poor appetite; diarrhea	Rarely causes severe disease; treat with anti-tapeworm medication

Table 26.1 Diseases and Disorders of Hamsters (*Continued*)

Disease or disorder	Clinical signs	Treatment and comments
Skin diseases		
Streptococcosis, staphylococcosis	Enlarged lymph nodes, abscesses	Often secondary to fight wounds; treat with antibiotics; lance
Mange (mites)	Hair loss, scaling, especially along back and face	Often appears secondary to other diseases; treat with insecticidal products as in cats
Musculoskeletal diseases		
Cage paralysis	Weakness; inability to move or lift head	Caused by nutritional deficiency; treat with vitamin supplementation
Other diseases		
Neoplasia	Variable signs, depending on organ systems involved; weight loss; loss of appetite	Tumors are not uncommon in hamsters; often affect glands within the body; treatment depends on organ system involved
Amyloidosis	Weight loss, dehydration, loss of appetite	Causes kidney failure in affected hamsters; common disease

Table 26.2 Diseases and Disorders of Gerbils

Disease or disorder	Clinical signs	Treatment and comments
Digestive system diseases		
Malocclusion of incisor teeth	Depression; inability to eat; weight loss	Trim incisors every 8–12 weeks as needed
Tyzzer's disease ("wet tail")	Weight loss; diarrhea; ruffled fur; dehydration	Can be rapidly fatal; treatment generally unrewarding once signs appear
Salmonellosis	Weight loss; diarrhea; ruffled fur; dehydration	Treatment is generally unrewarding
Skin diseases		
Mange (*Demodex*)	Hair loss, scaling, especially at base of tail and rear legs	Often appears secondary to other diseases; treat with acaricides as in cats
Dermatitis	Moist skin lesions, abscesses; hair loss, abrasions on nose	Usually secondary to poor husbandry and sanitation; self-induced trauma; parasites; antibiotics might be needed for secondary bacterial infections
Respiratory system diseases		
Upper respiratory infection and pneumonia	Sneezing; breathing difficulties; chattering; conjunctivitis	Often caused by stress and poor husbandry; treat with appropriate antibiotics

Table 26.2 Diseases and Disorders of Gerbils (*Continued*)

Disease or disorder	Clinical signs	Treatment and comments
	Urinary system diseases	
Kidney disease	Weight loss; increased water consumption; increased urination	Common in older gerbils; no effective treatment
	Nervous system diseases	
Epilepsy	Spontaneous seizures	Certain strains of gerbils highly susceptible; no treatment necessary
	Other diseases	
Neoplasia	Variable signs, depending on organ systems involved; weight loss; loss of appetite	Tumors are not uncommon in older gerbils; treatment depends on organ system involved

27

Mice and Rats

Although more popular as laboratory research animals, mice and rats are occasionally kept as pets. They are relatively easy to care for, and most have gentle dispositions, making them easy to handle. The mouse, *Mus musculus,* and the rat, *Rattus norvegicus,* originated from the Asian continent, but soon spread with man throughout the world. They are both nocturnal creatures, becoming most active during the twilight hours. However, some mice may choose to be quite active during the day as well. Both have hairless tails, a fact that helps differentiate the mouse from its rodent cousin, the gerbil. While most pet rats are pure white or white with black or brown "hoods," pet mice can be found in a variety of colors, including white, black, brown, and tan. The captive life span for mice and rats is around 2 to 4 years.

Restraint

Mice and rats are usually quite gentle and can be handled without much trouble. Feistier pets can be picked up and restrained by grasping the base of the tail with one hand and, as you lift, encircling the back and ribcage with the other hand. For mice, you can also use your thumb and index finger to grasp the scruff of the neck. Be ready: Most rodents will urinate and/or defecate when handled (Fig. 27.1).

477

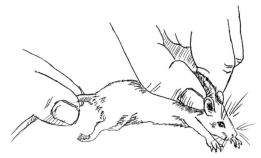

FIGURE 27.1 Restrain a mouse by grasping the scruff of the neck and the base of the tail.

DR. P'S VET TIP

When handling a belligerent rodent, use a paper towel or cloth to protect your hands as you grasp the neck region. In this way, if the rodent turns its head to bite, it won't be able to reach your fingers.

Housing

Mice and rats can be housed in any type of cage or container, provided there is enough room to maintain good sanitary conditions and to allow for an exercise wheel, nesting area, and feeding area. Mice tend to be escape artists, so the enclosure must be secure. Rats are social creatures and can be kept together, regardless of sex, with minimal hostilities (Fig. 27.2). Male and female mice usually can be housed together, but male mice should not be housed together because of their tendency to fight.

You can buy wire-mesh rodent cages for your pet mouse or rat at your favorite pet store. A 5- to 10-gallon aquarium-type enclosure with a wire-screened top can be used as well. Smooth plastic or metal floors are preferred over wire mesh, as the latter can pose hazards to both feet and tails. The floor of the cage should be lined with 2 to 3 inches of aspen shavings or commercial bedding. This bedding should be changed at least twice weekly to maintain good sanitation. Nesting material offered can consist of facial tissue, pieces of cloth, or cardboard.

DID YOU KNOW?

Cedar shavings should not be used as bedding for exotic pets, as the oils contained within the wood can be quite irritating to the skin and mucous membranes of these pets.

Exercise wheels, toys, and makeshift huts or sleeping quarters should be installed for your pet's enjoyment. When choosing a wheel for mice and rats, try to select one constructed of plastic. Avoid metal wheels with

spokes, since they can cause
serious injuries to tails that
become intertwined.

Ideally, the temperature
of the room in which you
house your rodent should
be kept between 70 and 75
degrees Fahrenheit, with a

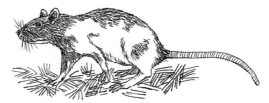

FIGURE 27.2 Rats are social creatures and
often enjoy human interaction.

humidity of around 55 to 60 percent. Twelve hours of both light and
darkness should be provided daily.

Nutrition

Rations for mice and rats should consist of commercial rodent pellets
with a few vegetables or fruit pieces added. However, these treats
should not exceed 5 percent of the total daily ration. Some mice and
rats may prefer the treats over the regular ration, leading to nutritional
imbalances. At the same time, be careful not to overfeed regular
rations, since obesity causes the same ill effects in these small animals
as it does in larger ones.

The average mouse will consume about 3 to 4 grams of food per
day; rats will consume 10 to 20 grams. Chew-resistant dispensers that
hang suspended from the side of the cage can be used to deliver water
and food. This method of delivery is much more sanitary than simply
placing a food or water bowl on the floor of the cage.

Be sure the sources of food and water are easily reachable and that
the delivery end of the water sipper remains accessible. Failure to
heed this advice could lead to death from starvation or dehydration,
especially in small or weak animals.

Natural wood blocks or sticks for chewing should be placed in the
enclosure as well to help keep the incisors worn down and healthy.

Reproduction

Male mice and rats can be differentiated from females on the basis of
their external genitalia and by the distance between the anal and genital openings (longer in males). Female mice and rats experience a heat

cycle every 4 to 6 days. Once they have been bred, the gestation period is approximately 21 days. Litter size normally ranges from six to twelve. Baby mice and rats, like other rodents, are born hairless and blind. New litters should not be disturbed for at least 3 days after birth. Weaning occurs at 3 to 4 weeks, with the young reaching sexual maturity close to 2 months of age.

Preventive Health Care

Strict sanitation, environmental control, and high-quality rations must be given top priority in order to prevent disease in mice and rats. Monitor behavior, eating habits, elimination habits, and physical characteristics closely and notify your veterinarian of any noticeable changes.

Diseases and Disorders

Table 27.1 lists some selected diseases and disorders seen in mice and rats. Stress, overcrowding, improper nutrition, and poor sanitation play important roles in the development of many diseases, especially infectious diseases. Exposure to insects, wild rodents, and other animals can lead to disease transmission to your rodent as well. Remember that with the appearance of any clinical signs, including changes in activity levels, food or water consumption, or character of droppings, a definitive diagnosis should be made by a qualified veterinarian. Identifying and treating diseases in their early stages are the keys to successful treatment and cure.

Table 27.1 Diseases and Disorders of Mice and Rats

Disease or disorder	Clinical signs	Treatment and comments
	Infectious diseases	
Bacterial infections	Enlarged lymph nodes; abscesses; breathing difficulties; conjunctivitis; weight loss; loss of appetite	Treat with antibiotics; lance abscesses

Table 27.1 Diseases and Disorders of Mice and Rats (*Continued*)

Disease or disorder	Clinical signs	Treatment and comments
Infectious diseases		
Sialodacryoadenitis	Swelling in neck region due to inflamed salivary glands	Seen in rats; caused by virus; antibiotics for secondary infections
Pox virus	Sloughing of tail and/or digits of feet	No treatment available
Skin diseases		
Ringtail syndrome	Ulcerated lesion at base of tail	Seen in mice; caused by low humidity; treat by maintaining humidity at 50%
Traumatic wounds	Sores and wounds on ear pinnae and tail	Usually caused by fighting between males; treat by separating males
Mange	Hair loss, scratching, especially around head and ears	Seen primarily in mice; treat with pyrethrin insecticide
Ringworm	Hair loss; scaliness	Treat with antifungal medications
Mammary tumor	Lumps; ulcerated tissue in mammary region of females	Must be surgically removed
Respiratory diseases		
Upper respiratory disease and pneumonia	Sneezing; chattering; nasal discharge; breathing difficulty; depression; eye discharge	Can be viral or bacterial in origin; treat with antibiotics; occasional sneezing may occur in healthy rats

Table 27.1 Diseases and Disorders of Mice and Rats (*Continued*)

Disease or disorder	Clinical signs	Treatment and comments
Gastrointestinal diseases		
Enteritis	Diarrhea; rectal prolapse	Pinworms, protozoal organisms, bacteria can all cause; treat according to source
Nervous system diseases		
Vestibular syndrome	Head tilt; circling	Often seen secondary to respiratory infections; treat with antibiotics

Chinchillas

Chinchillas (*Chinchilla lanigera; Chinchilla brevicaudata*) are members of the rodent family and close relatives of the guinea pig. These fascinating creatures boast compact bodies; squirrellike tails; large, batlike eyes; pronounced, thin, erect ears; and, of course, the famous thick, soft, velvety haircoats. Chinchillas were once native to the high, rocky slopes of the Andes Mountains, stretching from Peru to the tip of Chile. The Chincha Indians inhabiting these slopes valued the chinchilla's fur as clothing for protection against the bitter Andean cold. As Spanish influence spread across the South American continent, chinchilla fur soon became a valuable export item to Europe. As a result, chinchillas were harvested to near extinction up to the early part of the twentieth century. Today, Chile is the only country still harboring a native population of chinchillas, which is under government protection. Chinchillas first began to appear in the United States in the early 1900s, where they were and are bred and raised commercially for their valuable fur.

As the demand for natural fur declines in the United States, more and more chinchillas are finding

DID YOU KNOW?

Because their auditory apparatus is very similar to that of humans, chinchillas are popular laboratory models for hearing studies in people.

their way into homes as pets. As a rule, they are clean creatures and harbor little odor. Fun, active, and full of personality, they love to interact with people they know and trust. Chinchillas enjoy being petted and scratched and often emit a soft cooing sound when such attention is afforded them. Their long, heavily muscled hind legs enable them to sit up on their haunches while nibbling on a morsel, and hop around like a kangaroo when the feeling arises! Their acute sense of hearing can cause them to become easily frightened or startled when they are confronted with loud noises or high-pitched sounds. When frightened, a chinchilla may let out a cry and scurry for cover. In fact, if the fright turns into anger, this cry could actually turn into a surprisingly belligerent bark or growl.

The standard chinchilla is blue-gray to dark gray in color, although mutant color variations do exist. These include charcoal, black, brown, beige, and white. Chinchillas weigh in at approximately 400 to 800 grams (with females often weighing more than males) and average about 14 inches in length from head to tail. Their lifespan in captivity averages 10 years, although there have been reports of some living to be 20!

Restraint

Chinchillas are fairly easy to handle and require no special restraint techniques. They rarely bite when handled gently; however, they have been known to nip at a finger when frightened or startled. When picking up a chinchilla, grasp it gently at the base of the tail with one hand and scoop up the body under the belly using the other hand (Fig. 28.1). Chinchillas that are handled roughly can "slip" their fur, leaving large tufts of hair in the hands of the handler. This is a natural defense mechanism designed to leave potential predators with mouthfuls of hair!

Housing

When selecting living quarters for your chinchilla, keep in mind the dry, cool climate from where your friend originated. Ideal environmental temperature for chinchillas is between 55 and 65 degrees Fahrenheit. Temperatures can drop to as low as 32 degrees Fahrenheit for short periods of time without ill effects as long as the humidity

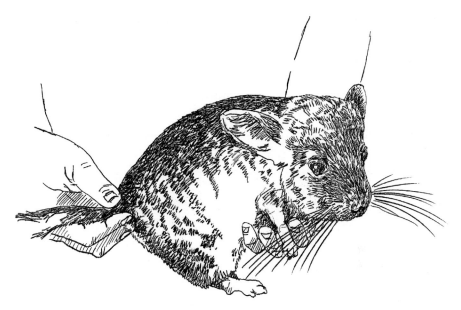

FIGURE 28.1 Method of restraint for chinchillas.

is kept low and the room is draft-free. Environmental humidity should be kept at 40 percent or lower. A humidity gauge attached to your pet's enclosure can help ensure that this requirement is being met.

Select a relatively remote, peaceful location within the home in which to place the cage. Since chinchillas are nocturnal creatures, distance the cage far enough from your family's sleeping quarters so as not to be disturbed by your chinchilla's nighttime activities.

Chinchillas need lots of room to move and roam in, so select a spacious enclosure. To prevent destruction due to chewing, your pet's cage should be constructed of metal instead of wood. Chinchillas love to climb. Providing multilevel cages or shelving within a single cage would make your chinchilla extremely happy (Fig. 28.2)! The smooth flooring of the cage can be lined

> **DR. P'S VET TIP**
>
> Chinchillas require lower environmental temperatures than do most other rodents, a factor that must be taken into account during hot summer months. Keep your chinchilla's cage in a portion of your home that can be closed off easily and kept well air-conditioned.

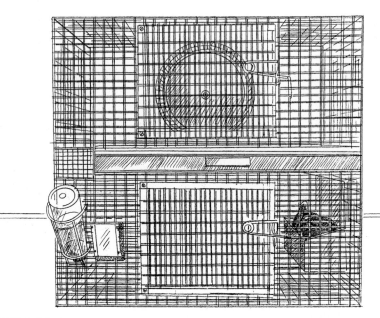

FIGURE 28.2 Because chinchillas love to climb, multilevel caging makes them extremely happy!

with aspen shavings or commercial rodent bedding. Cedar chips should not be used, as these can irritate the respiratory tract of rodents. Change this bedding at least twice per week to maintain proper sanitation. If you plan on owning more than one chinchilla, they need to be housed separately, as chinchillas housed together within a confined space (especially two males) can become quite bellicose to one another.

Provide your chinchilla with plenty of places in which to hide and burrow. Wooden hide boxes, ceramic enclosures, or a 4- to 6-inch portion of PVC (polyvinyl chloride) pipe works great. Even better, an actual arrangement of smooth-edged rocks can be configured within the cage to create crevices and hiding places that simulate your chinchilla's natural habitat. Obviously, make sure that the rocks are firmly seated and secured to prevent accidental injury to your pet from falling rocks.

Another important accessory you'll want to provide your unique friend on occasion is a dust bath. In the wild, chinchillas clean their coats by rolling or dusting in volcanic ash found along the mountain slopes. The purpose of such behavior is to rid their special coat of excess oils. Captive chinchillas also need to roll in dust for the same reason. An 8 × 10-inch pan or dust bin with edges high enough to prevent dust from flying out yet low enough to allow the chinchilla to easily enter is ideal. Fill the pan with 2 to 3 inches of sanitized chinchilla dust purchased from a pet store. This finely granulated dust is the closest you will come to mimicking volcanic ash. Some experts use a home mixture consisting of 9 parts silver sand and 1 part fuller's earth. Just know that regular sand or dirt won't do the trick .

Offer your chinchilla its dust bath three times per week. Leave the bath in the cage for 1 to 2 hours, then remove it. Dust baths should never be left as permanent fixtures within cages not only for sanitary purposes but also because overbathing can lead to eye irritation. Dust can be reused if it is free from fecal or urine contamination when removed from the cage. Because chinchillas are creatures of habit, offer their dust baths on set schedules each week.

Both hay racks and water delivery systems should be mounted on the sides of the cage and kept off the floor. Be sure to verify the patency of such devices on a daily basis. The entire cage should be thoroughly cleaned and sanitized weekly.

Nutrition

In the wild, the chinchilla's natural diet consisted of grasses, shrubs, roots, and the occasional berry. Fortunately, special food pellets designed for chinchillas are commercially available and make feeding a balanced diet quite easy. It should be noted that chinchillas like to grasp food pellets with their forepaws and eat from their hands. As a result, the size of the pellet offered is important. Short-pelleted foods are difficult for the average chinchilla to handle, and will lead to malnourishment.

Pellets should be offered in a sturdy, hard plastic, metal, or ceramic food dish. Feed your chinchilla approximately 1/2 ounce of pellets in the morning and again in the evening. In addition to pellets, you can supplement your pet's diet with nuts, raisins, or dried cherries. However, such supplementation should not exceed 15 percent of your chinchilla's daily dietary intake.

Because their digestive tracts are designed to ferment foodstuffs in the lower portion of the bowel, chinchillas require a good source of dietary fiber. For those kept as pets, hay provides the best source of this nutrient. The average chinchilla will consume up to one cup of hay per day. Chinchillas that are not provided adequate dietary fiber will develop potentially life-threatening enteritis. Hay racks should be hung from the sides of the cage and kept full at all times to help prevent such a problem.

Finally, because a chinchilla's teeth are in a constant growth mode, provide a hardwood chew block and/or tree branches (e.g., elm, maple, birch, apple, pear, peach) to help keep the teeth worn down properly and to satisfy the chinchilla's desire to chew. Avoid branches from trees such as cedar, redwood, cherry, and oleander, as these can be poisonous.

Reproduction

The age at which chinchillas reach puberty depends on the time of year they were born. For example, chinchillas born in spring will often reach puberty 4 to 6 months later, whereas those born in the fall months can take up to a year to reach sexual maturity. Breeding season runs between November and May each year. Females cycle every 6 to 7 weeks during this time.

When introducing male and female chinchillas to each other, always supervise the initial interaction. Females that feel uncomfortable with a potential mate can become aggressive and do much harm to him. This is especially true when a younger male is paired with an older female.

Gestation for chinchillas lasts an average of 111 days. A small nesting box containing straw may be offered to the pregnant female nearing parturition. However, when the time comes, she may simply choose to give birth directly on the floor bedding. The average litter size is two, although litters of up to five have been known to occur. Birth usually occurs in the morning hours. Newborn kits are born fully furred, with eyes and ears functional, and a full complement of teeth. Chinchilla kits are usually eating pellets as early as 7 days of age, although full weaning won't occur until 3 to 5 weeks of age. Note that once parturition has taken place, the female chinchilla will enter into heat again several days later.

Preventive Health Care

As with guinea pigs, routine vaccinations are not required for chinchillas, yet a routine annual visit to your veterinarian is highly recommended. Always pay attention to your pet's behavior, eating habits, elimination habits, and physical characteristics. Notify your veterinarian immediately of any changes. Obesity can be a problem in pet chinchillas, so monitor your pet's weight frequently.

As a rule, chinchillas are hardy creatures and rarely suffer health problems. Most unthriftiness and ill health seen are direct results of poor diet and poor housing conditions. Taking special care to ensure that these two husbandry factors are optimized is the best defense against illness or injury in chinchillas.

The chinchilla's soft, velvety haircoat requires little maintenance aside from its dust baths during the week. Weekly brushing using a soft cloth is also recommended to help remove any obvious dirt and shed hair from the coat. Your chinchilla will enjoy it as well!

Chinchillas enjoy exploring their environments with their mouths and will chew to maintain their long incisor teeth at proper length. As a result, don't allow your pet to roam the house unsupervised, as one encounter with an electrical cord or similar hazard could spell disaster.

As mentioned previously, chinchillas that don't receive adequate amounts of fiber in their diets are highly predisposed to serious digestive disturbances. Any abrupt changes in diet can also cause enteritis. If introducing a new food to your chinchilla, always do so gradually over several days. If diarrhea develops, contact your veterinarian immediately.

Hot, humid conditions can pose a definite health threat to chinchillas. The ideal environmental temperature for them is around 60 degrees Fahrenheit. Temperatures exceeding 85 degrees Fahrenheit can quickly lead to heat stroke.

Diseases and Disorders

Table 28.1 shows selected diseases and disorders seen in chinchillas. If your chinchilla shows signs of illness, do not give it any medications unless prescribed by your veterinarian. Remember that with the appearance of any clinical signs, a qualified veterinarian should be allowed to make a definitive diagnosis. Identifying and treating diseases in their early stages are the keys to successful treatment and cure.

Table 28.1 Diseases and Disorders of Chinchillas

Disease or disorder	Clinical signs	Treatment and comments
Bacterial enteritis	Diarrhea; listlessness; dehydration; rectal prolapse	Nonspecific, including antibiotics, fluid replacement, and increases in dietary fiber; often fatal condition; usually due to unsanitary living conditions, poor diets, or abrupt dietary changes
Pneumonia	Breathing difficulties; swollen neck; nasal discharge; depression	Treat with antibiotics and fluids; improve housing conditions, including ventilation and temperature
Fur chewing	Fur on lower portion of body short, "lion's mane" appearance (due to self-mutilation); moth-eaten appearance (barbering by cage mate)	Possible causes include boredom, poor nutrition, stress due to poor husbandry, heredity, hormonal disorders, and/or fungi; separate cage mates to prevent barbering; offer fatty acid and/or zinc supplements
Malocclusion (tooth overgrowth)	Drooling; weight loss; loss of appetite; crooked, curling teeth; runny eyes; bleeding from mouth	Trim teeth under sedation; allow access to chew blocks or other chewing material to help "file down" teeth

Table 28.1 Diseases and Disorders of Chinchillas (*Continued*)

Disease or disorder	Clinical signs	Treatment and comments
Paraphimosis (hair rings)	Male infertility; irritation and swelling of penis and prepuce due to hair wrapped around these structures	Manually remove ring using sterile lubricant; check for recurrence monthly
Heat prostration	Rapid, open-mouth breathing; extreme weakness	Immerse in cool water; seek veterinary care immediately; can occur when environmental temperatures exceed 80°F, especially with high humidity
Metal toxicity	Weakness; weight loss; seizures	Caused by excess consumption of lead and/or zinc; usually secondary to chewing on galvanized metal or objects containing lead
Abscesses	Swellings on or beneath skin	Surgical removal or drainage; treat with antibiotics; usually secondary to injuries or bite wounds
Bacterial encephalitis	Seizures; incoordination	Caused by poor sanitation or food contamination; poor prognosis, even with treatment with antibiotics

Table 28.1 Diseases and Disorders of Chinchillas (*Continued*)

Disease or disorder	Clinical signs	Treatment and comments
Ringworm	Hair loss, dermatitis	Oral antifungal drugs; antifungal agent added to dust bath
Bloat	Reluctance to move; recumbency; lethargy; loss of appetite	Decompress bloat using stomach tube; caused by overeating fruit or green feed; can also occur secondary to enteritis
Constipation	Straining; unable to defecate	Increase fiber in diet; administer laxative (i.e., mineral oil) to facilitate passage
Conjunctivitis	Red, irritated runny eyes	Caused by upper respiratory infection or irritation from dust; treat with antibiotics (oral and/or topical); reduce the number of dust baths offered each week

Prairie Dogs

Prairie dogs are members of the rodent family that once flourished across the western and southwestern portions of the United States. Each year, more and more of these unique, fun-loving creatures are finding their way into hearts and homes across the country as pets as their numbers in the wild decrease dramatically. In the wild, prairie dogs are viewed as pests by farmers and ranchers because they compete with livestock for food and dig holes and burrows that can make walking or running hazardous to livestock and horses. As a result, prairie dogs have been hunted and poisoned to the point where their numbers in the wild have decreased dramatically. In fact, the black-tailed prairie dog could become an endangered species, which could put their legality as pets in question (Fig. 29.1).

Four species of prairie dogs reside in the United States, including the Utah prairie dog, the white-tailed prairie dog, Gunnison's prairie dog, and the black-tailed prairie dog. Of the four, the black-tailed prairie dog (*Cynomys ludovicianus*) is the most popular choice as a pet. Whereas the other three varieties are native to the high plains, pastures, and mountainous slopes in and around the Rocky Mountains, the black-tailed prairie dog resides more in the lower plains and short grass prairies of the southwestern United States. As a result, it seems to adjust better to captivity than do the other three.

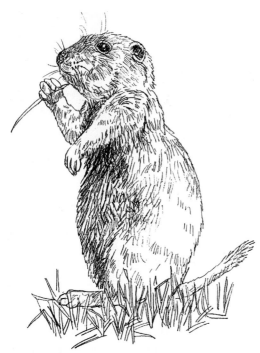

Depending on species, coat colors can range from red to brown to yellow buff, with all having black hairs interspersed throughout the coat. White patches on the tail and other coat patterns help distinguish one species from another. A close cousin of the squirrel, the prairie dog sports a stout body, relatively short legs, large black eyes, and small ears. The front paws possess remarkable dexterity and are used to grasp and hold food as it eats. Its short tail will flicker and flag if the prairie dog becomes agitated or threatened.

FIGURE 29.1 Labeled as pests and frequently exterminated by farmers and ranchers, an increasing number of prairie dogs are finding refuge as pets in homes across the country.

These unique creatures are diurnal in nature, being especially active in the early morning and late afternoon hours. Prairie dogs communicate with one another and with their owners through a series of chirps, chatters, yips, snarls, and squeals. Prairie dogs are social pets, and will often nudge noses with each other (or with their owners) as an outward sign of affection (Fig. 29.2). As far as their size is concerned, prairie dogs can grow to 15 inches in length and weigh up to 2 pounds when fully grown. When properly cared for, life span in captivity averages 8 years.

DID YOU KNOW?

Prairie dogs get their name from the shrill barking sound that they make when excited or alarmed.

Prior to purchasing one of these pets, be sure to contact your state's wildlife agency to be sure that it is legal to own a prairie dog in your particular state. Also,

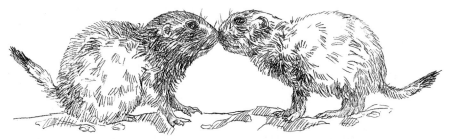

FIGURE 29.2 Prairie dogs like to nudge noses as an outward sign of recognition and affection.

realize that wild prairie dogs have been known to harbor hantavirus, tularemia, and fleas that carry bubonic plague. As a result, always purchase your prairie dog

DR. P'S VET TIP

If you want to win your way into your prairie dog's heart, rub or scratch its belly!

from a reputable source and be sure that it has been quarantined for at least 6 to 8 weeks before bringing it home.

Restraint

Prairie dogs that have been socialized to people possess sanguine personalities that make them relatively easy to handle. If a prairie dog has not been socialized or is acting nervous, roll it up in a towel with its head exposed before picking it up. This maneuver will not only protect you from being bitten but will also calm and relax your pet. An agitated prairie dog will emit a variety of sounds, including its characteristic "bark," and will flip its tail in annoyance. Wearing thick welder's gloves can also protect your hands against an overly aggressive prairie dog.

Housing

Because of their highly social nature, prairie dogs should ideally be kept in pairs rather than as solitary pets. When selecting housing for your prairie dog, keep in mind the natural habitat from where it came. Wild prairie dogs live in sophisticated underground tunnel systems.

As a result, the more you can simulate burrowing and tunneling conditions, the happier your prairie dog will be. Two or three large rodent or rabbit cages connected together via tunnels provide the ideal captive environment for prairie dogs. Also, your pet should have its own separate "apartment" somewhere within a cage into which it can retire if it so desires. Hay or aspen shavings deep enough for your pet to burrow should be supplied as well. Cedar chips should not be used, as these can irritate the respiratory tract of prairie dogs. Change this bedding at least twice per week to maintain proper sanitation.

The ideal environmental temperature at which to house your prairie dog is 70 degrees Fahrenheit. Although certain species of prairie dog that naturally live in the higher elevations hibernate during the cold, winter months, the black-tailed prairie dog does not. However, a decrease in activity may become apparent if your prairie dog is subjected to low environmental temperatures.

Nutrition

In the wild, prairie dogs eat grasses, cactus, shrubs, seeds, and the occasional insect. In captivity, prairie dogs should be offered a wide variety of food choices, including hay, alfalfa cubes, and commercial pellets formulated for squirrels and other rodents. Fruits can be offered as an occasional treat.

Both hay racks and water delivery systems should be mounted on the sides of the cage and kept off the floor. Be sure to verify the patency of water sippers on a daily basis. The entire cage should be thoroughly cleaned and sanitized weekly.

A hardwood chew block and/or tree branches (e.g., elm, maple, birch, apple, pear, peach) should be offered for your pet to chew on. These will help keep its incisors, which are in constant growth mode, worn down to proper length and prevent problems with overgrowth and malocclusion.

Reproduction

Prairie dogs will average one litter per year with a gestation lasting 27 to 33 days. Average litter size is five, with pups born blind, hairless, and helpless. However, they will begin to develop quite rapidly under their mother's nurturing care. Weaning takes place 3 to 6 weeks after birth. The average litter size is four. Young prairie dogs reach sexual maturity at 2 to 3 years of age.

DR. P's VET TIP

Have your prairie dog neutered at a young age to help reduce biting and aggression as an adult.

Preventive Health Care

Routine vaccinations are not required for prairie dogs, but an annual veterinary checkup is highly recommended. Always pay attention to your pet's behavior, eating habits, elimination habits, and physical characteristics. Notify your veterinarian immediately of any changes. Obesity can be a problem in prairie dogs kept as pets, especially during the winter months, so monitor your pet's weight closely.

Most unthriftiness and ill health seen in prairie dogs are due to poor diet and/or living environment. Taking special care to ensure that these two husbandry factors are optimized is the best defense against illness or injury in prairie dogs.

Offer your prairie dog plenty of attention each day. And keep your pet's nails trimmed to keep them from getting snagged and to keep you from getting scratched!

Neutering your prairie dog can help reduce anxiety as well as prevent reproduction-related health disorders as your pet matures. If surgery is to be done, however, your pet must not be obese. Slimming down obese prairie dogs prior to surgery reduces anesthetic and surgical risks, and makes the procedures much easier to perform.

Diseases and Disorders

Table 29.1 shows selected diseases and disorders seen in prairie dogs. If your prairie dog shows signs of illness, do not give it any medications unless prescribed by your veterinarian. Remember that with the appearance of any clinical signs, a qualified veterinarian should be allowed to make a definitive diagnosis. Identifying and treating diseases in their early stages are the keys to successful treatment and cure.

Table 29.1 Diseases and Disorders of Prairie Dogs

Disease or disorder	Clinical signs	Treatment and comments
Dietary-induced enteritis	Diarrhea; listlessness; dehydration	Often caused by change in diet, poor-quality diet, lack of fiber, or overeating; bismuth subsalicylate, yogurt, and/or antibiotics used to treat; fluid replacement to correct dehydration
Coccidiosis	Diarrhea; listlessness; dehydration	Treat parasite with sulfa drug; improve sanitation
Pododermatitis	Lameness; ulcerated feet	Due to rough flooring and/or poor sanitation; improve both conditions; treat with antibiotics
Malocclusion	Drooling; weight loss; loss of appetite; sores surrounding mouth	Caused by overgrown or poorly aligned teeth; clip or file teeth as needed
Rhinitis	Sneezing; nasal discharge; breathing difficulties	Usually caused by allergies; foreign matter in nasal passages, tumors or dental disease; treat with antihistamines and/or antibiotics; nasal flush
Prepucial occlusion	Swollen, painful prepuce; prepucial discharge, urine leakage	Seen in intact males; caused by an accumulation of debris within the prepuce; treat by douching prepuce with chlorhexidine or tamed iodine; antibiotics if necessary; prevent with castration

Table 29.1 Diseases and Disorders of Prairie Dogs (*Continued*)

Disease or disorder	Clinical signs	Treatment and comments
Osteochondroma	Swelling involving bone	If extremity is involved, amputation of affected limb; otherwise poor prognosis
Cardiomyopathy (heart disease)	Breathing difficulties; lethargy; weight loss; loss of appetite	Often seen in obese prairie dogs; other causes thought to include poor nutrition, tooth infections, genetics; treat with special medications designed to ease workload on heart
Ringworm	Nonitchy, patchy hair loss; flaky skin	This fungus can be transmitted to people; treat in prairie dogs with medicated shampoos and rinses; oral antifungal agents if needed
Fleas	Itching; reddened skin; hair loss	Fleas carried by wild prairie dogs can be vectors for bubonic plague
Odontoma (dental tumor)	Excessive salivation; strong mouth odor; nasal discharge; breathing difficulties	These tumors carry with them a grave prognosis for recovery

Hedgehogs

While pocket pets come in all colors, shapes, and sizes, there are none as unique-looking as the hedgehog. Sporting elongated snouts and coats covered with short spines up to $^3/_4$ inch in length, these small creatures can make delightful pets! Harboring a sweet, gentle, and even somewhat shy personality, hedgies love to interact with people they know and trust.

Hedgehogs are found naturally across the European, Asian, and African continents. Two types are generally kept as pets, the European hedgehog (*Erinaceus*) and the African hedgehog (*Atelerix*). The European hedgehog is a highly favored resident of British gardens, where it serves to protect precious flowers and plants from insects. The African hedgehog, on the other hand, is the preferred pet within the United States. It should be noted that in certain areas throughout Europe and the United States, hedgehogs are protected by law. As a result, if you are contemplating the purchase of one of these cute pocket pets, be sure to check local laws and ordinances prior to bringing one home.

The short, sharp spines of the hedgehog extend all along its head and back (except to a small band on the head). In contrast, the muzzle, chest, stomach, and leg regions are covered with a fine, soft white hair.

In the wild, hedgehogs are found in a wide variety of colors, ranging from cream to black, with multiple variations in between. Those kept as pets will usually have a mixture of white and gray-brown spines, giving them a characteristic salt-and-pepper color. Some individuals may sport white spines exclusively, giving them a snowflake appearance. Adult African hedgehogs are 5 to 8 inches in length, weighing in at around 300 to 600 grams. European hedgehogs are 12 to 14 inches long and can weigh up to 1200 grams. The average life span of the captive hedgie is 3 to 8 years.

Hedgies are inherently curious animals, loving to lumber and waddle around and stick their noses into any new place they can find. As they are nocturnal creatures, pet hedgehogs will tend to sleep during the daylight hours and emerge at night to eat and play.

Restraint

Gentle restraint is needed with these sensitive pets. When feeling frightened or threatened, hedgies may struggle when handled or simply tuck their nose and legs in tightly against their bodies and roll up into a compact "ball of spines." As you can imagine, this provides formidable protection against any interaction. Although they rarely bite, a few hedgehogs may hiss or squeal. Hedgies that are properly socialized to people as infants will rarely display this behavior if approached slowly and handled gently.

> **Dr. P's Vet Tip**
> If your hedgehog rolls up into a ball, a gentle stroking against the grain of the spines along the rump will usually entice your pet to uncurl itself.

Gloves may be worn to protect your hands from the sharp spines (Fig. 30.1). When lifting your pet, encircle the shoulder and chest regions with one hand and support the hind end with the other hand. Be sure to control the hedgehog's hind feet and rump to prevent it from scratching you. Because the spines are indeed sharp, care must be taken to resist the temptation to drop one of these pets if a finger accidentally gets pricked.

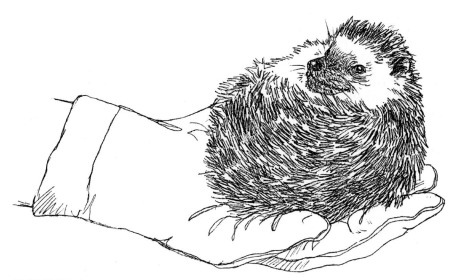

FIGURE 30.1 A glove may be worn when handling your hedgehog to protect your hand against its sharp spines.

Housing

Housing for your hedgehog can consist of a wire cage or hutch with solid flooring, or a glass aquarium. If the latter is used, it must be at least 20-gallon capacity and have a wire covering to prevent escape and to provide open-air ventilation. Bedding can consist of commercial pelleted bedding, aspen shavings (avoid cedar), or hay. It should remain clean and dry; as a result, plan on changing it at least twice weekly. For multiple hedgie households, plan on housing individuals separately to prevent fighting.

Situate the cage in a warm room free from drafts. Ideal room temperature should be around 80 degrees Fahrenheit. European hedgehogs kept in captivity may go into hiber-

> **DR. P's VET TIP**
>
> Large travel carriers make good homes for pet hedgehogs, offering portability, good ventilation, and easy maintenance.

nation if temperatures drop below 60 degrees Fahrenheit for any appreciable length of time. Keep your hedgehog's home out of direct sunlight, as temperatures over 90 degrees Fahrenheit can predispose it to heat stroke. Also, hedgehogs don't care for bright lights or loud noises, so situate your pet's abode away from brightly lit areas and noisy activity centers within the home. Offer plenty of hiding places for your hedgehog to frequent. A piece of PVC (polyvinyl chloride) pipe, wooden box, or ceramic enclosure can be placed in the cage to provide such a hiding area. Your hedgehog will enjoy an exercise wheel as well. Commercial exercise wheels designed exclusively for hedgehogs should be used, as wire-spoked wheels designed for rodents can cause leg injuries.

Nutrition

The elongated nose of these spiny creatures harbors a keen sense of smell that assists the wild hedgehog in rooting out insects, spiders, worms, snails, and other tasty morsels. For pet hedgies, commercial diets are now available and should be used. Enlist the help of your veterinarian if you have trouble locating a source for such diets. Contrary to popular belief, cat food by itself does not provide a nutritionally balanced diet for hedgehogs. Feed once daily, preferably in the evening. Discard any uneaten food the next morning. You can also supplement your pet's diet with a teaspoon of banana, apple, boiled egg, and/or the occasional cricket or mealworm. However, to prevent obesity, supplement the diet no more than twice weekly. Avoid feeding snails or slugs, for these can harbor parasites that can be harmful to your hedgehog. Fresh water should be available at all times, preferably contained within a sipper bottle mounted to the side of the enclosure. If your hedgie won't use a sipper, a small, sturdy tipproof water dish can be used as a substitute.

Reproduction

The mating season for African hedgehogs occurs year-round. Juvenile hedgehogs will reach puberty usually before 9 months of age. Following mating, the length of gestation is 35 to 37 days. The average litter size is four. Baby hedgehogs are born deaf and blind, with eyes and ears becoming functional between 14 and 20 days of age. Care must be taken not to disturb females with litters, as stress can lead to cannibalism of newborn hedgies by the mother. Weaning takes place between 4 and 6 weeks of age.

Preventive Health Care

Routine vaccinations are not required for hedgehogs, but an annual veterinary checkup is highly recommended. Always pay attention to your pet's behavior, eating habits, elimination habits, and physical characteristics. Notify your veterinarian immediately of any changes. Obesity can be a problem in pet hedgehogs, so monitor your pet's weight frequently.

Most unthriftiness and ill health encountered in pet hedgehogs is a direct result of a poor diet and poor housing. Taking special care to ensure that these two husbandry factors are optimized is the best defense against illness or injury in hedgies.

Offer your hedgehog plenty of attention each day. A great way to do this is to gently groom your pet's spiny coat using a soft cloth or a soft bristle tooth brush. Doing so will not only keep the skin and coat healthy but will also help tighten the bond of friendship between you and your spiny friend. Also, keeping your hedgie's teeth cleaned and nails trimmed are two other husbandry methods that will increase your pet's quality of life.

Hedgehogs exhibit a unique behavior known as "anting" or "anointing." Anting is often seen when new objects are placed within a hedgehog's cage. The hedgehog will approach the object and begin to produce copious amounts of saliva, which it then spreads onto its skin and spiny coat. The exact reason for this unusual behavior is not known. Some experts feel that it might play a role in territorial marking or predator avoidance; others feel it may simply be the way an excited hedgehog says "hello" to a new object! Regardless, it is normal behavior and is no cause for alarm (Fig. 30.2).

Diseases and Disorders

Table 30.1 shows selected diseases and disorders seen in hedgehogs. If your hedgehog shows signs of illness, do not give it any medications

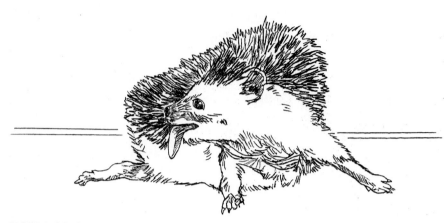

FIGURE 30.2 Normal "anting" behavior in a hedgehog.

unless prescribed by your veterinarian. Remember that with the appearance of any clinical signs, a qualified veterinarian should be allowed to make a definitive diagnosis. Identifying and treating diseases in their early stages is the key to successful treatment and cure. Sick hedgehogs are fragile creatures, and require prompt veterinary attention.

Table 30.1 Diseases and Disorders of Hedgehogs

Disease or disorder	Clinical signs	Treatment and comments
Bacterial or parasitic enteritis	Diarrhea; listlessness; dehydration	Antibiotics; antiparasitics, fluid replacement; improve sanitation
Obesity	Weight gain; listlessness; lameness	Evaluate diet; dietary portion control; eliminate "snacks"; pregnancy and neoplasia can cause weight gain as well

HEDGEHOGS **507**

Table 30.1 Diseases and Disorders of Hedgehogs (*Continued*)

Disease or disorder	Clinical signs	Treatment and comments
Musculoskeletal disease	Lameness; reluctance to move	Arthritis, fractures, overgrown nails, foot infections, obesity are among common causes; treat according to cause; keep nails trimmed
Dental disease; gingivitis	Drooling; weight loss; loss of appetite	Have teeth professionally cleaned, followed by daily brushing at home; antibiotics as necessary; normal "anting" behavior will also cause drooling
Fatty liver syndrome	Diarrhea; weight loss; loss of appetite; sudden death	Decrease amount of fat in diet; supplement diet with B complex vitamins
Rhinitis; pneumonia	Sneezing; congestion; breathing difficulties	Can be bacterial, fungal, or viral in etiology; treat with appropriate antibiotics or antifungal agents; fluid therapy; oxygen therapy in severe cases
Neoplasia	Nodules or masses on or beneath skin; ulcerations; abdominal enlargement; foul breath; drooling; weight loss	Increased incidence of tumors in hedgehogs over 3 years of age; treat according to type of tumor

Table 30.1 Diseases and Disorders of Hedgehogs (*Continued*)

Disease or disorder	Clinical signs	Treatment and comments
Skin parasites	Broken quills; flaky skin; irritability	Identify parasite and treat with appropriate medication; improve environmental sanitation and parasite control
Hypothermia	Listlessness; loss of appetite; lameness	Seen when environmental temperatures drop below 50°F; treat by warming pet with towel wrap or place on covered heating pad (low setting); increase environmental temperature appropriately

CHAPTER

31

Sugar Gliders

aving their roots deep within the rainforests of Australia, Indonesia, and New Guinea, sugar gliders (*Petaurus breviceps*) belong to the order Marsupialia, making them cousins to kangaroos, wombats, and opossums. Like their cousins, they come complete with an abdominal pouch used to carry their young. The unique creatures are clothed in soft, silky fur and sport big, black, doelike eyes that exhibit a natural aversion to sunlight and bright artificial lighting. Their forepaws are shaped much like our hands, and slender long claws allow them to climb with ease. Sugar gliders also possess a thin membrane that extends from the front leg to the ankle (tarsus) of the hind leg that enables them to launch themselves from a branch or limb and glide through the air, often for quite a distance. Their long, bushy tails act as an efficient stabilizer during flight. The average sugar glider is around 7 inches long (most of it tail!) and weighs in at about 3 ounces. Most are ash gray in color, with a black stripe running from nose to rump (Fig. 31.1).

Sugar gliders are very social creatures, and form loving bonds with their owners. They love to "body"-climb and hitch rides on arms and shoulders, as well as in shirt pockets and fanny packs. Realize that in order to from a strong bond with your pet, you'll need to keep some late nights and get up early in the morning (those are the times when your sugar glider will most want to interact with you).

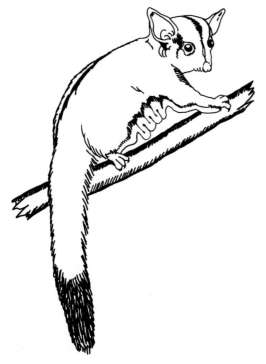

FIGURE 31.1 Sugar gliders are cousins to kangaroos, wombats, and oppossums.

As with other exotic pets, sound husbandry is essential for captive sugar gliders to flourish. With proper care, they can easily live 12 to 15 years in captivity. Note that in some states, it is illegal to own a sugar glider. As a result, check USDA regulations and contact your state's proper authority before purchasing one.

Restraint

Sugar gliders purchased from reputable sources will be fairly tame, so most are easy to handle and require no special restraint techniques. They rarely bite when handled gently; however, they have been known to get grumpy when handled during daylight hours. When frightened or alarmed, they can let out an ear-piercing scream. Keep this in mind when holding your sugar glider, being careful not to accidentally drop it if it decides to unload a volley on your eardrums!

Housing

Because sugar gliders are social creatures, they should be housed in pairs or larger groups. Sugar gliders that are raised in "solitary confinement" can suffer much stress and experience a decline in both mental and physical health. Housing should be spacious, allowing them plenty of room to climb and, yes, glide! Cages should be made out of wire, with horizontal bars (which allow for climbing) no more than 7/16 inch apart. Custom housing for sugar gliders is available commercially; a large birdcage can also be used.

Within the enclosure, an abundance of climbing branches is essential. Sugar gliders forced to spend their time on the ground will become quite stressed and more susceptible to disease. Also, because they are light-sensitive, they must be provided with plenty of enclosed, dark hiding places into which they can retreat during the day. An exercise wheel is optional. If one is provided, it must be a large one and solid in construction in order to prevent tail injuries.

Environmental temperatures should be kept between 72 and 85 degrees Fahrenheit for maximum comfort. Finally, a substrate made from recycled paper should be used to line the bottom of the cage. This should be changed at least once weekly. The entire cage should be thoroughly cleaned and sanitized weekly.

Nutrition

Sugar gliders are considered omnivores. Insects and sugary sap and nectars are their preferred sources of nutrition in the wild. Several dietary plans exist for sugar gliders that are kept in captivity. One such menu includes a one to one mixture of Leadbeater's mixture (10 tablespoons of warm water, 10 tablespoons of honey, 1 shelled hard-boiled egg, 25 grams of high-protein baby cereal, and 1 teaspoon of a multivitamin/mineral supplement) and an insectivore ration (available at most pet stores). Be sure to keep this mixture refrigerated until served.

Other good recipes can be found on Internet Websites. Live crickets and mealworms can be fed as the occasional snack, but be sure they are "gut-loaded" first to make them more nutritious. Small amounts of broiled chicken, diced fruits, and vegetables can be offered as snacks as well. Avoid seeds, as these can quickly lead to obesity.

Ideally, both food and water delivery systems should mounted on the sides of the cage and kept off of the floor. Keep plenty of fresh, filtered water available at all times for your glider. A large water sipper should be used to deliver a continuous source. Food bowls should be cleaned daily.

Reproduction

Sugar gliders breed year-round. The gestation period lasts 16 days, with an average litter size of one to three. The offspring are born hairless and helpless, and immediately on birth crawl into their mother's pouch to suckle. They will stay there for 8 to 9 weeks, and then will begin to crawl out and attach themselves to their mother's belly or explore their environment firsthand. Young sugar gliders become totally independent at 4 months of age. Sexual maturity is reached around a year of age.

Preventive Health Care

Routine vaccinations are not required for sugar gliders, yet a routine annual visit to a veterinarian is highly recommended. Always pay attention to your pet's behavior, eating habits, elimination habits, and physical characteristics. Notify the veterinarian immediately of any changes. Obesity can be a problem in sugar gliders, so monitor your pet's weight frequently.

As a rule, most unthriftiness and ill health seen in sugar gliders are direct results of poor diet and poor housing conditions. Taking special care to ensure that these two husbandry factors are optimized is the best defense against illness or injury in your pet.

Diseases and Disorders

Table 31-1 shows selected diseases and disorders seen in sugar gliders. If your pet shows signs of illness, do not give it any medications unless prescribed by your veterinarian. Remember that with the appearance of any clinical signs, a qualified veterinarian should be allowed to make a definitive diagnosis. Identifying and treating diseases in their early stages is the key to successful treatment and cure. Like many other exotic species that become ill, sick sugar gliders are very fragile, and require prompt veterinary attention.

Table 31.1   Diseases and Disorders of Sugar Gliders

Disease or disorder	Clinical signs	Treatment and comments
Obesity	Same	Avoid overfeeding; enlarge living space to encourage more climbing and exercise
Hyperparathyroidism	Weakness, muscle tremors, fractures	Caused by nutritional imbalance and calcium deficiency; review and correct diet; calcium supplements
Head alopecia	Hair loss in the center of the head	Normal in some males; identifies the location of a scent gland
Abdominal "lumps"	Apparent lumps on the stomach of a female glider	Again, this is normal; these "lumps" are baby sugar gliders in their mom's pouch!
Lack of or decline in appetite		Can be caused by stress (lack of companionship, too much light, temperature fluctuations), blindness, damaged teeth, other illness
Enteritis	Diarrhea	Caused by parasites and/or bacterial infections; treat accordingly; improve sanitation and reduce stress
Overeating/overdrinking; pacing; excess vocalization		Usually caused by boredom; insecurity (lack of adequate hiding places); lack of social interaction; housing too small; correct underlying cause
Blindness	Partial or complete loss of sight	Thought to be dietary in origin; often seen in obese gliders

Table 31.1 Diseases and Disorders of Sugar Gliders *(Continued)*

Disease or disorder	Clinical signs	Treatment and comments
Rear-end paralysis	Weakness or paralysis of the hindlimbs	Due to poor diet coupled with a lack of exercise; stress may also play a role; treat by correcting diet and increasing size of living quarters
Incoordination	Falling from branches; bounces into walls	Can be caused by blindness, rear-end paralysis, obesity, foot disorders, sprains and fractures; treatment should address the underlying cause

Ferrets

Ferrets are popular as pets in the United States, with thousands of households obtaining one or more of these curious, rambunctious creatures each year. Ferrets belong to the same family as do minks, skunks, and weasels. Several different species exist, yet *Mustela putorius furo* represents the most common pet species. This particular ferret is a direct descendant of the European polecat.

For centuries, ferrets have been used by humans for a variety of tasks, including pest control and, more popularly, hunting. Only in the past century has their role as house pet been established. Insatiably curious, ferrets love to roam and explore their environment, especially tight-fitting nooks and crannies. They also can be quite playful and mischievous. Ferrets love to gather up items and store them in predetermined hiding places. They are smart animals, and can be leash-trained quite easily (Fig. 32.1).

Ferrets exist in a variety of color patterns, including (but not limited to) sable, albino, siamese, cinnamon, cream, and silver mitt. Many sport black faces, tails, and legs as well. Male

DID YOU KNOW?

Ferrets are illegal to own or require ownership permits in many cities and states. Be sure to inquire about this prior to bringing one home.

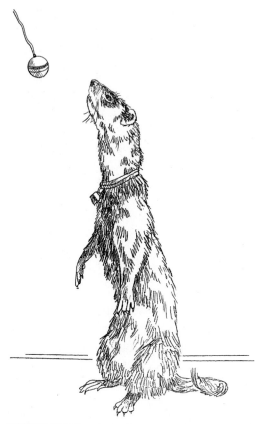

ferrets reach weights of up to 6 pounds; females average 2 to 4 pounds. Weight increases are common during the fall and winter months as ferrets store up fat for the winter. This weight is usually lost when spring arrives. The life span of a ferret in captivity is 5 to 9 years.

Restraint

Most ferrets are mild-mannered and can be handled with minimal restraint. One hand can be used to grasp the scruff of the neck or encircle the forequarters, pushing the forelegs together as the ferret is lifted from the cage or carrier. The other hand should support the hindquarters. Never lift a

FIGURE 32.1 Ferrets require plenty of daily exercise to allow them to expend their abundance of stored energy!

ferret solely by the scruff of its neck without supporting its hind end (Fig. 32.2). And never lift by its tail. Those are two good ways to injure your pet and/or get bitten!

Housing

Ferrets can be housed in any type of enclosure that allows them ample room to move about freely. You can house more than one ferret together, but be aware that males might fight with each other.

Wire cages of various sizes are readily available from most pet stores. Choose one with smooth flooring, as wire-mesh floor surfaces can be tough on ferret feet. The bottom of the cage can be lined with aspen shavings (no cedar) or commercial bedding material. A small box or hideaway constructed of plastic or wood can be placed in one corner of the cage to provide a place for seclusion and sleep. Ferrets also love blankets or old cotton undershirts in which to cuddle up and hide.

Ferrets can be trained to use a litterbox. As a result, a litter pan or tray can be placed at one end of the cage to help maintain cleanliness. Be sure to change this litter at least twice weekly.

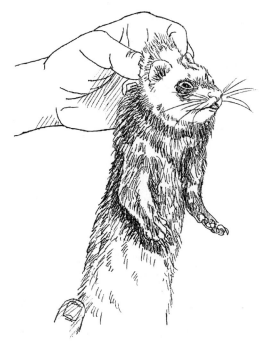

FIGURE 32.2 When lifting a ferret by its scruff, always support its hind end with your other hand.

For those ferrets kept exclusively in cages or pens, provide a daily exercise period to allow them to expend their abundance of stored energy. Offer plenty of safe toys to play with and play tunnels in which to explore.

Nutrition

Ferrets should be fed a commercial mink or ferret ration. Be sure the food you choose is not high in fiber because ferrets have difficulty digesting it. Fruits and vegetables should be offered as treats only sparingly, owing to their relatively high fiber content. Ferrets prefer six to eight meals throughout the day rather than one or two large meals. Water bowls should also be kept full at all times. Choose a water bowl weighted at the bottom to resist spilling. Also, because ferrets can develop hairballs, a feline hairball laxative should be administered to your ferret weekly.

Reproduction

Male ferrets are called *hobs*; females are referred to as *jills.* Sexual maturity for both occurs at approximately 8 to 10 months of age. The breeding season for ferrets runs from March to August, the time period in which the reproductive cycle of the jill is active.

Prior to breeding, place a wooden or plastic nesting box, complete with bedding material, within the cage or den. It should be large enough to allow the jill to move about freely and lie down comfortably. As jills come into heat, vulvular discharge and swelling will be noted. Female ferrets are induced ovulators; that is, the egg is ovulated only upon copulation. Hobs should be introduced to the jill only long enough for copulation to take place, and then they should be separated. Hobs and jills can inflict serious injury on one another if left together, and the former can even go so far as kill the offspring when they arrive.

The gestation period for ferrets is approximately 42 days. Litter size ranges from five to eight "kits." They are born blind and hairless. To prevent infant rejection or, worse yet, infanticide, try not to disturb or handle a jill and her box unnecessarily during the first 3 weeks after parturition except for cleaning and feeding purposes. Feline milk replacements should be added to the jill's diet to give an added nutritional boost during the lactation period. Starting at 6 weeks, kits can be gradually weaned off of the jill using canned cat food mixed one to one (1:1) with a commercial feline milk substitute.

Orphaned or abandoned kits can be raised by hand using the same feline milk substitute. Feedings should be performed at least every 2 hours for the first week and every 4 hours for the next 3 to 4 weeks. Orphans need to be stimulated to eliminate after each feeding. This can be accomplished using a warm, moist cotton ball and gently massaging the anal and genital region. Starting at 3 weeks of age, the orphan can be slowly weaned onto solid food using the formula mentioned above. As with any orphaned animal, warmth, sanitation, and lots of tender loving care are needed.

The reproductive cycle of jills is unique in that jills must be bred in order for estrogen levels within their

DID YOU KNOW?

Nonspayed female ferrets that are not bred when they come into heat can die from anemia!

bodies to decline, allowing them to go out of heat. This becomes significant because jills that are not bred can develop life-threatening ane-

DID YOU KNOW?

Pawing at the mouth can be a sign associated with nausea in a ferret.

mia and blood-clotting problems caused by persistently high estrogen levels. As a result, owners must be sure to have their jills bred each breeding season, or have their veterinarian administer a special injection each time to bring them out of heat. Another more preferable alternative is surgical spaying, which can be performed as early as 6 months of age.

Preventive Health Care

Ferrets should receive routine medical checkups just like dogs and cats (Fig. 32.3). For ferrets less than 4 years old, these visits to the veterinarian should be made annually. For ferrets older than 4 years, increase the visits to twice per year.

Ferrets are very susceptible to the canine distemper virus and should be vaccinated against this disease using a ferret-approved vaccine starting at 6 to 8 weeks of age. Booster immunizations should be administered at 12 weeks and 16 weeks, and then annually. A rabies vaccine should be administered on an annual basis as well.

The same types of intestinal parasites that can affect dogs and cats can infest ferrets. As a result, routine stool examinations should be performed annually by your veterinarian, and deworming medication should be administered if deemed appropriate.

Ear mites are very common in ferrets. As a result, owners need to be on constant lookout for these pests. Ferrets infested with these mites will shake their heads and have a brown-black discharge in the affected ear(s). Ear mite medication applied directly to the ears is the most effective method of eliminating an ear mite infestation.

Ferrets are also susceptible to heartworm disease. As a result, in those areas with large concentrations of this disease, a heartworm preventive medicine should be administered. Contact your veterinarian for his/her recommendations for your particular area.

Routine surgical procedures performed on ferrets include neutering and descenting. Neutering hobs will help reduce their aggressiveness and reduce body odor. If not to be bred, jills should be spayed as

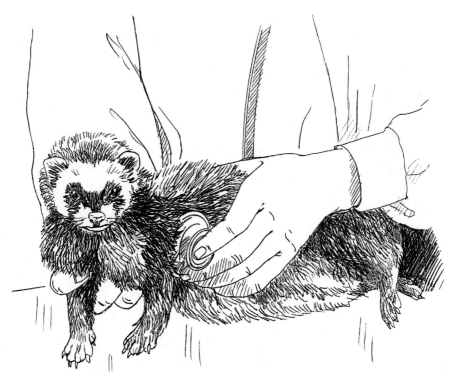

FIGURE 32.3 Ferrets should see their veterinarians for routine medical checkups as do dogs and cats.

well to eliminate the dangers of persistent estrus. Both procedures can be performed at 6 months of age.

Descenting can be performed at the same time as neutering to help reduce obnoxious odors emitted from ferrets. This involves the removal of the anal sacs. This procedure, combined with frequent baths using a hypoallergenic shampoo, can help control your ferret's odor.

Finally, because ferrets like to dig, their nails should be trimmed short on a weekly basis.

FACT *OR* **FICTION**

Descenting a ferret will remove its characteristic odor. **FICTION**. Descenting is really a misnomer, since the surgical removal of the anal sacs rarely eliminates odor completely. Secretions from glands in the skin beneath the tail also account for the characteristic odor of a ferret.

Diseases and Disorders

Some selected diseases and disorders seen in ferrets are listed in Table 32.1. Remember that others do exist, which is why definitive diagnosis should be made by a qualified veterinarian. Identifying and treating diseases in their early stages is the key to successful treatment and cure.

Table 32.1 Diseases and Disorders of Ferrets

Disease or disorder	Clinical signs	Treatment and comments
Infectious diseases		
Canine distemper	Fever; loss of appetite; nasal and eye discharge; convulsions	No treatment available; prevent by vaccinating
Human influenza	Fever; nasal discharge; sneezing; breathing difficulties	Can be transmitted by humans; treat with antibiotics and antihistamines
Retroviral infection	Signs vary with organ involved; can cause cancer; anemia	Some ill ferrets have tested positive for the feline leukemia virus
Skin diseases		
Skin parasites (fleas, mites, ear mites)	Itching; hair loss; inflamed ears	Treat with pyrethrin-type insecticide
Mast cell tumors	Itching; hair loss; reddened raised skin lesions	Can occur along with other tumors; surgical excision
Digestive system diseases		
Intestinal parasites (hookworms, roundworms, tapeworms, *Giardia*, coccidia)	Weight loss; loss of appetite; vomiting; diarrhea	Treat with dewormer similar to those used in cats

Table 32.1 Diseases and Disorders of Ferrets (*Continued*)

Disease or disorder	Clinical signs	Treatment and comments
Proliferative bowel disease	Green, mucoid diarrhea; weight loss; prolapsed rectum; incoordination	Age of onset is around 4–6 months; treat with antibiotics; might be zoonotic disease
Hairballs; gastric foreign bodies	Vomiting, loss of appetite	Treat hairballs as in cats; foreign bodies might need to be removed surgically
Insulinoma	Profound weakness; increased salivation; seizures	This tumor of the pancreas causes low blood sugar; surgical removal of tumor necessary
Reproductive system diseases		
Aplastic anemia	Weakness; loss of appetite; bruising; hemorrhaging; dark, tarry stool	Caused by persistent heat cycle; treat with hormones, blood transfusions, bone marrow stimulants; prevent by spaying at 6 months of age
Pregnancy toxemia	Lethargy; dehydration; black tarry stools; hair loss	Seen in jills on poor plan of nutrition; treat with cesarean section; fluids; antibiotics; improve nutrition
Urinary system diseases		
Urolithiasis	Blood-tinged urine; straining to urinate; depression	Treatment is the same as for cats

Table 32.1 Diseases and Disorders of Ferrets (*Continued*)

Disease or disorder	Clinical signs	Treatment and comments
Cardiopulmonary diseases		
Heartworm disease	Weakness; coughing; breathing difficulties	Treat and prevent the same as in dogs
Congestive heart failure	Weakness; coughing; breathing difficulties	Treat as in dogs
Eye diseases		
Juvenile cataracts	Cloudy eyes; vision difficulties	Seen in young ferrets; surgical removal of cataract might be needed to restore vision

Miniature Pot-Bellied Pigs

Miniature pot-bellied pigs (MPBPs) can trace their origins to the jungles of Vietnam and China. First introduced into the United States in 1985, they have gained a loyal following over the years. The popularity of miniature pot-bellied pigs can be attributed to the fact that they can make adorable, fun-loving pets. Not only are they relatively clean and odor-free (unlike domestic pigs) but miniature pot-bellied pigs are intelligent, affectionate, and easy to train and house-break (Fig. 33.1).

But miniature pot-bellied pigs are certainly not for everyone. For starters, they represent an initial purchase investment of hundreds, or even thousands, of dollars. Also, armed with a keen sense of smell, miniature pot-bellied pigs love to root, which can absolutely wreak havoc on carpets. Certainly those who pride themselves on expensively landscaped lawns should think twice about allowing a miniature pot-bellied pig access to their grounds!

Before making the decision to purchase a pot-bellied pig, check the laws of your particular city or municipality concerning these pets. In some areas, miniature pot-bellied pigs are still considered livestock rather than companion animals, and zoning restrictions may apply.

DID YOU KNOW ?

A pot-bellied pig is one of the cleanest pets you could own!

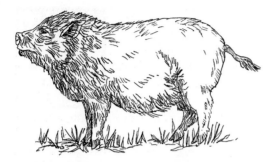

FIGURE 33.1 Miniature pot-bellied pigs are not only relatively clean and odor-free but are also intelligent and affectionate pets.

Miniature pot-bellied pigs come in basic black or black with white markings. The ideal standard for the pot-bellied pig calls for a weight of less than 50 pounds and a shoulder height of less than 14 inches. However, many pot-bellied pigs kept as pets in the United States exceed these standards. Maximum weight allowed for official registration of the adult pig is 95 pounds and maximum shoulder height is 18 inches. The snout of the pot-bellied pigs tends to be longer than those of domestic pigs, and their ears stand erect. Their eyesight is not as keen as that of dogs and cats, yet they have an exceptional sense of smell. The life span of a miniature pot-bellied pig is comparable to that of a cat or dog.

As with any pet, you will want to be sure the candidate that you are considering is healthy before purchasing it. Health problems to look for in miniature pot-bellied pigs include skin disorders, malformed snouts, breathing difficulties, retained testicles, lameness, hernias, and in newborns, *atresia ani,* or lack of an anal opening. To be safe, have your veterinarian perform a physical exam on your selection prior to purchase to evaluate your pig's health status.

Restraint

Because of a predisposition for hip and other musculoskeletal injuries, miniature pot-bellied pigs should be handled with care. When picking one up, be sure to cradle the pig's neck and hind end between your own body and forearm, just as you would a dog or cat. The legs of the pig should be allowed to hang free. Never grab or pick up a pig by its fore or hind legs, as this can cause joint dislocations. Get ready: Some pigs let out an ear-piercing squeal when restrained or picked up!

Housing

Miniature pot-bellied pigs can be housed just like a dog. However, whether kept indoors or outdoors, the ideal environmental temperature for a miniature pot-bellied pig is

> ## Dr. P's Vet Tip
> A small plastic kiddy pool filled with shallow water can not only help keep your miniature pot-bellied pig cool while outdoors but can also provide hours of wallowing enjoyment!

around 70 degrees Fahrenheit. If they get too cold, pigs tend to get irritable and stressed, tearing at their bedding and burrowing in order to get warm. On the other hand, if environmental temperatures get too hot, an MPBP can succumb to heat stroke quite rapidly. As a result, if a pig is to be kept outdoors, plenty of shade and fresh water should be provided. Finally, pigs love to root, so be sure to provide your porcine access to an area with soil or dirt to satisfy this craving.

Training

Miniature pot-bellied pigs are intelligent creatures that can be trained just like dogs. Training is most effective when a pig is acquired at a young age (less than 8 weeks of age) and allowed to form an emotional bond (socialize) with you. Using simple commands, rewards, and praises, you can teach your pig many things, including litter training, leash training, and even tricks.

Nutrition

Miniature pot-bellied pigs should be fed commercially available rations designed for pigs. Fruits, vegetables, and vitamins should be added as well to provide supplementation and variety. To avoid the dangers of salt toxicity, water must be easily accessible at all times. Obesity is a common health problem in pot-bellied pigs, yet can be avoided by adhering to strict dietary moderation.

Reproduction

Miniature pot-bellied pigs reach puberty at 6 to 7 months of age. Heat in the female occurs every 21 days and lasts 2 to 3 days. Your veterinarian can assist you in timing the breeding between the sow and boar to achieve best results. If the mating is successful, the gestation period for pot-bellied pigs is approximately 114 days.

Two weeks prior to parturition (farrowing), a noticeable "drop" in the abdomen of the sow will be noted. At this time, a farrowing crate for the sow should be provided. Contact your veterinarian for assistance in crate design and dimensions for your particular pig. Crates should be roomy enough to allow free movement of both sow and offspring. The sow can be kept in this crate until farrowing occurs. Be sure to remove her from the crate three to four times a day for exercise and eliminations.

Litter sizes can range from 4 to 12, depending on the maturity of the sow. At birth, piglets weigh about 16 ounces. Because of a predisposition to anemia, neonatal piglets should receive injections of an iron supplement daily for the first 3 days of life. The sharp needle teeth that these piglets possess should be clipped back as well to prevent inadvertent injury to the sow and other offspring.

Neonatal piglets are extremely susceptible to hypothermia. As a result, keep environmental temperatures maintained between 85 and 95 degrees Fahrenheit until weaning takes place at 4 to 6 weeks of age. In addition, piglets under 2 weeks of age should be observed for signs of hypoglycemia (low blood sugar). This condition, characterized by depression and coma, is a medical emergency and requires immediate veterinary intervention.

Preventive Health Care

Like dogs and cats, miniature pot-bellied pigs require routine preventive health care to keep them healthy and happy. MPBPs should be vaccinated against the common diseases seen in domestic pigs, including erysipelas (caused by *Streptococcus pyogenes*), transmissible gastroenteritis (TGE), atrophic rhinitis, and leptospirosis. Piglets should be vaccinated for these diseases starting at 6 weeks of age, and again at 9 weeks of age. Booster vaccinations should be given at six months of age, and then annually thereafter. If you intend to breed your pigs, contact your veterinarian for special vaccination schedules for sows and boars.

In addition to vaccinations, pigs need to have regular stool checks performed for internal parasites. Roundworms, whipworms, and nodular worms are the most frequently found parasites inhabiting the gastrointestinal tract of these pigs. If any worms are detected, appropriate medications can be administered and repeated in 3 weeks to ensure a complete kill.

Miniature pigs that are to be introduced to households containing dogs should be blood-tested for the pseudorabies virus. This virus is extremely deadly to dogs, which can contract the disease from otherwise healthy pigs.

Piglets less than 6 weeks of age are very prone to developing anemia and low blood sugar. Iron supplements and additional sources of glucose may be administered to prevent these problems. Since most piglets acquired as pets are older, this should not be a concern for most new pig owners.

Miniature pigs should be brushed daily with a soft-bristle brush to help control seborrhea and flaking. Hypoallergenic shampoos can be used if bathing is required. Periodic trimming of the tusks (if present) and hooves should be performed as needed.

Much to the jealousy of dog and cat owners, fleas have nowhere to hide on miniature pigs, so flea control is rarely necessary. However, the skin of miniature pot-bellied pigs is very sensitive to sunlight and cold temperatures, and owners should take care to shield their pig's skin from these environmental factors.

Routine surgical procedures performed on miniature pot-bellied pigs include spaying, castration, and removal of sharp canine teeth

DR. P'S VET TIP

Because pot-bellied pigs are prone to sunburn, use SPF-30 (sun protection factor level 30) sunscreen on yours if it is to be exposed to direct sunlight for a prolonged period of time.

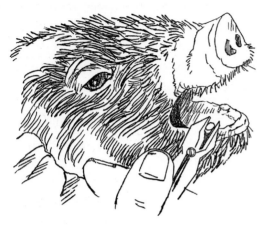

(Fig. 33.2). These procedures are generally performed
before 4 months of age.

Diseases and Disorders

The following are some
selected diseases and disorders seen in miniature
pot-bellied pigs. Remember
that others do exist, which
is why a definitive diagnosis by a qualified veterinar-

FIGURE 33.2 Clipping the sharp needle teeth on a miniature pot-bellied pig.

ian is always needed on a sick pig. Identifying and treating diseases
in their early stages is the key to successful treatment and cure
(Table 33.1).

Table 33.1 Diseases and Disorders of Miniature Pot-Bellied Pigs (MPBPs)

Disease or disorder	Clinical signs	Treatment and comments
Infectious diseases		
Erysipelas	Characteristic red, diamond-shaped skin lesions; depression; fever;lameness; conjunctivitis	Can lead to heart disease and arthritis if not treated early; treat with penicillin antibiotics
Transmissible gastroenteritis	Diarrhea; vomiting; fever; dehydration	Caused by a coronavirus (similar to that in dogs and cats); treat secondary problems with antibiotic and fluid support

Table 33.1 Diseases and Disorders of Miniature Pot-Belled Pigs (MPBPs) (*Continued*)

Disease or disorder	Clinical signs	Treatment and comments
Leptospirosis	Depression; fever; weakness	Causes anemia and kidney failure in affected pigs; treatment consists of antibiotics and blood transfusions if needed; zoonotic disease
Hemophilus	Breathing difficulties; blood-stained foam from mouth and nose; fever; coughing	Rapidly fatal if not treated promptly with appropriate antibiotics
Skin diseases		
Sunburn or frostbite	Reddening of the skin; ulcerations	MPBPs quite susceptible to environmental insults
Seborrhea	Dry, flaky skin	Caused by nutritional deficiencies, intestinal parasites, mange, environmental conditions; treat according to cause
Mange (mites)	Itching; small red raised bumps on skin	Oral ivermectin and topical dips used to treat
Greasy pig disease	Greasy skin surface; reddened wrinkled skin; scabs; dehydration	Caused by bacteria; highly fatal in young pigs; treat with antibiotics
Musculoskeletal diseases		
Posterior weakness or stiffness	Stiff gait; lameness; can't support weight on hind legs	Conformation of MPBP and improper restraint techniques make them prone to muscle pulls, ligament tears, hip dis-

Table 33.1 Diseases and Disorders of Miniature Pot-Bellied Pigs (MPBPs) (*Continued*)

Disease or disorder	Clinical signs	Treatment and comments
	Musculoskeletal diseases (*Continued*)	
		location, other musculoskeletal injuries; treat depending on problem
Infectious arthritis	Stiffness; lameness; fever	Can be caused by a variety of organisms; treat with appropriate antibiotics
Osteomalacia	Weakness; inability to stand	Caused by calcium deficiency; seen in nursing or postnursing sows
	Nervous system disease	
Bacterial encephalitis	Depression; circling; seizures; abnormal gait and posture; blindness; aggressiveness	Can be caused by a variety of organisms; treat with appropriate antibiotics
Shaker pig disease	Tremors, convulsions; shaking	No treatment needed; most recover spontaneously
Salt poisoning	Depression; circling; seizures; abnormal gait and posture; blindness; aggressiveness	Caused by water deprivation, then allowing free access to water; treatment generally unrewarding
	Respiratory system diseases	
Atrophic rhinitis	Snout deformity; sneezing; bloody nasal discharge	Associated with bacterial infections of the nasal passages in neonatal or newly

Table 33.1 Diseases and Disorders of Miniature Pot-Bellied Pigs (MPBPs) (*Continued*)

Disease or disorder	Clinical signs	Treatment and comments
Respiratory system diseases (*Continued*)		
		weaned pigs; infection can be treated with antibiotics yet clinical signs often persist
Pneumonia	Mouth breathing; bluish hue to skin	MPBP very susceptible to pneumonia; stress often leads to secondary bacterial infections; other causes include pseudorabies virus, roundworms, lung-worms, cleft palate; treat depending on cause
Digestive system diseases		
Motion sickness, excite-ment overeating	Vomiting	No treatment needed
Neonatal diarrheal disease complex	Severe diarrhea; dehydra-tion; abdominal disten-sion and pain	Can be caused by bacte-ria (colibacillosis), par-asites (coccidia), viruses (transmissible gastroenteritis virus); treat with antibiotics, fluids
Intestinal parasites	Bloody diarrhea; dehydration	Can include round-worms, whipworms, nodular worms, tape-worms; treat using appropriate dewormer

Table 33.1 Diseases and Disorders of Miniature Pot-Bellied Pigs (MPBPs) (*Continued*)

Disease or disorder	Clinical signs	Treatment and comments
Rectal prolapse	Prolapsed rectum; diarrhea; abdominal distention	Caused by parasitism, chronic diarrhea and straining, coughing; treatment involves replacing prolapse and antibiotic therapy; treat underlying cause
Atresia ani	Inability to defecate due to lack of external anal opening	Congenital disease; no effective surgical treatment
Urinary system diseases		
Cystitis or nephritis	Increased urination; straining to urinate; bloody urine	Can be caused by bacterial infections, kidney-worms, toxins; treat depending on cause
Prepucial diverticulum	Urine dribbling in male MPBPs	Small pocket in prepuce traps urine and leads to clinical signs; manually empty pocket, surgical correction of diverticulum
Urinary calculi	Straining to urinate; bloody urine	Surgical removal of calculi usually required
Reproductive system diseases		
Cryptorchidism	One or both testicles retained within the abdomen	Quite common; castration recommended
Vaginitis and uterine infections	Vaginal discharge; increased urination; fever; depression	Bacteria usual source of the problem; treat with medicated douches; antibiotics

Table 33.1 Diseases and Disorders of Miniature Pot-Bellied Pigs (MPBPs) (*Continued*)

Disease or disorder	Clinical signs	Treatment and comments
	Other diseases	
Hernias (umbilical, inguinal, scrotal)	Soft tissue swelling or lump on belly; swollen scrotum; diarrhea; painful abdomen	Surgical repair of hernia required

Reptiles

While the thought of keeping a snake or lizard as a pet might send shivers up the spine of some, most fanciers agree that reptiles can be enjoyable and fascinating alternatives to the more conventional pet species. The husbandry involved in keeping these scaly companions healthy is not difficult. In fact, just by knowing the proper nutritional and environmental requirements for the particular reptile species in question, most health problems can be avoided. By the way, captive-bred snakes make better pets and thrive in captivity much more so than do their wild counterparts.

Before obtaining a reptile as a pet, visit a local library or pet shop, or browse the Web to read up on your particular selection. Also, you can contact a local zoo and talk to an expert on reptiles. Finally, a veterinarian should be able to supply you with valuable information concerning the husbandry and health of the reptile species you are considering purchasing.

CARE OF SNAKES

Although thousands of snake varieties exist, the ones most commonly kept as pets include pythons, boa constrictors, garter snakes, milk snakes, king snakes, and corn snakes (rat snakes). Obviously, ownership of venomous snakes should be restricted to those persons having special training in the husbandry and handling of these species. As a result, the information contained in this section focuses on the more popular nonpoisonous varieties mentioned above. As with most other exotic pets discussed in this chapter, pet snakes will thrive in those environments that are climate-controlled, are sanitary, and offer high-quality sources of nutrition for their inhabitants. Many snakes kept in such conditions can live a healthy 10 to 20 years!

Restraint

Most snakes become accustomed to being handled by their owners without requiring any special restraint techniques. However, if a snake seems to be aggressive or hyperactive, restrain it by first gripping the snake just behind its head to gain control of this region. The body should then be supported with the other hand (Fig. 34.1). Gloves can be worn if necessary to protect the hands. Also, to be safe, never handle a very large constrictor snake, especially one with a belligerent attitude, if no one else is around.

Housing

Pet snakes can be categorized several different ways, depending on the type of living environment in which they are normally found in the wild.

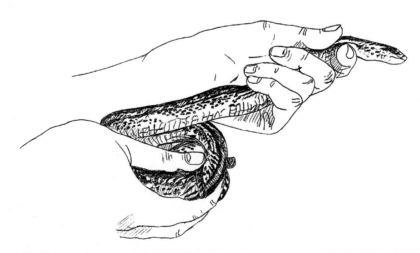

FIGURE 34.1 When holding your snake, gently support its body and control its head.

These can include arboreal snakes such as boa constrictors and Burmese pythons, which prefer living in trees; semiaquatic snakes such as garter snakes, which enjoy living both in water and on land; and terrestrial snakes like ball pythons and king snakes, which prefer solid ground.

DID YOU KNOW?

A snake flicks its tongue out of its mouth to pick up chemicals in the air, then returns it to a special structure within its mouth, called *Jacobson's organ*. This organ is the snake's "nose," helping it to scent nearby prey.

Most snakes kept as pets can be housed in converted glass aquariums or custom acrylic enclosures. As a rule, provide at least ¾ square foot of living area per foot of snake housed within. Secure, well-ventilated tops are needed as well to prevent premeditated escape. These tops should be constructed out of peg board, acrylic, or plastic instead of wire mesh, as the latter can cause snout abrasions. The configuration and setup provided within the enclosure itself should cater to your snake's individual preferences, whether they are arboreal, terrestrial, or semiaquatic. Regardless of the type, plan on thoroughly cleaning and disinfecting the floor, walls, and contents of your pet's home at least twice monthly.

Keep in mind that the two most crucial factors in providing a proper artificial environment for any reptile are temperature and humidity. In the wild, reptiles regulate their body temperatures (as necessary for various physiological functions) by changing their position in accordance with changes in environmental temperatures. As a result, snakes might choose to bask in the sun on a branch or rock to raise their body temperature, or to seek out shade to lower their body temperature. In captivity, such options should be available as well.

An incandescent lightbulb with a reflector can be positioned over one end of the cage containing a basking branch or rock. Temperatures in this "hot" region should remain a consistent 93 to 97 degrees Fahrenheit. (*Note:* Commercially available "hot rocks" should not be used within the enclosure, since these can burn the underside of snakes.) Temperature gradients elsewhere within the enclosure should range from 85 to 70 degrees Fahrenheit. Heating pads can be placed beneath selected sections of the aquarium to achieve these temperature gradients. Ceramic heating elements can be utilized as well.

Aquarium thermometers should be placed at multiple locations within the cage to monitor these temperatures throughout.

A humidity gauge should be centrally located in your snake's enclosure, away from heat and light sources. Relative humidity should be maintained between 40 and 70 percent. Environmental humidity kept too low can cause dehydration and shedding challenges. On the contrary, humidity kept consistently too high can predispose a snake to potentially harmful fungal and bacterial growth.

Artificial turf, indoor/outdoor carpet, aspen chips, or butcher-block paper can be used to line the floor of your snake's terrarium. If either of the first two are used, keep two or three clean pieces available as backups to quickly replace soiled ones. Excretions and any uneaten food should be removed daily, and the flooring should be changed at least every other day. A quaternary ammonium compound or chlorhexidine diluted 1:10 with water is an ideal disinfectant for cleaning and soaking soiled pieces of flooring. If you have only one piece of turf to work with, be sure to rinse and dry it completely before placing it back into the cage. Failure to do so could predispose your snake to skin irritation and disease.

For arboreal species, provide plenty of branches of different types and sizes on which your snake may climb. Smooth rock formations, hollow logs, or other hiding areas should be placed at different temperature locations within the enclosure. Burrowing snakes, such as sand boas, will also need a substrate into which they can burrow. Aspen shavings or other commercially available substrates designed for snakes serve this function quite nicely.

Another item needed for your snake's home is a sturdy ceramic or plastic water bowl large enough for the snake to crawl into. The bowl should contain a water level shallow enough as to not completely submerge the snake's body. Use filtered water as a water source to prevent chlorine irritation to your pet's skin. Change the water and clean the bowl on a daily basis.

Nutrition

Young, growing snakes should be fed at least twice weekly. As snakes mature, their feedings can be dropped to once every week or two. Standard food items for larger snakes include mice, rats, chicks, and rabbits. Smaller snakes can be fed insects (pesticide-free!), small mice, frogs, salamanders, small lizards, and earthworms. With the exception of smaller insects, do not serve live prey to your snake. Even the smallest of prey, if hostile enough, can cause serious, even life-threatening, injuries to a snake (Fig. 34.2). Instead, offer fresh prey that has been dispatched just prior to feeding. Frozen prey can be used as well; just be sure to thaw it out completely prior to feeding.

Don't handle your snake for several days following a meal to prevent a stress-related disruption of the digestive process. In addition, many snakes might become irritable and bite if disturbed following a good meal!

Keep careful records of the feeding activity of your snake. In this way, loss of appetite or any disruption in the normal feeding habits caused by illness can be noticed and addressed promptly.

Shedding

Shedding (*ecdysis*) is the process in which new skin is formed beneath the old and the latter is subsequently discarded. All reptiles (and amphibians) shed. In snakes, it usually occurs every 1 to 3 months depending on the age and size of snake involved. Snakes that are about to shed their skin will seem to lose their appetite and become somewhat lethargic a week or two prior to the event. As new skin develops beneath the old, the old skin will turn "opaque" for a few days, then return to its normal appearance. After several days, the old skin comes off. Keep accurate records of your snake's shedding activity (Fig. 34.3). Any changes in your snake's individual shedding pattern could be a sign of illness and warrants a trip to your veterinarian.

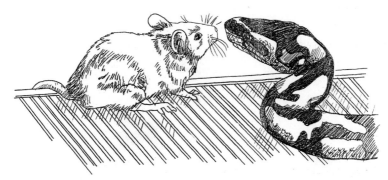

FIGURE 34.2 Live prey should be fed with caution, as it could seriously injure your snake.

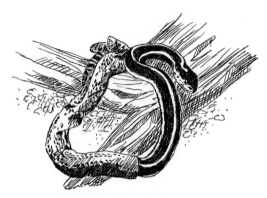

FIGURE 34.3 Shedding usually occurs every 1 to 3 months, depending on the age and size of snake involved.

To prevent inadvertent damage to the new skin, do not handle your snake while it is shedding until the process is complete. If an incomplete shed occurs, place your snake in a shallow water bowl and soak the nonshed regions for 1 to 2 hours. This should help the snake complete the shed.

Occasionally, the skin covering the eyes of a snake will fail to shed with the rest of the skin. These retained eyecaps might need to be manually removed. However, this should be performed only with the help of a qualified veterinarian, since, if done incorrectly, permanent damage to your snake's eyes could result.

CARE OF LIZARDS

Like snakes, a wide variety of lizard species adorn households across the country. Popular ones include geckos, chameleons, and, of course, iguanas. Iguanas belong to the Iguanidae family of reptiles. Out of this family, the most notable member to be kept as a pet is the green iguana.

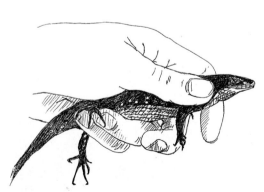

FIGURE 34.4 An effective method for restraining smaller lizards.

Fascinating creatures to observe, lizards are hardy and fairly easy to care for. This is assuming, of course, that an owner is well versed in the environmental and nutritional needs of these special reptiles.

Restraint

As a rule, handling of pet lizards should be kept to a

minimum. Lizards are incredibly strong for their size and can be difficult to manage if they put up a fight (Fig. 34.4)! When restraining large lizards, grasp the neck area and control the forelegs all with

> ## DID YOU KNOW?
>
> When the desire to change elevations hits, green iguanas will often purposely and recklessly hurl themselves down from great heights, yet rarely do they hurt themselves!

one hand, and with the other hand, encircle the belly of the lizard to lift. Never pick up a lizard by its tail. If you do, you might find yourself holding the tail as your reptile scurries off in the other direction!

Housing

Lizards may be kept in aquariums or similar enclosures with secure, mesh screening over the top to prevent escape (Fig. 34.5). As a rule, most lizards prefer to be housed alone, and may become aggressive toward any new additions. They can be arboreal (living on trees or plants) or terrestrial (living on land) in nature. The decor of the enclosure should reflect your lizard's personal preference.

Temperature and humidity are two crucial factors when providing a proper artificial environment for any reptile. In the wild, reptiles regulate their body temperatures by changing their body position and/or location in accordance with changes in environmental temperatures. As a result, a

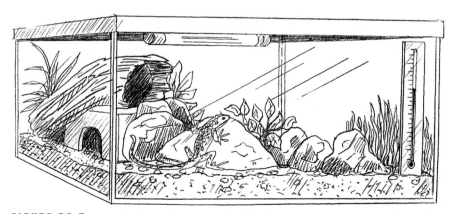

FIGURE 34.5 A typical terrarium setup for lizards.

DID YOU KNOW?

High levels of humidity in a vivarium necessitate good ventilation to prevent mildew and bacterial proliferation.

lizard might choose to bask in the sun on a branch or rock to raise its body temperature, or to crawl into the shade to lower the same. In captivity, these options should be available. For this reason, the cage you keep your lizard in should provide both warm and cool regions.

An incandescent lightbulb with a reflector can be positioned over one end of the cage containing a basking branch or rock. Temperatures in this "hot" region should remain between 93 and 97 degrees Fahrenheit. Commercially available "hot rocks" should not be used within the enclosure, since these can burn reptiles.

Temperature gradients elsewhere within the enclosure should range from 85 to 70 degrees Fahrenheit. Heating pads can be placed beneath selected sections of the aquarium to achieve these temperature gradients. Ceramic heating elements are most effective as well. Aquarium thermometers should be placed at multiple locations within the cage to monitor environmental temperatures throughout.

A humidity gauge should also be centrally located within your lizard's enclosure, away from light and heat sources. Relative humidity should be maintained above 50 percent for most arboreal lizards (including iguanas), and 20 to 40 percent for terrestrial species, such as the leopard gecko. High levels of humidity necessitate good ventilation within the enclosure to prevent bacterial and mold growth.

Although incandescent lighting may provide a source of heat and light, it does not supply the full spectrum of light that lizards require to maintain both their mental and physical health. The ultraviolet rays of the sun are required for the synthesis of vitamin D_3 in the skin of lizards. If not enough of vitamin D_3 is synthesized, nutritional bone disease can result. Most lizards kept in captivity are deprived of direct exposure to natural sunlight, and require an artificial source of "sunlight." Contrary to popular belief, placing your pet's enclosure next to a sunny window is not sufficient, since glass can interfere with the effective transmission and absorption of the sun's ultraviolet rays. Instead, an unfiltered black light fluorescent tube should be mounted approximately 2 feet above your reptile's basking site to provide these much needed rays. These tubes are readily available at most pet stores. [*Note:*

These are different from black light blue tubes, which are of little value and should not be used. Approximately 10 hours of this light should be provided for your lizard on a daily basis. Be sure no glass or plastic comes between the light source and the reptile (mesh

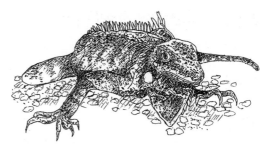

FIGURE 34.6 Iguanas and other lizards require special lighting in order to keep them healthy.

screen is okay).] To ensure maximum effectiveness, black lights should be replaced every 6 months (Fig. 34.6).

Butcher-block paper, which is inexpensive and easy to change, can be used to line the floor of your lizard's home. If used, it should be changed daily. As an alternative, artificial turf or indoor/outdoor carpeting can be used as well. Keep two or three clean pieces available as backups to quickly replace soiled ones. Excretions should be picked up daily, and the flooring should be changed and cleaned at least three times a week. A quaternary ammonium compound or chlorhexidine diluted 1:10 with water is an ideal disinfectant for cleaning and soaking soiled pieces of flooring. If you have only one piece to work with, be sure to rinse and dry it completely before placing it back into the cage. Failure to do so could predispose your reptile to skin irritation and disease.

For arboreal species, provide plenty of branches of different types and sizes on which your lizard can climb. Smooth rock formations, hollow logs, or other areas in which your lizard can hide should be placed at different temperature locations within the enclosure.

Some lizards enjoy substrate into which they can burrow. Pelleted, recycled newspaper (available at most pet stores) or commercially available substrate designed for reptiles serves this function quite nicely.

Another item needed for your lizard's home is a water bowl with easy access. The bowl should be large enough to hold your lizard and contain a level of water that would cover approximately two-thirds of its body. Use filtered water as a water source to prevent chlorine irritation to your pet's skin. Change the water and clean the bowl on a daily basis. Note that chameleons will rarely drink water from a bowl. They will, however, lick up water droplets from the sides of the enclosure. As a result, keep the sides of the cage well misted throughout the day. Even better (and less labor-intensive), consider installing a drip system (available commercially) to provide a constant source of water to your finicky pet. To maintain proper sanitation, give your lizard's cage flooring, walls, and contents a thorough cleaning and disinfecting at least twice monthly.

Nutrition

Nutritionally related bone disease due to poor feeding practices is common in captive lizards, especially green iguanas (Fig. 34.7). For herbivores like the green iguana, feed a varied diet consisting of

85 percent dark, leafy green vegetables, such as mustard greens, cilantro, collards, grape leaves, spinach, broccoli, etc.

5 percent fruit, such as bananas and pears

10 percent protein source, such as dry dog food, monkey chow, or hard-boiled eggs

In addition, a balanced vitamin-mineral supplement designed for herbivorous lizards should be sprinkled on the vegetables for added protection against nutritional bone disease.

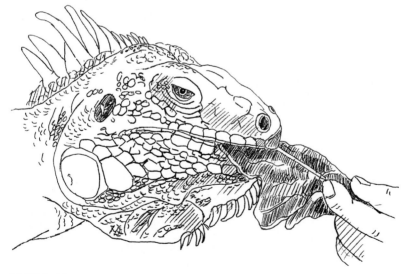

FIGURE 34.7 Nutritionally related bone disease due to poor feeding practices is common in captive iguanas.

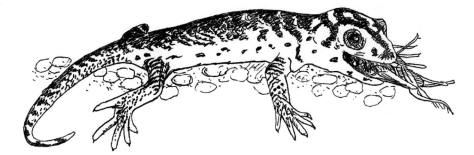

FIGURE 34.8 Crickets provide an excellent meal for most small reptiles.

The daily diet of a carnivorous species of lizard should consist of prey such as baby mice (pinkies), chicks, rabbits, insects, and/or mealworms, depending on the size of the reptile (Fig. 34.8). With the exception of insects (ants, crickets, grasshoppers) and mealworms, all prey should be prekilled prior to feeding. If insects are offered, make certain they are pesticide-free. Like their herbivorous cousins, these lizards should receive daily balanced vitamin-mineral supplement as well.

Plan on feeding both herbivorous and carnivorous lizards at least once daily. Remove and discard all uneaten food at the end of the day. Water should be offered free-choice at all times. Many lizards will eliminate in their water dishes. As a result, be sure to change them daily.

CARE OF THE PET CHELONIAN

Turtles and tortoises are also popular reptiles kept as pets. They belong to the reptilian order Chelonia, with hundreds of different species existing. The most common chelonians kept as pets include box turtles, snapping turtles, and various aquatic turtles. If well cared for, some turtles can live over 20 years in captivity (Fig. 34.9)!

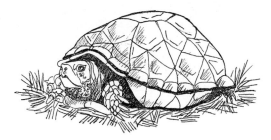

FIGURE 34.9 Certain turtles can live over 20 years in captivity with proper care!

Restraint

Most turtles can be easily and safely handled by grasping the edges of the shell with one hand and supporting the underside of the turtle, or plastron, with the other. Note, however, that snapping turtles and certain other species of turtles do require special precautions when lifting or handling to avoid being bitten and/or scratched. For instance, a snapping turtle should be picked up only by the base of its tail. Since turtles are unable to reach around and bite effectively because of their shell, this approach is the safest. Less aggressive turtles can be handled safely by grasping the sides of the shell near the hind end, as far away from the head as possible.

Housing

Turtles can be kept in 10- to 20-gallon aquariums or other similar enclosures. Semiaquatic turtles require both water to swim in and land to crawl on within their artificial environment. Both regions need to be easily accessible. Large, round gravel can be used to create the "land" portion of the environment. Sand, aquarium gravel, or wood chips should not be used, as these may be ingested by a bored pet. A hiding spot should also be provided at one end of the land mass. Aquatic turtles obviously need less land and more water in which to swim and feed. It needn't be deep, just enough for the turtle to be able to submerge itself. The only water that terrestrial turtles need is that provided within a shallow water dish (Fig. 34.10).

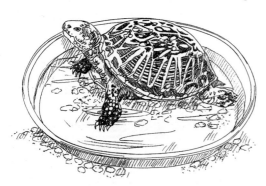

FIGURE 34.10 Turtles should have free access to water at all times.

All water should be filtered prior to adding to the vivarium to avoid the hazards of contamination. In addition, plan on complete water changes twice per week. A filtration system can be installed to help keep the water clean; however, this does not replace essential twice-weekly water changes. Environmental temperature, including water temperature, should be kept between 75 and 85 degrees Fahrenheit at all times (this includes any new water added). Abrupt changes in water temperature can be harmful to turtles. Also, if environmental temperatures fall too low, most turtles will go off feed and could become malnourished. As a result, be sure to use an aquarium thermometer to help monitor this important parameter.

Smooth rocks or branches suitable for climbing and basking should be provided for both aquatic and semiaquatic turtles. Floating platforms are appealing to these pets as well. Plenty of hiding places should be offered, and situated at various locations within the vivarium or terrarium. Enclosures, including fixtures, should be thoroughly cleaned and disinfected weekly using soap and water or a 1:10 dilution of chlorhexidine. After cleaning, rinse thoroughly to be sure no chemical residues are left that could be harmful to your turtle.

Turtles, like other reptiles, regulate body temperature according to physiological needs. As a result, a simple setup including an incandescent light bulb and reflector situated over a basking site within the terrarium should be used to create a "hot spot" of around 85 to 90 degrees Fahrenheit. Also, a heating pad can be placed beneath one section of the enclosure to create a thermal gradient within the enclosure. Thermometers can be placed in strategic locations within the enclosure to monitor temperatures.

Chelonians, like their lizard cousins, also require a source of ultraviolet light in order to synthesize vitamin D within their bodies, thereby preventing nutritionally related bone disease (see section on care of lizards).

Nutrition

The diet of aquatic turtles should consist of a variety of foodstuffs, including small fish, worms, insects, water plants, and dark green, leafy vegetables. Aquatic turtles like to eat their meals while in the water. Box turtles, on the other hand, prefer to eat on land. They, too, enjoy and need the same type of well-balanced diet as do their aquatic cousins, with the addition of some dark green or yellow vegetables and fruit. A balanced vitamin-mineral supplement should be added to the diet of all turtles for added protection against nutritional bone disease.

DR. P's VET TIP

The humidity within your reptile's environment can be raised by increasing the size of the water container within the enclosure, partially covering the screen top (if present) to reduce ventilation, misting the sides of the enclosure, and/or moistening the substrate. On the contrary, to reduce the humidity, use spot lamps or fans to promote evaporation, replace moist substrate with dry substrate, and/or increase ventilation within the enclosure.

PREVENTIVE HEALTH CARE FOR REPTILES

Pet reptiles can benefit from annual veterinary checkups just like other pets. In addition to a physical examination, stool checks and/or cultures should be performed to ensure that your pet is and remains free of infection or parasitism.

Reptile owners should realize that the pet reptiles can be carriers of salmonella, a bacterium that can cause food poisoning and severe diarrhea in humans. A commonsense approach to handling and hygiene is essential to prevent zoonotic transmission (see Chap. 44).

Strict sanitation, environmental control (including temperature and humidity), and high-quality rations must be given top priority in order to prevent disease in reptiles. Keep a close eye on your pet's behavior and movements, eating habits, elimination habits, and physical characteristics. Notify your veterinarian of any changes you see.

Diseases and Disorders

The vast majority of diseases and disorders seen in reptiles kept as pets are caused by improper sanitation, inadequate lighting, and/or poor nutrition. If your pet is exhibiting clinical signs or any type of strange behavior, take it to your veterinarian immediately for a checkup. If your veterinarian does not work on reptiles, ask for a referral to one in your area who does. Identifying and treating diseases in their early stages is the key to successful treatment and cure. Some of the more common diseases and disorders seen in reptiles are listed below. Others do exist, which is why a definitive diagnosis should be made by a qualified veterinarian (Table 34.1).

Table 34.1 Diseases and Disorders of Reptiles

Disease or disorder	Reptiles primarily affected*	Clinical signs	Treatment and comments
Vitamin D deficiency	L, T	"Rubber jaw"; limb and spine deformities; fractures; paralysis	Review and correct diet—vitamin-mineral supplement; provide source of ultraviolet light
Vitamin D excess	L	General malaise; bone abnormalities	Overuse of vitamin D supplement; treat by discontinuing supplement
Nutritional secondary hyperparathyroidism	L, T	Same as above	Caused by calcium-phosphorous imbalances; treatment same as above
Gout	L	Lameness; general malaise	Caused by improper diet, water deprivation, kidney disease; no treatment
Vitamin A deficiency	T	Swollen eyelids; eye and nose discharge; breathing difficulties	Seen in turtles on all-meat or all-vegetable diets; treat by changing diet, vitamin A supplement, antibiotics
Pneumonia	L, T, S	Gaping and breathing difficulties; nasal discharge; swollen eyelids	Can be caused by bacteria, fungi, or parasites; treatment depends on cause
Skin parasites (mites, ticks, etc.)	L, T, S	Variable, including weakness, loss of appetite	Can cause anemia; treat locally with safe insecticide

Table 34.1 Diseases and Disorders of Reptiles (*Continued*)

Disease or disorder	Reptiles primarily affected*	Clinical signs	Treatment and comments
Retained eye cap	S	Eye opacity, irritation	May be retained after shedding; moisten, then peel off gently
Mouth rot (infectious stomatitis)	S	Loss of appetite; open-mouth gaping; white discharge within the mouth	Occurs secondary to mouth trauma and other diseases; treatment involves local flushing and antibiotics
Amebiasis	L, T, S	Loss of appetite; regurgitation; loose, abnormal stool; weight loss	Seen in reptiles kept in groups; can be spread by cockroaches; treat with amebicide and antibiotics
Septicemia	L, T, S	Loss of appetite; weakness; lack of muscle tone	Often secondary to stress and other diseases; treat using antibiotics and correcting underlying cause
Lumps and bumps	L, T, S	Abnormal body shape; lumps and bumps	Suspect food ingestion, eggs, abscesses, tumors

*L = lizard; T = turtle; S = snake.

Amphibians

mphibians have always been highly favored as pets. The word *amphibios* means "double life," as these creatures are adapted for life both on land and in water. Adult amphibians will spend most of their time on land, only to return to water to reproduce. The offspring that result will, in turn, remain in their aqueous surroundings until maturity. Amphibians, like reptiles, are cold-blooded, meaning that their internal body temperatures fluctuate with environmental temperatures.

Over 2500 varieties of frogs and toads exist throughout the world (Fig. 35.1). The class Amphibia includes frogs, toads, salamanders, and newts. Frogs and toads are tailless amphibians that possess long, strong hindlimbs. Those that dwell in trees also sport prominent suction disks on the digits of their toes to be used for climbing and clinging. Salamanders and newts, on the other hand, possess short, relatively weak legs that protrude almost perpendicular to their bodies (Fig. 35.2). They also possess a long tail that assists them in their movements. Instead of walking or jumping like frogs, salamanders wiggle and slither toward their intended destinations.

Although the toad is considered a type of frog, they differ in a number of ways. Frogs possess bodies that are more streamlined and elongated than those of toads. The legs of frogs are elongated and ideal for

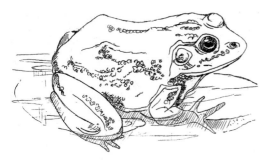

FIGURE 35.1 Over 2500 varieties of frogs and toads exist worldwide.

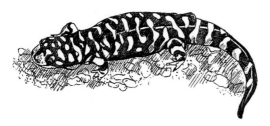

FIGURE 35.2 Salamanders have short legs that protrude almost perpendicular to their bodies.

leaping and swimming, whereas those of toads are shorter and used for walking and stalking prey. The skin of the frog is smooth and shiny, in contrast to the thick, dry, and knobby skin of the toad. When laying eggs, frogs will do so in clusters, while toads will lay their eggs in long chains. Finally, frogs come in a wide variety of shapes and colors, including black, various shades of green, and the bright oranges, reds, and yellows of the tropical varieties. Most toads, on the other hand, sport a basic brown color or shades thereof, providing them with the optimum camouflage within their terrestrial surroundings.

Like frogs and toads, salamanders and newts come in all sorts of shapes, sizes, and colors. Over 300 species exist worldwide. The major difference between the salamander and the newt (which is actually a type of salamander) is that the salamander prefers to dwell on land, returning to water only to breed. On the contrary, newts like to spend the majority of their time in aquatic settings. Realize, of course, that when speaking of any type of amphibian, there are always multiple exceptions to the rule!

The top two goals in the life of any amphibian are to (1) find food and (2) keep from drying out. Adult amphibians not only breathe through a set of lungs but also respire through their skin and mucous membranes. For this reason, the outer surfaces of most amphibians

DID YOU KNOW?

The body slime of the slimy salamander is almost as sticky as glue!

are coated with slimy mucus that allows them to retain the skin moisture necessary for proper oxygen exchange. Loss of surface moisture due
to dehydration, low humidity, and/or high environmental temperatures
can be deadly. This is why amphibians are primarily nocturnal creatures, seeking out food during the nighttime hours and retreating to
cool, sheltered areas during the day.

Amphibians can be purchased from pet stores or gathered from
their natural habitats. However, before doing the latter, familiarize
yourself with local laws and ordinances regarding ownership of native
amphibian species. If you accidentally grab hold of an endangered
species, you could be faced with a stiff penalty. Remember also that if
you purchase or obtain an amphibian that is not native to your region,
under no circumstances should you release it back into the wild. Placing such an individual into a foreign habitat could lead to the spread
of new diseases and parasites that could potentially wipe out your
local ecosystem!

Restraint

If you want a pet that you can cuddle and carry around with you all
day long, an amphibian is probably not the right choice for you. There
are three good reasons for this: (1) the skin of frogs and salamanders is
a sensitive, delicate organ and can be easily traumatized by repeated
handling; (2) certain frogs, toads, and salamanders can release toxins
from their skin that can be quite irritating to eyes and mucous membranes; and (3) amphibians can be carriers of bacteria and parasites
that can be transmitted to humans through close contact.

If you must pick up your amphibian, don a pair of disposable
gloves. Be sure the gloves are free of surface powder, as this can be
quite irritating to the sensitive skin of amphibians. For best results,
moisten your gloved hands prior to handling. Use cupped hands to
gently scoop up your pet. Avoid squeezing it to prevent its escape. That
act alone probably causes more injuries to captive amphibians and reptiles than all other sources combined! Because of their slimy skin,
amphibians can easily slip out of your hands and fall to the ground,
causing serious injury or death. As a result, always keep your hands
near a supporting surface just in case you lose your grip (Fig. 35.3).

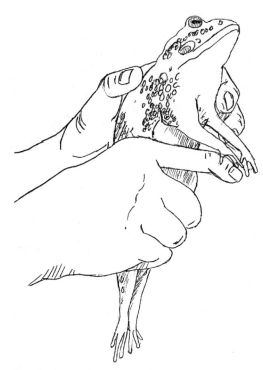

FIGURE 35.3 Method of restraint for larger amphibians.

DID YOU KNOW?

Frogs will sometimes urinate when handled. Their purpose for doing so is to reduce their body weight as much as possible, allowing them to jump farther and swifter should the opportunity to escape arise!

If transporting your amphibian more than a few yards, use a small container filled with moss as your means of transport. Be sure your container has a lid containing holes to allow for ventilation. If transporting for a prolonged period of time, mist your traveler every 20 minutes to prevent dehydration.

Housing

Although amphibians are quite adaptive to any environment in which they are placed, do your best to duplicate the environment from which your pet originated. Keep in mind that maintaining a constant environmental temperature and proper humidity within the living quarters are essential to your amphibian's health and well-being. If in doubt, ask for housing advice from your local pet store that sells amphibians. They will be able to assist you in a design of a functional and fun habitat for your amphibious friend.

The type of setup needed will obviously depend on the type of amphibian owned. For instance, tree frogs will need homes that are taller than those of their ground-loving peers, complete with plenty of tree branches and foliage on which to climb. "Gilled" aquatic amphibians will require an aquarium environment very similar to that of tropical fish, complete with water filtration systems. Terrestrial species may require a terrarium that consists of only a small container of water. For those in between, commercial kits are available that can transform any enclosure into a vivarium containing both aquatic and land areas (Fig. 35.4). All water added to an amphibian's abode should be filtered, salt-free, and chlorine-free, with a pH somewhere between 6.5 and 8. Salt (as found in "soft" water), chlorine, and an improper pH can be extremely irritating to the sensitive skin of these animals. Aquarium water test kits available at pet stores can be used periodically to ensure the water quality within your pet's habitat.

Most amphibians are typically housed in glass aquarium-type enclosures fitted with secure tops that prevent escape and allow for adequate ventilation. Acrylic tops containing multiple ventilation holes and secure fasteners are ideal, as these allow for visual pleasure while helping to maintain temperature and humidity within the enclosure. Plastic snap-on lids available at most pet shops can also be used as inexpensive alternatives to acrylic, yet are not quite as effective at regulating internal environment.

The size of the aquarium used will depend on the size of the amphibian in question, as well as the number of them to be kept therein. If you are planning on housing more than one amphibian within a particular enclosure, make certain that they are of the same species and of the same size. Never house frogs and salamanders together and never house a larger amphibian with a smaller one, even if they are of the same species. If you do, you may wake up one morning and find the smaller of the two missing and the larger one with a satisfied smirk on its face!

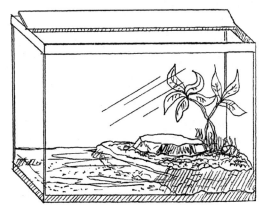

FIGURE 35.4 An example of a vivarium setup for amphibians. Note both the land and water portions.

Sphagnum moss is ideal for lining the floor of your pet's living quarters. Moss helps contain moisture and humidity within the enclosure, while providing your amphibian with a soft surface and an ideal medium in which to burrow. Even better, placing a 1-inch layer of gravel beneath the moss will allow water and waste to filter through the moss, helping to keep it clean. Adorn the mossy floor of the living space with smooth rocks, simulated wooden branches, and silk plants (these latter two items are easier to clean and maintain than the real things), thereby providing plenty of places to hide or climb.

To prevent accidental dehydration in an unsuspecting frog or salamander, situate the enclosure within your home so as to keep it out of direct sunlight and well away from incandescent heat sources. Fluorescent lighting provides the ideal light source, as it gives off very little heat. Since amphibians are nocturnal, they should be provided with at least 12 hours of darkness each day.

A thermometer and humidity gauge are always standard equipment when housing amphibians. Temperate amphibian species require temperatures ranging between 60 and 70 degrees Fahrenheit, with humidity around 75 to 80 percent. Tropical varieties need temperatures between 75 and 80 degrees Fahrenheit, with humidity at 85 to 90 percent. If environmental temperature is too high and/or humidity is too low, dehydration becomes a definite threat. On the contrary, if temperatures drop too low, overall activity, including eating, will diminish.

For land portions of a vivarium, a heating pad placed under the tank can help regulate temperatures. Standard aquarium heaters can be used to heat the water within the tank. Do not use heat lamps, as these will quickly dehydrate your pet. Humidity can be maintained by lightly misting the sphagnum moss with water at least two times per week. Don't overmist, as this can lead to harmful fungal growth.

Clean your pet's home on a daily basis. [*Note:* Always wear disposable gloves when performing these duties to protect yourself against diseases that can be spread by these types of pets (see Chap. 44).] Remove any uneaten food or debris left over from the day before and change the water in the water bowl (if used) daily. Remove soiled moss as needed, and plan on replacing the entire moss bedding every 3 weeks. For those enclosures with water reservoirs, perform a complete water change twice weekly. All wastewater should be siphoned from the bottom in order to remove organic debris that has settled to the bottom of the tank. Thoroughly clean the walls and fixtures inside the enclosure on a monthly basis. Use a mild soap when doing so and be sure to rinse all areas thoroughly, as soap residues can irritate and damage the skin of amphibians.

Nutrition

Feeding live food to your frog or salamander is recommended in order to stimulate and promote normal natural feeding behavior. Crickets are the ideal food, as they are inexpensive and easy to obtain. Crickets can be purchased from most pet stores or can be gathered from around your home. Just be sure, however, that all crickets you feed are pesticide-free. One day prior to offering them to your pet, feed the crickets tropical fish food or a commercial cricket diet loaded with nutrients to booster their nutritional value.

Terrestrial amphibians can also be fed fruitflies, mealworms, and aphids. Some of the larger toads may even make a meal of baby mice if offered to them! Aquatic amphibians enjoy earthworms, insect larvae, and small fish. Obviously, their food should be fed to them in the water. Feeding your amphibian once a day should be sufficient. Remove any uneaten food from the previous day prior to feeding a fresh meal.

You will soon discover that each frog or salamander will develop its own individualized eating habits. Some will prefer slow-moving prey while others enjoy the thrill of the chase. For instance, toads usually prefer to wait passively for prey to cross their paths, whereas frogs often take a more aggressive approach.

Preventive Health Care

Pet amphibians can benefit from annual veterinary checkups just like other pets. In addition to a physical examination, stool checks and cultures should be performed to ensure that your pet is and remains free of infection or parasitism. Because amphibians can be carriers of zoonotic organisms, special precautions should be taken when handling these pets (see Chap. 44).

Strict sanitation, environmental control (including temperature and humidity), and high-quality rations must be given top priority in order to prevent disease in amphibians kept as pets. Keep a close eye on your pet's behavior and movements, eating habits, elimination habits, and physical characteristics. Notify your veterinarian of any changes that you see.

Diseases and Disorders

Improper sanitation, inadequate environmental parameters (such as temperature and humidity), and/or poor nutrition cause the vast majority of diseases and disorders seen in amphibians. If your pet is exhibiting clinical signs or any type of strange behavior, take it to your veterinarian immediately for a checkup. If your veterinarian does not work on amphibians, ask for a referral to one in your area who does so. By identifying and treating diseases in their early stages, successful treatment and cure is much more obtainable. Below are some of the more common diseases and disorders seen in amphibians. Others do exist, which is why a veterinary diagnosis is essential (Table 35.1).

Table 35.1 Diseases and Disorders of Amphibians

Disease or disorder	Clinical signs	Treatment and comments
Red leg disease	Reddened skin on underside of pet; ulcers on toes; bloating; cloudy eyes	Treat with antibiotics; salt baths; sanitize amphibian's environment
Edema syndrome	Generalized swelling or bloating of the body; breathing difficulties; weakness	Can occur because of liver disease, skin disease, toxins; also seen in amphibians living in and around distilled water; treat by veterinary removal of fluid with needle and syringe; salt baths; treat underlying cause

Table 35.1 Diseases and Disorders of Amphibians (*Continued*)

Disease or disorder	Clinical signs	Treatment and comments
Water mold disease	White to brown cotton-like lesions on skin; weight loss; lethargy; breathing difficulties	Seen in amphibians housed in water kept below 70°F; diagnose with skin scraping; elevate water temperatures to above 70°F; salt baths
Dehydration	Weight loss; emaciation; lethargy; dull, dark skin; sunken eyes; incoordination	Seen in terrestrial amphibians kept in high temperatures; also in amphibians with skin disease; treat with water and electrolyte baths
Parasitic disease	Skin ulceration and lesions; diarrhea; weight loss; breathing difficulties	Due to poor husbandry and stress; treat with antiparasitic drugs and antibiotics; clean and sanitize enclosure; improve nutrition
Hypothermia	Listlessness; loss of appetite	Maintain proper environmental temperatures
Poisoning	Skin lesions; seizures; skin color change; bloating; breathing difficulties	Sources can include disinfectant residues, vegetation or food contaminated with insecticides; contaminated water; remove inciting cause; support through good nutrition and husbandry

Table 35.1 Diseases and Disorders of Amphibians (*Continued*)

Disease or disorder	Clinical signs	Treatment and comments
Bacterial skin infection	Nodules on skin; weight loss; skin ulcers	Treat with appropriate antibiotics; improve sanitation
Metabolic bone disease	Deformities of jaws and/ or limbs; limb fractures	Due to imbalance of calcium, phosphorus, and other vitamins and minerals in diet; treat or prevent by feeding or dusting food source with supplement prior to feeding to amphibian

Invertebrates

"Invertebrate" is the term used to describe any animal that is devoid of a backbone. Among the countless numbers that exist, the most popular ones kept as pets are tarantulas, scorpions, and hermit crabs. Spiders and scorpions both belong to the class Arachnida, whose members sport two body segments and four pairs of legs. Hermit crabs are members of the class Crustacida, and are cousins of lobsters and shrimp.

Prior to getting an invertebrate as a pet, do your homework first. Check out books and Websites to become an expert on your favorite type. Also, talk to pet-store owners who specialize in the sale of these type of animals. Their knowledge and experience in husbandry practices are invaluable. Look at the different living arrangements they have set up for the invertebrates that they sell. This will give you some great ideas that you can apply to your own pet's housing setup.

TARANTULAS AND SCORPIONS

Certainly the most popular of all arachnids kept as pets are tarantulas. With their hairy legs and bodies, multiple eyes, and quick, sudden movements, tarantulas are formidable in appearance. Yet despite their scary features, tarantulas make great pets. They are relatively easy to maintain and can display unique and entertaining personalities. In the wild, tarantulas can be found resting within foxholes deep within the ground or clinging to tree trunks and branches. Those persons living in "tarantula country" know that you can also find them climbing the sides of homes and buildings after a drenching rain! As a rule, tarantulas are hearty pets, with some living to be as old as 15 years with diligent care.

When selecting your tarantula, there are many species from which to choose. If you are a beginner, consider purchasing a Mexican redleg or Chilean rose tarantula, both known for their docility. Four other popular pet tarantulas include the pinktoe, redrump, whitecollared, and the curlyhaired tarantulas. Purchase a captive-bred tarantula versus capturing your own so that you will have some idea of the spider's temperament ahead of time.

As far as scorpions are concerned, thousands of species live in the deserts, semiarid regions, and tropical climates across the world. They can be found burrowed underground or hiding under rocks or fallen logs. Scorpions possess powerful pinchers that can deliver a mighty pinch if they latch onto a finger. They also have that infamous stinger attached to the end of their tails that can inflict painful wounds in a blink of an eye. Some scorpions deliver highly toxic poisons that can be quite dangerous to humans. As a result, always obtain your scorpion from a reputable source to ensure that the variety you are choosing is safe to handle.

The large emperor scorpion is a popular choice among beginners. Black in color, these scorpions can reach over 5 inches in length! When selecting yours, choose one that appears active, alert, fat, and healthy, not one that is thin and lethargic. If well cared for, scorpions can live 10 to 12 years in captivity.

Restraint

As a rule, arachnids should be handled as little as possible. When you do it, gentle restraint is needed.

Tarantulas that are handled roughly or startled could bite! Although their venom usually produces no more of a reaction than would a bee sting (depending on species), some persons can be allergic to the venom and suffer more severe reactions. It is always a good idea to wear gloves when handling your spider, not only to protect against bites but also to prevent irritation to the hands. The body and legs of tarantulas are covered with tiny hairs that act not only as sensors but also as defense weapons. This is particularly true of the barbed hairs covering the spider's abdomen. By scraping their abdomen with their hind legs, tarantulas can actually flick these tiny hairs at a perceived threat, including your hands. If these hairs embed themselves in the skin, they can be quite irritating and cause a rash. Tarantulas that are stressed or threatened are the ones most likely to exhibit this type of behavior when handled.

To hold your spider, place your hand down flat palm-up in front of it, then gently coax it onto your hand using your other hand to tap the rear end and push it forward. You can also gently lift your tarantula by its abdomen with its head facing away from you, keeping your free hand beneath your spider to create a platform on which it can stand (Fig. 36.1).

As a rule, gloves should be worn whenever handling a scorpion to protect your hands against being stung should your scorpion become agitated or frightened (Fig. 36.2). They will also protect your scorpion, as you are less likely to drop your pet if it lashes out at you. Coax your scorpion into your outstretched gloved hand as you would a tarantula, or you can pick it up by the base of the tail.

If you do get bitten or stung by your arachnid, by all means do not panic and drop it to the floor. Instead, gently place your pet down onto a stable surface, then

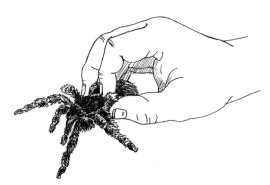

FIGURE 36.1 The proper way to lift your tarantula. Always keep it close to a supporting surface to prevent injury if it is accidentally dropped.

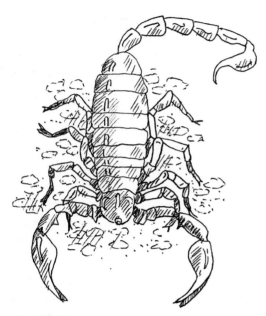

FIGURE 36.2 Scorpions can inflict nasty stings with their tails if they feel threatened.

treat your wound as you would any other sting or wound (don't hesitate to contact your physician for further directions). Note that abdominal rupture due to fall-induced trauma is one of the most prevalent injuries seen by veterinarians in these types of pets.

Housing

Arachnids can be housed in glass terrariums or simply clear plastic storage containers with snap-on lids. If you plan on owning more than one tarantula, they will need to be housed separately to prevent fighting or worse yet, cannibalism!

When choosing an enclosure, keep in mind that length is more important than height. The shorter the walls are, the less chance of injury from falling. Covers must provide adequate ventilation and prevent escape. Screen tops should not be used, as these can injure delicate legs and appendages.

As with all invertebrates, maintaining proper temperature and humidity within any enclosure is of the utmost importance. Standard equipment for all enclosures will include a thermometer and a humidity gauge. For most arachnids kept as pets, temperatures should not be allowed to fall below 72 degrees nor exceed 85 degrees Fahrenheit. Also, the humidity should be kept above 55 percent. Hot rocks should not be used as heating devices within your pet's enclosure, as these can cause serious burns. Instead, a heating pad placed one-third of the way under the enclosure (kept on low setting and covered with a towel for extra insulation) can be used to provide a temperature gradient within the enclosure that your arachnid will enjoy. In order to maintain proper humidity, lightly mist the substrate (until it barely clings to your finger when touched) and the sides of the enclosure with filtered water every few days. Housing facilities should be kept out of direct sunlight and away from drafts to prevent uncontrollable temperature and humidity fluctuations. No special lighting is required for your eight-legged friend!.

(*Note:* Depending on species, wild tarantulas and scorpions can live in habitats ranging from tropical rainforests to dry, arid deserts. As a result, to be sure the abovementioned guidelines fit for your particular species, consult your pet store professional.)

The best substrate to use on the floor of a terrestrial arachnid's home is vermiculite. It can be found at most lawn and garden centers. In most instances, a 3- to 4-inch layer of vermiculite will suffice to allow your pet to burrow into if it so desires. Vermiculite is also excellent at retaining moisture, thereby helping to maintain proper humidity within the enclosure. For tropical or forest dwelling varieties, a layer of sphagnum moss should line the bottom of the terrarium to provide an excellent cushion in case of an accidental fall.

Regardless of the substrate used, be sure to keep your arachnid's home pristine by removing any soiled substrate and uneaten food every day. A complete substrate replacement should be done every 6 weeks, or any time mold growth or substrate discoloration is detected. Before adding new substrate, give the inside of the enclosure a thorough cleaning with soap and water. Be sure to rinse and dry well to eliminate any residues.

For your arachnid's pleasure, you can further adorn its abode with smooth-edged rocks, silk plants, and plenty of places to hide. Cork bark, PVC piping, and/or an inverted clay flower pot with an entry hole in the bottom can provide excellent shelter into which your pet can retreat if it feels like doing so. Small caves made out of rock are also appreciated by most arachnids. Just be sure that there are no sharp edges on any items you place inside the enclosure. If you own a tree-dwelling species, you'll need to provide it with plenty of branches and foliage onto which it can climb.

Provide a shallow water dish for your spider or scorpion. Be sure that it is easily accessible and contains a water level shallow enough to prevent accidental drowning.

Nutrition

The basic meal plan for the captive tarantula or scorpion consists of crickets or grasshoppers (pesticide-free, of course), with the occasional moth, beetle, or mealworm thrown in for variety (Fig. 36.3). Larger species may even enjoy the occasional lizard or baby mouse. Regardless of what is fed, remove any uneaten prey if it has not been dispatched within 3 hours of feeding. For prey that has been killed by the spider or scorpion, remove any eaten or undigested portions from the enclosure within 24 hours after feeding.

Adult tarantulas and scorpions should be fed about every 3 days, whereas immature ones should eat at least every other day to provide proper nutrition for growth. Also, the warmer the environment in which your invertebrate is kept, the faster it will grow and consequently, the more food it will require.

Four to five crickets per week will be sufficient for most arachnids. For best results, feeding should be done at night to satisfy your pet's nocturnal hunting habits. Offer one or two crickets per meal. Never put more than two crickets at a time in with your tarantula, because they may collectively "gang up" on your pet and harm it. The same holds true for scorpions, although their pinchers allow them to defend themselves much more effectively. Again, keep in mind that no food is to be offered during the molting process, as this is the time when your arachnid is most vulnerable to attack.

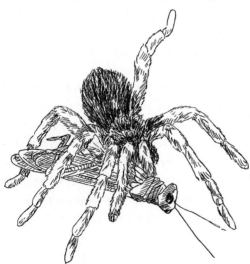

FIGURE 36.3 Tarantulas will crush their prey and cover them with digestive juices.

Molting

From time to time arachnids will molt and shed their outer skeletons (exoskeletons). This is how they grow in size and keep their protective coverings fresh. In younger individuals, molting may take place every month or so. In adults, molting occurs less frequently, usually every 12 to 18 months.

Prior to beginning a molt, your tarantula's color will darken, becoming almost black in appearance. Activity and appetite also diminish 1 to 2 weeks prior to the event. Avoid handling your spider once these signs appear, and during the actual molting process. The same rule holds true for offering live food. Regardless of size, live prey can seriously injure a spider that is in active molt. As your spider starts its molt, it may turn on its side or back and appear almost dead. Don't panic, as this is normal. Proper humidity within your spider's enclosure is essential for a successful molt. As a result, check the humidity gauge within the tank daily and, if needed, apply a light mist to the vermiculite and to the side of the enclosure. Avoid misting your spider directly.

Molting is considered complete once your arachnid's new exoskeleton has tanned and hardened. At this time, you can resume feeding your pet live food.

Preventive Health Care

Healthy tarantulas and scorpions should appear alert and active and have all appendages intact. (*Note:* If your pet does happen to lose a leg to an accident, don't fret. Otherwise healthy arachnids will regenerate the lost appendage after several molts.)

The abdomen should be plump and the legs fully functional, not curled in on themselves. In tarantulas, hair should not be missing except perhaps on the abdominal surface. The skin of an arachnid should not be blotchy in appearance or have any white spots on it. Those arachnids that move slowly, appear emaciated, and remain antisocial are probably harboring an illness. Always remember that dehydration due to poor environmental management and abdominal rupture caused by falling are the two most common causes of death in tarantulas and scorpions. Take care to protect your pet against both of them.

HERMIT CRABS

Hermit crabs are fascinating pets that can provide hours of enjoyment just observing their behavior and antics. It quickly becomes apparent that

DID YOU KNOW?

Some hermit crabs live on the ocean floor some 2000 meters below the surface!

each crab possesses a distinct and unique personality. They are fairly easy to maintain as pets, assuming, of course, that proper care and nutrition is afforded them.

Restraint

When picking up your crab (which should be done infrequently), grasp it by the shell with its front end pointing away from you. If your pet happens to latch onto you with its claw, by all means do not let go! Instead, make a gentle attempt to pry open the claw in order to release your finger. If this doesn't work, run lukewarm water over the claw until your crab releases its grip. (*Note:* Never attempt to extract your crab from its shell. If you try to do so, it will resist with all its might and more than likely injure itself in the process.)

Housing

Hermit crabs are usually housed in 10- to 20-gallon glass aquarium enclosures, with securely fastened acrylic tops containing multiple air vents. Large plastic boxes with tops containing plenty of ventilation holes or slits can also be used. Three to four inches of sand can be used to line the bottom of the enclosure. This should allow your crab enough room to burrow. Be sure to spot-clean this sand on a daily basis. As mentioned previously, keep an eye out for food buried beneath the surface. A complete change in substrate should be performed every 2 weeks. Because hermit crabs are mostly active at night, there are no special lighting requirements. Environmental temperature should be kept between 72 and 85 degrees Fahrenheit. Humidity within the enclosure should be kept above 80 percent. A moist sponge can help maintain humid conditions within your pet's home, as well as provide an alternate source of drinking water. Natural sponges are preferred over the artificial ones. Also, keeping your crab's living quarters out of direct sunlight and drafts will help prevent unpredictable changes in temperature and humidity.

Keep in mind that hermit crabs also love to cruise, climb, and jump, so the inside of your crab's home should provide amenities that cater to these needs. Smooth rocks and/or pieces of driftwood can be used to provide for places for your crab to climb and hide. Silk plants can also be added to spruce up the surroundings. Keep climbing surfaces low enough in elevation to prevent accidental injury if your pet slips and falls. If you want to go the extra mile for your crab, mist its sand with saltwater (available from your local pet store or aquarium shop) daily to more closely simulate its natural environment. This will also help to maintain proper humidity within the enclosure.

Hermit crabs enjoy company, so keeping two or more together will help prevent boredom. Just remember to provide at least three shells (of varying sizes) per crab to allow for plenty of new home choices. Avoid painted or decorated shells as these can be harmful to hermit crabs.

Nutrition

Hermit crabs will eat just about anything you put in front of them. However, to ensure a high plane of nutrition, they should be fed only commercial rations designed for hermit crabs. These are available at most pet stores specializing in exotic and aquatic animals. These commercial diets can be supplemented with cornmeal, oats, apples, bananas, grapes, beans, and lettuce and even moist dog food. In addition, most hermit crabs love peanut butter!

Whatever you use for food and water dispensers, they should be easily acces-

> **DR. P's VET TIP**
> Do not give bread to hermit crabs, as it can clog their gills and cause them to suffocate.

sible. Metal jar lids should not be used, as these can rust and can contaminate your crab's food and water. Clam shells can make ideal food and water bowls, and can also act as a source of calcium for your crab. Just be sure to keep water levels shallow enough to prevent drowning.

All uneaten food should be removed prior to the next fresh meal. Be aware that a crab will bury food just as a dog will bury a bone. As a result, you may have to do some digging in order to accomplish this task!

Molting

Your hermit crab will undergo a molt every 12 to 18 months (or more frequently if immature) in order to shed its exoskeleton. Molting is necessary for continued growth and for regeneration for any limbs they may have been lost since the previous molt. As an impending molt approaches, you may notice your pet becoming less active or less social. It may bury itself in the substrate a week or two prior to the actual molt. Molting hermit crabs are quite susceptible to attacks by pugnacious cagemates; therefore, all cagemates not undergoing molt should be removed until the process is complete. It is also vital that the humidity in the enclosure be kept at a proper level to assist your crab in its molt. Realize that every time your crab undergoes a molt, it will require a bigger shell. As a rule, the rounder the shell is, the better. Be sure it has plenty from which to choose.

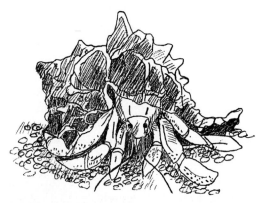

FIGURE 36.4 A good diet, a clean habitat, and plenty of shells from which to choose a home will allow your hermit crab to lead a happy and healthy life.

Preventive Health Care

Hermit crabs are relatively easy to care for and keep healthy. If provided with a good diet, a clean habitat, and plenty of shells from which to choose a home, your hermit crab will lead a happy, contented, and healthy life. In fact, when well cared for, it is not unusual for these pets to exceed 10 years of age in captivity (Fig. 36.4)!

DISEASES AND DISORDERS OF INVERTEBRATES

The vast majority of diseases and disorders seen in invertebrates kept as pets are caused by improper sanitation, poor nutrition, and excessive or improper handling. Table 36.1 lists some of the more common diseases and disorders seen.

Table 36.1 Diseases and Disorders of Invertebrates

Disease or disorder	Clinical signs	Treatment and comments
Dehydration	Gaunt, thin appearance; legs curled inward	Lower temperature and increase humidity accordingly; mist pet every 4 hours; move cage if exposed to direct sunlight; treatment often unrewarding if dehydration severe
Lethargy; loss of appetite	Same	Could be due to impending molt or illness; look for signs of illness, such as emaciation, dehydration, skin lesions; treat as appropriate
Malnutrition	Gaunt, thin appearance	Review and correct nutrition; be sure food is easily accessible
Skin infections	Blotchy skin; white patches	Usually due to unsanitary living conditions or improper temperature and/or humidity; treat by correcting underlying problem; apply antibiotics and antifungals
Injured or lost appendages	Same	No treatment needed; will be replaced after several molts

Table 36.1 Diseases and Disorders of Invertebrates (*Continued*)

Disease or disorder	Clinical signs	Treatment and comments
Dark color change	Same	Impending molt; normal
Circular hair loss on abdomen	Same	Normal in tarantulas; due to "throwing" hairs
Abdominal rupture	Obvious trauma to abdomen; protruding contents	Often occurs when dropped from a height; no treatment
Insecticide poisoning	Seizures; lethargy; death	Usually occurs when pet comes in contact with an insecticide sprayed in close proximity to its enclosure or fed insects contaminated with insecticide

Tropical Fish

$\mathbf{L}$ooking for a pet that doesn't eat much, requires no training whatsoever, will not bring fleas into your house, and can actually lower your blood pressure? Welcome to the world of tropical fish. More and more, these fascinating aquatic creatures are finding their way into the hearts of pet lovers all across the country. In fact, it is estimated that aquariums adorn approximately one out of three households in the United States alone.

Another key indicator of the popularity of tropical fish in this country is the amount of money spent on them each year. Retail sales of tropical fish and supplies are in the hundreds of millions of dollars per year, with no signs of stopping. So what makes these scaly creatures so fashionable as pets? What's the attraction to owning an aquarium filled with tropical fish?

To begin, aquariums, especially the freshwater variety, are really fairly easy to care for, regardless of what some people might say. With a basic knowledge of aquarium management and tropical fish husbandry, anyone can successfully create and propagate a self-contained aquatic environment. Tropical fish themselves are virtually maintenance-free, requiring only food and a clean, suitable environment in which to live. Unlike dogs, they don't require lots of attention on your part, yet you'll find that once you have your aquarium started, they'll

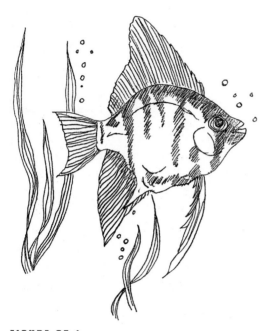

FIGURE 37.1 Aquariums and tropical fish can provide hours of enjoyment and relaxation.

receive loads of it nonetheless (Fig. 37.1).

Maintaining an aquarium filled with tropical fish is a relatively inexpensive endeavor when compared to other types of pet ownership. Aside from initial start-up costs needed for equipment and supplies, the yearly cost of food, maintenance, and new fish rarely places a strain on the average household budget. Fish do not require yearly trips to the veterinarian to keep them healthy, which, as any responsible dog or cat owner knows, can add considerably to the owner's yearly pet expense account.

Finally, people who own tropical fish as pets can plan on reaping the same benefits and sharing in the same joy and satisfaction that come with owning a pet. Aquariums can provide their caretakers with entertainment for hours on end and can contribute to our knowledge of an environmental ecosystem so very different from our own. As educational tools for children, aquariums can't be beat. They are a fun way to teach kids about aquatic life and also provide a means of teaching responsible pet ownership at an early age.

There is one more benefit to owning an aquarium that you might find fascinating. Medical research has actually shown that aquariums can be effective stress-management tools. That is, reduced anxiety levels and lowered blood pressure can result from spending just a few minutes each day observing the steady, flowing movement

DID YOU KNOW?

Fish can hear, even though they have no ear canals!

of aquarium life. Considering today's hectic world, this benefit alone is a good enough reason to rush out and get an aquarium started right away!

Getting Started

There are two types of aquarium environments that tropical fish hobbyists have to choose from: freshwater and saltwater. Since the latter variety requires a greater level of care and expertise (and expense) to ensure success, our discussion, for all practical purposes, is limited to the freshwater aquarium. This is by far the most popular and practical type for children and beginning hobbyists.

In order to create a first-rate freshwater aquarium for yourself or for your kids, you'll need to spend some money on proper equipment and supplies. Of course, you'll need a tank, along with ancillary supplies such as substrate for the bottom of the tank, plants (real or artificial), aquarium cover with fluorescent lighting, thermometers, tank cleaning equipment, and fixtures for your fish to use for shelter. In addition, a good water-quality control system, including water filtration and aeration devices, is a must.

Aquarium Tanks

Aquarium tanks are available in all shapes and sizes, from small goldfish bowls to 200-gallon reservoirs. Obviously, the size of the aquarium will dictate how many fish will be allowed to dwell within, as well as the amount of time necessary for care and cleaning. Regardless of the gallon capacity that you choose (the 10- and 20-gallon varieties are the most popular), it is best to select a tank that is rectangular in shape instead of one that is round or one that is tall and narrow, since the amount of oxygen exchange that occurs between the outside air and the water in the tank is directly proportional to the size of the air-water interface dictated by the shape of the tank (Fig. 37.2). Tropical fish thrive much better in tanks with large surface areas on top, simply because the oxygen levels in these tanks are greater. If a bowl-type aquarium is to be used, be sure to fill it only to the halfway mark with water, in order to achieve the greatest possible surface area for this exchange of oxygen between the air and the water to take place.

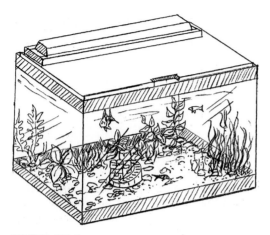

FIGURE 37.2 A rectangular tank allows for better surface-to-air interface than does a round tank.

Avoid aquarium tanks that use metal in their frame construction. Metal, if exposed to water over a period of time, could corrode and become a major source of contamination of your tank water. The more glass in the tank, the better. In fact, aquarium tanks composed entirely of glass with silicone-sealed edges and corners are preferred over others. Some enthusiasts prefer acrylic over glass, simply because of its durability, but the major disadvantage to acrylic is that it tends to scratch easily when cleaned and can become quite unsightly over time.

You will need to equip your aquarium tank with a cover, preferably one with a hinged access door. The purpose of aquarium covers is to keep dust, silt, and other airborne contaminants out of the water, and to keep the fish in! Some of the fancier models come equipped with fluorescent light sources and reflectors, which not only play a useful role in the temperature regulation within the tank but are also desirable if you choose to propagate live plants and vegetation within your aquarium.

Finally, you will need to establish a location within the house to place your new aquarium. Any location will do as long as the tank is not exposed to direct sunlight or environmental pollution. Be sure that the table or stand on which you place your aquarium is sturdy; a 10-gallon aquarium filled with water and ancillary supplies can weigh in excess of 80 pounds!

Ancillary Supplies

Two inches of gravel, stone, pebble, or sand can be used as a bottom lining for your tank to provide an anchoring substrate for plants and shelters and to serve as anchoring points for the tank's biological filter (explained later) (Fig. 37.3). If the gravel or substrate you are planning on using was used in a previous aquarium, be sure to boil it thoroughly to disinfect it before placing it into your tank. The choice between real and artificial plants is entirely up to you. The main advantage of artificial over natural is ease of maintenance and durabil-

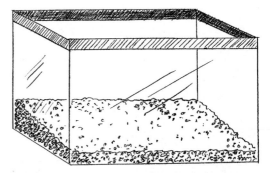

FIGURE 37.3 Sloping the gravel within the tank will cause waste to drift and accumulate at one side of the tank, where it can be more easily removed.

ity. However, for a more aesthetic and natural look to your aquarium environment, live flora can't be beat.

If you'll recall Biology 101, live plants can act as a source of oxygen for your fish through the process called *photosynthesis.* They also provide a source of food for some fish, as well as a place to lay their eggs. If you desire real vegetation over the artificial kind, you'll need to be sure to match it with the type of fish you want to keep in the aquarium. For more information about proper matching, ask a local tropical fish dealer or aquarium shop, or consult your local library, bookstore, or the Internet.

Using live plants also means that you'll need to provide a light source for them. Many aquarium covers contain built-in lighting. Ideally, artificial light sources such as fluorescent lighting (approximately 3 watts per gallon of water) should be used instead of natural lighting, since the latter can be difficult to regulate properly. Eight to ten hours of light each day should be enough to allow your plants to thrive in their watery environment. Be aware, however, that too much lighting is not good and can cause harmful temperature fluctuations within the tank, leading to algae growth.

Finally, every aquarium needs a variety of fixtures and structures designed to provide shelter and security for its finned inhabitants. You can certainly be creative in this department; however, you must also use some caution. If the object you're placing in the aquarium is made of plastic instead of glass or ceramic, be sure that it is nontoxic (including

Table 37.1 Equipment and Supplies Needed for a Freshwater Aquarium

Tank (size based on preference)
Lighted tank hood
Water heater
Thermometer
Gravel
Undergravel filter
Air pump and tubing
Plants, rocks, and decorations
Fish net
Pitcher or bucket

artificial plants!). The same goes for painted fixtures. To be safe, these items should be purchased from an aquarium supply house or pet store instead of trying to supply them yourself from everyday household items (Table 37.1).

Water-Quality Control

Before introducing any fish into your new aquarium, you must make certain that the water you are putting them in is of the highest quality possible. Now this doesn't mean that you'll need to invest in an expensive purification system or purchase stock in a bottled water company. On the contrary, ordinary tap water from the kitchen faucet works just fine as a water source for your aquarium. However, you need to take certain measures to ensure that this water is (and, once in the aquarium, remains) of satisfactory quality to ensure success.

Ordinary tap water is classified as being either "hard" or "soft," depending on the amounts of minerals dissolved within. Test kits are available from aquarium shops that can tell you whether your water supply is hard or soft. Most tropical fish prefer water that is on the soft end [about 40 to 60 ppm (parts per million)]. If you live in an area with hard water, make sure that it is softened before being introduced into the tank. There are several ways to do this. First, the most efficient way (and the most expensive way) is to purchase a water softener that can be hooked into your house's water supply, and will provide a continuous supply of soft water. Other alternatives to purchasing one of these machines or filters include boiling the water first to remove the mineral deposits, or mixing distilled water in with your untreated water to effectively dilute out the hardness.

In addition to correcting water hardness, you must also neutralize or remove the chlorine or chloramine normally added to most water supplies. This is achieved by adding commercially available tablets or powders to the water that are designed specifically for this purpose.

Water temperature is a vital parameter that warrants a fish owner's special attention. In fact, improper maintenance of water temperature is one of the more common causes of aquarium failure that many amateurs encounter. Just because fish are called "tropical" fish doesn't necessarily mean that they automatically thrive in warmer temperatures. In fact, warmer water carries less oxygen, and some of the more sensitive species of tropical fish will do quite poorly in excessively warm water. As a general rule, most tropical fish do well with water temperatures maintained around 75 to 80 degrees Fahrenheit. However, before purchasing many different types of fish for your tank, it would be wise to find out what the ideal temperature is for each species. If the temperature ranges differ significantly, then one species will thrive at the expense of another.

Rapid temperature fluctuations should be avoided at all costs, since these can be quite harmful to fish. Keep this in mind when replacing water within the aquarium. Be sure the water you add is at the same temperature as the existing tank water. And don't worry about the natural thermal layers associated with water. Your aerator pump will keep the water circulating enough to prevent significant temperature gradients from being established.

The best way to maintain narrow temperature margins within your tank is to invest in an aquarium water heater and a quality thermometer. If possible, avoid mercury thermometers. Although they are quite accurate, should the thermometer break and the mercury enter the water, your entire fish population could be fatally poisoned within a matter of minutes.

Fish, like people, rely on oxygen to sustain life. And since fish rely on their water supply for this source of oxygen, it stands to reason that the aquarium enthusiast be sure that the oxygen supply remains adequate. The most common method of ensuring well-oxygenated aquarium water is to install an aerator pump within the tank. These water aerators draw in air from the outside and "bubble" it into the water, helping to stimulate oxygen exchange. The circulating action of these pumps also helps increase total water contact with the outside air at the surface of the tank, thereby allowing greater amounts of oxygen to be absorbed into the system. An efficient aerator pump should exchange about 2 liters of air per 1 liter of water every hour. One interesting point to remember is that the fish are literally breathing the air you breathe; nicotine, fumes, and other pollutants in the air being pumped into the aquarium can have adverse effects on the health of some fish. As a result, take care to shelter your aquarium away from those obvious sources of air pollution.

Live plants, which release oxygen into their surrounding environment through photosynthesis, can also make a significant contribution to the oxygen levels within the aquarium. Also, keeping water temperatures from becoming warmer than the desired ranges and preventing fish overcrowding can both have a positive impact on this aspect of water quality.

Again, the very shape you choose for your aquarium tank (remember the air-water interface) can directly affect the oxygen content of the water, and hence, its overall quality

Filter Systems

In addition to water aeration pumps, a filter system is needed within the aquarium to remove solid and chemical contaminates from the water before they build up to harmful levels. These filters can be classified as either mechanical filters or biological filters. *Mechanical filters* hook onto the outside (or sometimes inside) of the aquarium and actively pump water through a filtering substance, such as filter wool or activated charcoal. Ideally, the capacity of the filter should be such that the entire water content of the tank can pass through it and be filtered every 2 hours. If mechanical filters are used, it is important to replace the filter material on a regular basis, preferably every 3 weeks.

The other type of filter is the *biological filter.* Compared to the cost of a good mechanical filter, the cost of a biological filter is negligible. Yet it can be an even more effective weapon at waste control than its mechanical, more expensive counterpart. A biological filter consists of nothing more than a porous plastic tray that is placed beneath 2 to 3 inches of gravel or substrate lining the bottom of the aquarium. This tray serves as a gathering site for bacteria found within the tank. These bacteria are "biological garbage gobblers" and break down organic wastes that are passively carried through the filter by the normal water circulation within the tank created by the air pump. In this way, Nature does the cleaning for you, the natural way!

Aquarium filters function to keep levels of ammonia and nitrites, two highly toxic substances derived from organic waste, within acceptable ranges. Ideally, the pH of the water should be kept between 6.8 and 7.5, and nitrite levels should be kept to an absolute minimum. Special test kits are available from aquarium shops and should be used to monitor these parameters. Unhealthy rises in pH and nitrite levels in newly established aquariums can often be traced back to an underdeveloped biological filter. Overcrowding and overfeeding can play a significant role as well, and these conditions should be corrected promptly.

When setting up a biological filter in a new tank, start with no more than four small fish as your pioneer population. Because new biological filters can take 3 to 6 weeks to become fully established and functional, daily water rotations (in which 20 percent of the tank water is removed and replaced) should be performed during this time to dilute out offending substances. After 6 weeks, you can begin to add more fish.

For established tanks, regardless of whether you use a mechanical filter, a biological filter, or both, plan on removing and replacing 25 to 30 percent of the water within the tank with seasoned tap water (hardness and chlorine removed) every 4 weeks. This rotation will help eliminate impurities that can't be filtered properly, as well as help ease the burden on the filters themselves (Fig. 37.4). A simple bucket or pitcher can be used to accomplish this task. Remember: Change no more than 30 percent at a time instead of the entire tank to prevent upsetting the environmental equilibrium that has already been established in the aquarium.

Cleaning your Aquarium

How often does an aquarium need to be cleaned? The answer to this is "almost never," assuming, of course that the water-quality control measures above are kept in force. Aeration, filtration, periodic partial water changes, and scavenger fish (explained below) should do the cleaning for you on a continual basis. Keeping the cover closed on your aquarium will help prevent dust and dirt from the outside from soiling the water.

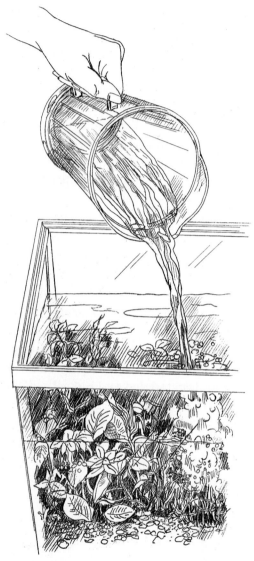

Water that appears gray and cloudy has too much bacteria in it. Such a presentation is caused by a poor filter, overcrowding, or overfeeding, or by failure to properly rotate the water each month. On the other hand, water that appears green and cloudy indicates too much algae. This is caused by excessive exposure to light and by an increase in nitrogen in the water. In both instances, the frequency of water rotations performed must be temporarily increased to regain water quality. Soap-free cleaning pads are useful for scraping off any algae that may have accumulated on the aquarium glass, artificial plants, or stationary fixtures within your tank. Avoid using soaps or detergents to clean your aquarium. Of course, to prevent a recurrence of either problem, the underlying causes must be addressed as well.

FIGURE 37.4 Water rotations help eliminate impurities and support the tank's biological filter.

Selecting Fish for Your Aquarium

As you know, there are countless varieties of tropical fish to choose from when populating your aquarium. The choice is really a matter of your preference and taste. Some people prefer ones with exotic coloring or patterns; others prefer larger varieties over the smaller ones. In addition, some species are more sensitive and delicate than others, and might require more attention and maintenance than you are willing to devote.

One thing you'll want to be very careful of is not to overstock your aquarium with fish. Tank overcrowding is right up there with poor water quality and temperature fluctuations as a major cause of aquarium failures. As a general rule, you should have no more than one inch of fish per one gallon of water. Exceed this ratio, and oxygen content and water quality will suffer.

The various tropical fish species can be classified into groups according to their aggressiveness toward other fish. For instance, goldfish, guppies, and mollies are all known for their mild-mannered temperaments, whereas angelfish can be considered semiaggressive, sometimes making a meal of fish small enough to swallow. Bettas and paradise fish are highly aggressive fish and won't hesitate to pick a fight with any fish in the tank. Regardless of which species you prefer, obviously you don't want to mix aggressive or semiaggressive fish with nonaggressive fish. In fact, if you decide to stock your tank with more aggressive varieties, you'll need to be observant of individual personalities to prevent your serene, peaceful aquarium setting from becoming a battleground!

Besides the more ornamental varieties, you'll want to stock your aquarium with one or more scavenger fish. These fish will inhabit the bottom of the tank or cling to its sides and feed on the algae and leftover food particles. As a result, these scavenger fish play an important role in maintaining water quality. Some of the more popular names include the *cory catfish,* the *suckermouth cats,* and the *coolie loach.* Large, freshwater snails are effective scavengers as well and can be introduced into an aquarium setting for this purpose.

Each type of fish you choose will often have its own little idiosyncrasies as to ideal food, water temperature, pH, and other water conditions. For best results when selecting tropical fish (keeping your desires in mind as well), ask your tropical fish retailer or specialist for recommendations on which tropical fish varieties will work best for you.

What to Look for

When selecting your fish at the aquarium shop or pet store, there are a few items to look for to ensure that you receive healthy pets. First, observe the way a particular fish behaves in its current aquarium setting. It should be active and alert and glide smoothly through the water when swimming. Fish that act lethargic or swim in a crooked or sideways pattern should be avoided.

Anatomically, all fins should be erect and intact, and the fish's belly should be slightly rounded versus sunken. Look for blotchy, discolored skin, ulcerations, or any other obvious signs of disease or parasitism. Eyes should be bright, not cloudy. If one fish in a particular tank is showing signs of illness, assume that all within that tank have been exposed to the disease, and avoid selecting fish from that tank altogether.

DR. P's VET TIP

When purchasing fish from a pet store, check out the water color in the tank containing your potential selections. Water that appears yellow, blue, or green could be medicated, indicating a disease outbreak in the tank. If so, move along to the next tank!

Your Pets' New Home

Once you've purchased your new friends, you'll want to slowly introduce them to their new home. Again, be sure all pumps and filters are in place and in working order. The transport container containing the fish should be lowered into the tank water, which should already be at the desired temperature (check your thermometer). Leave the container suspended like this for a good 15 to 20 minutes to allow for a gradual temperature equalization between the two water compartments. Once this is accomplished, open the transport container and allow the fish, at their leisure, to enter into their new domain.

Aquarium owners should make it a point to keep handling and disturbances to a minimum once the fish are set in their environment. The common urge among many beginners to tap on the aquarium glass to get a particular fish's attention should be suppressed! Avoiding this type of behavior will help keep stress levels low and make for a much healthier, happier environment.

If for some reason a fish needs to be removed from the tank, a small net should be used. As an alternative, a plastic storage bag with small holes punched in its bottom makes an excellent fish-catcher. Regardless of which you use, be as slow, deliberate, and patient as possible when trying to capture a fish, thereby keeping stress to an absolute minimum.

Feeding Your Fish

Prepackaged fish food is readily available, and comes in all forms and fashions, such as processed, frozen, or freeze-dried. As a general rule, you should feed only that amount of food that will be consumed within a 3- to 4-minute period. Leftovers are not good, and will eventually build up to such levels at the bottom of the tank as to start adversely affecting the water quality within the tank. Two feedings, one in the morning and one in the afternoon, should suffice to satisfy even the heartiest of appetites!

Diseases and Disorders

Selected diseases and disorders seen in tropical fish are listed in Table 37.2. Healthy fish should have smooth, glistening skin surfaces and should exhibit steady, controlled movement within the aquarium. Diseased fish, aside from exhibiting obvious external signs, will exhibit unusual swimming and behavioral patterns. For instance, excessive drifting, circling, hiding, curling, or bottom-sitting are all signs of disease and should alert you to a potential problem.

Stress, poor water quality, and failure to quarantine new additions to the aquarium are the three leading factors leading to disease outbreaks within aquariums. If disease does rear its

Dr. P's Vet Tip

When treating tropical fish suffering from white spot or velvet parasites, gradually raise the water temperature to 82 degrees Fahrenheit to speed up the life cycle of these parasites and expedite the cure.

Table 37.2 Diseases and Disorders of Tropical Fish

Disease or disorder	Clinical signs	Treatment and comments
Diseases related to water quality		
Ammonia and nitrite toxicity	Death of existing fish; inability to keep new additions alive	Caused by improper biological filters; treat by establishing filter; daily water change for 2–3 weeks to keep ammonia and nitrite concentrations low
Diseases		
Velvet	Yellow pollenlike spots on skin; scratching against rocks	Purchase commercial velvet treatment; raise water temperature to 82°F (slowly)
Ich (ichthyophthirius)	White spots or pustules on skin; fish scratch against rocks	Known as "white spot disease"; purchase commercial treatment; slowly raise water temperature to 82°F
Chilodenella; other protozoans; flukes	Excessive body mucus production; damaged gills; irritable behavior; gill rubbing	Treat by adding formalin to water (1 milliliter per 10 gallons of water), then changing water 8 hours later; fish in terminal stages of illness could die from treatment
Hexamita	General unthriftiness; white, stringy feces; thinning	Common in angelfish; treat with metronidazole (250 milligrams per 10 gallons of water)

Table 37.2 Diseases and Disorders of Tropical Fish (*Continued*)

Disease or disorder	Clinical signs	Treatment and comments
Diseases		
"Hole in the head"	Ulcerations on head and sides of body	May be associated with *Hexamita*; treat with frequent water changes, metronidazole; rarely causes death
Tapeworms	General unthriftiness; thinning	Treat by adding the drug praziquantel to water (90 milligrams per 10 gallons of water)
Bacterial diseases		
Aeromonas, Pseudomonas	Ulcerations on skin; unthriftiness	Often occur secondary to parasites or other diseases; treat with antibiotics added to water
Columnaris disease	Gray-white patches on skin; fraying or loss of fins and tail	Treat with frequent water changes and antibiotics added to the water
Septicemia	Reddish hue to skin; lethargy; unthriftiness; bulging eyes; bloat (dropsy)	Treat with antibiotics; generally unrewarding; improve water quality
Viral diseases		
Lymphocystis disease	White, raised plaques on surface of skin and tail	No treatment available; isolate infected fish; sanitize aquarium

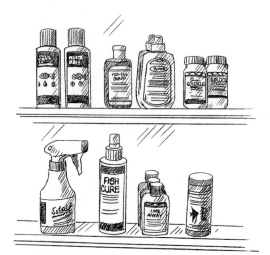

FIGURE 37.5 A number of over-the-counter remedies are available to treat tropical fish diseases.

ugly head within your aquarium, it is important that the disease be identified and treated quickly. Treatment for disease outbreaks generally consists of isolation of infected fish, partial or complete water changes performed on a prescribed schedule, and/or the addition of specific medications to the water within the tank (Fig. 37.5). If you seem to be having chronic problems keeping your fish healthy, contact your local veterinarian for advice or, if your vet is not versed in aquarium management and fish diseases, for referral to the proper resources that you need to answer your questions and find a solution.

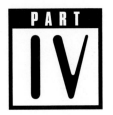

Other Interesting Pet Topics

First Aid for Dogs and Cats

Would you know the correct way to perform cardiopulmonary resuscitation (CPR) on your cat, how to administer first aid to your dog if it is hit by a car, or what to do if your pet swallows a poisonous substance? If not, here is your opportunity to learn. Note that this section is designed to instruct you on first aid for dogs and cats, and on the recognition of clinical signs and true emergency situations that involve your pet. By no means is this chapter intended to replace professional veterinary care. On the contrary, it simply provides a reference source for temporary management of minor and major emergencies until a veterinarian can see your pet.

All drugs, medications, and dosages contained herein are based on the author's recommendations, and are not necessarily the recommendation of the product's manufacturer or distributor.

The Five Goals of First Aid for Pets

- Keep your safety in mind at all times.
- Attend to any arterial or severe venous hemorrhage present.
- Administer CPR if needed.
- Immobilize injuries and/or pet for transport.

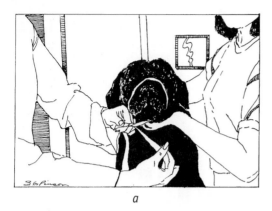

a

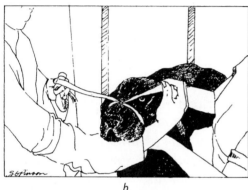

b

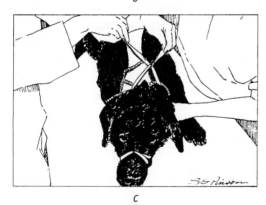

c

Figure 38.1 *(a–c)* Applying a muzzle.

- Transport to a veterinarian as soon as possible. Never delay in seeking professional help. Delay increases treatment costs and decreases treatment success rates.

What to Do When You Encounter an Emergency Situation

- Don't panic!

- Assess your surroundings, including environmental hazards such as
  Moving vehicles
  Broken glass
  Chemical spills
  Fire and electrical hazards

- Approach injured or ill animals slowly and with caution.

- Use a calm, reassuring voice.

- Apply a muzzle (see Fig. 38.1):
  Injured or ill animals will often bite out of pain or fear—don't take it personally!

A sturdy gauze roll, necktie, leash, belt, or cell phone power cord can be used .

Never use a muzzle on an animal that is vomiting, choking, convulsing, or having breathing difficulties. For these pets, for cats, and for dogs that have facial conformations that render muzzles useless, use heavy-duty gloves or drape a blanket or thick towel over the animal's head prior to handling.

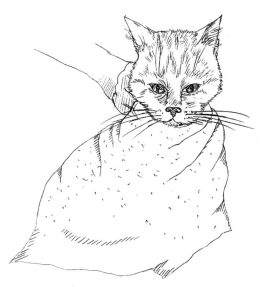

Figure 38.2 A towel wrap and a firm neck grip can be useful when restraining an anxious cat.

■ For injured or ill cats, restrain front and hind legs to prevent scratches. Duct tape, gauze, or leashes can be used to tie legs together, or a towel can be draped over the cat's body (Fig. 38.2).

■ Determine whether a life-threatening situation exists and render appropriate first aid.

Look, listen, and feel for abnormalities and obvious problems.

Unconsciousness, shock, hemorrhage, breathing difficulties, any HBC (hit-by-car) or other trauma, poisoning, and air leakage from chest are all life-threatening.

Once the major challenges have been addressed, you can then direct your attention to other, less serious problems.

■ Transport the pet to a veterinarian or to a veterinary emergency hospital.

Transport securely—use a travel kennel, box, or pillowcase (cats).

If head or spinal injury is suspected, use a board, plywood, window screen, or any flat, firm surface to transport. If this flat support is not available, gently transport the pet in a large towel or small blanket (Fig. 38.3).

Telephone the veterinarian or emergency clinic in advance of your arrival.

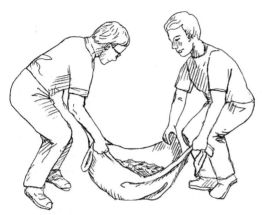

Figure 38.3 Use extreme care when transporting a pet with a suspected spinal injury.

Planning for the Emergency

Read and rehearse ahead of time; chances are that you won't have time to consult a book when a true emergency occurs.

- Gather important fingertip information:
  Preferred veterinary hospital
  Two of the closest 24-hour veterinary emergency clinics
  ASPCA Poison Control Center: (800) 548-2423

- Assemble or purchase a pet first aid kit (many of these items can be purchased from a veterinarian):

Muzzle	Hydrogen peroxide
Leash	Kaolin-pectin
Welder's gloves	Activated charcoal
Stretch bandage	Triple antibiotic ointment
Roll gauze	Splint
Solar blanket	Forceps and/or tweezers
Bandage tape	Scissors
Sterile nonstick wound pads	Bulb syringe
Clean hand towel	Plastic digital thermometer
Cotton balls and/or swabs	Reusable cold pack
Chlorhexidine wash (0.5%)	12-milliliter syringe
Saline solution	Disposable gloves
Sterile eye ointment	Feeding tubes
Lubricating jelly	Commercial pet piller
Clotting powder	

■ Home remedies:

Certain over-the-counter (OTC) medications (see Tables 38.1 to 38.3) can be used for emergencies in select instances. Always consult the veterinarian before administering any OTC medication to your injured or ill pet, as doing so may affect the vet's treatment plan.

Table 38.1 Useful Over-the-Counter Medications for Dogs and Cats

Medication	Indication	Dosage
3% hydrogen peroxide	To induce vomiting; general wound cleanser	1 teaspoon per 10 pounds
Syrup of ipecac (dogs only)	To induce vomiting	1 teaspoon per 20 pounds
Bismuth subsalicylate (dogs only)	Vomiting; mild diarrhea	1 teaspoon per 15 pounds 1 tablet per 40 pounds
Kaolin-pectin	Mild diarrhea	1 teaspoon per 10 pounds
Buffered aspirin (dogs only)	Fever and inflammation; mild to moderate pain; arthritis	1 adult tablet (5 grains) per 40 pounds
Diphenhydramine	Mild cough; allergies; allergic reactions	1 milligram per pound
Vegetable oil	Constipation; hairballs	1 teaspoon per 5 pounds mixed in food
Epsom salts	Constipation (dogs only); as a soak to reduce swelling and inflammation; do not give orally to cats	For constipation, 1 teaspoon per 10 pounds, dissolved in water and given orally; same dilution for soaks
Milk of magnesia	Vomiting; constipation; deactivate poisons	2 teaspoons per 10 pounds
Activated charcoal	Deactivate poisons	$1/2$ gram per pound
Petroleum jelly	Hairballs; constipation	$1/2$ teaspoon per 10 pounds

Note: Always consult your veterinarian before administering any of these over-the-counter medications to your pet.

Table 38.2 Useful Conversions

1 milliliter (mL)	=	1 cubic centimeter (cc) (cm³)
1 teaspoon (tsp)	=	5 milliliters (mL)
1 tablespoon (tbs)	=	15 milliliters (mL)
1 ounce (oz)	=	30 milliliters (mL)
1 pound (lb)	=	454 grams (g)
1 kilogram (kg)	=	2.2 pounds (lb)

Table 38.3 Drugs and Medications That Can Be Highly Toxic to Cats

Aspirin

Acetaminophen

Ibuprofen

Iodine

Coal tar shampoo

Organophosphate insecticides

Phosphate enemas

Primidone

General First Aid Procedures

Administering Oral Medications

ADMINISTERING ORAL TABLETS

- Lubricate the tablet with a small dab of butter or margarine.

- Place your hand over the pet's top jaw, with your thumb and fingers situated behind the upper canine teeth.

- Tilt the head back while pressing inward and upward with your thumb and fingers, causing the pet to open its mouth.

- With fingers of your free hand (the one holding the pill), pull down gently on the lower jaw (see Fig. 38.4).

- Place or, for cats, pop the pill far back on the center of the tongue, using your fingers or better yet, a pet-piller (available from a veterinarian).

- Close the pet's mouth and gently stroke its throat or blow on its nose to encourage swallowing.

ADMINISTERING ORAL LIQUIDS

For Dogs

- Hook your finger between the skin at the corner of the mouth and the teeth and "tent" the skin of the cheek out away from the gumline (Fig. 38.5).

- Insert the syringe, dropper, or spoon into the pocket formed.

- Pointing the pet's muzzle upward at a 45-degree angle, deliver the medication slowly.

- Gently stroke the throat to encourage swallowing.

- Do not deliver a liquid medication directly onto the tongue or into the back of the throat, as the pet may choke on it.

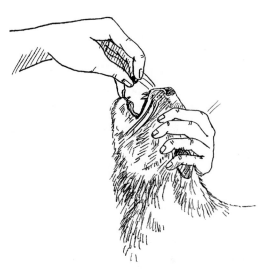

Figure 38.4 Administering a pill to a cat.

For Cats

- If the cat is rambunctious, wrap tightly in a towel with only the head exposed.

- Grasp and squeeze the skin on the neck just behind the head (this does not hurt cats; on the contrary, it usually has a calming effect).

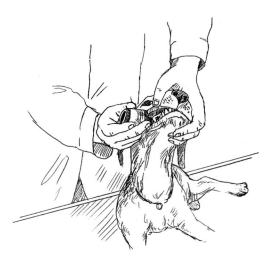

Figure 38.5 When administering liquid medication to a dog, "tent" the skin of the cheek to form a pocket, then insert the medication into the pocket.

- Insert the syringe tip, dropper, or spoon into either side of the mouth (Fig. 38.6).

- Deliver the medication slowly.

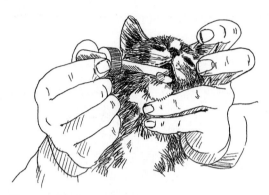

Figure 38.6 Administering liquid medication to a cat.

Obtaining and Assessing Vital Signs

OBTAINING A PET'S TEMPERATURE

■ Lubricate the tip of a plastic digital thermometer with a water-soluble lubricant—do not use glass thermometers, as these can break and damage rectal tissue.

■ Insert the digital thermometer into the anus and hold it in place until a final reading is obtained.

■ Elevated temperatures (see normal values in Table 38.4) can be caused by increased physical activity, high environmental temperatures, inflammation, and/or infection.

■ If your pet's temperature reading is higher than 102.5 degrees Fahrenheit and your pet seems lethargic or showing signs of illness, call the veterinarian for advice.

OBTAINING A PULSE READING

Several different methods can be used:

1. In the lower chest region, just behind the point of the elbow

2. In the groin region, or more specifically, in the middle of the inner portion of either leg just below its junction with the abdomen

3. Along the groove formed by the trachea and the muscles of the neck

Keeping an eye on your watch, simply count the number of pulses or heartbeats you detect over a 20-second period, then multiply this number by three to obtain a per-minute rate.

Table 38.4 Normal Values

Species	Temperature (degrees Fahrenheit)	Pulse (beats per minute)	Respirations (per minute)
Dog	99.5–102.5	60–120	12–22
Cat	100–103.2	80–140	20–30
Small bird	108–112	600–800	75–100
Large bird	108–112	200–300	30–50
Rabbit	102–103.5	175–210	50–75
Guinea pig	100–102.5	250–300	80–90
Small rodents	95–101	350–600	80–150
Chinchilla	102–103	200–350	45–80
Prairie dog	97–102.5	85–300	50–100
Hedgehog	97–100	200–300	45–100
Ferret	100–103	200–250	80–100
Pot-bellied pig	100.5–103	80–100	15–30

OBTAINING A RESPIRATORY RATE

Simply observe the rise and fall of the ribcage as the pet breathes. Count the number of breaths taken over a 15-second interval, then multiply that figure by 4.

The Physical Exam

- Perform routinely on all pets each month.
- The physical exam is helpful for assessing an injured or ill pet.
- Early detection of health problems increases treatment success rates.
- See physical exam checklist in Chap. 4.

Addressing Immediate Life-Threatening Conditions

Active Hemorrhage

To control active hemorrhage:

- Apply direct pressure over the source of the bleeding using any absorbable material or object available, such as a shirt, towel, or gauze.

- For minor bleeding, maintain this pressure with your hands for a good 5 minutes before releasing.

- For major hemorrhage, including those instances where blood spurts from the wound (indicating a damaged artery), secure the compress tightly over the wound using gauze, a belt, pantyhose, or a necktie and seek veterinary help immediately. If an extremity is involved, pressure applied to the inside, upper portion of the affected leg (near its attachment to the body; see Fig. 38.7) will also reduce blood flow to the limb.

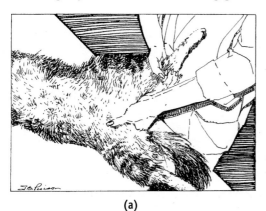

(a)

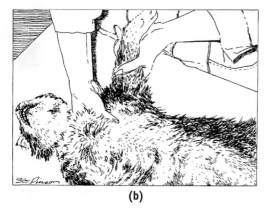

(b)

Figure 38.7 (*a, b*) Applying pressure to stop bleeding from an extremity.

- A tourniquet can be applied above hemorrhage point if all other efforts fail (tie and twist); loosen every 10 minutes to minimize tissue damage.

Circulatory Shock

- *Circulatory shock* is a life-threatening situation often associated with trauma and other serious medical disorders in animals, so prompt attention to this condition is vital.

- With shock, the blood fails to circulate properly throughout the body; as a result, the tissues and organs do not get enough oxygen to maintain their normal functions.

- Causes of shock can include excessive bleeding, heart disease, infection, and severe stress and pain due to trauma or any major illness.

- Symptoms are rapid heart rate; weak, thready pulse; cold, pale mucous membranes (gray to white in color); dry, shriveled tongue; weakness; stupor or unconsciousness; panting; and subnormal body temperature.

- Unfortunately, there are no specific first aid techniques to counteract this condition in pets, other than keeping the animal calm and warm.
  Blankets, towels, or hot-water bottles (empty 2-liter soda bottles filled with warm water) can be used to provide warmth.
  A solar blanket is useful as well for keeping the pet warm.

- Shock needs to be treated with intravenous fluids, colloids, and medications administered by a veterinarian; therefore, the sooner you get a shocky pet to a veterinarian, the better are its chances of survival.

Breathing Difficulties, Choking, and Chest Wounds

Signs of breathing difficulties and choking include:

- Coughing
- Gagging
- Wide-base stance with head and neck extended
- Open-mouth breathing
- Pale or purple (cyanotic) gums and mucous membranes
- Forceful expansion and contraction of the ribcage

Choking can be caused by foreign bodies, trauma to mouth or trachea, laryngeal swelling or paralysis, tracheal stenosis, and allergic reactions. To relieve choking caused by foreign bodies

- Carefully open the animal's mouth.

- Place your hand over the pet's top jaw, with your thumb and fingers situated behind the upper canine teeth.

- Tilt the head back while pressing inward and upward with your thumb and fingers, causing the pet to open its mouth.

- Use a tongue depressor or pen to flatten the tongue—do not use your finger.

- If you see a foreign object, attempt to dislodge and remove it with a pair of tweezers or small needle-nose pliers. *If the animal is conscious, do not use your hands.*

If these attempts are unsuccessful:

- Place a hand on each side of the chest and abdomen (near the last three ribs; see Fig. 38.8) with your fingers facing toward the pet's head.

- Apply a forceful, upward-and-inward compression.

- Repeat until the foreign object is dislodged.

For sucking chest wounds, characterized by a rush of air from the wound opening and breathing difficulties:

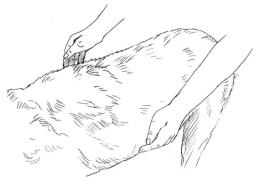

Figure 38.8 Applying quick, forceful pressure on either side of the chest near the last three ribs can be used to dislodge a foreign object caught in the airways.

1. With a piece of gauze, a clean cloth, or article of clothing, seal the wound by applying firm pressure.

2. Secure the seal and compress to the site with a belt, duct tape, or other wraparound object, making sure that the bandage does not interfere with normal chest expansion needed for breathing (see Fig. 38.9).

3. Transport to a veterinarian immediately.

Cessation of Breathing or Heartbeat

Cardiopulmonary resuscitation (CPR) involves artificial respiration and external heart massage. The ABCs of CPR are as follows:

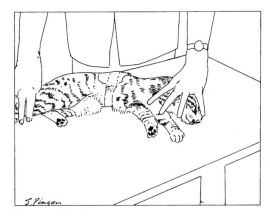

Figure 38.9 Bandaging a chest wound in a cat.

Airway—should be clear and patent

Breathing—artificial respiration

Circulation—external heart massage

Artificial respiration is used to supply oxygen to the lungs and tissues in those instances when a pet has stopped breathing. If the heart has stopped beating, external heart massage is needed as well to help maintain circulation. The following guidelines are

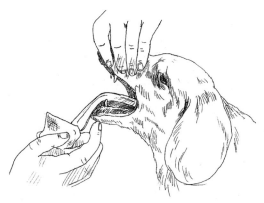

Figure 38.10 Ensure a patent airway by extending the neck, gently pulling out the tongue, observing the oral cavity, and, if necessary, sweeping the mouth with your fingers.

recommended for applying artificial respiration:

1. If the pet is unconscious and has stopped breathing (no evidence of chest wall expansion; pluck a few hairs from the coat and hold in front of nostrils), look inside the mouth and sweep the mouth with your finger (Fig. 38.10) to clear it of any blood, mucus, vomitus, or other debris that may be present. Foreign objects may also be removed with tweezers or needle-nose pliers.

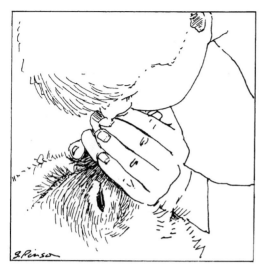

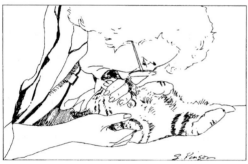

Figure 38.11 Artificial respiration is performed by blowing air directly into the nostrils.

2. If needed, perform abdominal thrusts to clear the airway of debris.

3. Tilt the head back to straighten the airway, then clasp the mouth shut with your hand and place your mouth over your pet's nose and mouth, forming a tight seal (Fig. 38.11).

4. Blow into the nose until you see the chest expand (if a small puppy or kitten is involved, deliver gentle puffs of breath to inflate the lungs).

5. If the chest doesn't expand, repeat the first two steps, then try again. If there still is no expansion, probe the back of the throat for a foreign body obstructing the airway.

6. Release the seal, allowing your pet to fully exhale.

7. Deliver three more breaths in rapid succession, then check for a pulse.

8. Repeat this sequence once every 3 seconds until the pet is breathing on its own, or until veterinary assistance is obtained.

If these attempts are unsuccessful, apply external heart massage:

1. If no pulse is detected, institute external heart massage.

2. Administering three breaths in rapid succession, lay the pet on its right side and place the heel of one hand on the ribcage just

behind the elbow and place the other hand on top of the first (Fig. 38.12).

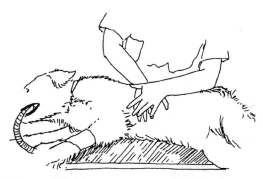

3. Using a smooth, rhythmic movement, compress the chest about 30 to 40 percent with your hands.

Figure 38.12 When giving CPR, perform two chest compressions per second (120 compressions per minute). After every 10 compressions, perform artificial respiration.

4. Each compression should last no more than 1/2 second.

5. Perform these chest compressions at a minimum rate of one per second (two per second is ideal).

6. After every 5 seconds (5 to 10 compressions), administer a breath.

7. Check for a heartbeat after every second cycle; if still no heartbeat, resume CPR.

8. Discontinue external heart massage when a heartbeat is detected.

Acupressure can also be employed in life-threatening situations (see Fig. 45.6).

Managing Trauma in Pets

Common Sources of Trauma

- Automobiles (tires, fenders, fan belts)
- Bullets, pellets, arrows, and other foreign bodies
- Fights with other animals
- Falls or jumps from elevations (high-rise syndrome) or automobiles
- Blows from blunt objects

See also Table 38.5.

Table 38.5 Injuries and Disorders Commonly Resulting from Hit-by-Car Trauma

Fractures—limbs, pelvis, jaw, skull
Lung contusions and fluid buildup
Ruptured organ or internal bleeding
Concussion
Diaphragmatic hernia
Shock
Spinal injuries

Priorities

1. Ensure safety first.
2. Ensure a patent (open, unobstructed) airway.
3. Control bleeding.
4. Check respiration rate and pulse.
5. Perform CPR if needed.
6. Manage chest wounds.
7. Bandage wounds and/or immobilize fractures.
8. If spinal injury is suspected, slide the pet onto a board, piece of plywood, stiff piece of cardboard, window screen, or taut blanket before transporting.
9. If a head injury is suspected, keep head level with body or elevated at a 20-degree angle.
10. Transport to a veterinarian as soon as possible.

Wounds: Applying Dressings and Bandages

A *dressing* is a protective covering that is placed directly over a wound (Fig. 38.13). It can be made of any material but should always be sterile or at least very clean. It can be used to control bleeding, to absorb blood and other fluids, and to minimize wound contamination.

Dressings are held in place by bandages:

■ Gauze, stretch, and elastic bandages can be used.

■ All types can be secured with tape, safety pins, or clips.

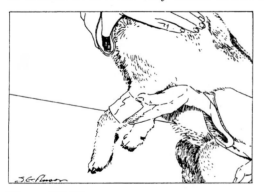

Figure 38.13   Applying a dressing to a wound.

- The bandage should be tight enough to keep the dressing in place, yet not so tight that it interferes with circulation; swelling and discoloration at the affected site should prompt you to loosen the bandage.
- Bandages applied across joints can impede circulation; monitor closely for tissue swelling.

To apply a bandage:

1. If indicated, clean the wound first.
2. Apply a nonstick absorbant wound pad (dressing).
3. Secure the dressing with a layer wrapping of roll gauze or cotton.
4. Secure the wrapping with an elastic, gauze, or stretch bandage.
5. Secure the bandage (i.e., with tape).

See also Fig. 38.14.

Fracture Management

Signs of a fracture are as follows:

- Abnormal limb position or mobility
- Localized pain
- Bruising and/or swelling

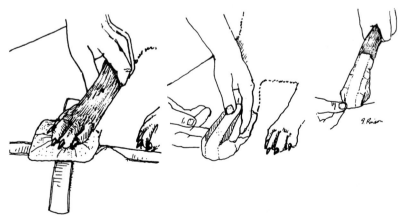

Figure 38.14 Bandaging a lacerated paw.

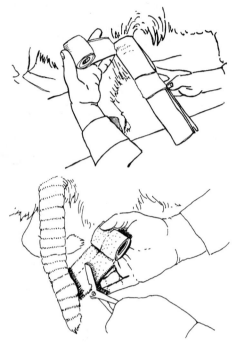

Figure 38.15 One method of temporary fracture stabilization using a rolled-up magazine.

- Crepitation (the crackling feel made when two ends of bone rub together)
- Exposed bone (open fracture)

For open fractures:

1. Control bleeding

2. Do not attempt to replace the exposed ends of bone or to clean the wound

3. Apply a dressing or bandage

For closed fractures:

1. If the fracture is located below the elbow or knee, immobilize the fracture with a splint made of a rolled-up magazine (Fig. 38.15), stick, thick towel, ruler, bubble packing wrap, or sturdy cardboard.

2. Affix the splint to the limb with a belt, necktie, duct tape, or other wraparound material.

3. Do not tape or tie directly over the fracture site.

Managing Poisoning in Pets

Common Sources of Poisoning

- Antifreeze
- Over-the-counter medications (e.g., aspirin, acetaminophen, and naproxen are highly toxic to cats)
- Prescription medications (antidepressents, cardiac medications, arthritis medications)
- Rat, snail, roach, and predator poisons
- Food (chocolate, salt, etc.)

Table 38.6 Ornamental Plants That Can Be Hazardous to Pets

Aconite	Hydrangea
Amaryllis	Iris
Azalea	Jerusalem cherry
Bittersweet	Jonquil
Caladium	Larkspur
Castor bean	Laurel
Common box	Lily-of-the-valley
Crown-of-thorns	Narcissus
Daffodils	Nightshades
Daphne	Oleander
Dumbcane	Philodendron
Elephant ear	Pine needles
English holly	Precatory bean
English ivy	Rhododendron
Euonymous	Rose bay
Foxglove	Skunk cabbage
Honeysuckle	Wisteria
Hyacinth	Yew

- Frogs, toads, salamanders
- Pesticides and insecticides
- House plants (see Table 38.6)

Signs of poisoning

- Vomiting
- Diarrhea
- Depression

- Unconsciousness
- Seizures
- Muscle tremors
- Abdominal pain
- Drooling
- Panting

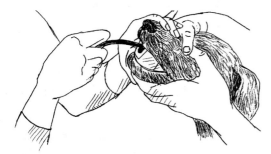

Figure 38.16 A veterinarian administering activated charcoal via a stomach tube to neutralize a poison.

Table 38.7 Poisonings in Which Vomiting Should *Not* Be Induced

Bathroom cleaners
Drain cleaners
Dry-cleaning fluids
Fire extinguisher fluids
Fuels (gas, oil, kerosene)
Furniture polish
Glues and adhesives
Laundry bleach
Metal cleaners
Oven cleaners
Paint and varnish removers
Rust removers

Rapid Management of the Poisoned Pet

The goal of treatment is to eliminate, dilute, or neutralize the poison as quickly as possible prior to veterinary intervention (e.g., as shown in Fig. 38.16). If the poison came from a container, read and follow the label directions concerning accidental poisoning; be sure to take the label and container with you to the veterinarian. If the pet has ingested a caustic or petroleum-based substance, or is severely depressed, seizuring, or unconscious, waste no time in seeking veterinary help.

For other types of poisons that were ingested, induce vomiting (however, see list in Table 38.7) using a teaspoon per 10 pounds of body weight of hydrogen peroxide or $1/2$ milliliter per pound syrup of ipecac (dogs only):

- Repeat the dosage of hydrogen peroxide in 5 minutes if needed.

- If the pet does not vomit within 10 minutes, abandon your efforts and transport to a veterinarian.

- Once the pet vomits, administer activated charcoal ($1/2$ gram per pound of body weight) to help deactivate any residual poison, then take the pet to the nearest veterinarian immediately.

- If the poison was applied to the skin, flush the affected areas with copious amounts of water.

- If the offending substance is oil-based, a quick bath using water plus a mechanical hand cleanser or dishwashing liquid should be given to remove any remaining residue.

- In all instances of poisoning, specific antidotes may be available at the veterinarian's office; as a result, always seek out professional care following your own initial first aid efforts.

Other Common Emergencies in Pets

Allergic Reactions

Allergic reactions (e.g., see Fig. 38.17) can occur following administration of medications or vaccinations, or exposure to chemicals and environmental irritants or snake and insect bites. The degree of reaction can vary considerably with each incident. Signs can show up minutes to hours (usually no more than 6 hours) following exposure to the offending substance and can include intense itching, skin rash, facial swelling, hives, vomiting, and lethargy.

A severe allergic reaction (called *anaphylactic shock*) constitutes a true medical

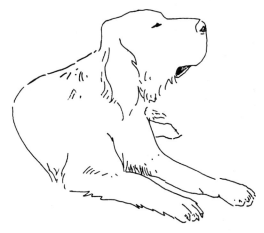

Figure 38.17 Acute allergic reactions are often accompanied by intense facial swelling.

emergency. This type of reaction most often appears seconds to minutes after exposure to the offending agent, and signs include breathing difficulties, protracted vomiting, shock, collapse, and unconsciousness. If the reaction was caused by application of a topical substance, wash off as much of the offending substance as possible. For mild to moderate reactions, a cold-water bath or oatmeal bath often helps relieve itching. Diphenhydramine can be administered orally at a dosage of 1 milligram per pound of body weight.

Bleeding Toenails

Apply direct pressure to the nail for 5 to 10 minutes. Then apply commercially available clotting powder, flour, or toothpaste to the exposed end of the nail (see Fig. 38.18).

Bloat (Gastric Dilatation–Volvulus Complex)

Gastric dilatation–volvulus complex (GDV), or bloat, is a serious, life-threatening disorder that usually affects large, deep-chested breeds such as Great Danes, Saint Bernards, Irish setters, Standard poodles, Rottweilers, and English sheepdogs. Dachshunds and Pekinese also have a higher incidence of GDV than do other similar-sized breeds. Regardless of the size and age of the dog, death can quickly ensue if the condition is not recognized and treated with speed. Genetic predisposition, as well as rapid ingestion of a large amount of food and water, followed by exercise, is an important predisposing cause for this disorder.

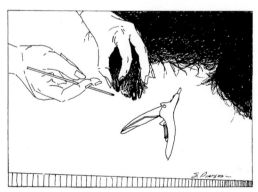

Figure 38.18 Bleeding from a toenail can be easily controlled and is no cause for alarm.

GDV results when the stomach dilates following food, water, gas, and stomach secretions. This dilatation, in turn, puts pressure on the large blood vessels located within the abdomen and seriously reduces blood flow through them, placing almost every major organ within the abdomen in serious jeopardy. Cardiac arrhythmias and irregular heartbeats often occur and can prove fatal. Once dilated, the stomach may rotate or twist (volvulus) on its long axis, blocking off all entry into and exit from the stomach. The condition worsens as the stomach contents are not allowed to escape and more gas and secretions fill the stomach.

Signs of GDV includes distended, bloated abdomen, vomiting (often unproductive), excessive salivation, rapid breathing, abdominal pain, restlessness, weakness, and shock. Prompt veterinary treatment, including surgery, will be needed to save the life of the pet.

For dogs predisposed to GDV, consider preventive surgery. GDV can be prevented by feeding small meals multiple times during the day, with no exercise after feeding, and controlling water consumption after exercise.

Bruises, Strains, and Sprains

For minor bruising and orthopedic injuries resulting from trauma:

1. Apply a cold pack or ice pack (wrapped in towels) to the affected area for 15 minutes every 4 hours following the injury (for up to 72 hours).

2. Restrict your pet to leash-only activity for 2 weeks.

3. Do not administer pain relievers; these could encourage excess activity, which could make the injury worse.

If lameness does not steadily improve over the next 14 days, seek veterinary assistance.

Burns

THERMAL

Signs of thermal burns include skin redness, blisters, charred skin, and singed haircoat.

If skin is not blistered:

1. Run cold water over the affected area for 15 minutes or wrap an ice pack in a towel and place on the burn for 15 minutes.

2. Apply a small amount of topical anesthetic cream to help soothe the burn.

If skin is blistered:

1. Do not immerse in water or apply any medication to the burned surface.
2. Apply a sterile, nonadherent dressing and bandage.
3. Transport to your veterinarian.

CHEMICAL

Signs of chemical burns include skin redness, blisters, oral ulcers, and moist skin and haircoat (where chemical contact was made).

Neutralize or remove the offending chemical:

1. Flush the affected site thoroughly with water for 5 minutes, even if the skin is blistered or broken.
2. Do not apply any topical medication to the burn site.
3. If the offending substance is acidic, mix 1 teaspoon of baking soda into 1 cup of water and apply to the affected region.
4. If the offending substance is basic, mix 1 teaspoon of vinegar into 1 cup of water and apply to the affected region.
5. Flush the region with water for 5 minutes.
6. Apply a sterile dressing and bandage.
7. Prevent the pet from licking or chewing at the affected region.
8. Transport to your veterinarian.

Constipation

Isolated incidents of simple constipation can be treated at home, yet if the problem persists, recurs frequently, or is accompanied by lethargy, abdominal pain, or vomiting, a medical exam is warranted.

Constipation can be mistaken for colitis, intestinal foreign bodies, and urinary disorders. For simple constipation:

1. Administer a hairball laxative or petroleum jelly orally at 1 teaspoon per 10 pounds; repeat in 4 hours.
2. Vegetable oil may also be used to relieve constipation; dose at 1 teaspoon per 10 pounds (mixed with food).

3. Do not attempt to give an enema at home.

For long-term management, consider adding fiber to your pet's diet.

Cuts and Abrasions

1. If minor bleeding is occurring, apply direct pressure to the wound for 5 minutes, using a sterile gauze pad or clean cloth.

2. If clippers are available, apply a water-soluble lubricating gel to the wound, then clip the hair from around the wound before cleaning.

3. Use a mild hand soap and water or hydrogen peroxide to clean the wound.

4. Rinse the wound thoroughly with tap water.

5. Gently blot the wound dry, preferably with a sterile gauze pad.

6. Apply a triple antibiotic ointment or cream to the wound three times a day for 5 to 7 days to help prevent infection.

7. Bandaging is optional, yet it might help prevent the pet from licking or chewing at the wound.

8. Monitor daily for signs of infection including swelling, heat, pain, redness, and/or pus.

Dehydration

A state of dehydration can occur in dogs and cats whenever there is excessive fluid loss from the body. Conditions that predispose the animal to dehydration include water and food deprivation, burns, large wounds, increased frequency of urination, vomiting, diarrhea, bleeding, increased salivation, and excessive panting.

When a pet becomes dehydrated, its blood becomes very thick because the heart is forced to work extra hard in order to pump blood through the blood vessels to the organs throughout the body. In severe cases of dehydration, circulatory shock and subsequent organ failure can result.

Signs of dehydration include weight loss, loss of skin elasticity, dry mucous membranes, sunken eyeballs, depression, weakness, breathing difficulties, and lack of urination or extremely dark urine.

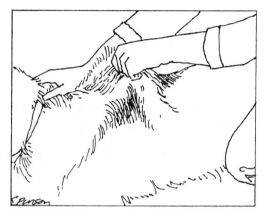

Figure 38.19 Tent the skin along the back to determine dehydration status. If it does not snap back into place within 2 seconds after you release your grip, your pet is dehydrated.

Skin elasticity, as a measure of dehydration, can be tested by gently lifting the skin along the pet's back or neck, and then releasing it. If it fails to return to its normal position immediately (see Fig. 38.19), then the pet is dehydrated. Older pets may naturally lose skin elasticity because of age and may not actually be dehydrated.

All suspected cases of dehydration should receive prompt veterinary care. Simply allowing your pet unlimited access to water will not correct the condition. Intravenous fluids and/or colloids administered by a veterinarian will be needed to stabilize your pet while the underlying cause of the dehydration is determined.

Diarrhea

Diarrhea can rapidly dehydrate a pet. See a veterinarian when:

- Diarrhea lasts more than 48 hours.
- The pet appears depressed, dehydrated, or in pain at any time.
- Vomiting accompanies the diarrhea.
- Blood is present in the stool.

For minor flare-ups where the pet is acting normal otherwise:

1. Take away all food for 24 hours.
2. Administer a kaolin-pectin mixture orally.
3. Bismuth subsalicylate can be used in otherwise healthy dogs (do not use in cats, as it contains aspirin).

Drowning

If physically possible, hold the pet upside-down by the hind legs for 20 seconds to allow the water to drain from the lungs.

For large dogs:

1. Place a hand on each side of the chest and abdomen near the last three ribs with your fingers facing toward the pet's head.

2. Apply a forceful, upward-inward squeeze to help expel water from the lungs.

3. Administer CPR as needed.

4. Using a solar blanket or other means, keep the pet warm until veterinary assistance can be obtained.

Electrical Shock

1. Remember: Your safety comes first!

2. Disconnect the power supply to the appliance or turn off the main electrical switch.

3. Use a long pole or similar item to safely move the pet away from the electrical source.

4. Signs of electrical shock can include burns on lips, tongue, and corners of the mouth and breathing difficulties.

5. Administer CPR as needed.

6. Transport to a veterinarian.

Eye Emergencies

PROLAPSE (EYE OUT OF SOCKET)

1. Do not attempt to push the eye back into its socket.

2. Apply a sterile ophthalmic solution (such as contact lens solution), ophthalmic ointment (if available), or plain tap water in order to keep the eyeball moist.

3. Immobilize the pet's front legs to prevent further self-trauma.

4. Transport to a veterinarian.

CHEMICAL BURNS

1. Flush the affected eye(s) thoroughly with copious amounts of water for 5 minutes.

2. Keep the pet from rubbing the affected eye(s)—immobilize the front legs if necessary.

3. Do not apply any ointments to the eye(s), as these can seal in the caustic agent and cause further damage to the eye.

4. Transport to a veterinarian.

FOREIGN BODIES, SCRATCHES, AND/OR BLEEDING

1. Prevent the pet from further traumatizing the eye; immobilize the front legs if necessary.

2. If there is a foreign body penetrating the eye, do not attempt to dislodge it.

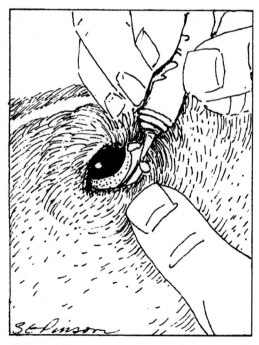

Figure 38.20 A sterile ointment can be applied to an injured eye to provide additional protection until veterinary help can be obtained.

3. If there is active bleeding from the eye or eyelid, apply direct yet gentle pressure to the site of the bleeding using a sterile ointment (Fig. 38.20) or dressing, a soft clean cloth, or an article of clothing.

4. If there is foreign matter in or discharge from the eye, gently flush the eye liberally with an ophthalmic solution or tap water to clear the eye of foreign matter. Use a tissue or soft cloth to dab (do not rub) any discharge or remaining foreign matter from the eye.

5. Transport to a veterinarian.

Fishhooks

1. If the fishhook is embedded in the-mouth or eye, do not attempt to remove the hook.

2. If it is embedded in the skin

Advance the hook until the barbed end is exposed.

Snip off the end of the barb with wire cutters (see Fig. 38.21).

Remove the remaining portion of the hook by gently backing it out of the entry site.

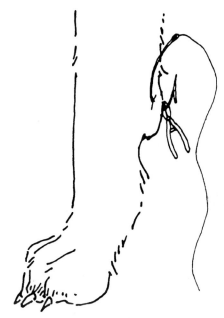

Figure 38.21 Remove a fishhook by first snipping off the barbed end, then backing the shaft back out of the wound.

3. All puncture wounds should be seen by a veterinarian to help prevent infection.

Heat Stress and Stroke

Most cases of heat stroke seen in dogs and cats are due to owner neglect:

- Pets left in cars
- Pets kept outdoors or overexerted without adequate shelter, shade, and/or water
- Obesity and poor conditioning can predispose to heat stroke

Other predisposing causes can include seizures, hyperthyroidism, heart disease, lung disease, and flat noses.

Signs of heat stroke include elevated body temperature, often exceeding 106 degrees Fahrenheit; rapid respirations; bright red mucous membranes; thickened saliva; vomiting; diarrhea; recumbancy; and unconsciousness. At 109 degrees Fahrenheit, multiple organ failure can occur. Take the pet's temperature with a digital thermometer. If the body temperature is less than 105 degrees Fahrenheit:

1. Move your pet indoors or to a cool, shady area outdoors.

2. Offer plenty of cool (not cold) water, in small portions only.

3. Place cool, moistened towels over pet's neck and back or spray down the pet with a water hose.

If the body temperature is greater than 105 degrees Fahrenheit:

1. Immerse your pet in a bathtub filled with cool (not cold) water or spray down with water from a hose; cold packs or ice packs (wrapped in towels) can also be used.

2. Monitor rectal temperature every 5 minutes.

3. When the temperature reaches 103 degrees Fahrenheit or if more than 10 minutes elapses from the time first aid is instituted (whichever comes first), discontinue the cooling procedure.

4. Seek immediate veterinary care.

Hypothermia and Frostbite

Hypothermia is often seen in neonatal puppies and kittens that are not properly kept warm by their mother. Frostbite usually affects the tips of the ears, tail, and/or scrotum; blisters may or may not be present.

Signs of hypothermia include:

- Lethargy
- Drowsiness
- Unconsciousness
- Weak pulse
- Shallow breathing
- Shivering
- Subnormal body temperature

Signs of frostbite include those listed above, plus pale skin, blisters, and hair loss.

Obtain a rectal temperature using a lubricated, digital thermometer. If the body temperature is below 98 degrees Fahrenheit:

1. Cover the pet with a blanket or towel and apply hot-water bottles (if available) or a heating pad (set on low and wrapped in a towel) to the torso of the pet. *Do not apply heat to the extremities!*

2. A solar blanket works well to conserve body heat.

3. Minimize movement of the pet to reduce chances of cardiac arrhythmias.

4. Monitor rectal temperature every 15 minutes.

5. Once body temperature reaches 100 to 102 degrees Fahrenheit, remove any external heat sources.

If signs of frostbite are evident:

1. *Do not rub the affected area.*

2. Keep the injured body part elevated if possible.

3. Apply a dressing and bandage to the region and seek veterinary help.

Intestinal and Abdominal Injuries

In all cases of abdominal injury or pain consult a veterinarian at once, even if no signs of internal injuries are present. Signs might not show up for 12 to 24 hours after an injury.

If abdominal contents are exposed:

1. Gently rinse the exposed organs with tap water.

2. Carefully place any exposed organs back into the abdominal cavity.

3. Pack the wound with a moist towel or cloth.

4. Using a T-shirt or other article of clothing, apply an encircling bandage to the abdomen to keep the pack in place (see Fig. 38.22).

5. Administer CPR if needed.

6. Transport to a veterinarian.

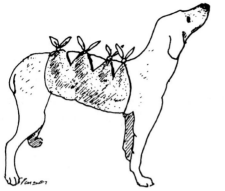

Figure 38.22 **Support sling for an abdominal wound.**

Insect Stings and Spider Bites

Signs associated with a bite or sting from an insect or arachnid include:

■ Localized redness, swelling, and pain

■ Lameness

■ Excess salivation

■ Breathing difficulties

Treatment is as follows:

1. If a stinger is evident in the wound, remove it with a pair of tweezers.

2. Apply a cold pack or ice pack (wrapped in a towel) to the affected area for 15 minutes to control swelling and pain.

3. Apply baking soda, calamine lotion, or anesthetic cream to the site.

4. Monitor the site for infection.

5. If the pet is having breathing difficulties, vomiting, or abdominal pain, obtain veterinary care as soon as possible.

Nosebleed

Apply pressure to the openings of both nostrils with your thumb and forefinger and maintain for 5 minutes. Depending on the size or the nostrils, gauze may be packed within the nostrils to control the bleeding.

Seizures

Seizures are characterized by an alteration in mental acuity and/or involuntary, rapid muscle contraction. If a pet experiences a seizure, don't panic; wrap the pet in a thick blanket or towel to prevent it from hurting itself. Also:

1. Do not apply a muzzle.

2. Do not attempt to give anything orally to the pet.

3. Do not reach into the mouth of a seizuring pet; it will not swallow its tongue.

4. If applicable, administer anticonvulsant medication per rectum according to the veterinarian's instructions (for pets with previously diagnosed conditions).

5. Transport the pet to a veterinarian if:

   It is the first time the pet has had a seizure.

   More than two seizures have occurred within a 24-hour period.

   If the seizure lasts over 3 minutes.

   If severe depression, breathing difficulties, or unconsciousness occurs following the seizure. (*Note:* Temporary disorientation may normally occur following a seizure episode.)

Snakebite

Clinical signs associated with snakebite are related to the type of snake involved, the amount of venom injected into the animal, and the location of the bite wound.

The venom of pit vipers, such as rattlesnakes and water moccasins, causes tissue damage and destroys red blood cells. Coral snake venom often causes little pain or swelling; however, it does affect the animal's nervous system, and difficulty swallowing, depression, paralysis, and death are common sequels to the bite of this snake.

Snakebites are more toxic in spring following hibernation. The venom of young snakes can be especially toxic because it is more concentrated than that of older snakes. Also, snakebites that occur on the head, neck, tongue, or torso are more serious than bites on the extremities:

Signs of snakebite include:

- Fang puncture wounds
- Localized severe pain
- Localized swelling and bruising

- Breathing difficulties
- Neurologic disorders/paralysis

The recommended treatment is:

1. Keep the pet as calm as possible to prevent the rapid spread of venom throughout the bloodstream.
2. Clean the bite wound with soap and water.
3. Apply an antibiotic ointment to the area.

If the bite is on an extremity, affix a tight pressure compress directly over the site of the bite with a bandage:

1. *Use caution, as the site will be painful.*
2. A piece of cloth or clothing can be used as bandaging material.
3. Do not apply a tourniquet and do not incise the skin.

In all cases of snakebite, seek veterinary care immediately.

Urinary Tract Obstruction

Male cats and dogs can suffer from urinary obstruction. In dogs, mineral crystals coalesce into actual stones within the bladder, ranging from the size of a small pellet to the size of a baseball.

Bladder stones are not as common in the cat, yet the crystals themselves are large enough to create a life-threatening obstruction to urine outflow in male cats. Obstructions are more likely to occur in males than in females, as the urethra of the male is much narrower than that of the female.

If a urinary obstruction is not relieved promptly, death can result because of toxin buildup within the bloodstream, kidney failure, and/or ruptured bladder. Seek veterinary care without delay.

Signs of urinary obstruction include:

- Frequent attempts at urination with minimal or with no results
- Bloody urine
- Enlarged, painful abdomen

- Panting
- Pet may appear constipated

Vomiting

Vomiting, the forceful expulsion of food or stomach secretions through the mouth, is a symptom of some underlying disorder. Vomiting should be differentiated from *regurgitation,* which can be defined as the effortless expulsion of food or saliva from the mouth due to a disorder of the esophagus.

Puppies and kittens will dehydrate seven times faster than adult animals; as a result, any case of persistent vomiting, especially in a young animal, should be regarded as a medical emergency.

You cannot rehydrate vomiting pets by force-feeding water, as they will always lose more than they take in. Seek veterinary help if:

- The pet is depressed.
- The pet vomited more than two times in the past 24 hours.
- Diarrhea is present.

For minor stomach upset in dogs, bismuth subsalicylate or milk of magnesia may be administered.

Pregnancy and Labor Challenges

During the spring and summer months, whelping will often occur during the morning hours, whereas during the fall and winter months it commonly occurs in late afternoon or early evening.

Up to 36 hours prior to delivery, the body temperature of the female will drop to about 98.5 degrees Fahrenheit. Once labor begins, the temperature will rise up back to normal. A green to clear vaginal discharge may be noticed just prior to the beginning of labor.

The birthing process can be divided into three segments:

1. Prelabor
   - Prelabor can last anywhere from 2 to 36 hours.
   - Signs include anxiety, panting, a loss of appetite, and nesting behavior.

2. True labor

   ■ Actual birth occurs.

   ■ Signs include panting, muscular contractions of the abdomen, obvious straining, and the eventual appearance of the placental sac.

   ■ Once labor begins, the female's environment should be kept as stress-free as possible; some dogs and cats can actually delay the parturition process if they feel uncomfortable with their surroundings.

3. Expulsion stage

   ■ This stage marks the passage of the placenta either with the newborn or soon afterward.

   ■ A dark green fluid will normally accompany this passage.

   ■ Although the female will sometimes instinctively eat the afterbirth, it is best to prevent this from happening; if the female is allowed to do so, bacteria within her digestive tract may start producing toxins that in turn can cause milk toxicity in her newborns.

Newborn puppies and kittens are usually born covered with placental membrane sacs. If the mother fails to remove the sac:

1. Remove it and then tie off the umbilical cord approximately 1¹/₂ inches from the newborn's body using string or dental floss.

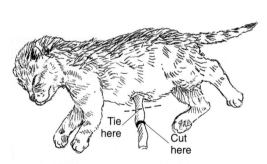

Tie here
Cut here

Figure 38.23 Correct placement of ligatures when severing the umbilical cord.

2. Snip the cord in half on the side of the knot closest to the placenta, not the body wall (see Fig. 38.23).

3. Treat the stump with tamed iodine and put the puppy or kitten back with its mother.

Birthing difficulties are seen most often with first

litters involving smaller breeds of dogs; Himalayan and Persian cats can also be predisposed.

Contact a veterinarian if:

- Over 70 days has elapsed since breeding occurred.

- A pet is in true labor for more than three hours without the appearance of a placental sac.

- More than 45 minutes has elapsed since the appearance of a placental sac and there is still no birth.

- More than 3 hours elapse between births.

If a newborn doesn't appear to be breathing:

1. Place it in a soft towel and rub it vigorously to help stimulate respiration.

2. Cradle and support the newborn's body and head upside-down in your hands (Fig. 38.24) or a towel (have the nose facing you and the top of its head pointing to the

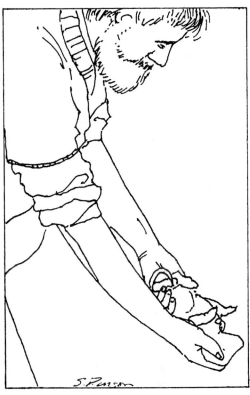

Figure 38.24 To stimulate a newborn to breathe, hold it upside-down in your hands and supporting its head, swing your arms up and down several times to help clear fluid from its lungs and airways.

ⒻACT *OR* *FICTION*

Females eat the placental membranes following birth for their nutritional value. **FICTION.** It is instinctive for the female to eat the afterbirth in order to hide any signs of recent birth from predators.

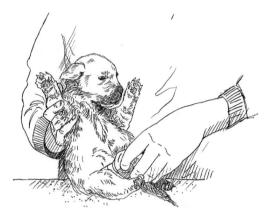

Figure 38.25 Puppies and kittens that are hand-nursed need to be stimulated to eliminate. This can be achieved by gently rubbing the anal region with a warm, damp cloth or cotton ball following each meal.

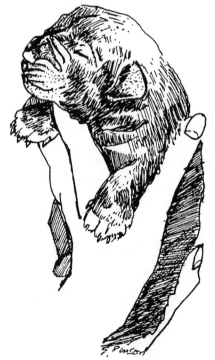

Figure 38.26 A newborn puppy or kitten that continues to cry even after it has eaten could be ill and warrants a call to a veterinarian.

floor), firmly rocking it up and down to help clear secretions from its lungs.

3. If a bulb syringe is available, use it to suction out any accumulated fluid and mucus from the mouth and nostrils to help facilitate normal airflow into the lungs.

Watch for rejection by the mother. Rejection can occur if the newborn's body temperature is lower than it should be or if it is harboring any physical abnormalities. If you suspect rejection, try warming the puppy or kitten by wrapping it in a blanket and holding it close to your body, and/or by filling a latex glove or water bottle with warm (not hot!) water and placing it next to the newborn's body. Once rewarmed, place the newborn back with its mother and observe her actions closely. If she still rejects it, then you may be forced to hand-feed the newborn.

A dark red discharge coming from the vulva usually signifies the end of the birthing process. Usually an entire litter is born within 15 hours after the onset of true labor; however, this can vary between individuals. Have your female pup checked out by your veterinarian as soon as you feel that the birthing process is complete (see also Figs. 38.25 and 38.26).

Caring for Injured and Orphaned Wildlife

A t one point in our childhood, no doubt each of us had encountered the baby bird that had fallen from its nest; the injured squirrel, rabbit, or raccoon that failed to outrun the family cat; or the frightened fawn lying crouched beneath a cluster of trees deep within the woods, with its mother nowhere in sight. Our inherent curiosity and compassion often prompted us to come to the rescue of the poor, unfortunate creature, yet we quickly discovered that caring for a wild bird or animal is not like caring for our family pet, and can become a stress-filled endeavor, not only for us but also for the animal we are trying to help.

If you do encounter an injured or abandoned wild animal or bird, your number one goal is to get that creature into the hands of a trained wildlife specialist as soon as possible. Failure to seek professional help in a timely manner only decreases survival rates, even in those animals and birds that seem healthy otherwise. Although your intentions may be pure, keeping a wild bird or animal as a pet or as a long-term houseguest is not acting in that individual's best interest, and greatly decreases their chances for survival. There are three good reasons to resist the temptation to nurse or raise the animal on your own:

1. It greatly decreases their chances for long-term survival.

2. The ultimate goal of rendering assistance to injured or orphaned wildlife is to care for it in such a way as to accomplish release back into the wild as soon as possible. This requires professional training that is far beyond the scope of this book.

3. State and federal wildlife agencies protect many wild animals and birds. If you are found in possession of wildlife without a permit, you could be subject to fines or worse. This is especially true for threatened or endangered species. For more information on those species requiring a possession permit, contact your federal and state wildlife agencies (including the U.S. Fish and Wildlife Service) or visit their Websites.

Gather a database of phone numbers and contact persons for state wildlife agencies, local nature and wildlife centers, wildlife rescue organizations, zoos, local county or city animal control departments, veterinary specialists, and licensed wildlife rehabilitators in your area that you can turn to in the event of a wildlife emergency. By all means, talk to them ahead of time, before you actually need them, and obtain their valuable input as to what you should do and whom you should call if you indeed encounter such an emergency.

Caring for Injured or Ill Wildlife

Wild animals and birds most commonly fall victim to automobiles, family pets, wild predators, gunshots, infectious diseases, and (human-made) structures such as fences and windows. Poisonings can also occur, with heavy metals (such as found in lead shot), pesticides, and contaminated foodstuffs.

Extreme caution should be used whenever interacting with injured or ill wildlife. Injured wildlife that seem otherwise lethargic or stupefied may instinctively come alive when approached or touched by a perceived threat, lashing out with teeth, claws, talons, or hooves in a severe fight-or-flight response. If you do get bitten or injured while attempting to render assistance, it will more than likely mean an expensive trip to the emergency room for you and euthanasia for the frightened animal.

It is important to remember also that interacting with wildlife can pose other risks as well besides traumatic bites and scratches. For instance, rabies is always a potential threat when dealing with skunks, raccoons, bats, foxes, and other wild carnivores. Deer can carry tuberculosis and brucellosis, two diseases that can affect humans. Rabbits can act as reservoirs for tularemia and for ticks that harbor the Lyme disease organism. The raccoon roundworm, *Baylisacaris procyonis,* can be especially nasty, causing cerebral larval migrans, a severe and often fatal brain disease in humans. Wild reptiles pose a risk for salmonella bacteria that can cause severe gastrointestinal disease in humans. And even starlings and other wild birds can harbor histoplasmosis, a serious fungal disease that can affect people.

Wildlife that you take into your home can also pose a threat to your existing pets. For example, raccoons can transmit the distemper virus to dogs, as well as a variety of parasites. Wild birds can harbor diseases that can threaten other birds within a house that are kept as pets. And the opposite is true as well. A curious housepet may suddenly have its predatory fire stoked by the presence of "perceived prey" within their territory and quickly dispatch the intruder.

Unfortunately, you are limited in what you can do to help a wild animal or bird recover from an injury or an illness. First aid and rehabilitation efforts should be left to the professionals; your job is to seek their help as soon as possible. However, here is some advice for the interim:

- If you must move an injured or ill wild animal, avoid touching it directly. Instead, use a board, branch, or other object to move the animal into a container, box, or bag suitable for transport. If hands-on interaction is simply unavoidable, extensive protection for your hands and arms will be needed. Thick, sturdy welder gloves along with a thick blanket or towel are the minimum equipment requirements.

- If feasible, keep the animal in a warm, dark, stress-free environment. This means protecting it against loud noises (including televisions and radios), drafts, temperature fluctuations, and the curiosity of children and other pets in the household. A heating pad set on low or hot-water bottles can be placed beneath the box (not in the box) to provide a source of warmth.

- Interaction with humans is extremely stressful for wild birds and animals, especially if injured or ill, so keep it to a minimum. And whatever you do, avoid the temptation to cuddle or kiss a wild animal or bird, no matter how cute it may appear. Remember that their survival instincts are telling them to avoid contact with you at all costs!

- Do not attempt to feed the animal until you've spoken with a wildlife specialist. A small portion of water can be offered (free choice; do not force) in the meantime.

- Do not administer any medications, such as antibiotics, to injured or orphaned wildlife unless instructed to do so by a veterinarian.

Caring for Orphaned Wildlife

Most wildlife species give birth to their young between March and September. As a result, this is the time when you are most likely to encounter a baby bird or animal in the woods or in your backyard. If this happens, don't automatically assume that the baby has been orphaned. Every year, countless animals and birds are made orphans by well-meaning individuals who take it on themselves to "rescue" the hapless creatures. Unfortunately, most act prematurely and unknowingly snatch these offspring away from their mothers, who are hiding nearby. For example, a doe will often leave her young fawn alone in thick brush or near clumps of trees while she forages for food during the early morning and evening hours. This is to protect the fawn from falling easy prey to a predator that may choose to stalk his prey while the latter feeds. The doe rarely travels too far from her offspring. As a result, if you happen upon a fawn in the woods, leave it alone and keep your distance. If the doe senses your presence, she won't return.

Contrary to popular belief, a mother in the wild won't abandon her young if humans have touched them. However, if this same mother senses that humans are loitering around her nest, den, or offspring, she may keep her distance as long as the perceived threat is present.

There are times when legitimate abandonment will occur. Perhaps a cat or a dog kills the parents. Or a den or nest is inadvertently destroyed by a storm, commercial development, or felled tree, leaving offspring homeless and exposed. Sometimes, the young are abandoned if they harbor some congenital defect or sustain an injury early in life. Or, as in the case of baby opossums, they may accidentally fall out of their mother's pouch and get left behind. In these instances, your intervention may mean the difference between life and death for these helpless creatures.

What to Do if You Find a Baby Mammal

For small mammals such as baby squirrels, rabbits, and raccoons, your best course of action if you find one is to leave it laying in the same place where you found it and wait patiently at a distance to see if its mother will return to it. To help minimize exposure to environmental hazards, you can place the baby in an open shoebox or small plastic container lined with a soft cloth or towel. Be sure that the sides of the container are short enough to allow the returning mother to enter, yet not so short that the baby can climb or fall out. Scan the nearby trees for a nest that the baby squirrel or raccoon may have fallen from and, if possible, return it to the original nest. If the nest is out of reach, secure your (human-made) nest to a branch closest to the real nest and place the baby in it.

Do not offer food or water to the neonate at this stage. Often, the cries and complaints of a hungry or thirsty child will entice the parents to return.

If mom hasn't returned by nightfall, go ahead and bring the baby inside for the night. Keep it warm and isolated, minimizing stress as much as possible. Offer it a teaspoon or two of water by dropper or syringe; just give it slowly. If it seems weak, offer it a teaspoon of Karo syrup.

Get up early in the morning and return the baby to its original location, preferably just before daybreak. If mom fails to appear by noon, contact a local wildlife specialist for further instructions.

If for some reason you are not able to reach a wildlife specialist before nightfall, feed your houseguest. Again, use extreme caution when handling wildlife, even babies, for they, too, can inflict serious bite and/or scratch wounds. Commercial puppy formulas or other milk replacers can be used as emergency rations for orphaned baby squirrels, opossums, and rabbits. Kitten milk replacers work best for baby raccoons. Follow label directions as you would for feeding puppies or kittens. Plan on feeding every 2 to 4 hours, with the exception of baby rabbits, which should be fed no more than every 8 hours. Remember to stimulate the baby to urinate and defecate after it has finished its meals by gently rubbing its anal and genital areas with a warm, moist cotton ball.

What to Do If You Find a Baby Bird

If you find a hatchling (pink, with eyes closed, featherless) or nestling (eyes partially opened, covered in down and sparsely feathered) on the ground, look for a nest in the trees branches above you. If you locate it, go ahead and place the baby back into it. Again, you don't need to worry about the parents rejecting it because you touched it with your hands. If the nest is unreachable, create a new nest by placing the bird into a small shallow cardboard box lined with leaves or grass and secure it to the highest branch you can reach. If you can't find the nest, put your (human-made) nest beneath the tree closest to the point where you found the bird. Chances are that the mother and/or father will adopt the new nest as their own and resume care of their offspring. Stay a good distance away to encourage the parents to return.

If you find a fully feathered baby bird (a fledgling), it may have jumped from its nest or have been pushed from it by its parents in order to learn to fly and to feed itself. It is best not to intervene with the learning process. More than likely, the parents are nearby, scoping out food and shelter for the fledgling. If the bird appears to be in immediate harm's way, feel free to move it to the edge of a nearby bush or shrub.

Realize that some species of birds normally nest on the ground in fields, brush, and tall grass. These birds may leave their young for hours at a time in search of food, so don't automatically assume these offspring have been orphaned and accidentally raid a nest.

If the mother bird hasn't returned by nightfall, and the baby cannot be returned to its nest in a tree, go ahead and bring it inside for the night. Keep it boxed in a warm, dark, noise-free location within the house. Offer it a small amount of water and food by dropper or syringe (see Care for Sick Birds in Chap. 23 for instructions on feeding baby birds). Arise before daybreak and return the box and baby to its location beneath the tree. If mom fails to appear by noon, contact a local wildlife specialist for further instructions.

CHAPTER 40

Geriatrics: Caring for Your Older Pet

It is estimated that in the United States alone, over 35 percent of all pets owned are geriatric. Depending on which veterinarian you talk to, dogs and cats are considered geriatric when they reach 7 years of age (5 years of age for larger dog breeds). Understand, though, that breed, genetics, nutrition, and environmental influences will all ultimately affect the aging process in a particular pet (see Tables 40.1 and 40.2).

Cats and smaller dogs tend to age more slowly and live longer than do larger dogs. However, different breeds of large dogs can vary vastly in their life spans and the age at which they are considered geriatric. For instance, German shepherds can easily live to be 13 to 15 years, while a 10-year old Great Dane would be considered ancient. Likewise, bulldogs and boxers are thought to age at an accelerated rate.

The overall care that a dog or cat receives throughout its life will also have a great impact on the rate of aging. Pets that are well cared for during adolescence and throughout their adult lives tend to suffer fewer infirmities as they grow old. Furthermore, through diligent preventive health care measures, age-related health problems can be detected early, greatly diminishing their impact. In contrast, neglecting a pet in husbandry or in preventive health care will greatly accelerate the aging process.

Table 40.1 Chronological versus Biological Age of Dogs Compared to Humans

Age of dog, years	Age of human, years
1	12
2	22
3	30
4	35
5	40
6	45
7	50
8	55
9	60
10	65
11	70
12	75
13	80
14	85
15	90

Physical changes seen as dogs and cats age are related to wear and tear on all body systems. Again, these are variable between individuals and breeds, and can be greatly influenced by an owner who provides good environment, proper nutrition, and routine veterinary care throughout the pet's life.

Physical Challenges in Older Pets

As with people, the overall metabolism of a pet has a tendency to slow as the years advance. This, combined with a decrease in the amount of exercise, can easily predispose a geriatric pet to obesity and all its dangerous ramifications. As dogs and cats age, they don't suffer from many of the cardiovascular challenges that humans do, such as hardening of the arteries and atherosclerosis. Yet, as aging occurs, the heart does become less efficient at pumping blood during exercise or stressful situations that can arise. In addition, heart valve disease caused by wear and tear from years of normal use is common in older pets, especially dogs. This type of heart disease can sometimes be related back to untreated periodontal disease during the pet's younger years. The major changes are as follows:

1. *Bone and joint challenges.* Arthritis is one of the more common ailments affecting dogs as they grow old. In addition, many of the larger breeds can suffer from the painful condition of the back known as

vertebral spondylosis. Furthermore, as intervertebral disks mature and become less resilient, the risk of disk rupture in these older pets increases at the same time. Arthritis can affect older cats as it affects their canine counterparts. Since cats are relatively lightweight, joint degeneration from age-related wear and tear is rarely as profound as it would be in a dog the same age. However, it will slow an older cat down, and limit its desire to jump on and off of objects as it used to do.

2. *Muscular challenges.* The muscles of older dogs and cats tend to atrophy due to a decrease in muscle activity and due to age-related protein loss from the body. A loss in flexibility can also occur, causing upwardly mobile canines and felines to slow down.

3. *Disorders of the skin and hair.* These can increase in prevalence in the geriatric pets due to aging effects on the hair cycle and due to metabolic and endocrine upsets.

Table 40.2 Chronological versus Biological Age of Cats Compared to Humans

Cat age, years	Human age, years
1	16
2	23
3	27
4	31
5	35
6	39
7	43
8	47
9	51
10	56
11	60
12	64
13	69
14	73
15	77

DID YOU KNOW?

Dogs and cats experience accelerated biological aging during their first few years of life, which allows for hastened sexual maturity. This feature allowed their ancestors, who had much shorter life expectancies in the wild, to raise litters while chronologically young and strong, thereby ensuring speedy and effective propagation of the species.

4. *Aging kidneys.* It is a well-known fact that as a dog or cat matures, its kidneys become less efficient at filtering the blood and ridding the body of waste products. As a result, care taken early on to help ease the burden placed on the aging kidneys using special diets and medications will greatly enhance the longevity of a pet. Also, a special test that detects low levels of protein in the urine is available from veterinarians and can greatly assist in the early detection of kidney disease in dogs, even before clinical signs occur. This test is recommended for all geriatric dogs.

5. *Urinary incontinence.* Older dogs, especially spayed females, may begin to lose control of their bladders as they enter into their teens. This is usually the result of weakened sphincters that normally prevent the involuntary outflow of urine from the bladder. Medications are available that can increase sphincter tone and help curb this problem.

6. *Reproductive challenges.* Female dogs and cats that were not spayed at an early age are prone to uterine diseases and mammary cancer as they enter into their geriatric years. At the same time, most older male dogs are afflicted with some degree of prostate enlargement. Furthermore, as one might expect, fertility and reproductive performance in both dogs and cats tend to decrease with advancing age.

7. *Intestinal challenges.* The aging gastrointestinal tract might begin to show signs of reduced efficiency and intolerance to excesses. For this reason, flare-ups of gastritis, colitis, and constipation can become more prevalent as a pet enters into its golden years. At the same time, liver function can decrease, making it more difficult to metabolize nutrients and detoxify wastes within the body.

8. *Weakened immune systems.* It is well documented that the efficiency and activity of the immune system are compromised with age. As a result, geriatric pets are more susceptible to disease, especially viruses and cancer. For this reason, preventive health care takes on an even more important meaning in these pets.

9. *Endocrine challenges.* As dogs mature, the activity of the glands within the body may start to decrease, leaving the pet with hormone-related challenges. For example, hypothyroidism is a com-

mon condition seen in maturing dogs. Diabetes mellitus, seen in both dogs and cats, can occur secondarily to aging of the insulin-producing cells within the pancreas, or to repeated bouts of pancreatitis over the years. In contrast, age-related tumors affecting glands within the body can lead to oversecretion of hormones, resulting in illness. Canine Cushing's disease and feline hyperthyroidism are prime examples.

10. *Vision challenges.* Most older dogs and cats will likely develop a slight grayish white or bluish haze to the lenses of both eyes. This change, termed *nuclear sclerosis,* is brought on by a complex deposition of body metabolites into the eye lenses. It is a normal change and should not be confused with a cataract. Unlike cataracts, nuclear sclerosis only mildly affects vision. Dogs and cats with decreased visual ability might not be able to focus on an object rapidly, so they might react suddenly if approached. Don't confuse this with crankiness or irritability. A slow approach with a gentle hand accompanied by a calm voice will allow a pet with failing vision to hear and smell the familiar person approaching.

11. *Hearing loss.* Partial or total hearing loss is common in geriatric pets. It is often related to long-term, irreversible nervous changes in the inner ear. Further hearing loss occurs with senile changes or damage to the eardrum or ossicles (the bones of vibration conduction) housed within the middle ear. Wax accumulation within the ears can play a role in deafness as well.

12. *Dependence on sense of smell.* The sense of smell is usually the last sense to fail in dogs and cats. For this reason, the geriatric pet depends more and more on its sense of smell to identify people, objects, and food. Also, the senses of taste and smell are highly dependent on one another. As a result, the appetite of older pets may taper off as the sense of smell becomes compromised. This can be especially dangerous in cats, as a loss of appetite can lead to secondary liver disease. As a result, pay close attention to your cat's appetite.

13. *Cognitive dysfunction syndrome (senility).* Signs of senility in older dogs can include changes in sleep patterns, changes in the levels and types of social interaction desired, increased house soiling, increased anxiety, and disorientation. Senility is rare in older cats, but it can occur. If diagnosed in your pet, your veterinarian can prescribe medications to help ease the symptoms of senility and improve your pet's quality of life.

TABLE 40.3 Common Medical Conditions Seen in Older Pets

Kidney disease
Heart disease
Osteoarthritis
Periodontal disease
Cancer
Cognitive dysfunction syndrome

The changes that occur with aging (see also Table 40.3) warrant special adjustments in husbandry practices and preventive health care for geriatric pets. The following are five steps you can take to be sure your pet's geriatric years are filled with health and happiness:

1. Adjust your pet's diet to match its health needs. A veterinarian can assist you with this switch. If your pet suffers from a specific ailment, such as heart disease, special diets can be prescribed to reduce the wear and tear on the affected organ systems. For the otherwise healthy pet, feed a diet that is higher in fiber and reduced in calories. Don't forget to weigh your dog or cat on a regular basis. Obesity is an enemy, and can significantly shorten your pet's life.

2. Maintain a moderate exercise or play program to keep your pet's bones, joints, heart, and lungs conditioned. Always consult your veterinarian first as to the type and amount of activity appropriate for your particular pet.

3. Be sure to brush your pet daily. Skin and coat changes secondary to metabolic slowdown or adjustments within the body can often be managed with a stepped-up home grooming program. In addition, keep those canine toenails trimmed short. Older dogs suffering from arthritis don't need the added challenge and pain of having to ambulate on nails that have grown to the floor.

4. Along with grooming and brushing, be sure to give your geriatric pet plenty of attention and petting each day. As the senses start to fail, pets can become frightened by the gradual loss of sensory contact with their owners. As a result, you need to reinforce the care and companionship you are offering.

5. Semiannual veterinary checkups, monthly at-home physical examinations, and annual blood and urine screens for aging pets

are a must. Remember: Early detection of a disease condition is the key to curing or managing the disorder. Frequent checkups are also important if your older pet is taking medication for a chronic condition, as periodic dosage adjustments may be needed to keep the condition under control. For information on how to administer medications to your pet, see Chap. 23.

Saying Good-bye to an Older or Terminally Ill Pet

Inevitably, every pet owner is faced with the difficult decision concerning euthanasia of a beloved pet. It is certainly an act not to be taken lightly or performed without extensive forethought. When does euthanasia become a consideration or option when dealing with a pet? When is it time to say good-bye?

Certainly if a pet suffers from a terminal illnesses or irreparable, painful injuries, euthanasia becomes a viable option when compared to a life of continued discomfort and pain. Still, how can we be sure that the time has come to make the difficult decision? If a pet is suffering from acute obvious pain that cannot be brought under control, then euthanasia will provide the only humane relief from the pain. But what about those older or terminally ill pets that outwardly don't seem to be in pain? Fortunately, Nature has given us this answer. In the wild, animals that are nearing death and are suffering from less noticeable pain or discomfort will stop eating and seek solitude for themselves. Older or terminally ill dogs and cats will do the same. If your pet is showing both of these signs, it may be time to say good-bye. A veterinarian can help you verify that your decision is the correct one. Rest assured the vet does not take the task of euthanasia lightly; it is a heavy and sometimes disturbing responsibility of the profession. As a result, if the vet feels that it is time, then it probably is and you should take solace in the fact that your decision was indeed justified.

Grieving for a Lost Pet

Although many might try to deny its existence, a psychological "bonding" does occur between people and their pets. Researchers have even given a name, referring to this phenomenon as the *human–companion animal bond.* In fact, veterinary colleges across the country teach courses devoted only to this subject. It certainly makes sense that such a bonding exists. Pets are bundles of love and friendship that add that much touch of happiness and companionship to our sometimes unfriendly and hectic world. Pets are always ready to listen to our problems, never interjecting their own problems or opinions along the way. Instead, we receive a responsive wag of the tail or a friendly purr.

So why is this so important? The proven existence of the human–companion animal bond should help pet owners realize that grieving for a lost pet is perfectly natural. There is a stigma in our society about grieving openly for a pet that has died or has been put to sleep. Failure to do so only causes a strong buildup of emotion and sometimes confusion within the pet owner. This is not only psychologically unhealthy, but also—and most health care professionals will point this out—physically unhealthy as well.

Stages of Grieving

With the loss or impending loss of a loved one, whether animal or human, there are stages of grief that we all experience. Some will experience all four stages sequentially; others might find that one or two stages predominate. Understanding that these stages are natural and should not be suppressed can help you better cope with the impending death of a pet.

1. *The denial stage.* In this stage of grieving, a pet owner has yet to come to grips with the fact that their pet is going to die. In terms of the euthanasia decision, some pet owners find themselves refusing to believe that making such a serious decision should even be presented as an option. This can lead into the second stage of grief, the anger stage.

2. *The anger stage.* Anger can be vented at a veterinarian for even suggesting euthanasia as an option. In other instances owners will be angry at themselves for even considering euthanasia.

3. *Depression.* The third stage of grief is *depression*—the thought of losing a loved one and how life will be afterward.

4. *The resolution stage.*   In this stage, an owner finally comes to accept a pet's death, and has learned to cope with it. It is usually in this stage that the burden of the euthanasia decision is finally, and correctly, lifted.

When the grief is just too overwhelming, don't be afraid to contact a psychologist or other professional specializing in grief counseling for help. Support groups do exist which can help pet owners overcome the loss of their loved one. Again, what you are experiencing is very real and very natural, and a trained, understanding ear can be great comfort and relief at times of such emotional distress.

Increasing Your Pet's Longevity

t goes without saying that eating right, getting plenty of exercise, and eliminating bad habits can add years to our lives. Well, believe it or not, the same principles apply to our pets. As a result of recent advancements in veterinary medicine and a growing public awareness concerning responsible pet ownership, pets are living longer today than at any time in the past (Fig. 41.1). Want to find the fountain of youth for your pet? Here are some proven tips that can lead you and your pet right to it!

Avoid Junk Food

No matter what the pet food companies tell you, you can't beat the new premium-type diets on the market today. Lots of research and little filler go into these products, making them popular recommendations of veterinarians across the country. Regardless of the type of pet you own, you have many types and brands to choose from. The choice is yours. However, when in doubt as to which one would be best for your pet, don't hesitate to ask your veterinarian. And though the expense of such rations may seem inflated at first, most pet owners find that the amounts consumed per feeding are much less than those for nonpremium foods, making the actual per-feeding cost for the two types of rations about the same.

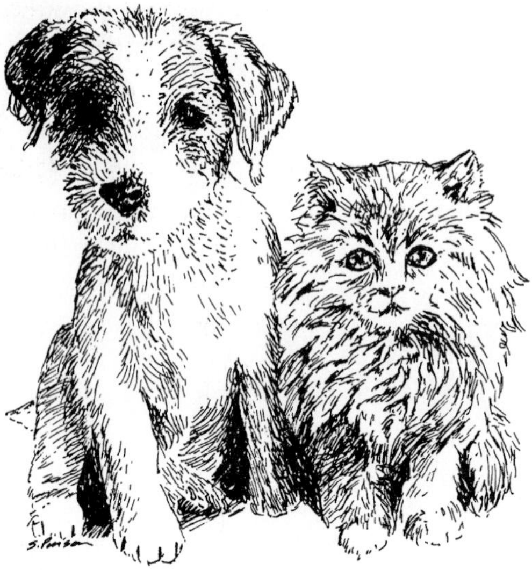

FIGURE 41.1 The key to boosting your pet's longevity is to practice responsible pet ownership from the time your pet is young.

Think Thin

Obesity causes the same ill effects in pets as it does in people. Pets pushing the scales to their maximums are more prone to, among other things, heart disease, kidney disease, liver disease, and diabetes. They also become sluggish, tire easily, and seem to just crave more and more food (sounds familiar, doesn't it?).

The two biggest culprits underlying obesity in pets are indiscriminate feeding practices and lack of exercise. Feeding table scraps, too many snacks, or in the case of birds, too many seeds, is probably the worst thing you could do for your pet. Not only do these upset the

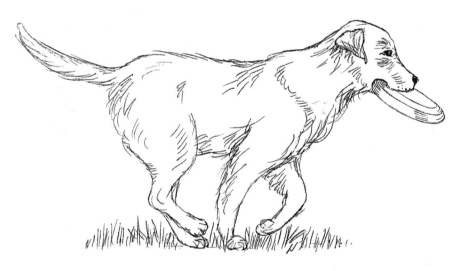

a

FIGURE 41.2 (*a, b*) Daily exercise will help your pet live longer.

nutritional balance of your pet's daily requirement, they often cause gastrointestinal upset as well. Not only that; you're going to create a pet that constantly begs or scavenges for food, which always goes over big when you're entertaining guests for dinner.

If your pet is indeed fat, simply cutting back on snacks and the amount of food you feed might not be enough. There are, however, some great weight-loss diets available that can help your pet lose the added poundage while at the same time satisfying its appetite. Ask your veterinarian for a recommendation on such a diet, since requirements could vary depending upon the age of your pet.

Exercise, Exercise, and More Exercise

Exercise offers the same benefits to pets as it does to humans: cardiovascular fitness and weight control. Twenty to thirty minutes of moderate exercise daily (walking, chasing the Frisbee or toy mouse, running on an exercise wheel) will help keep your pet slim, trim, and healthy (Fig. 41.2).

For dog owners, walking or jogging is an excellent way to keep canines fit and trim. Just remember that unless you own a Russian wolfhound, stride-for-stride, your dog is going to have to work harder than you do, so be sure you don't overdo it. Heat stroke and/or musculoskeletal injuries can be unfortunate side effects to such marathon exercise sessions.

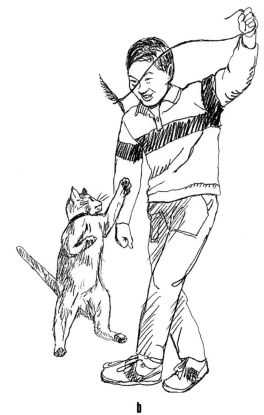

b

FIGURE 41.2 (*a, b*) Daily exercise will help your pet live longer.

Cats that are leash-trained from the start can also benefit from controlled exercise. For those that are not, a designated daily play session will help elevate the heart rate and burn calories. The same holds true for pot-bellied pigs. Just don't allow your porcine to get overheated!

Getting a bird or exotic pet to willfully exercise can be a challenge, and requires a great deal of creativity on your part. However, it can be done. Certainly birds whose feathers have not been clipped can be offered free flight time each day. Just be sure that all windows and doors are closed and secured, all stove burners are off, access to mirrored surfaces has been denied, and other household hazards have been isolated. In addition, for all birds, including those with clipped feathers, installing several perches, each at a different height within the cage, can provide exercise value by encouraging them to move from perch to perch. However, for sanitary reasons, avoid situating one perch directly beneath another.

For rodents, an exercise wheel should always be provided. Most will catch the exercise fever right away without any coaxing from you! Other pocket pets can be taken from the confines of their cages and, for a defined period of time, allowed free access to a room or a portion thereof. This allows them to scurry and explore with their movement unimpeded by the bars of a cage. Of course, make sure that such a room or space is escape-proof and free of potential hazards.

As a corollary to this longevity tip: Give your pet plenty of attention each day. The easiest way to stress out your pet is to ignore it. So keep this in mind the next time you come home from work. Take some time to interact with your faithful companion.

Work on That Smile

Excessive dental tartar and gingivitis play important roles in heart and kidney disease in pets. To make matters worse, most dogs and cats show signs of periodontal (tooth and gum) disease by the time they're only 3 years of age! This is why it's so important to keep your pet's dental tartar under control (Fig. 41.3).

Simply feeding your pets hard food or biscuits won't do the trick alone. In fact, many of these foodstuffs may actually promote plaque and tartar formation, and subsequent periodontal disease. Surprised? You shouldn't be. Just think about what your teeth would look like if you never brushed your teeth or had a dental cleaning performed, and you'll get the picture.

You should have a dental checkup performed on your pet every time you visit your veterinarian (at least annually). If it's necessary, have your pet's teeth professionally cleaned and polished while you're there. When you get your pet home, make it a point to incorporate some type of dental care into your pet's daily routine, whether brushing with toothpaste specifically formulated for pets or using special pet mouthwashes containing

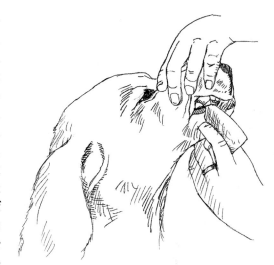

FIGURE 41.3 Cleaning your pet's teeth daily is not difficult and yields tremendous health benefits!

chlorhexidine. Also, there are a plethora of toys and chew items available on the market today that are designed to assist in pet tartar control. The more of these your pet has access to, the better!

Let Them Know Who's Boss

Proper obedience training will keep your dog off the streets—literally. Dogs that dart off despite their owner's commands to the contrary, or dig escape tunnels out of their backyards, are prime candidates for being hit by a car.

Pet owners need to teach their dogs to respond to the basic commands to stop, sit, stay, and heel. No dog is too old to be taught these commands, yet for those old, crusty canines set firmly in their ways, a good obedience school might be just what the doctor ordered.

Carpet versus Concrete

Make no mistake about it: Pets kept indoors are healthier than those kept outdoors. For instance, indoor dogs are psychologically healthier because of the increased contact with their pack members (their owners). In addition, they are less prone to physical illnesses such as infectious diseases, skin disorders, gastroenteritis induced by dietary indiscretions, and environmental afflictions such as heat stroke and car fenders.

Along the same lines, making your cat an indoor pet will keep it safe from car tires, and significantly reduce its risk of contracting deadly diseases such as feline leukemia, feline infectious peritonitis, and feline AIDS.

Finally, birds kept indoors escape the risk of exposure to infectious diseases such as avian pox and internal parasites, as well as stealthy feline predators.

An Ounce of Prevention Is Worth a Pound of Cure

Preventive health care is a proven boost to longevity in pets. Such care includes keeping your pet current on its vaccinations and parasite preventive medications (if applicable), having routine checkups performed, adhering to sound grooming and husbandry principles, and heeding those longevity tips previously mentioned.

Also, if you haven't already done so, consider having your pet neutered. Besides the advantage of population control, there can be health benefits as well. For example, female dogs neutered prior to their second heat have a reduced risk of mammary cancer as they get older. In addition, male dogs that are neutered may have a reduced incidence of certain cancers as they mature when compared with their intact peers. In fact, neutering totally eliminates the possibility that these dogs will develop testicular cancer as they age. Finally, because neutering can reduce aggressiveness and anxiety in select instances, it may help reduce the chances of injury from fighting or self-inflicted trauma.

CHAPTER
42

Reducing Stress and Promoting Mental Wellness in Dogs and Cats

*M*ental wellness can be defined as emotional contentment and satisfaction, in other words, a state of persistent happiness. Unfortunately, we humans have enough trouble agreeing on what constitutes a state of happiness. So, how are we to know what it means to our four-legged friends? To help us figure this out, let's take a look at what causes them to be unhappy.

Animal behavioral experts agree that most unhappiness and mental distress in dogs and cats is caused by fear, anxiety, and/or frustration, emotions that invariably lead to behavioral challenges. Grief and despondence at the loss of a companion or separation from pack members can also lead to stress and mental illness, as can anger and aggression, especially if the source inciting the belligerent behavior is not removed.

Physically, stress affects dogs and cats just as it does us, causing a marked increase in heart rate, blood pressure, and nervous output. If the stress is chronic, the immune system can become depressed, leaving the body susceptible to a wide variety of diseases, including cancer.

Promoting mental wellness in our pets means reducing stress in their lives as much as possible. Doing so has key implications for our own health as well. The importance of the human–companion animal bond and its positive effect on human health has been studied extensively in recent years. No one will argue that we form deep emotional attachments to our pets. It stands to reason that if our pets become stressed, we will experience stress as well. As a result, by promoting mental wellness in our companions, we enhance not only their quality of life, but ours as well.

So how do we do it? We do it by ensuring that the emotional and physical needs of our pets are being met. To encourage positive emotions, our pets need positive mental stimulation on a daily basis, predictability and control in their lives, and dependable social companionship. Physical needs include ready access to food, water, and shelter, and the ability to eliminate when the need arises. These needs also include freedom from illness and/or pain.

That said, here are some positive steps we can take to promote mental wellness in our pets:

1. Go to extra lengths to make sure your dog or cat is properly desensitized and socialized in its first few months of life. Doing so will dramatically decrease fear, anxiety, and stress as your pet matures.

2. Daily walks, exercise sessions, play periods, and/or grooming sessions will all contribute to overall mental wellness and contentment of your pet while promoting physical vibrancy at the same time. This is especially true for older pets, whose diminished sensory awareness and physical deterioration may burden them with feelings of detachment and isolation. Without a doubt, the comfort of continued interaction with the ones they love will help ease the stress and burden associated with the aging process.

3. Dogs kept fenced up outdoors with limited social companionship, cats confined to limited space for long periods of time, or any pet that perceives its environment as monotonous and unstimulating, may turn to nuisance vocalizations, inappropriate

eliminations, destructive activities, and even self-mutilation as a way to spice up their lives and cope with their boredom and stress. As a result, make your dog an indoor (or at the very least, an indoor-outdoor) pet, and provide your cat with plenty of space to roam and explore.

4. Allowing dogs and cats to engage in problem solving and decision making will invariably provide high levels of mental satisfaction. When designing games and activities for your pet, get creative and think of ways you can stimulate its thinking process. For instance, when playing fetch with your dog, try throwing two sticks at once instead of just one. Forcing your dog to make a decision on which stick to go for first provides healthy positive mental stimulation.

5. Dogs and cats are creatures of habit. Although they need positive mental stimulation in the form of variety, they also need predictability in their lives in order to keep stress levels to a minimum. For example, a dog or cat will come to expect that evening meal (regardless of the type of bowl you use), or that daily hour of play (regardless of the activity), and if missed, will stress over it. Pencil your pet into your busy schedule and stick to a daily routine.

6. Catering to your pet's instinctive cravings will help prevent boredom and the stress that it causes. For example, if you own a terrier, provide it with its own place to dig, whether this is a sandbox or designated area of the yard. If you own a hunting dog, yet you don't hunt, design games and "hide and seek" activities that will stimulate your dog's instinctive juices to flush out or give chase to game. If you own a cat, use interactive toys to play "cat and mouse," thereby satisfying its urge to stalk and hunt. Provide enough variety, novelty, and interaction to allow your dog to be a dog and your cat to be a cat!

7. Be sure to properly establish a dominance hierarchy between you and your pet through proper training. Failure to do so will lead to a continual power struggle that will increase stress levels for both of you.

8. A houseful of visitors can be stressful to both dogs and cats, who often view the human visitors as territorial intruders. It may be less stressful to temporarily isolate your pet from the crowd rather than force them to hide from or unwillingly interact with strange people.

9. Introducing a new puppy or adult dog into a household already containing an adult cat can be highly stressful for the latter, who may never fully warm up to the new addition. On the contrary, introducing a new kitten into a home containing an adult dog is usually less traumatic; in fact, most kittens will be "adopted" by their canine housemates over time. Although this is not a hard-and-fast rule, it should be kept in mind whenever planning new pet additions to your home.

10. Have your pets neutered. This is especially true for male dogs and cats, who can become quite stressed and frustrated if not allowed to roam, fight, and satisfy their territorial and sexual urges.

11. If your pet becomes highly stressed when traveling or boarding, consider hiring a pet sitter to take care of your pet at your home while you are away. Not only will your pet feel more comfortable in its own environment, but you'll also reap the peace of mind knowing that someone is watching over your house in your absence.

12. Provide fresh food and water to your pet on a daily basis.

13. For cats, avoid disturbing them while they are using or thinking about using their litterbox. Also, remain consistent with the type of cat litter you buy. Cats can be quite finicky about their litter, and will stress out if you fill the litterbox with one they don't like.

14. Obviously, pain, injury, and illness can all wreak havoc on a pet's mental health. As a result, prioritize your pet's preventive health care program and observe the rules of longevity. Preventing injuries or catching illnesses early in their development will keep your pet happy, both mentally and physically.

As mentioned earlier, stress in a pet will manifest itself most often as a behavioral challenge. As a result, if your pet is exhibiting such behavior, attempt to uncover the underlying source of stress and eliminate (or minimize) it. This is where the veterinarian can help, by assisting in rooting out the source and recommending an appropriate solution. Occasionally, antianxiety medications and behavioral modification agents may be prescribed for controlling stress in select patients. However, most veterinarians will use these only as a last resort, when all other modes of behavior modification have been exhausted.

Promoting mental wellness is the job of everyone who chooses to take on the responsibility of pet ownership. Our dogs and cats rely on us to help satisfy both their emotional and physical needs, and by so doing, we automatically improve their quality of life. After all, the old saying "To live without stress is to live" is as true for our pets as it is true for us!

Cancer in Companion Animals

n recent years, veterinary medicine has made tremendous advances in the diagnosis, treatment, and prevention of disease in pets. For instance, because of public education and sophisticated vaccines, the incidence of viral disease in companion animals has decreased dramatically. Another frequent cause of death—bacterial disease—can now be combatted more effectively with new generations of antibiotics. In addition, both veterinarians and breeders have learned much about the control and elimination of genetic defects through selective breeding, and leash laws and responsible owners have greatly decreased the incidence of pets killed by trauma. Indeed, pets, like their owners, are living longer lives.

Yet there is one disease that, despite our efforts, remains one of the leading causes of death in older pets. That disease is cancer. Fortunately, veterinarians know a great deal more about the diagnosis and therapy of neoplastic disease in small animals than they did 20 years ago. In fact, the field of veterinary oncology (the study of cancer) is one of the fastest-growing segments of the profession today. However, there is still much to be learned about the origins and susceptibilities of this notorious killer.

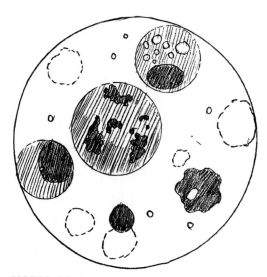

FIGURE 43.1 A cancer cell undergoing uncontrolled division.

Tumor Definition and Types

A *tumor* or *neoplasm* is an abnormal growth of tissue containing cells that proliferate more rapidly than those of the normal tissue from which they originated. These cells are not subject to the same control mechanisms that keep normal cell growth in check (Fig. 43.1). Normal cells grown in a laboratory tissue culture medium will cease growing when they have made contact with surrounding cells and/or filled their container. This is called *contact inhibition,* and it explains, for instance, why our liver grows to a certain size and doesn't keep growing until we burst. Tumor cells, on the other hand, don't display the same respect for boundaries. For example, in laboratory tissue cultures, they grow relentlessly, tumbling over each other and spilling over the edges of their containers.

Benign Tumors

Benign tumors are "well differentiated" tumors, differing only slightly in appearance and behavior from their tissue of origin. These tumors are slow-growing and noninvasive, do not spread throughout the body, and will often have a fibrous tissue capsule surrounding them.

All of these characteristics make benign tumors easy to surgically remove in most cases. Unless allowed to grow to a huge size, they seldom pose a threat to life. However, they might cause significant problems if they are located within a vital organ. In fact, the most significant alteration that a benign tumor makes in its host organism is that of encroachment on surrounding normal tissue, leading to obstruction or replacement of the innocent (nontumorous) tissue by the tumor.

To identify a benign tumor, the suffix *-oma* is used. For example, a benign tumor of osseous (bone) tissue would be called an *osteoma,* and a benign tumor of fibrous tissue would be called a *fibroma.* The term *adenoma* is used to describe a benign tumor of a glandular structure, such as a mammary gland (mammary adenoma) or the thyroid gland (thyroid adenoma). The term *papilloma* or *polyp* is applied to wartlike projections originating from epithelial surfaces such as skin or intestinal lining.

Malignant Tumors

Malignant tumors, in contrast to benign tumors, grow rapidly. Malignant tumors send spreading fingers into the surrounding normal tissue, making it difficult to surgically remove the entire tumor. As a result, they frequently regrow after surgery. Malignant cells demonstrate marked *dedifferentiation,* or *anaplasia.* In other words, they do not look like the cells from which they originated.

Malignant tumors are commonly referred to as *cancer.* Cancers of epithelial or glandular structures are referred to as *carcinomas,* while cancers of other tissues are referred to as *sarcomas.* The major danger of a malignant tumor rests in its ability to metastasize, or spread throughout the body. Vital organs in distant locations can be invaded, often resulting in rapid death.

Carcinomas, as a rule, spread via the lymph vessels, although some can skip the lymph nodes and go directly into blood vessels. An example of a carcinoma in dogs that can metastasize either by lymphatics or blood is the mammary carcinoma.

Sarcomas usually metastasize via the bloodstream. Organs that are frequent sites of bloodborne metastasis include the liver and lungs, both of which can be rapidly overwhelmed by the tumors.

We have all seen or heard of people who have been seriously debilitated by cancer, and pets are affected similarly. A malignant tumor can cause what is called the *cachexia* of cancer. With cachexia, the animal literally starves as the tumor grows and steals the body's nutrition. Hemorrhage, pain, fever, and infection are also frequent secondary effects of cancer.

Some tumors produce side effects on the host through the production and release of hormones. These tumors cause the secretion of dangerously high levels of hormones. For example, an *insuloma* of the pancreas produces excessive amounts of insulin. Animals with this tumor will experience very low blood sugar levels, resulting in weakness and/or seizures. Also, thyroid adenomas in cats can produce excessive amounts of thyroid hormone, leading to nervousness, weight loss, and diarrhea in affected animals.

Causes, Occurrence, and Diagnosis of Cancer in Pets

What do we know about the occurrence of cancer in pets? Most people are very surprised to learn that dogs and cats have a higher incidence of many tumors than do humans. For example, dogs experience 35 times as much skin cancer as do humans, 4 times as many breast tumors, 8 times as much bone cancer, and twice the incidence of leukemia.

Only a few types of cancer are seen more frequently in humans than in small animals. For instance, the rate of occurrence of lung cancer is 7 times higher in humans, and gastrointestinal malignancies occur 13 times more frequently in humans than in dogs and cats.

Breed Predilections (Dogs)

Through careful statistical evaluation by veterinary researchers, certain breed predilections for cancer have been noted. If asked which breed of dog has the highest incidence of cancer, a veterinarian would undoubtedly reply "the boxer." When a sick, aged boxer turns up at the hospital, the attending veterinarian suspects a tumor almost immediately. Other dog breeds that can have a high incidence of cancer include Boston terriers, cocker spaniels, and wire-haired fox terriers. Breeds with a relatively low incidence of cancer include beagles, poodles, collies, and dachshunds.

Why do some breeds have a high incidence of cancer while some are rarely affected? The answer to that question is still elusive. One hypothesis deals with the immune system of these pets. The boxer's immune system is thought to be less able to mobilize resistance against cancer cells than the immune systems of many other breeds. It is also hypothesized that the high incidence of cancer in breeds such as the cocker spaniel and boxer is related to heavy inbreeding decades earlier that effectively weakened the breed's immune capabilities.

Some types of tumors are more prone to develop in one type of dog than in others. For example, the giant breeds, such as the St. Bernard and the Great Dane, have a much higher incidence of osteosarcoma (a very malignant bone tumor) than does the general canine population. Dogs with lightly pigmented noses are prone to develop carcinomas in that area, probably due to long-term exposure to the ultraviolet rays of the sun. Finally, black dogs have a comparatively higher incidence of melanomas (pigmented malignant tumors) than do their light-colored peers.

Finally, the sexual status of a dog can predispose to certain types of cancer. The female dog that is not spayed has a sevenfold greater chance of developing mammary tumors than does the dog that is ovariohysterectomized early in life. Intact male canines are more likely to develop certain types of cancers, such as perianal and testicular tumors, as well.

Age Predilection

It is well noted that the incidence of cancer increases with advancing age. Cells that continually divide throughout life have a greater chance of undergoing a spontaneous genetic mutation due to cell-division "accidents" and the effects of carcinogens, or cancer-causing agents. Also, age-related depression of the normal immune response interferes with its ability to kill cancer cells that may spontaneously arise within the body. As a result, older pets will, by nature, have a higher incidence of cancer than will their younger neighbors.

Other Causes of Cancer in Pets

Some tumors affecting pets are contagious. For instance, the transmissible venereal tumor in the dog is spread by implantation during breeding, and

DID YOU KNOW ❓

Second-hand cigarette smoke, either inhaled or licked from the fur, has been linked to cancer in cats!

a virus is known to cause the canine oral papilloma tumor of young dogs. In cats, cattle, mice, and poultry, a virus causes lymphosarcoma, but no virus has as yet been recovered from the lymphosarcoma of canines or humans. Finally, research has revealed that second-hand cigarette smoke can cause lymphoma in cats!

Unfortunately, the causes of most types of tumors still remain a mystery. This is one area in which more research is desperately needed. Until veterinary professionals know the cause of a disease, attempts at "shotgun" treatment will be symptomatic at best and will seldom lead to a cure.

Diagnosing Cancer in Pets

The diagnosis of cancer is not always as straightforward as it would seem. Some animals may exhibit clinical signs for months before the actual cancer can be found. However, several methods are available that can be used to pinpoint and diagnose neoplastic disease in pets:

1. *Physical examination.* Many tumors can be diagnosed on physical examination alone using visual observation and/or manual palpation.

2. *Radiography* (*X rays*). Both plain films and contrast techniques can be used to demonstrate tumors of the lung, gastrointestinal tract, bladder, and other internal organs. Sometimes a radiograph can be pathognomonic (completely typical) for a particular type of tumor, as in the case of bone tumors. Multiple nodular masses in the lung would suggest bloodborne metastasis of a malignant tumor somewhere else in the body. However, in most cases, a tumor visualized on a radiograph must be biopsied to rule in or rule out malignancy.

3. *Ultrasonography.* The use of ultrasonic waves to visualize structures within the body is commonplace in modern veterinary medicine, and is a valuable tool for diagnosing internal cancers. Ultrasound is a very reliable method to help differentiate tumors from benign cysts. It is also useful in evaluating the sizes of internal organs. One area in which ultrasonography is not of much value is in the evaluation of the lungs, since ultrasound waves cannot effectively pass through air-filled structures.

4. *Cytology.* Examination of cells pulled from body cavities, mammary gland secretions, nasal exudates, respiratory secretions, bone marrow, lymph nodes, or various "lumps and bumps" is a popular method of diagnosing neoplastic disease. Cytological examinations are especially effective in ruling out other causes of lumps and bumps, including abscesses, cysts, and granulomas.

5. *Biopsy.* Biopsy is the most common and the most definitive way to make the diagnosis of cancer in animals. Gross and microscopic examination of a neoplasm by a competent veterinary pathologist can be expected to yield an accurate diagnosis 90 percent of the time. Misdiagnosis can occur if the sample of tissue submitted is too small or if an area of the tumor that was selected for biopsy does not contain viable cells. For example, osteosarcoma is frequently misdiagnosed because these tumors contain a great deal of dead tissue and reactive fibrous tissue. If these "benign" areas of the tumor are inadvertently biopsied, the pathologist will not find malignant cells.

6. *Endoscopy or laparoscopy.* Fiberoptic endoscopes are valuable diagnostic tools in the fight against cancer. With these instruments, tumors in the esophagus, stomach, bronchi, liver, spleen, and other organs can be visualized without dangerous exploratory surgery. Biopsies of tumors can also be obtained with these instruments.

7. *Nuclear medicine.* Nuclear scans of the liver, thyroid, lung, spleen, kidney, and bone are used in veterinary colleges and highly specialized veterinary hospitals to diagnose cancer. Radioisotopes with short half-lives are used, and anesthesia of the pet is rarely required. These scans have few adverse effects on the pet.

8. *Blood tests.* The diagnosis of certain types of neoplastic disease can be assisted by results obtained through the microscopic and biochemical analysis of a pet's blood (Fig. 43.2). For example, an increase in serum cholesterol and the enzyme alkaline phosphatase is typically found in canine Cushing's disease, which is caused by a tumor of the adrenal gland or pituitary gland. Similarly, cancer of the bone marrow (leukemia) can be diagnosed by finding tumor cells in the bloodstream. Finally, specific blood tests can be used to confirm or discount suspected cases of feline leukemia or feline immunodeficiency virus infections in sick cats.

Prognosis

Once cancer has been diagnosed in a pet, the prognosis for survival with treatment versus without treatment must be considered. One factor to consider is that these pets will frequently be older, and other diseases, such as heart and kidney disease, might be present. Therefore,

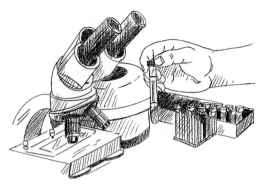

FIGURE 43.2 Certain types of neoplastic disease can be diagnosed through the microscopic and biochemical analysis of a pet's blood.

the first objectives in deciding whether to treat a pet with cancer should be to identify all the underlying conditions that may be present, and assess the severity of those conditions. If a pet has progressive kidney or heart disease, it is unlikely that it will live through major surgery. Even the animal's small secondary problems can become major primary problems once cancer treatment has started. For example, a pet might be coping well with hookworm infestation until chemotherapy depresses its immune system. At this point, a raging bloody diarrhea might develop. As a result, before initiating treatment, other problems must be taken care of first if at all possible.

Another factor that figures into the prognosis is the behavior of the particular tumor afflicting the pet. Ideally, biopsies should be performed on all tumors to determine information about growth patterns and likelihood of metastasis.

Finally, if a tumor is malignant, the extent of the disease's spread must be determined. With most sarcomas, chest radiographs are necessary because the lungs are frequent sites of bloodborne metastasis. With carcinomas, both lymph nodes and lungs should be evaluated closely, since either or both sites can be involved at the time of presentation to the veterinarian. With tumors that affect the oral and nasal cavities, skull radiographs are necessary, since prognosis is not as good if there is much bone destruction and invasion. Finally, if a lymph node is enlarged, cytology should be performed on it to determine whether it is enlarged due to tumor metastasis. Tumors that have metastasized throughout the lymphatic system carry with them a grave prognosis.

Treating Cancer in Pets

Treatment techniques for cancer have multiplied rapidly in recent years. Previously, a pet with a malignant tumor received surgery, and if that tumor grew back or spread to other organs, the pet was probably put to sleep. However, other options are now available. A combination of therapies, including chemotherapy, radiation therapy, immunotherapy, and/or surgery, is now the optimum protocol to achieve control of a malignancy (Fig. 43.3).

Surgery

If a tumor is localized and easily accessible, surgery is still the best method to effect a cure. If a highly malignant tumor involves an extremity, amputation of the affected limb may be needed to save the life of the pet. The goal of all cancer surgeries is to remove all malignant cells (or as many as possible) before any spread occurs to regional lymph nodes or other organs. With some malignancies, however, total removal may not be possible. In these instances, surgery must be combined with other forms of therapy in order for treatment to be effective.

Radiation

Many tumors are controllable, if not curable, through the use of radiation. Radiation can be administered using radioactive implants (brachytherapy), or externally, using radiation beams (teletherapy). Regardless of method used, radiation will destroy the DNA (deoxyribonucleic acid) of cells so that they can no longer reproduce. To be affected by radiotherapy, a tumor should

1. Be of a radiosensitive cell type
2. Involve no vital radiosensitive organs, such as the gastrointestinal tract
3. Have readily definable borders
4. Be slow to metastasize

Frequently, radiotherapy is combined with surgery to ensure that residual microscopic foci of disease that might have been left by the surgeon are killed.

Chemotherapy

In the past, the expense of chemotherapy had prohibited its widespread use in veterinary medicine. However, today a multitude of

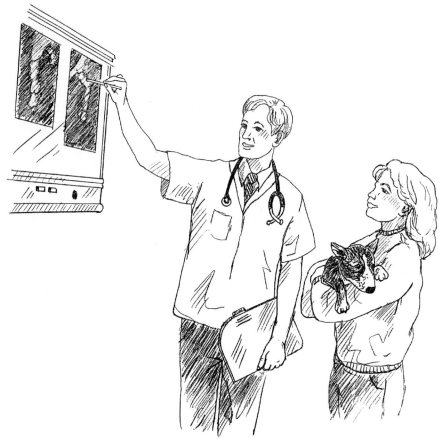

FIGURE 43.3 Be sure to discuss all cancer treatment options thoroughly with your veterinarian.

affordable anticancer drugs are readily available for use in pets. These drugs work to kill tumors by several mechanisms, including fragmenting the chromosome strands within the tumor cells and inhibiting cell division.

Of course, the actions against tumor cells also cause changes in normal cells, with significant side effects in the animal being treated. These side effects can include severe bone marrow depression, nausea, vomiting, hair loss, and hemorrhage. The objective of the veterinarian is to achieve a drug dosage that is strong enough to control or cure the tumor while minimizing these side effects.

Some tumors are very responsive to chemotherapy. For example, the average life span after diagnosis of a lymphosarcoma in a dog is 56 days; however, with chemotherapy, the life expectancy can be increased to about a year.

On the other hand, tumors such as fibrosarcomas and osteosarcomas are notoriously resistant to chemotherapy. Human oncologists are controlling many of these highly malignant tumors with expensive drugs that cost hundreds of dollars per treatment, but these agents have had (understandably) very limited use in pets.

One disadvantage of chemotherapy is that it is relatively ineffective against large tumors. With these tumors, the number of neoplastic cells must first be reduced by either surgery or radiation therapy before chemotherapy can be effective.

Immunotherapy

Immunotherapy is a newer form of cancer therapy that shows great promise in the fight against this disease. This type of therapy is based on the premise that in many cancers, growth of the tumor is a result of a defect in the pet's immune system. Had immunity been normal, the tumor growth should have been suppressed early in its development. As a result, immunotherapy utilizes various drugs and vaccines (biological response modifiers) to stimulate the pet's immune system to fight the cancer. One form of immunotherapy, monoclonal antibody therapy, has shown promise as an effective adjunct therapy in the treatment of canine lymphoma and other cancers. *Monoclonal antibodies* work by binding to cancer cells and triggering the body's immune system to destroy the cells to which they are attached. Since these antibodies are very specific in the types of cells they bind to, normal cells within the body remain unharmed. Research is currently focusing on even newer applications for monoclonal antibody therapy, as well as newer forms of immunotherapy in general, such as gene therapy.

Treatment Summary

Both surgery and radiation therapy are excellent treatments for localized cancers. However, even if only a few tumor cells have escaped beyond this local area, the treatment will fail. If this is suspected, then chemotherapy will be used in combination with surgery and/or radiation therapy. Chemotherapy is also recommended if the tumor is of the type that readily metastasize. The combination of all the above-mentioned therapies can pack a powerful "one-two punch" against neoplastic disease in animals. Adding immunotherapy to the fray will further enhance remission in select cases.

Nutritional support of the cancer patient can play a key role in the success of any treatment protocol. Scientific diets are available from veterinarians that can help reverse cancer cachexia, enhance immune function, and may actually inhibit tumor growth in certain instances. For example, studies have shown that high levels of omega-3 fatty acids in the diet of animals can help inhibit the growth and spread of tumors. As a result, if you have a pet with cancer, be sure to provide it with the proper nutritional support, including omega-3 fatty acids, to help combat the disease.

Even with the advances made in the fields of cancer therapy and support, there is still much to learn about cancer, its origins, and its behavior. As we become more knowledgeable in these areas, more effective treatments can be developed. Perhaps 30 years from now, veterinarians and pet owners alike will be able to look with amazement (and a little disdain) at the "primitive" methods now used to control cancer in pets.

Specific Types of Neoplasia in Dogs and Cats

As mentioned previously in this chapter, countless types of neoplasms can arise in dogs and cats; however, certain types appear more frequently than others.

Adenomas are tumors affecting glandular structures within the body. Adenomas arising from the sebaceous glands of the skin account for the largest percentage of tumors affecting dogs. There is no sex predilection for these tumors, and most occur in animals over 9 years of age. Sebaceous gland adenomas are cauliflower, wartlike growths and are pink to orange in appearance, although some may be pigmented. Sites most commonly affected include the limbs, trunk, eyelids, and head. In most cases, they are benign in character and pose little threat to the health of the pet.

Diagnosis of sebaceous gland adenomas is based on physical appearance and biopsy test results. Treatment consists of surgical excision, cryotherapy, and/or heat therapy. Once removed, they rarely recur in the same location. However, they may appear elsewhere on the body. In those instances in which multiple adenomas exist on a particular pet, treatment is sometimes bypassed altogether, unless the tumors appear to be growing extraordinarily fast or become ulcerated or traumatized.

Adenomas can also arise from modified skin glands in the region of the anus (perianal glands) and anal sacs of dogs. Seen most often in dogs over 11 years of age, perianal gland adenomas are nine times more likely to occur in male dogs than in females. The reason for this is that the activities of these glands are normally modulated by sex hormones, mainly the male hormone testosterone. Interestingly, female dogs afflicted with Cushing's disease may be predisposed to these tumors because disease-induced elevated levels of testosterone are produced by the adrenal glands.

Most tumors involving the perianal glands are benign in nature; however, malignancy (adenocarcinoma) can occur, especially if the tumor involves the anal sac. As a result, diagnosis of these tumors should always include biopsy evaluation to determine their status. The treatment of choice for benign adenomas is castration to remove the source of hormonal influence. In addition, in extensive cases, surgical excision, chemotherapy, and even radiation therapy can be used to attempt a cure. Therapy with estrogen compounds is often used to treat malignant adenomas and also female dogs that may be afflicted with benign or malignant tumors. Prognosis for recovery is good to excellent with benign tumors, but guarded to poor with malignancies.

Cats can be affected with several different types of adenomas as well. Two of the more common forms of adenomas and adenocarcinomas seen in cats include ceruminous gland tumors, which affect the ears and ear canals, and thyroid adenomas, which are responsible for the development of hyperthyroidism.

Tumors involving the mammary glands, including mammary adenocarcinomas, are quite common among both canines and felines. Owing to the hormonal influences on mammary tissue, female dogs and cats are more likely to develop such tumors than are males. These neoplasms can arise from a number of cell types within the mammary tissue itself, and can be benign or malignant in nature. Malignant mammary neoplasms grow quite rapidly, and tend to invade and cause inflammation in and around surrounding tissue. Metastasis to other organs such as the lungs, liver, bone, and kidney can occur as well. Mammary tumors appear as hardened, sometimes painful swellings usually involving the last two glands of the mammary chain, although the others may also be affected. Local lymph node enlargement, especially in the groin region, may become noticeable as well. A fluid discharge from the affected nipples may occur, and, if metastasis takes place, breathing difficulties, coughing, swollen limbs, vomiting, and/or diarrhea may arise.

The treatment of choice for any type of mammary tumor is surgical excision. This may involve simply removing the mass if only one location along the mammary chain is affected, or in the case of multiple locations, the entire gland or a large portion thereof may need to be removed. Since mammary tumors are usually highly malignant in cats, radical mastectomies are indicated in all cases. Regional lymph nodes are removed as well if metastasis is suspected. On biopsy of the affected tissue, subsequent chemotherapy is recommended if the tumor is deemed malignant.

It should be noted that female dogs that are spayed prior to their first heat cycle experience a dramatically reduced incidence of mammary cancer when compared to those females that were allowed to go through one or more heat cycles. As a result, this is a great way to prevent this devastating form of cancer.

Lipomas are relatively common tumors in dogs that can arise from fatty tissue anywhere in the body. Dachshunds, cocker spaniels, poodles, and terriers seem to be especially predisposed to this type of tumor. The most prevalent sites of occurrence include the subdermal (beneath the skin) fatty tissue on the belly and chest regions. Lipomas present as soft, fluctuant round masses that are adhered tightly to surrounding tissue. As a rule, lipomas rarely pose a health risk to a dog, unless they become secondarily infected or achieve such a size as to mechanically interfere with normal body functions. This can occur within the body cavities, where lipomas arising from fat adhere to body organs or from membranes lining the cavities form large space-occupying masses that can impinge on surrounding organs.

Surgical removal is the treatment of choice for lipomas, yet they can sometimes be difficult to completely excise because they tend to infiltrate into surrounding muscles and tissues. As a result, recurrences following surgery are not uncommon. In many instances, if tumor growth is minimal and there is little to no interference with normal body function, lipomas are left untreated.

The malignant form of fatty tumors, *liposarcomas,* are rare in dogs, yet must be ruled out whenever a fatty mass is discovered. Veterinarians can distinguish lipomas from liposarcomas through cytology and biopsy procedures. If a malignancy is diagnosed, liberal surgical excision of the mass and a portion of the surrounding tissue is indicated in an effort to completely remove the cancer. Chemotherapy is indicated as well.

Another prevalent form of neoplasia in cats and dogs is malignant *lymphoma-lymphosarcoma* (LSA). In fact, this is by far the most common form of neoplasia found in cats. This type of cancer involves the neoplastic proliferation of lymphocytes in sites throughout the body, including the lymph nodes, digestive tract, skin, spleen, liver, and kidneys.

In dogs, the primary clinical sign associated with malignant lymphoma typically includes a generalized swelling of the lymph nodes throughout the body, especially noticeable on the neck, shoulder, hindlimb, and inguinal regions. Other nonspecific signs may appear as organ systems within the body are adversely affected.

In cats, LSA is usually seen concurrently with FeLV infections. There are a number of different presentations or forms of this particular neoplastic condition in felines. *Alimentary LSA* affects primarily the intestines and associated lymphatic tissue. Other organs within the abdomen can be affected as well. Symptoms commonly seen with alimentary LSA include loss of appetite, weight loss, vomiting, diarrhea, bloody stool, jaundice, and/or constipation. The *mediastinal* form of LSA presents itself as the proliferation of a large tumor within the chest cavity. As one might expect, prominent signs seen with this form include breathing difficulties, coughing, pleural effusions, chest wall incompressibility, and swallowing difficulties. *Multicentric LSA* affects lymph nodes and tissue in multiple sites throughout the body, all at one time. The signs seen with this type are variable, depending on the organs most heavily involved. Prominent swelling of the lymph nodes, including those situated beneath the skin, is usually seen with this form of LSA. *Atypical LSA* is a form of LSA that is limited to solitary organs or organ systems within the body. Such solitary sites may include the skin, eyes, spinal cord, muscles, brain, and kidneys. Obviously, symptoms exhibited will reflect the organ(s) involved. Finally, *lymphocytic leukemia* is a type of LSA characterized by the growth and proliferation of neoplastic lymphocytes within the blood and bone marrow, often affecting secondary structures such as the spleen and liver. Symptoms associated with lymphocytic leukemia tend to be nonspecific in nature, and can include anemia, jaundice, loss of appetite, weakness, fever, and organomegally (enlargement of internal organs).

Diagnosis of malignant lymphoma in dogs and cats can be achieved through lymph node cytology and biopsy, radiographs of the abdomen and chest, and ultrasonography of the same. FeLV testing of affected cats will often yield positive results, although not always.

Treatment for malignant lymphoma for both dogs and cats involves chemotherapy, radiation therapy, and in select cases, immunotherapy. Unfortunately, the prognosis for a long-term remission (extending beyond 6 months) is poor for most patients.

Myeloproliferative disorders and *leukemia* are a family of disorders seen primarily in cats and characterized by a neoplastic proliferation of the cellular components of the bone marrow, including the white blood cells, red blood cells, and platelets. Again, the feline leukemia virus is the culprit responsible for most myeloproliferative disorders seen in cats. Symptoms associated with these disorders are often related to anemia and blood clotting disorders (weakness, labored breathing, pale mucous membranes, loss of appetite), as the proliferating cells, especially white blood cells, within the bone marrow interfere with the normal production of red blood cells and platelets. In addition, certain myeloproliferative disorders are characterized by the abnormal production of the red blood cells and platelets themselves, leading again to those signs mentioned previously, and also to an enlargement of the spleen and liver. Definitive diagnosis of a myeloproliferative disorder or leukemia is made on evaluation of the blood and a biopsy sample of the bone marrow. Chemotherapy is the treatment approach of choice. Bone marrow transplants, although not readily performed on cats, can be useful as well.

Melanomas are neoplasms seen most often affecting the integument of dogs, with a special predilection for the lips, tongue, gums, oral cavity, eyelids, and the digits of the feet. Arising from pigment-producing epithelial cells, melanomas may be either benign or malignant in nature. In fact, the degree of malignancy exhibited by these tumors seems to be directly correlated with where they are located. For example, melanomas involving the mouth and oral cavity tend to be more malignant than those affecting the digits or eyelids. Male dogs seem to have a higher occurrence of this type of skin tumor than do females.

Benign melanomas appear as darkly pigmented nodules or skin blotches with well-defined borders. Rarely do they exceed 1 inch in diameter. Malignant melanomas, on the other hand, appear as rapidly growing, often ulcerated masses or nodules that may or may not be pigmented and can reach greater sizes. These cancers often metastasize via the blood and lymph to various organs throughout the body, including the liver, lungs, spleen, brain, spinal cord, heart, and bone. As with other tumors, definitive diagnosis of a melanoma and whether a malignancy exists is accomplished through biopsy and microscopic examination of the tumor. Radiography, ultrasonography, and lymph node biopsies may all be used to help determine the extent of metastasis if a malignancy is diagnosed. Treatment involves the surgical removal of the tumor and radiation therapy. Chemotherapy has proved to be of limited use in the treatment of malignant melanoma. Unfortunately, malignant melanomas have usually undergone metastasis by the time they are first recognized, and tend to recur after surgical removal. As a result, an overall prognosis for cure is poor.

Although melanomas are not common in cats, *basal cell tumors* are. In fact, these are the most prevalent skin tumors seen in cats. These tumors, which are usually benign in nature, present as a firm, raised nodule with or without an ulcerated surface. They may also be heavily pigmented, appearing brown to black in color. Basal cell tumors originate from the deeper layers of the skin, hair follicles, and/or sebaceous glands. Sites most often affected include the skin of the head, neck, ears, and shoulder regions. These tumors can usually be treated quite successfully with surgical removal of the tumor, chemotherapy, and/or radiation therapy.

Still another type of neoplasia that can arise from the skin epithelial cells of dogs and cats are *squamous cell carcinomas* (SCCs). Areas of skin lacking pigment or subject to repeated trauma or irritation are especially susceptible to SCC development. The oral cavity, tonsils, lips, nose, eyelids, external ear, and limbs are common sites of occurrence. SCC can involve the nails and toes as well.

A squamous cell carcinoma may appear as a slightly raised mass, often with an ulcerated surface, or it may actually resemble a papule or wart. As a rule, these tumors are slow to spread to other organs, yet usually readily invade surrounding tissue. Diagnosis is achieved through biopsy evaluation of the actual tumor. Surgery, cryotherapy, hyperthermia, chemotherapy, and radiation therapy are the most effective ways to treat SCC in dogs and cats.

Mast cell tumors (*mastocytoma*) may present as solitary or multiple skin nodules, some of which may be ulcerated and pigmented. Seen primarily in dogs, such tumors may be located anywhere on the body, yet those located around the reproductive structures and on the digits of the feet seem to exhibit a higher degree of malignancy than do those in other locations.

Mast cell tumors are especially significant because the cells making up the tumor are filled with granules containing histamine and several other powerful chemicals that can have profound effects on the body if released from the cells. Some of these effects include gastrointestinal ulcers, interference with normal blood clotting, and kidney inflammation. Diagnosis of a mast cell tumor can often be made on cytological examination and biopsy of a tumor sample. In addition, evaluation of the blood often reveals abnormalities related to the release of histamine and other granules, such as low platelet counts, anemia, and elevations in white blood cells.

Treatment for mast cell tumors employs a wide variety of techniques because of the stubborn nature of this neoplasia. Surgical excision of the visible mass along with a generous portion of healthy tissue surrounding the mass (to ensure complete removal) is usually the first step taken. Veterinary surgeons must exercise extreme care when handling these tumors, since excessive handling could cause a massive release of granules from the tumor that can induce shock and collapse. Following surgical recovery, radiation therapy and chemotherapy may be employed to help reduce the chances of recurrence and metastatic growth. Cryotherapy is also employed in those instances in which surgical excision of the tumor is incomplete or impossible.

Osteosarcoma (OSA) is a highly malignant tumor involving the bones and joints. This tumor is quite destructive in nature and metastasizes readily to other organs of the body, especially the lungs. Locally, bone destruction with infiltration of surrounding tissues occurs in most cases. The most common site of involvement in dogs is the forearm, yet the tumor can also appear on the hindlimbs and even facial bones. In cats, the hindlimbs and skull are the areas most often affected.

Clinical signs associated with OSA include limb swelling and lameness. Coughing, breathing difficulties, and other signs related to internal organ involvement may also be seen if metastasis has occurred. Diagnosis can usually be made with clinical signs and with radiographs of the affected bones. Of course, biopsy evaluation is needed to confirm such a diagnosis.

Treatment for an osteosarcoma invading the bone of a limb involves aggressive surgical intervention, including amputation of the affected limb or special surgical techniques designed to preserve limb integrity while allowing for tumor removal. Chemotherapy should follow surgery to slow or eliminate metastatic disease. If chemotherapy is not instituted, most pets diagnosed with OSA and treated with surgery alone will die within 1 year following diagnosis.

Fibrosarcomas are malignant tumors arising from the fibrous tissue located just beneath the skin. They usually present as solitary, irregular masses on or protruding from the skin. Their surfaces may or may not be ulcerated. In addition, fibrosarcomas have been known to develop at sites of vaccine administration along the back and flank regions of cats. When they occur, fibrosarcomas aggressively invade local tissue, and secondary metastasis to the lungs and lymph nodes is not uncommon.

Diagnosis of fibrosarcomas is made through biopsy evaluation. Treatment usually involves a combination of surgery, radiation therapy, and chemotherapy; surgery is the most important of the three.

Hemangiomas and *hemangiosarcomas* are neoplasms seen primarily in dogs that arise from the cells within the blood vessels. Common sites of occurrence include the spleen, heart, liver, and skin, although any organ within the body can be affected if metastasis via the blood takes place. Hemangiosarcomas tend to be very malignant and often ulcerate as a result of rapid growth. German shepherds, boxers, Scottish terriers, and Airedale terriers seem to have the highest incidence of this tumor type.

Clinical signs associated with hemangiomas and hemangiosarcomas involving the skin include the appearance of soft, friable masses, usually on the chest or extremities. If the spleen or other internal organs are involved, symptoms seen include weakness and depression, abdominal swelling, breathing difficulties, progressive emaciation, enlarged lymph nodes, and/or nosebleeds. Overt collapse and shock can occur secondary to excessive bleeding typically from the spleen.

Diagnosis of these blood vessel tumors is based on clinical signs and tumor biopsy results. Surgical excision or cryotherapy can be utilized on hemangiomas with favorable results. Hemangiosarcomas, on the other hand, provide a greater treatment challenge because of their invasive and metastatic nature. Often, amputation of an entire limb may be required because of the tumor's invasiveness. Removal of the spleen is indicated in cases of splenic hemangiosarcoma. Chemotherapy can be employed postsurgically, yet the prognosis for a lasting recovery still remains poor.

Bladder tumors are relatively common in dogs. They can arise from a variety of different tissues that constitute this organ. The two most prevalent bladder neoplasms include transitional cell carcinomas and squamous cell carcinomas. Female dogs seem to be affected more than males.

Tumors present within the urinary bladder can predispose to secondary infection and urolith formation. In instances where the tumor is especially large, it can obstruct the outflow of urine and cause associated complications. Clinical signs of a bladder tumor include bloody urine, straining to urinate, and painful urinations. Diagnosis is achieved through an evaluation of the urine as well as contrast radiographs or ultrasonography of the bladder. Biochemical evaluation of the blood may reveal elevated kidney enzymes if the kidneys have been damaged by an obstruction to urine flow.

Benign and malignant bladder tumors are best treated by surgical excision if their location and involvement permit. Unfortunately, most malignant bladder tumors are highly metastatic; as a result, the chances of recurrence after surgery are high. For this reason, both chemotherapy and radiation therapy may be employed after surgery to help reduce the chances of this recurrence and to attack any spread that may have taken place.

Zoonotic Diseases

"Doctor, I think my dog has a cold. Can I catch it?" In veterinary practices across the country, questions such as this one are common. And although the answer to this particular question is "no," there are numerous other diseases that can indeed be transmitted from family pets to their owners. Such diseases are properly termed zoonotic diseases.

Children are at greatest risk of contracting a disease from the family pet, primarily because of their inherent curiosity and often less-than-desirable hygiene habits (Fig. 44.1). However, adults are susceptible as well. Failing to provide adequate preventive health care for pets greatly increases the chance of exposure to one or more of these diseases. Refer to Table 44.1 for a listing of some of the zoonoses carried by dogs, cats, birds, and exotic pets.

Animal Bites and Scratches

Besides the potential for rabies transmission, a bite (Fig. 44.2) from a pet can also lead to severe bacterial infections and tissue damage in the affected individual. Likewise, scratches, especially those inflicted by cats, can be just as bad as, if not worse than, those injuries caused by teeth. For instance, cat-scratch fever, a disease that can cause fever and swollen, painful lymph nodes (lymphadenopathy), can be transmitted to an unsuspecting owner by the mere scratch of a cat harboring the organism on its nails.

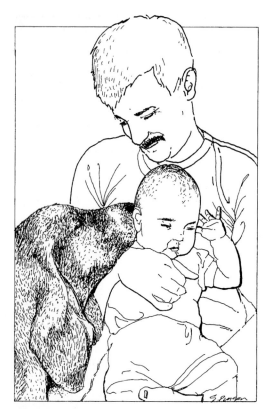

FIGURE 44.1 Children are especially suscepti-ble to zoonotic diseases.

FACT *OR* *FICTION*

Rabbits, opossums, armadillos, and rodents are resistant to the rabies virus. **FICTION.** While these animals can get rabies, they are considered very low risk, since they rarely survive an attack by a rabid animal in the first place.

If your pet bites you or a member of your family, don't delay! Seek medical attention immediately.

Rabies

Certainly the most infamous of all zoonoses is rabies. This is an incurable, fatal viral disease that attacks the nervous system of its unfortunate host. The rabies virus is excreted in the saliva of infected animals and transmitted to other animals and to people via bite wounds and through contamination of open wounds or sores. Although rabies is restricted primarily to wild or feral carnivores, cases occasionally spill over into the domestic and stray dog and cat population, thus providing the important link between wildlife rabies and human rabies.

Because rabies cannot be cured, the key here is prevention. Obviously, it's very important to keep all dogs, cats, and ferrets current on their rabies vaccinations. In addition, don't allow your pets to roam free outdoors at night, since this is the time when they are most likely to interact with wild animals. Use common sense: Discourage your children from playing with or petting stray animals. Avoid touching dead or dying bats that may be lying on the ground (Fig. 44.3). And don't keep wild animals such as descented

Table 44.1 Zoonotic Potential of Various Pet Species*

Dogs	Rabies
	Dermatophytes
	Roundworms
	Hookworms
	Tapeworms
	Leptospirosis
	Bacterial enteritis (*Giardia, Salmonella*)
	Tickborne illnesses
	Mites
	Heartworms
	Fleas
Cats	Rabies
	Dermatophytes
	Roundworms
	Hookworms
	Tapeworms
	Bacterial enteritis (*Giardia, Salmonella*)
	Tickborne illnesses
	Mites
	Cat-scratch fever
	Toxoplasmosis
	Heartworms
	Fleas
Birds	Psittacosis
	Bacterial enteritis
	Yersinia pseudotuberculosis
	Erysipelothrix dermatitis

Table 44.1 Zoonotic Potential of Various Pet Species* (*Continued*)

Reptiles	*Salmonella*
	Bacterial enteritis
	Bacterial dermatitis
	Various fungal diseases
	Tickborne illnesses
Amphibians	Bacterial enteritis
	Salmonella
	Leptospirosis
	Trypanosomiasis
Ferrets	Bacterial enteritis (*Giardia, Salmonella*)
	Dermatophytosis
	Tuberculosis
	Influenza A
	Mites
	Rabies
	Heartworms
	Fleas
Rabbits	Bacterial enteritis
	Dermatophytosis
	Tularemia
	Rabies
	Tapeworms
	Mites
	Fleas
Rats, mice, hamsters, gerbils	Tapeworms
	Dermatophytosis

	Meningitis	
	Allergies	
	Fleas	
	Bubonic plague (rats)	
Guinea pigs	Dermatophytosis	
	Mites	
	Allergies	
	Fleas	
Chinchillas	Dermatophytosis	
	Meningitis	
	Fleas	
	Bacterial enteritis	
Prairie dogs	Bubonic plague	
	Dermatophytosis	
	Rabies	
	Meningitis	
	Monkey pox	
	Fleas	
	Mites	
	Bacterial enteritis	
	Hantavirus	
Pot-bellied pigs	Bacterial enteritis	
	Roundworms	
	Hookworms	
	Tapeworms	
	Leptospirosis	
	Rabies (rare)	

Note: The majority of these diseases are rare in pets born and raised in captivity.

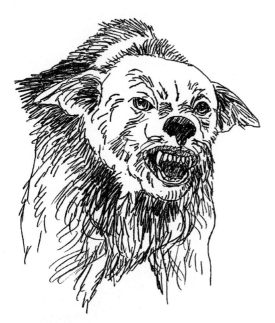

FIGURE 44.2 Animal bites are the most common "zoonotic" encounters experienced.

skunks or raccoons as pets. Because of their high susceptibility to rabies, to do so is to ask for trouble!

Intestinal Worms

Hookworms, roundworms, and tapeworms can pose serious health threats to humans if exposure to infective eggs or larvae occurs. For example, certain types of hookworms can be transmitted from pets to people by contact with soil or sand contaminated with infective hookworm larvae. These larvae have the ability to penetrate and burrow into the outer layer of exposed skin, usually the feet, legs, and/or hands, causing intense itching. The term for this condition is *cutaneous larva migrans.* Adult hookworms have also been known to infect the human intestinal tract, leading to a chronic enterocolitis.

Roundworms can be transmitted by contact with soil contaminated with egg-laden feces. If these eggs are consumed, the larvae hatch within the gut and begin to migrate throughout the organs and tissues of the body. The disease caused by these larvae, called *visceral larva migrans,* is much more serious than that caused by the hookworm. In fact, blindness, seizures, and other serious maladies can result. This is especially true in children, or in those individuals with compromised immune systems. If there is one good reason for having your family pet routinely dewormed and checked for parasites, this is it!

Dipylidium caninum, the most common tapeworm seen in dogs and cats, can infest the intestinal tract of people who accidentally consume a flea that contains the tapeworm larva. Pet owners can avoid such exposure by controlling fleas on their animals. More seriously, though, hydatid cyst disease, caused by the tapeworm *Echinococcus* (Fig. 44.4), can be contracted by humans through contact with tapeworm eggs shed by dogs and cats harboring the adult form of these worms. On ingestion, the tapeworm larvae emerge from the eggs and migrate throughout all tissues and organs of the body, including the brain. The resulting damage can be deadly if not detected and managed soon enough. Dogs can become infested with adult *Echinococcus* tapeworms by eating meat

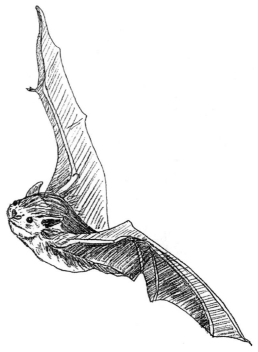

FIGURE 44.3 The bat is an important vector for the rabies virus.

from cattle, sheep, or pigs infected with the larval form of the disease. As a result, prohibiting the consumption of raw meat and offal by pets is the surest way to keep the risk of this disease low.

Heartworms

Rarely, humans can be infected with *Dirofilaria immitis,* the canine and feline heartworm. The heartworm larvae, which gain entrance into the body via a mosquito bite, do not migrate to the heart as they do in pets, but rather to the lungs. Here, they can form coinlike lesions that have been mistaken on human chest radiographs for tuberculosis or cancer. Fortunately, the actual inflammation and disease caused by these lesions are rarely severe.

Besides using mosquito repellents and practicing environmental control, you can reduce the chances of exposure to heartworm-laden

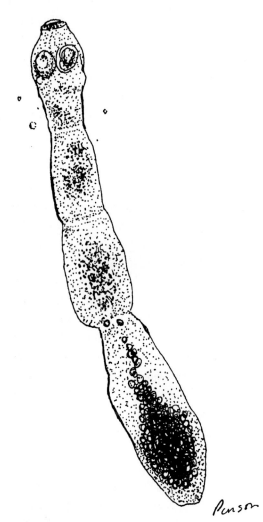

FIGURE 44.4 The *Echinococcus* **tapeworm is the cause of hydatid cyst disease.**

mosquitoes by keeping your dog and cat current on their heartworm preventive medication and encouraging other pet owners to do the same as well.

Ringworm

Ringworm (dermatophytosis) is not a worm at all; it is a fungus that attacks the skin, hair, and nails of both humans and animals. In humans, it typically causes red, itchy skin lesions. Pets can transmit this disease to owners by direct contact with their infected skin and coat. An outbreak of ringworm within a household can often be traced back to the family cat, since felines are common carriers of this disease.

Because of its zoonotic potential, ringworm must always be ruled out as the cause of distinct hair loss in the family pet. An exam and/or fungal culture performed by your veterinarian can verify or dispel such suspicions.

Infectious Diarrhea

Campylobacteriosis, salmonellosis, and giardiasis are three infectious diseases among many that can cause diarrhea in pets. They also happen to be three major infectious causes of diarrhea recognized in people. Transmitted via infected feces, these organisms have the ability to cause severe cramping, nausea, and diarrhea in exposed people. As a result, protect yourself and your family from such diseases by observing good hygiene practices when handling pets, especially exotics. In addition, always seek prompt veterinary care for any diarrheic animal.

Toxoplasmosis

Shed in the feces of infected cats, toxoplasmosis is one of the most common zoonotic diseases around. In the United States alone, up to 40 percent of the adult population have already been exposed to this disease. The majority of cases occurring in people are subclinical in nature (don't show any signs) and often pass undetected.

However, if a pregnant woman who has never been exposed to toxoplasmosis contracts this parasite, it could pose a serious threat to the health of the fetus. If infection occurs early enough in pregnancy, mental retardation in the unborn child can occur. For this reason, if you are pregnant, avoid activities that involve working with soil or sand (your garden might serve as a litterbox for a neighborhood cat), and avoid changing or cleaning cat litterboxes. Contact your obstetrician for more detailed information regarding this disease.

Leptospirosis

The leptospirosis organism that infects dogs can infect humans as well, causing severe chills, fever, anemia, kidney damage, eye damage, and occasionally brain damage. Exposure to infected urine and other secretions or tissues is the primary method of transmission to people. Since the efficacy of the canine vaccine is questionable, keeping dogs away from potential sources of the disease, including livestock and farm tanks or water pools, is the best way to guard against this disease.

Flea- and Tickborne Illnesses

Fleas and ticks have proven to be effective vectors for a variety of diseases that infect humans (Fig. 44.5). Because pets can be reservoirs for fleas and

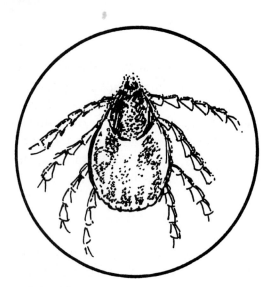

FIGURE 44.5   Ticks are notorious vectors for zoonotic diseases.

ticks within households, owners who fail to undertake adequate external parasite control measures could be placing their own health and their family's in jeopardy.

As mentioned previously, fleas are important vectors for tapeworms in dogs and cats. The chances of a person developing tapeworms following ingestion of tapeworm-infested feces are low; nonetheless, it can occur, especially in children. As a result, minimizing exposure to fleas is a must.

Fleas are also the primary mode of transmission for the plague organism *Yersinia pestis,* the same disease that achieved historical infamy during the Middle Ages. In the southwestern portions of the United States, plague still occasionally rears its ugly head. Cats and prairie dogs carrying the organism or plague-laden fleas pose the greatest threat to human health in these areas. In humans, signs of plague include sore, swollen lymph nodes, fever, seizures, and/or coughing due to pneumonia. Fortunately, if detected early enough, plague can be treated quite effectively with modern medicine. Again, an ounce of prevention is worth a pound of cure, and flea control is the key to protecting your family against this serious disease.

Three of the more infamous tickborne illnesses that can affect people include Rocky Mountain spotted fever, ehrlichiosis, and Lyme disease. Again, pets can act as reservoirs for ticks carrying the causative organisms. Clinical signs of these diseases in humans can include malaise, headaches, chills, painful muscles and joints, and organ failure. Owners wishing to reduce their chances of exposure to these diseases should practice strict tick control, and never remove a tick from a pet with bare hands.

Mites

The *Sarcoptes, Notoedres,* and *Cheyletiella* mange mites that normally infest housepets can also cause disease in people. As in pets, these mites can cause itchy, irritated skin lesions in exposed individuals. Fortunately, such infestations rarely last long and will usually clear up on their own. Pet owners can help shield themselves from such infestations by having all skin lesions involving itching and/or hair loss that might appear on a pet properly diagnosed and treated by their veterinarian.

Psittacosis

Psittacosis is a serious zoonotic disease of pet birds that can cause severe respiratory and flulike illness in humans. Complicated cases can even result in life-threatening inflammation of heart and brain tissue. Caused by the organism *Chlamydia psittaci,* psittacosis is transmitted from birds to humans through the ingestion or inhalation of dried particles from infected feces or discharges. Birds that are smuggled into the United States pose the greatest threat to those unsuspecting pet owners who purchase their birds from roadside stands and other questionable sources. To protect yourself from this disease, be sure that you purchase only birds that have been legally imported and have passed the mandatory quarantine procedures. For additional peace of mind, a laboratory test available from your veterinarian can help confirm the negative status of your new pet.

Control Summary

Although the diseases listed above represent some of the more important zoonoses that parents and pet owners should be aware of, it is certainly not all-inclusive. The following guidelines reiterate and expand on those preventive measures previously mentioned and will help protect you and your family from zoonotic diseases. Be sure that your children understand why these measures are important. By doing so, you can ensure that your family's relationship with your pet will remain a healthy one (Fig. 44.6).

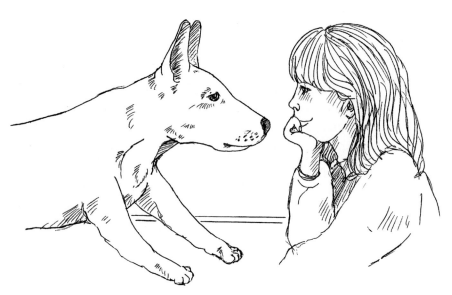

FIGURE 44.6 Be sure that your pet's relationship between you and your family remains a healthy one!

- Purchase your pets (especially birds and exotics) from reputable sources only.

- Insist on a veterinary checkup before finalizing a purchase on any pet.

- Parents and children alike should always wash their hands thoroughly after handling family pets, especially prior to meals.

- Avoid "kissing" pets or being licked on the face by them. After all, you don't know where their mouths have been!

- Avoid interactions with stray or wild animals, alive or dead!

- Clean up and dispose of all animal waste promptly. Waste left unattended in a yard can be a source of infection to pets and people for years to come!

- Keep children's sandboxes covered when not in use, and keep other play areas free of animal excrement.

- Wear disposable gloves when handling reptiles and amphibians.

- Control fleas and ticks on your pet.

- If the area in which you live is at high risk for Lyme disease, consider having your dog vaccinated against this disease.

- If a pet becomes ill, minimize handling and seek veterinary help immediately. Always separate ill animals from young children.

- Have pets routinely examined, vaccinated, and checked for worms by your veterinarian. Birds and exotics should be checked for both external and internal parasites, and their stools should be checked for infectious organisms. New puppies and kittens should be routinely dewormed starting at 3 weeks of age. If applicable, be sure that your pet is on heartworm preventive medication.

An Introduction to Holistic Pet Care

Just imagine having the best of both worlds when it comes to your pet's health care! That's exactly what you get when you merge conventional Western medicine with holistic or "alternative" medicine. When over 40 percent of Americans utilize alternative medicine for themselves and spend billions of dollars each year on holistic treatments and remedies, it's no wonder that the popularity of veterinary holistic treatments for pets and their ailments is increasing as well. And as this popularity rises, so does the need for continued education and research in order to identify and refine specific indications, techniques, benefits, and limitations of holistic treatments in our furred, scaled, and feathered friends.

The philosophy of holistic veterinary medicine is one of wellness and disease prevention. Holistic approaches are geared toward stimulating the body's own natural resources and internal mechanisms to afford self-healing and self-protection against disease. Holism not only targets the physical needs of a particular pet but also takes into account the emotional and mental needs of that pet. These needs can be influenced by such factors as breed characteristics, individual personalities, socialization, environmental influences, and disease states that may alter the biochemistry within the body and adversely affect emotional and mental well-being.

To many followers of holism, this school of thought is in direct contrast to the traditional Western approach to veterinary medicine, namely, to target and treat diseases or symptoms only as they arise. Such treatments are felt to be too standardized, failing to take into account patient differences other than those of species, breed, and/or body weight. In conventional veterinary medicine, patients are grouped together by species according to their reaction to disease and to the pharmacological, medical, and/or surgical management of such reactions. In contrast, holistic philosophy theorizes that no two individuals have identical responses to disease manifestations. Therefore, treatment approaches must be customized to each individual patient.

However, to close one's mind on traditional veterinary medicine is to naively discard the facts that they stand true. Let's face it—because of conventional veterinary preventive and therapeutic approaches, a multitude of infectious diseases that at one time killed countless pets have been eradicated or controlled through conventional vaccination programs. Injuries and illnesses that just a few short years ago meant certain death or disability to an unfortunate pet so affected can today be cured or managed with remarkable conventional therapies and techniques. Life span and quality of life are on the increase for today's pet, primarily because of the advances made in traditional veterinary medical knowledge and its application.

Holistic opinions have certainly had their influence on traditional veterinary medicine. For instance, veterinarians have been prescribing aloe vera for years for the treatment of burns and skin irritations. Curricula within veterinary schools and teaching hospitals across the country are placing greater emphasis on the understanding of animal mental health and its role in disease creation, prevention, and cure. And the use of nutraceuticals and dietary management for disease prevention and treatment has become highly favored among traditional veterinary practitioners in recent years.

It goes without saying that both traditional medicine and holistic medicine have their inherent strengths as well as their weaknesses. And this brings up a great point: When traditional and holistic medicine are used in synergy, their combined strength serves to diffuse any weaknesses that one or the other may possess! The use of both traditional and holistic approaches to patient care has been coined "complementary" veterinary medicine. Make no mistake about it: Acute life-threatening injuries or illnesses are still best handled by traditional methods. However, chronic, long-term health challenges that have responded poorly to traditional methods can and should be approached holistically.

To find a holistic veterinarian in your area, contact your local or state veterinary associations. You can also contact the American Association of Holistic Practitioners, the official licensing board of veterinary holistic practitioners. Whenever choosing a veterinary holistic practitioner for your pet, ask the following questions:

- Is your veterinarian a licensed veterinarian who has specific training in the holistic specialty you are seeking?
- How extensive is your vet's holistic training?
- How long has your vet been practicing holistic medicine?
- Can references or success stories be provided with whom you can make contact or follow up?
- What are your vet's feelings toward conventional veterinary medicine? Does he/she practice complementary medicine?
- Is your vet able to explain the reasoning behind any procedure that may be prescribed or performed?

The more popular types of holistic medical approaches or tools used in veterinary medicine include botanical (herbal) medicine, nutritional medicine, homeopathy, chiropractic care, and acupuncture.

Botanical (Herbal) Medicine

The use of herbs to fight disease dates back far beyond the advent of modern medicine as we know it. Ancient people throughout the world, especially the Chinese and other Eastern cultures, utilized herbs to treat illnesses and injuries arising from hunting and gathering, armed conflict, and recreational activities. Written documentation on the use of herbs for medicinal purposes apparently first appeared in ancient Egyptian culture. By 1000 B.C., this knowledge had made its way across the ocean to Greece, whereupon Greek scholars such as

Socrates, Pliny, Dioscorides, and Krateus expanded on it, refined it, and recorded their findings in a *Materia Medica.* During the Middle Ages, European and Middle Eastern practitioners continued to expound on the works of the Greeks and helped solidify the foundation of the modern herbal *Materia Medica.*

Certainly the usefulness of an herbal remedy in the past depended on that herb's availability in a particular geographic location. Unfortunately, herbal practitioners within the United States found many of the herbs contained in the Old World *Materia Medica* could not be found in the New World. However, thousands of years before Columbus set foot on the shores of the Americas, local herbs had been used by Native American tribes to prevent and combat disease. This knowledge of New World herbal remedies was quickly assimilated into the new EuroAmerican culture and ultimately grew with subsequent westward expansion, leading to the formation of a *Materia Medica* dealing specifically with native New World herbs.

Thanks to the knowledge imparted by these pioneers in botanical medicine, today's veterinarians have valuable weapons at their disposal. Indeed, herbs can provide a powerful formulary against disease in pets (see Table 45.1). In fact, many of the active ingredients found in herbs are the same ones used in today's modern drugs. These active components include tannins, polysaccharides, glycosides, alkaloids, turpoids, and essential oils. Drug companies extract and isolate these constituents from the whole plant, then potentiate their strength in a laboratory, rendering them highly effective (and highly toxic). However, there has been a paradigm shift in recent years regarding herbs and their active ingredients. Scientists are now recognizing the therapeutic importance of certain "phytochemical" constituents found in whole plants that are absent in isolated extracts. Research is finding that these constituents may not only improve the effectiveness of the active ingredients within a patient's body but also lessen the risk of harmful side effects that the ingredients may cause.

Herbal remedies may be eaten, ingested as/or with liquids, or applied externally as poultices. Both fresh and dried herbs can form the foundation for a particular remedy. However, with the exception of topical poultices (such as aloe vera poultices for burns), most herbal products used in veterinary medicine are made from dried herbs.

Table 45.1 Herbs Commonly Used in Veterinary Medicine*

Common name	Scientific name	Used to treat or prevent
Aloe	*Aloe barbadensis*	Burns; dermatitis
Astragalus	*Astragalus membranaceous*	Immune system depression and stress
Bilberry	*Vaccinium myrtilis*	Diseases of blood vessels and eyes
Bitter melon	*Momordica charantia*	Diabetes mellitus
Black cohosh	*Cimicifuga racemosa*	Inappropriate urination behavior in cats
Black walnut	*Juglans nigra*	Heartworms and other internal parasites
Boswellia	*Boswellia serrata*	Arthritis
Calendula	*Calendula officinalis*	Skin and ear irritations; stomach ulcers
Cranberry	*Vaccinium macrocarpon*	Urinary tract infection
Echinacea	*Echinacea purpurea*	Immune system depression and stress
Eleutherococcus	*Eleutherococcus senticosus*	Weakness; age-related "slowing down"
Eyebright	*Euphrasia officinalis*	Eye inflammation
Garlic	*Allium sativum*	Infections, parasites, cancer
Ginger	*Zingiber officinale*	Carsickness; nausea
Ginkgo	*Ginkgo biloba*	Senile changes, diseases of heart and vessels
Goldenseal	*Hydrastis canadensis*	Infections; liver disease; cancer
Green tea	*Camellia sinensis*	Cancer
Gymnema	*Gymnema sylvestre*	Diabetes mellitus
Hawthorn	*Crataegus oxycantha*	Heart disease

Table 45.1 Herbs Commonly Used in Veterinary Medicine* (*Continued*)

Common name	Scientific name	Used to treat or prevent
Maitake	*Grifola frondosa*	Cancer; immune system depression
Milk thistle	*Silybum marianum*	Liver disease
Red raspberry	*Rubus idaeus*	Pregnancy support
Reishi	*Ganoderma lucidum*	Immune system depression and stress
Saw palmetto	*Serenoa repens*	Prostate disease/enlargement
St. John's wort	*Hypericum perforatum*	Mental/behavioral disorders
Tea tree	*Melaleuca alternifolia*	Ringworm; skin disorders
Turmeric	*Curcuma longa*	Inflammation; liver disease; cancer
Valerian	*Valeriana officinalis*	Mental or behavioral disorders

Note: When used improperly, many herbal remedies can be harmful to pets. As a result, all herbal preparations should be administered by (or under the guidance of) a licensed veterinarian trained in herbology.

These dried herbs are crushed and formed into pills or enclosed within gelatin capsules, made into tealike preparations, or pulverized and mixed with alcohol to form elixirs (Fig. 45.1). Herbal elixirs can be administered to pets in the same way as any other liquid medication, or they can be added directly to a pet's food. Pills and gelatin capsules can be administered directly or cleverly disguised in a treat.

Factors that can affect herbal potency include the method of drying used, the age of the herbal preparation, and the stage at which the plant was originally harvested. For example, dandelion leaves are most effective if harvested before flowering, whereas blue violet is best collected after flowering. Herbs that have not been dried properly may be contaminated with mold, which can certainly adversely alter their effectiveness. Also, the older the herbal preparation, the greater is the chance of a loss in potency due to natural degradation or mishandling. As a rule, potency of herbal remedies will tend to diminish rapidly after 1 year on the shelf. In order to improve shelf life, herbal products should be stored in dark, airtight containers and in cool, dry locations away from direct light.

When addressing an illness, veterinary herbalists rarely use only a single herb, but rather use a combination of herbs. Doing so offers two powerful advantages: (1) Combining certain herbs will create a synergistic attack against the targeted disorder, and (2) herbal combinations

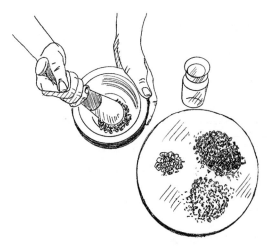

FIGURE 45.1 Dried herbs are first crushed and then formed into pills, enclosed within gelatin capsules, or further pulverized and mixed with alcohol to form elixirs.

can be used to help dilute out undesirable side effects that may be caused by one or more herbs in the formula.

Herbal treatments in animals are usually prescribed for no more than 2 to 4 weeks at a time. Standard dosages are usually continued for 2 to 3 days following the disappearance of clinical signs, and then slowly tapered off over a week's time.

Herbal remedies cannot be used indiscriminately, nor, as mentioned above, should they be used on a long-term basis. Realize that adverse interactions can occur with existing medications that your pet may be taking. Also, certain herbal remedies, given at improper dosages, can cause significant bodily harm. For instance, white willow and white oak bark contain salicylates and can be highly toxic to cats. With more people turning to the Internet as their source for information, it is vital to remember that although this resource and others can indeed provide valuable information concerning herbs and their application in pets, they can also be the source of dangerous misinformation concerning dosages, duration of treatment, and applications of herbal treatments. For your pet's sake, always validate any information you may gather with a veterinian professionally trained in botanical medicine and, of course, never administer a herbal preparation without first consulting a veterinarian.

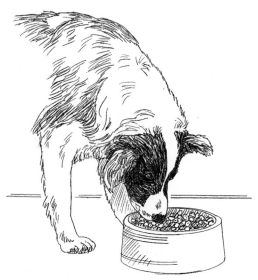

FIGURE 45.2 The holistic mindset strives for finding and feeding the most natural diet available.

Nutritional Medicine

A holistic approach to nutrition includes the feeding of a "natural"-type food ration and/or the use of nutraceuticals (Fig. 45.2). Many advocates of alternative veterinary medicine believe that many of the health challenges seen in pets today are the result of processed diets loaded with preservatives and by-products.

As emphasized in previous chapters, good nutrition is the foundation for any preventive health care program designed for pets. The holistic mindset strives for finding and feeding the most natural diet available. This ideal ration should

- Be cooked utilizing low temperatures. This will help preserve the food's nutritional value and prevent vital nutrients from being destroyed by high heat.

- Undergo minimal processing, again helping to retain as many of the original nutrients as possible.

- Consist of high-quality, fresh ingredients, including meats, grains, and vegetables. These ingredients should be highly bioavailable (easily digested and assimilated) and contain no by-products.

- Contain no artificial colors or flavorings, as these are viewed as potentially harmful agents when used on a long-term basis.

- Use only natural preservatives such as vitamins E and C. Artificial preservatives such as butylated hydroxytoluene (BHT) and ethoxyquin should be absent from the ingredient statement.

■ Contain no refined sugar or excess amounts of salt, both of which are used primarily as flavor enhancers.

From a holistic point of view, a high-quality ration will contain multiple protein sources, and have all protein sources utilized within the food specifically identified on the ingredient statement. In other words, if beef is used as the primary protein source, it will be stated as such on the label. On the contrary, the words "meat" or "beef by-products" indicate that parts other than high-quality muscle tissue were used in the food's formulation. The holistic veterinary nutritionist also wants a protein source that is free from hormone or antibiotic residues. Unfortunately, the only way to be certain whether this is the case is to do your research on the particular supplier in question. Many pet owners even go so far as to have samples of the food independently tested for such residues (although significant costs are usually attached to such a procedure). Also, ethoxyquin is a chemical preservative used to prevent rancidity in pet foods. Holistic rations should have the statement "ethoxyquin-free" printed on the bag.

Many holistic pet owners prefer homemade diets for their pets, often using raw sources of protein. However, with the tremendous number of natural pet food products reaching the market every day, such homemade preparations are not necessary. In fact, there are several disadvantages to preparing homemade diets, including the time it takes to prepare them, the potential for spoilage or nutritional imbalances, and parasite transmission from tainted ingredients.

Nutraceuticals are defined as food compounds that have scientifically proven health benefits when used at predetermined therapeutic dosages. When used properly, these nutritional supplements can help support healing processes within the body and even help prevent disease (Fig. 45.3). Just some of the nutraceutical agents commonly used in veterinary medicine include glandulars (actual extracts of glandular tissue), antioxidants, bioflavonoids, sulfated glycosaminoglycans, omega-3 fatty acids, probiotics, DHEA (dehydroepiandrosterone), coenzyme Q, *dl*-phenylalanine, creatinine, lactoferrin, vanadium, and DMG (dimethylglycine). Refer to Table 45.2 for a more complete listing of popular nutraceuticals used in veterinary medicine and their indi-

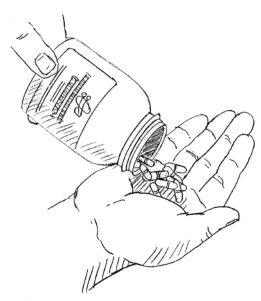

FIGURE 45.3 The use of nutraceuticals in veterinary medicine is on the rise.

cations for use. Because dosages are empirical, consult your veterinarian prior to giving any nutraceutical agent to your pet.

Homeopathy

Homeopathy is considered by many to be the most controversial of all alternative medical practices. The homeopathic movement found its origins in eighteenth-century Europe. Its founder, a German physician by the name of Samuel Hahnemann (1755–1843), promoted homeopathic medicine as an alternative to the conventional medical approaches of that day. Indeed, back then, these conventional orthodox methods of treating disease were in themselves quite crude and sometimes brutal. Blistering, purging, blood letting, heavy-metal treatments, and crude surgical procedures were all accepted practices of the day, and often did more harm than good. Hahnemann viewed homeopathy as a less risky alternative. He also felt that orthodox medicine was being driven by symptomatic treatment of disease rather than by the treatment of the patient as a whole being. As one can imagine, Hahnemann received harsh criticism from his more orthodox peers.

The homeopathic movement made its way to the United States in the early part of the nineteenth century, and slowly gained a loyal following. Well-known proponents of the day included Mark Twain, Daniel Webster, William Cullen Bryant, and John D. Rockefeller. In 1844 the American Institute of Homeopathy was founded. In fact, this was the first national medical society formed in the United States. Interestingly, the American Medical Association was founded 2 years later. One reason for this was to counter the threat that the homeopathic movement posed to conventional medicine!

Table 45.2   Popular Nutraceuticals Used in Veterinary Medicine*

Nutraceutical	Used to treat or prevent
Blue-green algae	Viral infections; cancer; immune depression
α-Lipoic acid	Eye disorders; diabetes; circulatory disturbances
Arginine	Heart disease; liver disease; cancer; diabetes
Bioflavonoids (pycnogenol, rutin, etc.)	Eye disorders, age-related degeneration; allergies
Carnitine	Heart disease; liver disease, submaximum athletic endurance
Creatinine monohydrate	Submaximum athletic performance and endurance; muscle wasting
Coenzyme Q10	Heart disease; tooth and gum disease
Dehydroepiandrosterone (DHEA)	Immune disorders; obesity
dl-Phenylalanine (DLPA)	Arthritis; generalized or specific pain
Dimethylglycine (DMG)	Epilepsy
Enzymes (bromelain, papain, etc.)	Pancreatic enzyme deficiency; inflammatory disorders
Fiber supplements	Constipation, diabetes, bowel inflammation; hairballs; anal sac impaction
Glutamine	Bowel inflammation
Chondroitin sulfate	Arthritis; bladder disease
Glucosamine	Arthritis; bladder disease
Lactoferrin	Feline stomatitis
Lysine	Herpes infections of the eye
Magnesium	Heart disease; neurologic disease

Table 45.2   Popular Nutraceuticals Used in Veterinary Medicine*
(*Continued*)

Nutraceutical	Used to treat or prevent
Omega-3 fatty acids	Allergic skin disease; heart disease; arthritis; cancer
Phosphatidylserine	Senility
Probiotics	Food allergies; immune system disorders and suppression; diarrhea
Taurine	Heart disease; liver disease; epilepsy
Vanadium	Diabetes mellitus
Vitamin C (ascorbic acid)	Allergies; immune system disorders; cancer; cataracts

*Note: When used improperly, some nutraceuticals can be harmful to pets. As a result, all nutraceuticals should be administered by (or under the guidance of) a licensed veterinarian trained in nutritional therapy.

Information regarding the various homeopathic remedies has been amassed through trial-and-error applications and case studies. These findings or "provings" can all be found in the *Homeopathic Pharmacopoeia*. Within this book, first published in 1897 and updated regularly, homeopathic remedies are listed in "rubrics," which are flowcharts or listings of particular disease symptoms cross-referenced with those homeopathic preparations that produce similar symptoms in the patient.

Classical homeopathy of the type promoted by Hahnemann emphasizes single remedies to be given for specific symptoms. In recent years however, classical homeopathy has been giving way to newer schools of thought that promote combination remedies versus single remedies. The theory behind combining homeopathic remedies is that in doing so, synergy is increased, resulting in a greater chance of treatment success.

Homeopathy was and remains so controversial because its principles have yet to be proved scientifically. One challenge that traditional veterinarians have with homeopathic approaches is that standards have yet to be established that take into account the species, breed, and size of the patient being treated. For example, a small kitten and a large horse may both be prescribed the same remedy at the same potency! Many medical doctors write off apparent homeopathic successes in humans as "placebo effects." Unfortunately, this does not explain the anecdotal successes achieved in certain clinical cases involving animals. Certainly any scientist or research practitioner would agree that when working with living organisms, countless variables exist that we do not understand or recognize. Perhaps it is one or more of these variables that accounts for homeopathic treatment successes when they occur.

Homeopathy is based on the *law of similars,* or "like cures like." This law contends that agents that cause disease symptoms at standard doses can cause the body to mimic those symptoms when introduced in extremely diluted doses and stimulate the body to cure the underlying disease.

The goal of the veterinary homeopath is to support and strengthen the pet's "vital force." This vital force is responsible for maintaining health and internal harmony within the body. According to homeopathic principles, clinical signs, which are recognized as simply outward expressions of disease and not diseases in themselves, are caused by imbalances affecting this vital force. As the vital force attempts to restore its own balance, clinical signs start to appear. Subtle clinical signs result from a weak vital force response. Severe, pronounced symptoms are indicative of a strong vital force response. Homeopathic treatment is designed to stimulate and strengthen the vital force into restoring its internal balance. When in balance, the vital force is able to effectively call on the natural body defense mechanisms to rise to the occasion and eliminate the disease from the body.

Homeopathic theory contends that focusing treatment efforts toward the elimination of symptoms will not adequately treat the underlying disease. In fact, treating symptoms without addressing the underlying disease is believed to drive the disease even deeper into the body, thereby strengthening the disease itself and weakening the vital force. Instead, if one will assist the body's vital force in regaining its balance, both the disease and the symptoms will disappear.

Veterinary homeopathic remedies are administered to animals either as tiny pellets (crushed and placed on the tongue) or elixirs. For best results, they should not be given with meals. Remedies are formulated

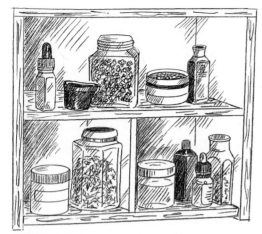

FIGURE 45.4 Homeopathic remedies are formulated using herbs, extracts, heavy metals, minerals, toxins, or any other substance that has the potential to stimulate the "vital force."

using herbs, extracts, heavy metals, minerals, toxins, or any other substance that has the potential to stimulate the vital force at homeopathic concentrations (Fig. 45.4). If administered at full strength, many of these substances could harm or even kill a patient! However, when diluted the homeopathic way, they purportedly stimulate the body to heal itself.

Dilutions are performed in a stepwise fashion, with the preparations succussed (shaken) after each dilution in order to increase potency and vibrational energy. This process of dilution followed by succussion is termed *potentiation.* According to homeopathic theory, the more dilute the remedy, the more powerfully it acts to stimulate natural healing. Because of their diluted and energized natures, homeopathic remedies are said to be very sensitive to temperature fluctuations, chemicals, strong odors, and light, and need to be stored carefully.

Homeopathy and Prevention of Infectious Disease

Homeopathic preparations designed as substitutes for vaccines to prevent infectious diseases in pets are called nosodes. These preparations consist of diseased tissue or substances produced by the disease condition. Like other homeopathic preparations, nosodes are diluted and succussed for potency. Homeopathic nosodes are available for most of the diseases that are routinely vaccinated for in dogs and cats. In addition to protecting against disease, nosodes are used by homeopathic practitioners to treat disease.

Nosodal therapy is viewed with much suspicion and concern by traditional veterinary medical researchers, who question its effectiveness against these devastating diseases in dogs and cats. Many homeopathic practitioners believe that vaccinations weaken the vital force of the patient, thereby actually increasing patient susceptibility to the disease agent. However, in defense of traditional thinking, such a view does not fit very well with clinical and research evidence. Vaccinations indeed do what they are intended to do: protect against infectious diseases. Because of diligent vaccination programs, diseases such as canine distemper have been virtually eliminated in the pet dog population. Are vaccinations always effective and safe? Of course not. Idiosyncrasies in the biochemical makeup of individuals, as well as variations in the types and qualities of vaccines utilized, can lead to unexpected and detrimental responses when a vaccine is administered. For various reasons, a vaccine could be rendered ineffective once introduced into the body. Or, a patient could experience an adverse response ranging from severe life-threatening anaphylactic shock or immune complex formation to the development of vaccine-related tumors, such as feline sarcoma. However, with extended vaccination schedules available for dogs and cats, and continuing improvements in vaccine quality, the incidence of such adverse reactions will continue to decrease. Certainly if a pet has displayed sensitivity to one or more conventional vaccines, it may be considered a candidate for an alternative approach to preventive health care. Yet the effectiveness of nosodal therapy as this alternative approach is still highly questionable.

Chiropractic Care

A rapidly growing segment of veterinary alternative health care is chiropractic care. Since chiropractic care is so popular among the human population, it is no wonder that many pet owners are seeking it for their pets as well. As far back a Hippocrates, spinal manipulations were used on people and pets to treat a wide variety of disorders. Modern human chiropractic medicine traces its roots back to Canada in the late nineteenth century to an individual by the name of Daniel D. Palmer (1845–1913). Palmer went on to establish a college of chiropractic in the United States in 1898 and subsequently published a textbook in 1910 entitled *The Science, Art and Philosophy of Chiropractic.* Information gleaned from Palmer and his predecessors has formed the foundation for modern veterinary chiropractic. Initially, chiropractic procedures on pets were performed by chiropractors working in collaboration with veterinarians. Today, however, you will find an increasing number of veterinarians themselves receiving actual training in chiropractic theories and techniques as they apply to animals.

Chiropractic philosophy maintains (and rightly so) that all organ systems within the body are controlled by the nervous system. It does so through elaborate control systems (including those responsible for hormone production and release) and complex feedback mechanisms that coordinate all body functions and responses, including those related to health and to disease. Any disruption of the free flow of nerve impulses throughout the body can disrupt homeostasis within the body and lead to poor immune function and subsequent disease.

The focus of chiropractic medicine is centered on the spinal column, that portion of the central nervous system through which nerves course to and from the brain. More specifically, chiropractors target motor units along the spinal column. Each motor unit consists of two adjacent vertebrae and all the nerves, muscles, ligaments, blood vessels, and ancillary structures associated with the joint formed by the two vertebrae. Either a *malarticulation* or a *fixation* of one or more of these motor units can disrupt the free flow of nerve impulses. Such deviations from the normal anatomy and/or structural mechanics of the spinal column put pressure on and irritate the spinal cord, causing pain and/or preventing the body from mounting an effective response against other diseases. In addition, loss of motor unit mobility can slow the flow of spinal fluid, leading to malnourishment and degeneration of vital muscles, nerves, and other structures associated with the motor unit.

Chiropractic adjustments are used to treat lameness, hip dysplasia, intervertebral disk disease, nonspecific joint pain, muscle spasms, and poor flexibility in pets. In addition, chiropractic therapy has been shown to be effective against gastrointestinal illness, musculoskeletal trauma, stress-induced exhaustion, and certain types of paralysis in pets (Fig. 45.5).

The type and extent of clinical signs seen are dependent on the site(s) and severity of malarticulation or fixation. If a primary pressure site is not relieved in a timely fashion, other sites may subsequently appear as the animal tries to compensate for the pain and lack of motion through altered posture and locomotion.

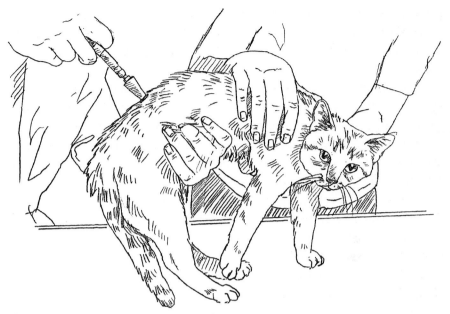

FIGURE 45.5 Chiropractic care has been used to treat certain types of paralysis in pets.

Chiropractic treatment consists of adjustments made to affected motor units. No drugs or surgery are used. An adjustment is defined as a sudden controlled thrust delivered at a precise direction and depth to a specific contact point along the vertebral column. The goal of such a maneuver is to realign the vertebra and to relieve pressure on the surrounding tissue.

The veterinarian will examine the gait and posture of the patient for obvious asymmetries and lameness. Hands-on palpation will be performed next in an attempt to localize regions of pain, muscle spasms, swellings, and or temperature variations along the spinal column and extremities. Afterward, the clinician will assess the overall alignment of the vertebral column and the range of motion and mobility of the various joints. Once the degree of malalignment(s) or joint fixation(s) has been assessed, the direction and point of contact for the adjustment can be determined. Adjustments are performed on animals by using thumb pressure, joint stretching, or a special instrument called an activator, designed to make the adjustment process easier. If a pet is in a great deal of pain, manipulations may need to be performed under sedation or anesthesia.

Following chiropractic adjustments, many animals become more active and playful, exhibit increased appetites, and desire more interaction with their owners. The number of chiropractic adjustments required will depend on the severity and duration of the problem and the age of the patient. As a rule, the younger the patient, the fewer the adjustments needed to correct a malarticulation or fixation.

Acupuncture

The word *acupuncture* is derived from the Latin word *acus,* which means "needle," and *punctura,* which means "to prick." Acupuncture involves the stimulation of specific points on the body in order to produce chemical and physical responses within the body. This ancient form of medical therapy is thought to have originated in the Far East over 7000 years ago. Because of the close interdependence of humans and animals throughout the ages, it has no doubt been used as a form of veterinary medicine for thousands of years as well. Ancient civilizations certainly practiced acupuncture on their animals, as evidenced by the antiquated acupuncture charts that exist for a wide variety of species, including horses, camels, water buffaloes, and even elephants!

The ancient Chinese explained acupuncture in terms of Ch'I, yin, yang, acupuncture points, and meridians. *Ch'I,* the life force or life energy, moves throughout the body via channels called *meridians.* These meridians run in pairs throughout the body and are associated with the major organ systems within the body. They also interconnect with hundreds of acupuncture points on the body surface. These points correspond to those areas where the meridians containing Ch'I course closest to the body's surface.

Ch'I is believed to be bipolar in nature, with the positive ("male") forces called *yang* and the negative ("female") forces called *yin.* In order for the health of an individual to be maintained, a balance between yin and yang is needed. Any imbalance, disruption, or disturbance in these forces will create disease. The purpose of acupuncture is to reestablish the normal flow of Ch'I throughout the body, thereby restoring the balance between yin and yang. This, in turn, will restore health to the individual.

In the Western orthodox world, acupuncture points are known to be electrically discrete entities located in predictable regions of the body. These include areas where nerves enter into deep-muscle tissue and where peripheral nerves emerge from openings in bone. Also, it has been observed that certain disorders of the internal organs, muscles, and bones can cause spontaneous "tender spots" to appear on the surface of the body. These tender spots are believed to correspond directly to acupuncture points. And although meridians have yet to be actually identified scientifically, tests utilizing special radioactive markers injected directly into select acupuncture points demonstrate a predictable flow within the body that could very well correspond to the meridians themselves.

Several theories have been proposed in an attempt to explain the effects that acupuncture can have on animals (and people). The first theorizes that stimulation of an acupuncture point directly blocks the transmission of pain sensation along select nerve fibers within the body. A second theory postulates that chemicals called *endorphins* are released on stimulation of an acupuncture point. Endorphins, which are up to 100 times more potent than morphine, effectively block pain sensation and can circulate in the bloodstream for several hours at a time, providing a lasting effect. Endorphins can also influence the body's hormonal system, stimulating the release of various hormones (including steroids and epinephrine) that can have positive effects on all organ systems within the body. Still another theory proposes that acupuncture stimulation causes select sensory nerve endings to transmit nerve impulses to the spinal cord and brain, and then back out again to glands located throughout the body. On stimulation, these glands release hormones into the bloodstream that can exert various influences on the organ systems within the body.

More than likely, the actual mode of action for acupuncture is created by a blend of two or more of these theories. Interestingly, for acupuncture to work, an animal's nervous system must be intact. Studies involving patients suffering from nerve damage have revealed that the beneficial effects normally gained by stimulation of a particular acupuncture are actually negated by the damage.

Scientific research such as this, coupled with innumerable clinical success stories, has rendered acupuncture an accepted therapeutic tool for today's veterinary practitioner. In fact, the American Veterinary Medical Association now recognizes veterinary acupuncture and veterinary acutherapy as legitimate forms of veterinary medicine. While acupuncture is certainly not a "magic pill," it can present a viable alternative in those medical cases where conventional therapy has failed.

Acupuncture has been used with success in pets to control pain associated with intervertebral disk disease, trauma, hip dysplasia, and other forms of arthritis. In addition, it may also help speed healing in animal patients stricken with conditions such as allergies, epilepsy, nerve injuries, chronic respiratory disease, and disorders of the stomach and intestines. Acupuncture has also been used as a source of local anesthesia for pets undergoing minor surgical procedures, and as a tool to help minimize blood loss during such procedures. One of the most exciting applications of acupuncture in small-animal medicine is the use of shock point GV-26, a governing vessel meridian point, for the treatment of shock and cardiovascular collapse. This point is located at the *philtrum,* that indented portion of the upper lip just below the nose. In those animals that have stopped breathing or have suffered cardiac arrest, stimulation of this point can be a lifesaver (Fig. 45.6)!

The International Veterinary Acupuncture Society (IVAS) establishes a *code of ethics* and provides acupuncture certification within the profession. To help ensure competency when choosing a veterinary acupuncturist, always select one who has been certified by a veterinary acupuncture specialty organization such as the IVAS.

The competent veterinary acupuncturist believes in integrating veterinary acupuncture with the practice of orthodox Western veterinary medicine and always makes a complete clinical assessment of the patient prior to using acupuncture. This is vital because acupuncture can mask or alter clinical signs, sometimes making an otherwise obvious diagnosis difficult to recognize.

Stimulation of an acupuncture point in a pet can be achieved using several different methods. These include the use of needles, heat sources, finger pressure, vacuums ("cupping"), electrical currents, or lasers (Fig. 45.7). Certainly needles are the most common tools used to stimulate acupuncture points; 25- to 34-gauge stainless needles, some

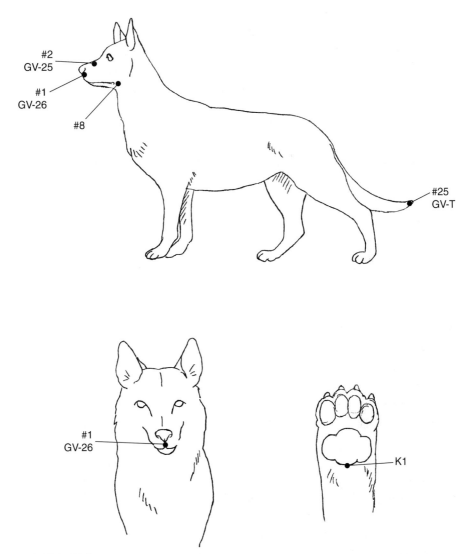

FIGURE 45.6 Acupuncture "shock" points often used in emergency situations.

up to 5 centimeters long, are used to perform acupuncture on dogs and cats. The acupuncture points needing stimulation and the condition being treated will determine the actual needle gauge and length selected. Needles are usually inserted $1/8$ to $1/2$ inch into the particular point on the skin. For added benefit, the needles, once inserted, can

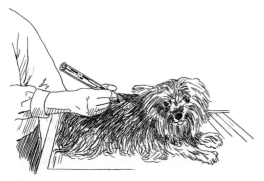

FIGURE 45.7 Laser acupuncture being performed on a patient.

be stimulated using a heat source (moxibustion) or electrical charge. Applying heat to an acupuncture point can be especially effective in treating arthritic conditions in dogs. Special electronic heating devices are available for such therapy in small animals.

The duration of a veterinary acupuncture treatment usually ranges from 1 to 30 minutes. During treatments, many pets become sedate and quite relaxed. Treatments are administered two to three times per week until desired results are seen. In chronic conditions, weeks or months of serial treatments may be necessary to effect positive results.

Implants may be inserted into specific acupuncture sites to provide continuous stimulation of those locations. For example, metallic beads implanted near the hip joints are said to be effective in select cases for treating pain associated with hip dysplasia. Also, gold beads implanted near the head region have been used to treat seizures in dogs (Fig. 45.8). *Aqua acupuncture,* performed by injecting liquid solutions containing sterile saline, vitamins, herbal preparations, or select therapeutic compounds directly into acupuncture points, is another popular method of achieving continuous stimulation.

Correctly locating a particular acupuncture point is much more important than the type of stimulation used on that point. When an acupuncture point is correctly identified and stimulated, initial reactions that may be seen in a pet include a bending at the waist, a raising of the tail, and sounds of relaxation, such as a heavy sigh. Some animals may even inadvertently eliminate on the spot!

There are few side effects associated with proper acupuncture therapy. Adverse effects could potentially occur if too many acupuncture points are stimulated at one time, if the wrong point is stimulated, or if a particular point is overstimulated. The most common side effect that could be seen with acupuncture is a temporary exacerbation of the disorder being treated, especially if the treatment is for pain. If this occurs, the adverse response will usually subside within a day or two. Other side effects of acupuncture therapy can include burns (if heat is used) or infections at the sites of acupuncture stimulation. Of course, accidental injury caused by an anxious or improperly restrained

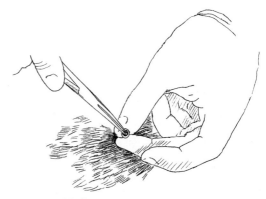

FIGURE 45.8 Implanting a gold bead into an acupuncture site using a hypodermic needle.

pet probably poses the greatest risk associated with acupuncture treatment.

Under the direction of a qualified veterinarian, you can safely perform a technique called *acupressure* at home on your pet. This form of acupuncture involves stimulating acupuncture points using finger pressure instead of needles. This can be quite helpful in helping to relieve muscle spasms and to eliminate localized pain. When stimulating such a point using acupressure, use a steady, massaging circular motion. Pressure should be maintained for 30 to 60 seconds prior to moving to the next point in the treatment sequence. An entire session should take no more than 5 to 6 minutes. Sessions can be repeated two to three times per day, or as often as directed by your veterinarian.

Ten Super Strategies for Reducing the Cost of Pet Ownership

I f you currently have a pet living at home, or have ever owned one in the past, you've no doubt discovered that pet ownership can be an expensive proposition. Between the cost of food, supplies, and medical care, expenses can run into the hundreds, if not thousands, of dollars each year, depending on the type of pet you own and how many pets adorn your household. However, there is good news! There are strategies that you can employ that can help soften the fiscal challenges you may encounter. Here are 10 of them that you can put to use immediately.

Strategy 1: Purchase Pet Health Insurance or Self-Insure Your Pet
Unexpected injuries or illnesses can rapidly generate hundreds of dollars in unanticipated expenses. Such costs can no doubt cause financial and emotional strain, leading to painful decisions that an owner

may regret later on. As a result, pet fanciers need to protect themselves against such circumstances

Years ago when pet health insurance first appeared on the market, it was too downright expensive for the extent of coverage it offered the consumer. Well, times have changed, and so has pet health insurance. Today, every owner should consider it as a viable option to help cover the costs of veterinary care. Obviously, when comparing the various pet health insurance programs available, look closely at the deductibles offered and services covered. A good policy should provide the option of covering not only major medical or surgical procedures, but preventive health care as well.

If you consider yourself financially disciplined, self-insuring your pet can save you even more money. By socking money away each month into a special interest-bearing account designated for your pet's health care, you can build up a resource that you can turn to in the event of an emergency. In the best-case scenario, your pet will glide through life unscathed, and you'll never have to touch the fund, leaving you with a nice savings account that you can use as you please. This is certainly in stark contrast to insurance premiums, which must be paid regardless of your pet's health status. On the flip side, if you indeed have to draw from the account, you will have the peace of mind knowing that the money is there and that any decisions that you must make in that moment of crisis will not be solely determined by the balance in your checkbook.

But you say, "Doc, I have enough trouble saving money as it is! How am I going to find money to set aside for such a fund?" Well, believe it or not, it's there if you look for it! Are you a slave to an expensive habit? Would you be willing to give it up temporarily until your pet's account is funded? Give up one soda a day or skip one meal per week and save over $200 per year, money that you can deposit into your pet's account! Check out your weekly movie entertainment from the local library instead of renting it from the video store, and add another $250 per year. Have a garage sale and use the proceeds you earn as a source of capital for your pet's personal health plan! As you can see, the possibilities are endless! Just take a close look at your own personal lifestyle and brainstorm possible sources of savings.

Strategy 2: Be Realistic by Planning Ahead   Whenever talking money and pets, it is vitally important to your family and to your financial well-being to determine ahead of time how much you are willing to pay for veterinary medical care in the event of an unexpected injury or illness involving your pet. Even if you have insurance, it may not pay the entire bill. No one should ever be emotionally "guilted" into a personal financial crisis. Yet spontaneous emotional decisions can prove to be very expensive. Obviously this does not mean that we are released from our obligations as responsible pet owners, but rather that we should prepare ourselves in advance of that unexpected moment, should it occur.

Strategy 3: Select Your Pet Wisely   Obviously, the type of pet you choose to share your life with will determine the level of financial commitment you'll need to make. This crosses not only species lines but also breed lines. For instance, owning a dog will no doubt cost more than owning a guinea pig. In addition, owning an African gray parrot will entail greater husbandry-related expenditures than would owning a budgie. Large dogs will consume more food than their smaller peers, and will be more expensive to medicate in the event of an illness.

When selecting a dog or cat, keep in mind that the more diverse the gene pool, the heartier the individual tends to be (a phenomenon known as *hybrid vigor*). This translates into a reduced chance of a genetically related illness rearing its ugly, expensive head later on. If this is of concern to you, stick to mixed breeds or to one of the top five purebred breeds of dogs and cats.

Be sure to set limits on the number of pets you own. While every stray dog or cat that crosses your path may pull your heartstrings, be realistic. Do you have the time and the financial resources to properly devote to so many pets? If so, then go for it. If not, then find good homes for your "lost and founds" before you become emotionally attached to them.

Strategy 4: Obtain Your Pet from a Reputable Source Only   That $10 puppy you purchased at the flea market or grocery store parking lot could be a carrier of a massive veterinary bill if it is harboring a virus, mange, or internal parasites. Also, the parrot you purchased from that roadside stand could be a carrier of psittacosis, a serious disease in both parrots and humans! Purchasing your pet from a breeder or pet store isn't an automatic guarantee of quality, either.

Always check references on potential pet vendors. And always insist on a prepurchase evaluation of the pet by a qualified veterinarian of your choice prior to exchange of any money. If the vendor is reputable, this won't be a problem at all. Have your veterinarian verify the shot and deworming records of your prospective purchase. Often pets that are sold as having "all of their shots" may in fact have missed an important booster or deworming, leaving you holding an unexpected bill.

Unless you are planning to enter your pet into AKC (American Kennel Club)-sanctioned competitive events, there is no need to pay the extra expense associated with purchasing a pet with "papers" unless you can verify the reputation and record of the breeder. Because the AKC has no real regulatory enforcement of quality standards outside of its sanctioned events, purchasing a pet with papers is not a guarantee of quality. If purchasing your pet from a breeder who is renowned for quality or from a reputable pet store, it may be worth paying more for an "AKC" puppy. However, if purchasing your pup from a backyard breeder, forget the papers. The mere fact that a dog is AKC-certifiable is no justification for jacking up the purchase price by hundreds of dollars!

Strategy 5: Be a Wise Pet Food Buyer For many pet owners, food purchases make up the majority of pet-related expenditures each year. As a result, using a little savvy when purchasing pet food can save you tremendous amounts of money. For starters, buy quality. Feeding your pet a high-quality diet versus a cheap low-quality brand can be compared to you eating plenty of fruits, vegetables, and whole grains versus eating a diet full of fast food. Feeding high-quality rations does not have to be more expensive, either. The feeding portions will be much smaller than those of a poorer-quality ration, making your food purchases last longer. Also, by comparing labels, you'll be able to discern which diets have similar ingredients and nutritional values, despite differences in price. Like human food producers, pet food manufacturers often market identical rations under several different labels and several different price points. And don't be influenced by advertising. For instance, avoid lamb-and-rice diets unless your veterinarian specifically prescribes one. Despite what pet food manufacturers may claim, most of these "hypoallergenic" foods found on the market today have limited use in the treatment of food-related skin allergies and itching. Yet they generally cost more than other formulations. Don't pay for something you don't need!

Here's another rule of thumb: Buy your pet food in bulk. You can realize significant savings by purchasing food this way. The larger the bag you buy, the lower the cost is per ounce. Once a bulk bag is opened, simply transfer the contents into resealable plastic containers to keep the food fresh and nutritious for later use.

By the way, while on the subjects of food and money, don't feed your pets table scraps or bones! These serve no nutritional purpose whatsoever and can lead to expensive bouts of pancreatitis, periodontal disease, and digestive disturbances.

Strategy 6: Become an Informed Pet Owner   With the wealth of information available at your fingertips via books, periodicals, and the Internet, there is no reason to plead ignorance when it comes to your pet's husbandry and health care. Two special questions to research and find answers for are (1) what constitutes a real veterinary medical emergency and (2) what, if any, over-the-counter remedies are available to treat the various conditions you may encounter with your pet. Verify any answers you find with your veterinarian. By gathering such information long before you need it, you can save yourself hundreds of dollars over the life of your pet in unnecessary trips to the veterinary hospital.

Strategy 7: Remember That Bigger Is Not Always Better   Veterinary hospitals come in all shapes and sizes. Just remember that in any business, fees charged are usually directly related to the amount of overhead involved. Indeed, if you opt to pay higher fees for pet care, just be sure you're paying for superior quality of care, not just superior real estate. Let's face it: There are not many differences in vaccine administration or spay/neuter skills between veterinarians. As a result, don't be afraid to price-shop for these routine procedures. Many clinics offer regular vaccination and spay/neuter clinics as a public service to their communities. If you are afraid that your veterinarian will get mad at you for shopping around, get over it. It's your money, not your vet's!

Strategy 8: Always Ask for an Estimate   Whether your pet is receiving routine preventive maintenance or being treated for an actual injury or illness, you have the right to know the costs associated with the procedures to be performed. The purpose is not to question your veterinarian's judgment or fees, but to avoid misunderstandings or unexpected financial surprises. The advantage of a written estimate is that it will reveal to you those areas that may lend themselves to cost savings. For example, is a hospitalization charge included on the estimate? If so, will there be somebody at the hospital throughout the night to monitor your pet's condition? If not, don't hesitate to question this charge. If your pet's condition is not life-threatening, there is no need for you to incur overnight hospitalization charges, since no one will be present to care for your pet, anyway. Take your pet home for the night with detailed instructions from your veterinarian on how to play nursemaid. This could save you anywhere from $10 to $30 per day, depending on the hospital. Will your pet require medications? Perhaps a written prescription could be a source of cost savings.

Estimates on preventive health care procedures are extremely important since the fees associated with these services can vary widely between veterinary practices. For instance, some clinics include an office charge with vaccination fees whereas others charge only for the vaccinations themselves. If your pet has already had a physical examination within the past 6 months, another one may not be necessary. Many clinics include a laboratory charge with their fee for teeth cleaning. Again, if routine bloodwork was performed within the last 6 months, repeating it on an otherwise healthy animal may be an unnecessary expenditure. If you have a question regarding a fee, don't be afraid to raise it. If your veterinarian becomes defensive, it may be time to look for another veterinarian. True veterinary professionals will not be offended by such questions; in fact, they encourage such open lines of communication with their clients.

Strategy 9: Form a Neighborhood "Pet Club" Associating yourself with other pet owners in your neighborhood can provide you with incredible informational and financial leverage. Have periodic meetings with your "club," either in person, by phone, or by email! Use the time to share information, ideas, and recommendations on pet husbandry, preventive care, veterinarians, groomers, trainers, and pet-supply retailers. Pool resources with club members to purchase food and supplies in bulk, taking advantage of volume discounts. You can also organize a pet-sitting cooperative with other club members and save megabucks in boarding fees. Get creative and brainstorm with your compadres. The possibilities of saving money by working together are extraordinary!

Strategy 10: Barter for Bucks Do you have a particular skill or training that would prove useful to your veterinarian or local pet supply owner? If so, talk to them about the possibility of setting up an equitable barter program. Bartering will help preserve your cash flow, and in most cases, save you money. For example, do you have sales and marketing expertise? For clients who can offer their veterinarians practical tips on how to market and promote their practices, a barter arrangement is probably only a handshake away. Are you skilled at carpentry, plumbing, or other types of handy work? If so, you are a valuable asset to any business. Considering this was the way our ancestors conducted business, the possibilities are endless. But there is only one way you'll ever become an effective barterer—learn how to ask!

APPENDIXES

Clinical Signs and Complaints in Dogs and Cats

The ability to recognize and distinguish what is normal and what is not is a critical key in determining a pet's longevity. As one may expect, timing is of the essence when it comes to effective treatment or management of disease. The sooner a clinical sign is detected and reported to a veterinarian, the better the chances are of identifying and halting the progression of a disease.

Clinical signs (symptoms) are not disease entities in themselves, but rather the outward manifestations of disease. Onset of symptoms may occur acutely (suddenly) or slowly and progressively over a period of time. In some instances, the underlying disease condition causing the clinical sign may be in advanced development before the symptom even appears. For example, pronounced weight loss, excessive thirst and urination, vomiting, and other signs linked to chronic kidney failure may not become readily apparent until at least 75 percent of the kidney tissue has been rendered nonfunctional. As a result, any delays in seeking professional help once symptoms appear could turn an otherwise manageable condition into a life-threatening crisis.

Note that the clinical signs and complaints presented here are not all-encompassing. In addition, the possible etiologies (causes) of each are certainly not limited to those listed. As a result, proper veterinary diagnosis is essential.

Abdominal Pain

Tumor

Bloat

Torsion

Constipation

Granuloma or abscess

Infectious gastroenteritis

Intestinal foreign body and/or obstruction

Kidney disease

Liver disease

Organ rupture

Pancreatitis

Poisoning

Ulcers

Urinary obstruction

Abdominal Swelling

Tumor

Fluid buildup (ascites)

Heart disease

Constipation

Bloat

Urinary obstruction

Granuloma or abscess

Hemorrhage within the abdomen

Intestinal parasites

Liver disease

Obesity

Pregnancy

Uterine infection (pyometra)

Appetite: Increased

Cushing's disease

Drug therapy (i.e., prednisolone)

Exocrine pancreatic insufficiency

Hyperthyroidism (cats)

Inadequate caloric intake (underfeeding)

Intestinal parasitism

Malabsorption or maldigestion of food

Appetite: Decreased

Infection

Anemia

Heart disease

Dehydration

Dietary boredom

Fever

Gastrointestinal disease

Kidney disease

Liver disease

Loss of smell

Nausea

Neoplasia

Pain

Pancreatitis

Trauma

Upper respiratory infection

Arched Back

Abdominal pain

Pancreatitis

Intestinal foreign body

Back pain

Kidney disorder

Breathing Difficulties

Allergic bronchitis

Anemia

Choking

Heart disease

Pneumonia

Heartworm disease

Neoplasia

Obesity

Pneumothorax

Respiratory foreign body

Pulmonary effusions

Hypothyroidism

Collapsing trachea

Constipation/Straining

Anal sac impaction or infection

Dehydration

Stool impaction

Fractured pelvis

Intestinal parasites

Intestinal neoplasia

Intestinal obstruction

Spinal cord trauma

Urinary obstruction

Coughing

Allergic bronchitis

Heart disease (pulmonary edema)

Kennel cough

Infectious rhinotracheitis

Metastatic lung cancer

Pneumonia

Respiratory foreign body

Tonsillitis

Diarrhea

Dietary indiscretions and changes

Autoimmune disease

Intestinal infections (viral, bacterial, fungal)

Food allergy

Intestinal parasites

Intestinal neoplasia

Intestinal obstruction

Intestinal foreign body

Kidney disease

Liver disease

Pancreatitis

Toxins or drugs

Discharge: Nose

Allergies (clear)

Bacterial infection (mucus, pus, blood)

Fungal infection (mucus, blood)

Tumor, polyp (mucus, pus, blood)

Trauma (blood)

Foreign body (clear, mucus, blood)

Blood clotting disorder (blood)

Periodontal disease (mucus, pus, blood)

Open socket due to tooth loss (mucus, pus, blood)

Viral infection (clear, blood)

Parasitic infestation (blood)

Discharge: Eyes

Allergies (clear)

Bacterial infection (mucus, pus)

Foreign matter (clear, pus, mucus)

Neoplasia or cyst (mucus, pus, blood)

Trauma (blood, clear)

Viral infection (clear)

Discharge: Reproductive Tract

Bacterial infection (mucus, pus, blood)

Neoplasia or cyst (mucus, pus, blood)

Tumor, polyp (mucus, pus, blood)

Vaginitis or metritis (mucus, pus, blood)

Discharge: Ears

Bacterial infection (pus, blood)

Ear mites (black, crusty)

Trauma (blood)

Yeast infection (brown, odorous)

Discharge: Skin

Bacterial infection or abscess (pus)

Fungal infection (brown, blood, granular)

Eye: Redness or Cloudiness

Allergies

Bacterial infection

Cataracts

Corneal pigmentation

Foreign matter

Glaucoma

Neoplasia or cyst

Trauma

Uveitis

Viral infection

Facial Swelling

Abscess

Allergic reaction to insect sting

Fungal infection

Jaw fracture or trauma

Lymphatic obstruction

Oral or bone tumor

Oral foreign body

Snakebite

Fever or Elevated Body Temperature

Infections (bacterial, viral, fungal)

Inflammation due to disease or injury

Autoimmune disease

Drug therapy (i.e., tetracycline antibiotics)

Neoplasia

Excitement or fear

Heat stroke

Overexertion

Seizures

Incoordination, Falling, and Circling

Ear infection

Viral infections

Fractures

Infection involving nervous system

Inflammation of brain or spinal cord

Poisoning

Seizure

Parasites

Trauma involving nervous system

Jaundice (Icterus)

Bile duct obstruction

Gallbladder disease

Internal bleeding and/or destruction of red blood cells

Infection

Autoimmune disease

Liver disease

Lameness

Arthritis

Bruised or traumatized footpad

Abscess

Deep fungal infection

Degenerative joint disease

Foreign body penetration

Torn nail

Fracture

Hip dislocation

Hyperparathyroidism

Infections involving bones, joints, or muscles

Joint sprain or muscle strain

Ligament tear

Muscle trauma/bruising

Neoplasia

Odors: Breath

Colitis

Kidney disease

Oral foreign body

Oral ulcer

Periodontal disease

Tumors involving the oral cavity

Odors: Body

Colitis

Ear infections

Haircoat contamination

Allergic dermatitis

Flea allergy

Seborrhea

Skin infections

Skin tumors

Anal sac infection or inflammation

Paralysis

Abscess or fight wound

Brain or spinal cord trauma or inflammation

Ear infection (facial paralysis)

Fractures

Neoplasia

Poisoning

Heart disease

Regurgitation

Esophageal foreign body

Megaesophagus

Esophageal infection

Esophageal ulcer

Salivation: Excessive

Esophageal obstructions

Foreign body within oral cavity

Jaw fractures

Nausea

Oral mass or tumor

Periodontal disease

Poisoning

Rabies (rare)

Reactions to noxious objects, chemicals, or medications

Seizures

Seizures

Brain inflammation secondary to trauma

Brain tumor

Infection of nervous system

Heat stroke

Idiopathic epilepsy

Kidney disease

Liver disease

Metabolic disease

Low blood sugar

Poisoning

Parasites

Low blood calcium (nursing mothers)

Skin: Hair Loss (Alopecia) and Itching

Abscess

Allergies (fleas, food, inhalant)

Any chronic illness

Bacterial skin infections

Cushing's disease

Diabetes mellitus

Hypothyroidism

Nutritional deficiency

Self-trauma

Skin parasites (fleas, mites)

Stress

Skin: Lumps and Masses on or Beneath

Abscess

Cyst

Fibrous nodular scar

Granuloma

Hematoma or seroma

Swollen lymph node(s)

Tumor—benign or malignant

Sneezing

Allergic rhinitis

Nasal infection

Nasal polyp or tumor

Nasal foreign body

Thirst: Excessive

Dehydration

Kidney disease

Bladder infection

Poisoning

Uterine infection (pyometra)

Urination: Excessive

Cushing's disease

Diabetes mellitus

Drug therapy (i.e., corticosteroids)

Bladder infection

Kidney infection

Hyperthyroidism

Increase in physical activity

Kidney disease

Liver disease

Mineral or electrolyte imbalances

Poisoning

Stress

Uterine infection (pyometra)

Urination: Incontinence

Age-related

Idiopathic (cause unknown)

Spinal cord injury or disease

Urinary tract infection

Urination: Straining (Stranguria)

Bladder infection

Urinary obstruction

Neoplasia

Spinal nerve damage

Trauma to bladder or urethra

Urolithiasis

Vomiting

Abdominal neoplasia

Bacterial gastrointestinal infections

Brain disorders

Diabetes mellitus

Dietary indiscretions or changes

Viral disease

Food allergies

Hairballs (cats)

Gastrointestinal obstruction

Ingestion of a foreign body

Intestinal parasites

Kidney disease

Liver disease

Pyometra

Stomach ulcers

Stress

Toxins or drugs

Vestibular disorders

Pancreatitis

Weakness or Collapse

Heart disease

Heat stroke

Trauma

Poisoning

Diabetes mellitus

Pain

Anemia

Arthritis

Fever

Low blood sugar

Neoplasia

Pleural effusion

Poisoning

Spinal cord disease

Weight Loss and Wasting (Cachexia)

Chronic infections

Diabetes mellitus

Pancreatic disease

Viral infections (FeLV; FIV)

Kidney disease

Gastrointestinal parasites

Malnutrition

Heart disease

Hyperthyroidism (cats)

Liver disease

Maldigestion of food

Neoplasia

Persistent fever

Stomatitis

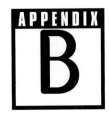

Medications for Dogs and Cats

Table B.1 Medications

Drug name (trade name)	Action or class	Commonly prescribed for
Acepromazine	Tranquilizer	Travel anxiety
Acetazolamide (Diamox)	Lowers intraocular pressure	Glaucoma
Albendazole (Valbazen)	Antiparasitic	Intestinal parasites
Albuterol (Proventil, Ventolin)	Dilates respiratory airways	Heart and/or pulmonary disease
Aluminum hydroxide (Amphojel)	Neutralizes stomach acid and binds phosphate	Stomach upset; vomiting; kidney disease
Aminophylline	Dilates respiratory airways	Heart and/or pulmonary disease
Amitraz (Mitaban)	Antiparasitic	Demodecosis
Amitriptyline (Elavil)	Antidepressant	Behavioral disorders
Amlodipine besylate (Norvasc)	Dilates blood vessels	High blood pressure

Table B.1 Medications (*Continued*)

Drug name (trade name)	Action or class	Commonly prescribed for
Amoxicillin (Amoxi Tabs, Biomox)	Antibiotic	Bacterial infections
Amoxicillin/clavulanic acid (Clavamox)	Antibiotic	Bacterial infections
Amphotericin B (Fungizone)	Antifungal	Fungal infections
Ampicillin (Omnipen, Principen)	Antibiotic	Bacterial infections
Amprolium (Amprol, Corid)	Antiprotozoal	Coccidia infections
Atenolol (Tenormin)	Stops abnormal heart rhythms and slows heart rate	Heart disease
Azathioprine (Imuran)	Suppresses the immune system	Immune-mediated diseases
Betamethasone (Celestone)	Steroid anti-inflammatory	Inflammation and immune-mediated diseases
Bunamidine hydrochloride (Scolaban)	Antiparasitic	Tapeworms
Buspirone (BuSpar)	Reduces anxiety	Urine spraying in cats
Butorphanol (Torbutrol Torbugesic)	Sedative; analgesic	Pain; coughing
Calcium carbonate (Tums)	Stomach acid neutralizer; phosphate binder	Stomach ulcers; kidney disease
Captopril (Capoten)	Dilates blood vessels	Heart disease and high blood pressure
Carprofen (Rimadyl)	Analgesic	Musculoskeletal and arthritic pain
Cefaclor (Ceclor)	Antibiotic	Bacterial infections
Cefadroxil (Cefa-Tabs, Cefa-Drops)	Antibiotic	Bacterial infections

Table B.1 Medications (*Continued*)

Drug name (trade name)	Action or class	Commonly prescribed for
Ceftiofur (Naxcel)	Antibiotic	Bacterial infections
Cephalexin (Keflex)	Antibiotic	Bacterial infections
Charcoal, activated	Adsorb drugs and toxins within gastrointestinal tract	First aid for poisonings
Chlorambucil (Leukeran)	Antineoplastic	Tumors and autoimmune diseases
Chloramphenicol and chloramphenicol palmitate (Chloromycetin)	Antibiotic	Bacterial infections
Chlorothiazide (Diuril)	Diuretic (promotes fluid excretion from the body)	Heart disease; high blood pressure; calcium uroliths
Chlorpheniramine maleate (Chlortrimetron, Phenetron)	Antihistamine	Prevents allergic reactions; itching
Chondroitin sulfate/ glucosamine (Cosequin)	Nutraceutical	Pain associated with degenerative joint disease
Cisapride (Propulsid)	Stimulates stomach and intestinal motility	Stomach reflux, bowel stasis, constipation
Clemastine (Tavist)	Antihistamine	Itching; skin allergies
Clindamycin (Antirobe)	Antibiotic	Bacterial infections
Clomipramine (Clomicalm)	Antidepressant	Behavioral disorders, including separation anxiety
Cloxacillin (Cloxapen)	Antibiotic	Bacterial infections
Codeine	Opiate analgesic	Pain; sedation
Cimetidine (Tagamet)	Decreases stomach acid secretion	Vomiting; stomach ulcers

Table B.1 Medications (*Continued*)

Drug name (trade name)	Action or class	Commonly prescribed for
Cyclophosphamide (Cytoxan)	Antineoplastic	Tumors and autoimmune diseases
Cyclosporine (Optimmune)	Suppresses the immune system; stimulates tear production	Keratoconjunctivitis sicca (dry eye); autoimmune diseases
Desmopressin acetate	Synthetic hormone	Diabetes insipidus; von Willebrand's disease
Dexamethasone (Azium, Dexasone, Decadron)	Steroid anti-inflammatory	Inflammation and immune-mediated diseases
Dextromethorphan (Benylin)	Antitussive	Coughing
Diazepam (Valium)	Sedative; anticonvulsant	Anxiety; seizures; appetite stimulant
Dichlorphenamide (Daranide)	Diuretic (promotes fluid excretion from the body)	Glaucoma
Dichlorvos (Task)	Antiparasitic	Intestinal parasites
Diethylstilbestrol (DES)	Synthetic estrogen hormone	Urinary incontinence
Difloxacin hydrochloride (Dicural)	Antibiotic	Bacterial infections
Digoxin (Lanoxin, Cardoxin)	Increases force of heart contraction and decreases heart rate	Heart disease
Diltiazem (Cardizem, Dilacor)	Lowers blood pressure; stabilizes heart rhythms	High blood pressure; heart disease
Dimenhydrinate (Dramamine)	Antihistamine	Vomiting; motion sickness
Diphenhydramine (Benadryl)	Antihistamine	Sedation; allergies; prevents allergic reactions
Diphenoxylate (Lomotil)	Regulates bowel motility	Diarrhea

Table B.1 Medications (*Continued*)

Drug name (trade name)	Action or class	Commonly prescribed for
Docusate calcium (Surfak, Doxidan)	Stool softener	Constipation
Doxycycline (Vibramycin)	Antibiotic	Bacterial infections; *Ehrlichia* infections
Enalapril (Enacard, Vasotec)	Dilates blood vessels	Heart disease and high blood pressure
Enrofloxacin (Baytril)	Antibiotic	Bacterial infections
Ephedrine	Stimulant; increases blood pressure	Low blood pressure; urinary incontinence
Epsiprantel (Cestex)	Antiparasitic	Tapeworms
Erythromycin	Antibiotic	Bacterial infections
Etodolac (Eto-Gesic, Lodine)	Nonsteroidal anti-inflammatory	Musculoskeletal and arthritic pain
Famotidine (Pepcid)	Decreases stomach acid secretion	Vomiting; stomach ulcers
Fenbendazole (Panacur)	Antiparasitic	Intestinal parasites and *Giardia* infestations
Fentanyl transdermal patch (Duragesic)	Opiate analgesic	Pain control
Fluconazole (Diflucan)	Antifungal	Fungal infections
Flucytosine (Ancobon)	Antifungal	Fungal infections
Fludrocortisone (Florinef)	Steroid hormone	Hypoadrenocorticism (Addison's disease)
Flunixin meglumine (Banamine)	Nonsteroidal anti-inflammatory	Moderate pain and inflammation
Fluoxetine (Prozac)	Antidepressant	Behavioral disorders
Furazolidone (Furoxone)	Antiprotozoal	*Giardia* infestations
Furosemide (Lasix, Disal)	Diuretic (promotes fluid excretion from the body)	Heart disease; high blood pressure; kidney disease

Table B.1 Medications (*Continued*)

Drug name (trade name)	Action or class	Commonly prescribed for
Glipizide (Glucotrol)	Oral hypoglycemic agent; increases insulin secretion	Non-insulin-dependent diabetes mellitus
Glucosamine	See *Chondroitin*	
Griseofulvin (Fulvicin)	Antifungal	Ringworm
Hydralazine (Apresoline)	Dilates blood vessels	Heart disease
Hydrocodone bitartrate (Hycodan)	Opiate antitussive	Coughing
Hydrocortisone (Cortef)	Steroid anti-inflammatory	Inflammation and immune-mediated diseases
Hydroxyzine (Atarax)	Antihistamine	Skin allergies; itching
Insulin (Regular, NPH)	Hormone responsible for glucose utilization	Diabetes mellitus
Interferon	Immune system stimulant	FeLV/FIV infections
Ipecac	Induces vomiting	Poisonings
Isosorbide dinitrate (Isordil, Isorbid)	Dilates blood vessels	Heart disease
Itraconazole (Sporanox)	Antifungal	Fungal infections
Ivermectin (Heartgard, Ivomec)	Antiparasitic	Intestinal and skin parasites; heartworm prevention
Ketoconazole (Nizoral)	Antifungal	Fungal infections; ringworm; yeast infections on skin
Ketoprofen	Nonsteroidal anti-inflammatory	Moderate pain and inflammation
Lactulose (Chronulac)	Laxative; lowers pH in colon	Constipation; liver disease
Levamisole (Levasole, Tramisol)	Antiparasitic	Intestinal parasites

Table B.1 Medications (*Continued*)

Drug name (trade name)	Action or class	Commonly prescribed for
Levothyroxine sodium (Soloxine, Thyrotabs, Synthroid)	Synthetic thyroid hormone	Hypothyroidism
Lincomycin (Lincocin)	Antibiotic	Bacterial infections
Lisinopril (Prinivil, Zestril)	Dilates blood vessels	Heart disease and high blood pressure
Loperamide (Imodium)	Regulates bowel motility	Diarrhea
Lufenuron (Program)	Antiparasitic	Flea control
Lufenuron + milbemycinoxime (Sentinel)	Antiparasitic	Flea, intestinal parasite, and heartworm prevention/control
Magnesium hydroxide (Milk of magnesia)	Neutralizes stomach acid	Vomiting; stomach ulcers
Marbofloxacin	Antibiotic	Bacterial infection
Mebendazole	Antiparasitic	Intestinal parasites
Meclizine (Antivert)	Antihistamine	Motion sickness
Meclofenamic acid (Arquel, Meclofen)	Nonsteroidal anti-inflammatory	Arthritic pain
Medroxyprogesterone acetate (Depo-Provera)	Sex hormone	Behavioral disorders; skin disease
Megestrol acetate (Ovaban)	Sex hormone	Behavior disorders, including urine spraying
Melphalan (Alkeran)	Anticancer agent	Cancer, especially myeloma
Meperidine (Demerol)	Analgesic	Pain
6-Mercaptopurine (Purinethol)	Anticancer agent	Cancer, especially leukemia and lymphoma
Methazolamide (Neptazane)	Diuretic (promotes fluid excretion)	Glaucoma

Table B.1 Medications (*Continued*)

Drug name (trade name)	Action or class	Commonly prescribed for
Methenamine hippurate (Urex)	Urinary antiseptic	Urinary tract infections
Methimazole (Tapazole)	Antithyroid agent	Hyperthyroidism
Methocarbamol (Robaxin-V)	Skeletal muscle relaxant	Muscle spasms; back pain
Methotrexate (MTX, Mexate, Folex)	Anticancer agent	Cancer, especially carcinomas, leukemia, and lymphoma
Methylprednisolone (Medrol)	Steroid anti-inflammatory	Inflammation and immune-mediated diseases
Methyltestosterone (Android, generic)	Male sex hormone	Testosterone deficiency; stimulates red blood cell production
Metoclopramide (Reglan)	Stimulates upper gastrointestinal tract	Vomiting; stomach reflux
Metoprolol tartrate (Lopressor)	Controls rapid heart rate and rhythms	Heart disease
Metronidazole (Flagyl)	Antibacterial and antiprotozoal drug	Intestinal infections
Mibolerone (Cheque-drops)	Androgenic steroid	Estrus suppression
Milbemycin oxime (Interceptor, Interceptor Flavor Tabs, and Safe Heart)	Antiparasitic	Prevention of intestinal parasites and heartworms; treatment of *Demodex*
Mitotane (o,p'-DDD) (Lysodren)	Chemotherapeutic agent	Pituitary-dependent hyperadrenocorticism (Cushing's disease)
Moxidectin (ProHeart)	Antiparasitic	Prevention of intestinal parasites and heartworms
Naproxen (Naprosyn, Naxen)	Nonsteroidal anti-inflammatory	Moderate pain and inflammation

Table B.1 Medications (*Continued*)

Drug name (trade name)	Action or class	Commonly prescribed for
Nitroglycerin ointment (Nitrol, Nitrobid, Nitrostat)	Dilates blood vessels	Heart disease
Norfloxacin (Noroxin)	Antibiotic	Bacterial infections
Olsalazine (Dipentum)	Anti-inflammatory agent	Colitis
Omeprazole (Prilosec)	Reduces stomach acid secretion	Gastrointestinal ulcers
Ondansetron (Zofran)	Antiemetic	Vomiting, especially when associated with chemotherapy
Orbifloxacin (Orbax)	Antibiotic	Bacterial infections
Ormetoprim	Antimicrobial	Bacterial infections
Ormetoprim plus sulfadimethoxine (Primor)	Antibacterial	Bacterial infections
Oxacillin	Antibiotic	Bacterial infections
Oxazepam (Serax)	Sedative	Sedation; appetite stimulant
Oxtriphylline (Choledyl-SA)	Dilates airways	Heart and lung disease
Oxybutynin chloride (Ditropan)	Smooth-muscle relaxant	Urinary tract spasms
Oxytetracycline (Terramycin)	Antibiotic	Bacterial infections
Pancrelipase (Viokase)	Pancreatic enzymes	Pancreatic exocrine insufficiency
Paroxetine (Paxil)	Serotonin modulator	Behavioral disorders
Penicillin V	Antibiotic	Bacterial infections
Phenobarbital (Luminal)	Anticonvulsant	Seizure control
Phenoxybenzamine (Dibenzyline)	Dilates blood vessels; relaxes urethral smooth muscle	Feline lower urinary tract disease

Table B.1 Medications (*Continued*)

Drug name (trade name)	Action or class	Commonly prescribed for
Phenylbutazone (Butazolidin)	Nonsteroidal anti-inflammatory	Moderate pain and inflammation
Phenylpropanolamine (Dexatrim, Propagest)	Decongestant; dilates airways; increases tone of urinary sphincter	Tracheobronchitis; rhinitis; urinary incontinence
Phenytoin (Dilantin)	Anticonvulsant	Seizure control
Piperazine	Antiparasitic	Intestinal parasites
Piroxicam (Feldene)	Nonsteroidal anti-inflammatory	Moderate pain and inflammation
Polysulfated glycosaminoglycan (Adequan)	Inhibits enzymes that erode joint cartilage	Degenerative joint disease
Potassium bromide (KBr)	Anticonvulsant	Seizure control
Praziquantel (Droncit)	Antiparasitic	Tapeworms
Prednisolone (Delta-cortef)	Steroid anti-inflammatory	Inflammation and immune-mediated diseases
Prednisone (Deltasone)	Steroid anti-inflammatory	Inflammation and immune-mediated diseases
Primidone (Mylepsin)	Anticonvulsant	Seizure control
Prochlorperazine (Compazine)	Tranquilizer	Vomiting
Promethazine (Phenergan)	Antihistamine	Allergies and motion sickness
Propranolol (Inderal)	Decreases heart rate, cardiac conduction, and blood pressure	Heart disease
Pseudoephedrine (Sudafed)	Decongestant; increases tone of urinary sphincter	Tracheobronchitis; rhinitis; urinary incontinence

Table B.1 Medications (*Continued*)

Drug name (trade name)	Action or class	Commonly prescribed for
Psyllium (Metamucil)	Laxative	Constipation; anal sac disease
Pyrantel pamoate (Nemex, Strongid)	Antiparasitic	Intestinal parasites
Pyrimethamine (Daraprim)	Antibacterial; antiprotozoal	Intestinal infections
Quinidine polygalacturonate (Cardioquin)	Stops abnormal heart rhythms	Heart disease
Racemethionine (*dl*-methionine, Uroeze, Methio-Form)	Urinary acidifier	Uroliths; feline lower urinary tract disease
Ranitidine (Zantac)	Suppresses stomach acid secretion	Gastrointestinal ulcers
Rifampin (Rifadin)	Antibacterial	Higher bacterial infections
Selegiline (Deprenyl, Anipryl)	Inhibits degradation of dopamine in the nervous system	Cushing's disease, senility (cognitive dysfunction)
Spironolactone (Aldactone)	Diuretic	Heart disease
Stanozolol (Winstrol-V)	Anabolic steroid	Kidney disease; muscle wasting
Sucralfate (Carafate)	Coating agent	Gastrointestinal ulcers
Sulfadiazine	Antimicrobial	Bacterial infections
Sulfadimethoxine (Albon, Bactrovet)	Antimicrobial	Bacterial infections; coccidia infestations
Tamoxifen (Nolvadex)	Anticancer agent	Cancer therapy
Taurine	Nutraceutical	Cardiomyopathy and retinal degeneration in cats

Table B.1 Medications (*Continued*)

Drug name (trade name)	Action or class	Commonly prescribed for
Terbutaline (Brethine)	Dilates respiratory airways	Heart and/or pulmonary disease
Tetracycline (Panmycin)	Antibiotic	Bacterial infections
Theophylline (Theo-Dur)	Dilates respiratory airways	Heart and/or pulmonary disease
Ticarcillin (Ticar, Ticillin)	Antibiotic	Bacterial infections
Triamcinolone (Vetalog, Trimtabs)	Steroid anti-inflammatory	Inflammation and immune-mediated diseases
Trimeprazine tartrate (Temaril)	Antihistamine	Allergies and motion sickness
Trimethobenzamide (Tigan)	Antiemetic	Vomiting
Trimethoprim + sulfadiazine (Tribrissen)	Antimicrobial	Bacterial infections
Trimethoprim + sulfamethoxazole (Bactrim, Septra)	Antimicrobial	Bacterial infections
Tylosin (Tylan)	Antibiotic	Colitis
Ursodiol (Actigall)	Promotes bile flow	Liver disease
Vancomycin (Vancocin)	Antibiotic	Bacterial infections
Verapamil (Calan, Isoptin)	Dilates blood vessels; lowers heart rate	Heart disease
Vitamin B_{12} (cyanocobalamin)	Nutraceutical	Anemia
Vitamin C (ascorbic acid)	Nutraceutical	Cystitis
Vitamin K (Mephyton, Veta-K1)	Nutraceutical	Blood clotting disorders; rodenticide poisoning
Warfarin (Coumadin)	Anticoagulant	Thromboembolism in cats
Zidovudine (AZT; Retrovir)	Antiviral	FeLV and FIV infections

Glossary

acariasis Mite infestation.

acupressure The stimulation of an acupuncture point using finger or instrument pressure instead of a needle.

acupuncture Ancient form of medical therapy that involves the stimulation of specific points on the body in order to produce chemical and physical responses that will treat specific illnesses, reduce or eliminate pain, and promote overall health.

acute Short-term, severe.

Addison's disease Also known as *hypoadrenocorticism*; reduced secretion of hormones by the adrenal glands.

adenoma Benign tumor involving glandular tissue.

aerobic Requires oxygen to live or function.

air sacs Structures attached to and surrounding the lungs of birds that serve as storage areas for air and contribute to a bird's ability to fly.

airsacculitis Inflammation of the air sacs.

albumin One of the major proteins normally found in the bloodstream.

allergen Substance capable of producing an allergic response.

allergy Exaggerated immune response to a foreign substance.

alopecia Hair loss.

anaphylactic reaction A dramatic fall in blood pressure caused by a massive release of histamine and other chemicals within the body.

anemia A reduction in the number of red blood cells within the body.

anorexia Loss of appetite.

antibiotic Chemical compounds used to treat bacterial infections.

antibody Protein produced by the body to fight infectious diseases and foreign invaders.

antifungal Chemical compounds used to treat fungal infections.

antigen Substance capable of stimulating an immune response.

antimicrobial Chemical compounds used to treat bacterial, viral, or fungal infections.

anting Unique behavior of hedgehogs characterized by the hedgehog producing copious amounts of saliva whenever a new object is placed within its cage.

aqueous fluid Special fluid found in the anterior chamber of the eye.

arboreal Living in trees or on plants.

arrhythmia Abnormal heart rhythm.

arteries Vessels that carry blood away from the heart.

arthritis Inflammation of a joint.

artificial respiration First aid procedure used on a pet that has stopped breathing.

ascarid Common roundworm found in the intestinal tract of birds and mammals.

ascites Fluid buildup within the abdominal cavity; often seen with liver and heart disease.

aspergillosis Fungal disease of birds affecting the respiratory system.

aspiration cytology Removal of fluid or cells from a mass, organ, or lesion using a needle and syringe, followed by microscopic examination of the fluid or cells on a slide.

associative learning Type of learning where a pet creates a link between a stimulus, response, and reward.

astringent Substance with drying capabilities when applied to a surface.

ataxia Incoordination.

atopy Allergies caused by pollens or other inhaled substances.

atria The upper chambers of the heart.

atrophy Shrinking or deterioration of an organ or tissue.

autoimmune disease Disease characterized by the body's immune system attacking its own tissues and organs.

autoimmune hemolytic anemia Autoimmune disease characterized by the destruction of red blood cells within the body by the body's own immune system.

avian pox Viral disease of birds causing severe respiratory and skin disease.

benign Noncancerous, nonmalignant.

bilirubin Pigment formed from hemoglobin that has been recycled from red blood cells.

biological filter A type of "natural" filter used in aquariums in which accumulated bacteria within the tank break down organic waste material.

biopsy Procedure involving the removal of a small portion of living tissue for microscopic examination.

botanical medicine Using herbal remedies to prevent and/or treat disease.

bowel Refers to the small and large intestines.

cachexia Loss of weight and tissue mass resulting from disease or malnutrition.

calculus Urinary stone; also refers to the hard brown buildup on the teeth of dogs and cats.

calicivirus Virus that infects the upper respiratory system in cats.

callus Region of thickened skin devoid of hair.

cancer Malignant tumor.

candidiasis A digestive system disease of birds caused by a yeast organism; causes characteristic ulcers covered by a white film or plaque.

canine cough complex Respiratory disease in dogs caused by a group of viral and bacterial organisms that attack the upper airways, causing inflammation and coughing.

canine distemper Multisystemic viral disease of dogs.

carcinogen Substance or agent capable of producing neoplastic changes in cells.

carcinoma Cancer involving epithelial or glandular tissue.

cardiac output A measure of the heart's ability to pump and circulate blood.

cardiomyopathy Abnormal thickening or thinning of the heart wall.

cardiopulmonary resuscitation (CPR) First aid procedure used on a pet whose heart has stopped beating.

cardiovascular Pertaining to the heart and blood vessels.

carnivore   Individual that feeds on other animals.

cartilage   Connective tissue found on joint surfaces.

castration   Surgical removal of the testicles.

cataract   Opacity of the eye lens.

CBC   Complete blood count.

CCDS   Canine cognitive dysfunction syndrome.

cellulitis   Inflammation involving the connective tissue located beneath the skin.

central nervous system   That part of the nervous system that includes the brain and the spinal cord.

cere   Soft-tissue structure located at the top portion of a bird's beak; sometimes used to determine the sex of a bird.

cervix   The portion of the female reproductive tract that separates the uterus from the vagina.

cestode   Tapeworm.

chemotherapy   The treatment of cancer using chemicals and drugs.

cheyletiellosis   Infestation with the mange mite *Cheyletiella.*

chiropractic medicine   A holistic medical approach that utilizes vertebral manipulations and adjustments to treat disease and promote health.

chronic   Long-term; persistent.

circovirus   Agent implicated as the cause of psittacine beak and feather disease.

circulatory shock   Life-threatening condition characterized by a gradual shutdown of vital body processes, including blood circulation.

cloaca   The terminal portion of the avian large intestine where the digestive and urinary systems meet.

clutch   A group of eggs.

colitis   Inflammation of the colon.

colostrum   Mother's milk produced in the first few days after birthing that contains high levels of protective antibodies.

complementary medicine   Medical approach to disease that involves the use of both traditional and holistic techniques and treatments.

compound fracture   A fracture that penetrates the skin.

congenital defect   Birth defect.

conjunctiva   The membrane lining the eye socket and sclera of the eyeball.

conjunctival worms   Parasites that infest the eyelids and eyes of birds.

conjunctivitis Inflammation of the conjunctiva.

connective tissue The type of tissue that connects and supports structures located beneath the skin.

contour feather The major type of feather seen on a bird's head, wings, body, and tail.

cornea The clear curved front portion of the eyeball.

coronavirus Virus causing mild enteritis in dogs and feline infectious peritonitis in cats.

corticosteroids Steroid hormones produced by the adrenal glands.

cortisone A steroid hormone; the synthetic variety is often administered by injection.

crepitus The grating sound made when the ends of a fractured bone rub together.

crop An outpouching of the esophagus in birds that serves as a temporary storage place for food.

cryotherapy Treatment of cancer by means of applications of extremely cold temperatures in order to freeze and kill the tumor cells.

cryptorchidism Retained testicle(s).

Cushing's disease Also known as *hyperadrenocorticism*; increased secretion of steroid hormones by the adrenal glands.

cuterebriasis Tissue infestation with the fly larva *Cuterebra*; most often seen in cats and rabbits.

cyclosporine An immunosuppressive drug often used to treat dry eye in dogs.

cystic endometrial hyperplasia Overgrowth of uterine lining, leading to the formation of cysts.

cystitis Inflammation of the bladder.

cytology The examination of cells and body fluids using a microscope.

definitive diagnosis A diagnosis that has been confirmed by physical examination or by specific diagnostic tests and procedures.

dehydration Condition in which the water level within the body is below that required for normal body function.

dermatitis Inflammation of the skin.

dermatophytosis Ringworm infestation.

descenting The removal of the anal sacs; usually performed on ferrets.

diabetes mellitus Metabolic disease characterized by a deficiency of the hormone insulin and subsequent elevated levels of glucose in the blood.

diaphragm   Muscular wall separating the thorax from the abdomen.

dietary indiscretion   The consumption of foodstuffs or substances that are not normal components of a pet's diet.

dip   Highly concentrated form of insecticide.

disseminated intravascular coagulation   Also known as DIC; the formation of small blood clots throughout the body in response to shock or severe disease.

diuretic   Drug that promotes urination.

down feathers   Small, soft insulating feathers located beneath contour feathers.

dry eye   Keratoconjunctivitis.

dysfunction   Abnormality in function.

dystocia   Difficulties in giving birth.

ecdysis   Term used to describe the shedding process in reptiles.

ECG   Electrocardiogram; test that measures electrical activity within the heart.

eclampsia   Calcium deficiency in a lactating pet; also known as "milk fever."

ectropion   Condition characterized by the outward rolling of the eyelid.

edema   Abnormal buildup of fluid within the tissues and/or spaces within the body.

efficacy   Competence; efficiency.

effusion   Escape of fluid into an open space or cavity.

electrolyte   Molecule found within the body that is able to conduct an electrical current.

ELISA   Enzyme-linked immunosorbent assay; laboratory test used to detect antibodies to or antigens of specific disease agents in the blood.

embolism   A clot usually composed of blood, tissue, air, or bacteria that plugs a blood vessels.

endocarditis   Inflammation of the heart lining.

endocrine organs   Organs that produce hormones within the body.

endoscope   Tubelike diagnostic device used to examine the interior of hollow body organs and spaces.

enteric   Involving the small intestine.

enteritis   Inflammation of the small intestine.

entropion   Condition characterized by the inward rolling of the eyelid.

enzyme   Chemical substance that enhances and increases the speed of metabolic reactions within the body.

epistaxis   Nosebleed.

erysipelas   Bacterial disease of the heart and joints in pigs.

erythrocyte   Red blood cell.

esophagus   The muscular, tubular digestive organ that attaches the pharynx to the stomach.

estrogen   Female sex hormone that stimulates estrus.

estrus   The period of "heat" during which the female becomes receptive to the male.

etiology   The cause of a particular disease or disorder.

exercise intolerance   Inability to engage in physical exertion without becoming weak or lethargic.

exotic Newcastle's disease   Also known as *avian distemper,* this viral disease can adversely affect the respiratory, intestinal, and nervous systems of infected birds; has been eradicated from the United States.

feather cysts   Skin nodules caused by abnormal feather shafts.

febrile   Having a fever.

feline enteric coronavirus   Virus found in the digestive system of cats.

feline immunodeficiency virus   A virus similar to the AIDS virus in humans that attacks and suppresses the immune systems of cats.

feline infectious anemia   Feline hemobartonellosis.

feline infectious peritonitis   Severe, usually fatal disease of cats caused by the overreaction of the cats' immune system to a coronavirus.

feline leukemia virus   Virus related to the feline immunodeficiency virus that suppresses the immune system and can instigate a number of diseases, including cancer.

feline panleukopenia   Also known as *feline distemper*; a disease caused by a parvovirus.

fibroma   Benign tumor involving the connective tissue beneath the skin.

fibrosarcoma   Cancer involving the connective tissue.

FLUTD   Feline lower urinary tract disease.

folliculitis   Inflammation of the hair follicles.

fracture   Cracks or breaks involving bone.

French molt   Disease of psittacine birds characterized by the abnormal development of tail and/or flight feathers.

frounce   Respiratory disease of birds caused by a parasitic organism.

FUS   Feline urologic syndrome; see *FLUTD.*

gapeworm   A parasite that can inhabit the trachea of finches and canaries and interfere with breathing.

gastrointestinal   Pertaining to the stomach and intestines.

geriatric   Senior; old.

gestation   The period of pregnancy.

giardia   Protozoa that infects the intestinal tract of animals; has also been implicated as a cause of feather picking in birds.

gingivitis   Inflammation of the gums.

glaucoma   Increased fluid pressure within the eye.

glomerulonephritis   Inflammation involving select portions of the kidney.

glucocorticoids   A particular class of corticosteroids used to treat allergies, autoimmune diseases, and shock.

gout   A disease in birds characterized by a buildup of uric acid within the tissues and joints, leading to lameness and other maladies.

granuloma   Hard lesion characterized by a buildup of inflammatory cells surrounding an infectious organism or a foreign body.

grit   The term given to any hard substance found within a bird's gizzard that helps crush and grind food, and thereby aids in digestion.

habituation   Basic type of learning seen in dogs and cats characterized by a diminishing response to a repeated stimulus over a period of time.

hairballs   The most common cause of vomiting in cats; also seen in guinea pigs.

halitosis   Bad breath.

hematoma   Localized swelling containing blood.

hemoglobin   The molecule found within red blood cells that binds with and carries oxygen.

hemoparasites   Parasites living within the bloodstream; up to 50 percent of all birds may harbor hemoparasites.

hemorrhage   Active bleeding.

hemostasis   The ability of the body to control internal or external bleeding.

hemostatic pathway Sequence of events that occur within the body whenever it is called on to control bleeding.

hemothorax Blood within the thoracic cavity.

hepatic lipidosis Abnormal fatty buildup within the liver; can be seen in malnourished cats.

herbal elixir Type of medicinal preparation made by mixing crushed herbs with alcohol.

herbivore Individual that eats only plants.

hernia Protrusion of an organ or tissue through the body wall or diaphragm.

hip dysplasia An inherited disease of dogs characterized by malformation of the hip joints.

histamine Chemical substance contained within special body cells; it is responsible for many of the signs seen with an allergic reaction.

hob Male ferret.

holistic Term indicating a natural approach to maintaining and restoring health.

homeopathy A holistic approach to medicine that employs highly diluted dosages of agents designed to stimulate the body to cure itself.

hormone Chemical produced by a specific endocrine gland that regulates the activity of other select organs within the body.

husbandry The general care given to a pet, including feeding, housing, grooming, and preventive health care.

hybrid vigor Genetic phenomenon seen in mixed-breed dogs and cats that tends to make them healthier and more vigorous than their purebred peers.

hydrocephalus Buildup of fluid within the brain and skull.

hyperadrenocorticism See *Cushing's disease.*

hyperplasia Proliferation of cells within a tissue.

hyperthermia Elevated body temperature.

hyperthyroidism Elevated levels of thyroid hormone within the body caused by an overactive thyroid gland.

hypertrophy Increased cellular size within a tissue.

hypoadrenocorticism See *Addison's disease.*

hypoallergenic Devoid of allergy-producing substances.

hypoglycemia Low blood glucose (sugar).

hypokalemia Low blood potassium levels.

icterus Jaundice.

ictus Seizure.

idiopathic Referrring to an unknown source or cause.

immunity-mediated Any disease caused by an overactive immune system.

immunization Artificial exposure of the immune system to the antigens of a disease-causing agent; designed to stimulate immune protection against the agent.

immunosuppressed Characterizing a condition in which the immune system fails to respond adequately to a foreign substance or disease agent.

immunotherapy Treatment of cancer by means of immune system components.

inappetence Loss of appetite.

incontinence Inability to control body eliminations.

inflammation Body response to disease characterized by heat, swelling, redness, and pain.

insulin Hormone that regulates the uptake and utilization of glucose within the body.

insulinoma Tumor of the pancreas that leads to excessive insulin production and low blood sugar.

integumentary Pertaining to the skin and associated structures.

interferon A chemical substance produced by the body designed to fight viral infections and tumors.

intervertebral disk Cartilaginous structure located between vertebrae that functions as a shock absorber.

intranasal Referring to the nose and nasal passages.

intravenous fluids Special solutions that are similar in composition to those fluids found naturally within the body; used to correct or prevent dehydration, replace electrolytes, and stimulate heart function and blood circulation.

intussusception Condition characterized by the prolapse of one portion of the intestine into another one.

invertebrates Those animals that do not possess a backbone.

IV Intravenous.

ivermectin Antiparasitic drug that is useful in treating and preventing a wide variety of parasitic diseases.

Jacobson's organ Organ found in the mouth of snakes that assists in the sense of smell.

jaundice A yellowing of the body's skin and mucous membranes caused by excessive bile pigments within the blood.

jill Female ferret.

keel bone The breastbone of a bird.

keratitis Inflammation of the cornea.

keratoconjunctivitis sicca Dryness of the eye(s) characterized by inadequate tear production.

ketones By-products of fat metabolism within the body.

lactose Sugar found in milk.

lenticular sclerosis Progressive clouding of the eye lenses due to the aging process.

leptospirosis Bacterial disease affecting primarily the kidneys and liver.

lethargy Listlessness; apathy.

leukocytes White blood cells.

leukopenia Abnormally low numbers of white cells within the blood.

ligament Fibrous band of tissue connecting two bones together within a joint.

lipoma Benign tumor of fatty tissue.

lufenuron Insect development inhibitor.

lumen The cavity of a tubelike structure.

lupus An autoimmune disease affecting the skin, mucous membranes, and various organs of the body.

luxation Dislocation of a joint.

Lyme disease Tickborne disease causing fever, arthritis, and other symptoms in affected hosts.

lymph Liquid substance within the body that contains immune cells, proteins, and fat molecules.

lymphadenitis Inflammation of the lymph nodes.

lymphocyte The type of white blood cell capable of responding by producing antibodies or mounting an immune response to a foreign invader within the body.

lymphosarcoma Malignant tumor of lymphoid tissue and lymphocytes.

macaw wasting disease Disease of psittacine birds characterized by an abnormal distension of the proventriculus, which disrupts the normal digestion of nutrients and leads to weight loss, muscle wasting, and nervous system disorders.

malaise Despondence; weakness.

malignant Characterized by uncontrolled, frenzied growth; cancerous.

mastitis Inflammation of the mammary glands.

mechanical filter A device that actively pumps and filters (cleans) the water in an aquarium.

melanoma Tumor involving pigmented epidermal cells.

meridians Acupuncture term for the channels that carry the life force throughout the body.

metabolism The sum of all chemical, life-sustaining processes that occur within the body.

metastasis The spread of tumor cells from their site of origin to other parts of the body.

metritis Inflammation of the uterus.

microfilaria Heartworm larva.

miliary dermatitis Name given to a skin condition in cats characterized by numerous crusty skin lesions, especially around the head, neck, and back.

modified live vaccine Vaccine containing live disease-causing agents that have been altered in such a way that they stimulate immunity without causing disease.

molting In invertebrates, the process of shedding exoskeletons periodically in order to grow in size and replace lost or damaged limbs. Also, the process of seasonal feather loss and renewal in birds.

monocyte Large white blood cell that responds to foreign material within the body.

mouth rot Bacterial and/or fungal disease of the mouth in reptiles.

moxibustion The stimulation of an acupuncture point using a heated needle.

multisystemic Affecting multiple organ systems.

mutation Genetic alteration.

myelin Fatty sheath that surrounds nerve cells.

myelopathy Degenerative disease of nerve fibers.

myocardial Pertaining to heart muscle.

myoglobin The molecule found within muscle cells that binds oxygen.

myopathy Degenerative disease of muscle.

myositis Inflammation of muscle tissue.

necropsy Visual examination of a dead animal's external and internal organs.

necrosis Death of cells and tissue.

nematode Roundworm.

neonate Newborn.

neoplasia Uncontrolled cellular growth and division.

nephritis Inflammation of the kidney.

neuron Nerve cell.

neuter To remove the testicles in a male or ovaries and uterus in a female.

neutering Performing an ovariohysterectomy or castration on a pet.

neutrophil White blood cell that acts as first line of defense against foreign invaders, especially bacteria; it is the major component of pus.

nosodes Homeopathic preparations containing diseased tissues or substances created by the disease condition; used as vaccine substitutes.

noxious Unpleasant; adverse.

nutraceutical Food compound with proven health benefits when given at a therapeutic dosage.

nystagmus Rapid involuntary movements of the eyes; can be horizontal, vertical, or rotary.

occult heartworm infestation Heartworm infestation characterized by the presence of adult worms but without circulating larvae.

ocular Pertaining to the eye.

odontoma Tumor originating from the teeth.

omega-3 fatty acids Fatty acids derived from cold-water fish that are used in veterinary medicine to treat allergies and inflammation.

omnivore Individual that eats both plants and animals.

opacity Cloudiness; opaque region.

organophosphate Insecticidal compound used to kill fleas and ticks on pets; can be highly toxic to cats.

osteomalacia Bone thinning and weakness caused by a calcium deficiency.

osteomyelitis Bone infection.

osteosarcoma Highly malignant neoplasia of bone.

otitis externa Inflammation of the external ear canal.

otitis interna Inflammation of the inner ear.

otitis media Inflammation of the middle ear.

ovariohysterectomy Surgical removal of the ovaries and uterus.

Pacheco's disease   Multisystemic avian disease caused by a herpes virus; often seen in birds smuggled illegally into the country.

palatability   The taste and flavor appeal of a food.

palliative   Serving to alleviate without curing.

palpation   Diagnostic technique used by veterinarians that involves probing and touching of a particular region of the body with the hands and fingers.

pancreatitis   Inflammation of the pancreas.

papilloma   Benign tumor involving epithelial surfaces.

papovavirus   The virus implicated in budgie fledgling disease, a highly fatal disease of young birds less than 4 weeks of age.

parasite   Organism that uses another living organism as its food source.

parathyroid glands   Two glands located on either side of the thyroid gland that are responsible for the regulation of calcium and phosphorus levels within the body.

paresis   Weakness.

parturition   The act of birthing.

parvovirus   A type of virus that primarily affects the gastrointestinal system of dogs and cats.

patella   Kneecap.

patellar luxation   Orthopedic condition characterized by a slipping or displacement of the patella.

pathogenesis   The mechanism by which a specific disease develops.

pemphigus   Autoimmune skin disease.

pericardium   The membrane that surrounds the heart.

perineum   The region of the body located between the external sex organs and the anus.

periodontal disease   Inflammation and infection of the teeth and gums.

periosteum   The outer tissue lining of bone.

pH   A measurement used to express the acidity or alkalinity of a solution.

physiologic   Pertaining to the body, its components, and their functioning.

pinna   Earflap.

pituitary gland   Major gland located at the base of the brain that secretes hormones controlling the activities of other glands throughout the body.

plasma   The fluid portion of the blood.

plastron   The ventral portion of a chelonian's shell.

platelet   Blood component that assists in the formation of blood clots.

pleura   Tissue membrane lining the chest cavity and outer surfaces of the lungs.

pleural effusion   Fluid buildup within the chest cavity.

pleuritis   Inflammation of the pleura.

pneumonitis   Inflammation of the lungs.

pneumothorax   Air within the chest cavity that is not contained within the lungs.

polydipsia   Increased thirst.

polyestrous   Refers to the continuous heat period of the female rabbit.

polyphagia   Increased appetite.

polyuria   Increased urination.

potentiation   The homeopathic process of diluting, then shaking a preparation in order to increase potency and vibrational energy.

preening   The self-grooming habit of birds designed to lubricate and smooth their feathers.

progesterone   The female sex hormone that functions to maintain pregnancy.

proptosis   Protrusion of the eye from the eye socket.

proventriculus   The glandular stomach of birds that secretes juices that aid in digestion.

pruritis   Itching.

psittacosis   An infectious disease of birds that affects the respiratory and other organ systems within the body; can cause serious disease in humans.

puberty   Age of sexual maturity.

pulmonary edema   Fluid buildup within the lungs.

purulent   Consisting of pus.

pus   An accumulation of dead neutrophils and tissue debris.

pyometra   Pus-filled uterus.

radiograph   Pictorial representation of a structure or region of the body created by placing that structure or region over special photographic film and then passing X rays through it.

rectrices   Flight feathers located on a bird's tail.

red leg disease   Inflammation and infection of the skin in amphibians.

regurgitation   The passive expulsion of food or water from the esophagus.

remiges   The primary and secondary flight feathers located on the wings.

residual   Long-acting; prolonged in effect; remaining.

rhinotracheitis   Respiratory disease in cats caused by a herpes virus.

ringtail   Skin disease in mice characterized by ulcerations near the base of the tail; caused by low humidity.

sanguineous   Blood-tinged.

sarcoma   Cancer involving connective tissue.

scabies   Mange mite infestation.

sclera   The white outer surface of the eyeball.

sebaceous gland   Oil glands attached to hair follicles within the skin.

seborrhea oleosa   Condition characterized by excessively oily skin.

seborrhea sicca   Condition characterized by dry, flaky skin.

sedative   Chemical agent that, when administered to a pet, exerts a calming and relaxing effect.

semiaquatic   Living both in water and on land.

sensory   Pertaining to the senses.

serum   The fluid portion of the blood, minus fibrinogen, the blood protein involved in clotting.

sialodacryoadenitis   Viral disease of the salivary glands in rats.

slobbers   Refers to excess salivation in rodents and lagomorphs caused by dental malocclusion.

snuffles   Bacterial respiratory infection in rabbits.

sour crop   Inflammation of the crop leading to the regurgitation of food; usually occurs secondary to a bacterial or fungal infection.

spay   Ovariohysterectomy.

sphincter   Muscular band of tissue that regulates entrance into or out of an organ.

splayleg   Musculoskeletal disease in rabbits characterized by lameness and an inability to walk.

splenectomy   Surgical removal of the spleen.

spondylosis   Degeneration and spurring of the vertebral column.

sprain   Abnormal stretching of a ligament.

stiff wrist syndrome   Bone deformities seen in guinea pigs caused by a magnesium deficiency.

stomatitis   Inflammation and infection involving the mouth.

strain   Abnormal stretching of a tendon.

stress bars   Abnormal feather markings or streaks caused by improper molting.

struvite   A specific type of crystal or stone that forms within the urinary tract.

subcutaneous   Beneath the skin.

subluxation   Partial dislocation of a joint.

substrate   Any substance lining the bottom of a tank or cage used to absorb moisture and waste, and/or to provide for bedding or nests.

supplement   To add to; enhance.

symmetry   Balance; congruity.

synergism   The effect of enhanced potency obtained when one herb is combined with one or more other herbs.

syrinx   An organ of the avian respiratory tree responsible for a bird's vocalization abilities.

tachycardia   Rapid heart rate.

tapetum   Reflective layer located beneath the retina of the eye.

tendon   Fibrous structure that connects muscle to bone.

tenesmus   Straining to defecate.

tentative diagnosis   An unconfirmed diagnosis that is usually based on history, clinical signs, physical examination, and preliminary laboratory findings.

terrestrial   Living on land.

TGE   Transmissible gastroenteritis; a viral digestive system disease seen in pigs.

thorax   The chest cavity.

thrombocytopenia   Presence of an abnormally low number of platelets within the blood.

thyroidectomy   Surgical removal of the thyroid gland.

titer testing   The measurement of specific antibody levels in a blood sample.

toxin   Poison.

tracheobronchitis   Inflammation of the trachea and bronchi.

ulcer   An erosion in the lining or surface of an organ.

ultrasound   The passing of sound waves through the body to create a picture of internal organs and structures on a special screen.

urethra Tubelike organ that carries urine from the bladder to the exterior of the body.

urolith Mineralized stone within the urinary tract.

uropygial gland A gland located near the base of a bird's tail that produces oils used for preening.

vaccination See *immunization.*

vaccine Synthetic (human-made) preparation of antigenic substances designed to elicit an immune response when introduced into the body.

vaginitis Vaginal inflammation.

veins Vessels that carry blood to the heart.

vent The external opening of the cloaca.

ventriculus That portion of the avian digestive tract responsible for grinding digesta before it enters the small intestine; also known as the "gizzard."

viremia The presence of viral organisms in the blood.

vital force The homeopathic term for the energy that is responsible for maintaining health and internal harmony within the body.

vitamin Organic substance needed for many physiologic processes within the body.

vitreous humor Fluid found within the posterior chamber of the eye.

vomiting The forceful expulsion of ingesta from the stomach.

wet tail Name given to bacterial enteritis in rodents.

zoonose Disease capable of spreading from animals to people.

INDEX

So that you will find it easier to use, the index for this book is divided into five sections: *General*, *Birds*, *Cats*, *Dogs* and *First Aid*.

General Index

Birds

Cats

Dogs

First Aid

U
Umbilical cord, 628
Urinary tract obstruction, 626–627

V
Vital signs, assessing, 600–601
Vomiting, 597, 612–613, 627

W
Water moccasins, 625
Wildlife, 634–636
Wounds:
  birds, 442
  cats/dogs, 603–605, 608–609

ABOUT THE AUTHOR

Chris C. Pinney, D.V.M., is the author of eight books and has served as veterinary host and advisor for television news magazines and syndicated radio talk shows. He currently practices veterinary medicine in Houston, TX.